SURGERY OF THE AORTA AND ITS BODY BRANCHES

Grune & Stratton Rapid Manuscript Reproduction

SURGERY OF THE AORTA AND ITS BODY BRANCHES

Edited by

John J. Bergan, M.D.

Magerstadt Professor of Surgery
Chief, Division of Vascular Surgery
Northwestern University Medical School
Chicago, Illinois

James S. T. Yao, M.D., Ph.D.

Associate Professor of Surgery
Director, Blood Flow Laboratory
Northwestern University Medical School
Chicago, Illinois

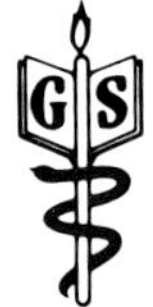

Grune & Stratton
A Subsidiary of Harcourt Brace Jovanovich, Publishers
New York London Toronto Sydney San Francisco

Library of Congress Cataloging in Publication Data

Main entry under title:

Surgery of the aorta and its body branches.

Bibliography: p.
Includes index.
1. Aorta–Surgery. 2. Arteries–Surgery.
I. Bergan, John J. II. Yao, James S. T.
[DNLM: 1. Aorta–Surgery–Congresses. WG410 S961
1979]
RD598.5.s88 617'.413 79-21919
ISBN 0-8089-1240-2

Grune & Stratton, Inc.
111 Fifth Avenue
New York, New York 10003

Distributed in the United Kingdom by
Academic Press, Inc. (London) Ltd.
24/28 Oval Road, London NW 1

Library of Congress Catalog Number 79-21919
International Standard Book Number 0-8089-1240-2

Printed in the United States of America

Contents

SURGERY OF THE THORACIC AND ABDOMINAL AORTA

AORTOILIAC OCCLUSIVE DISEASE

Foreword

This book is the product of a successful annual symposium which Dr. John J. Bergan and Dr. James S. T. Yao have organized with consummate skill. Devoted to papers concerned with surgery of the aorta and its body branches, it is particularly effective to have this volume available at the time the symposium is held. Dr. Bergan and Dr. Yao are to be congratulated for their selection of participants, the systematic organization of the symposium, and the careful combination of clinical and basic topics. The advantages provided by the concentration of effort on a particular area of vascular surgery are evident from a perusal of the list of participants and their topics. Such a multidisciplinary approach enhances the value of this book. Not only are surgeons included who are known for their contributions in cardiac and vascular surgery, but representatives from cardiology, anesthesia, and radiology are included as well. The comprehensive nature of the symposium assures the reader of this book that the volume contains the current status of surgery of the aorta and its branches.

John M. Beal, M.D.

Contributors

John Anderson, M.D.
Vascular Fellow
University of Tennessee Center for the Health Sciences
Memphis, Tennessee

William H. Baker, M.D.
Associate Professor of Surgery and Chief
Section of Peripheral Vascular Surgery
Loyola University Medical Center
Maywood, Illinois

Victor M. Bernhard, M.D.
Professor of Surgery
Medical College of Wisconsin
Milwaukee, Wisconsin

Eugene F. Bernstein, M.D., Ph.D.
Professor of Surgery
University of California School of Medicine
San Diego, California

F. William Blaisdell, M.D.
Professor and Chairman
Department of Surgery
University of California—Davis School of Medicine
Sacramento, California

Scott J. Boley, M.D.
Professor of Surgery and Chief of Pediatric Surgical Services
Albert Einstein College of Medicine
Montefiore Hospital and Medical Center
New York, New York

Lawrence J. Brandt, M.D.
Associate Professor of Medicine
Associate Director
Division of Gastroenterology
Albert Einstein College of Medicine
Montefiore Hospital and Medical Center
New York, New York

S. N. Carson, M.D.
Assistant Professor of Surgery
University of California–Davis School of Medicine
Veterans Administration Medical Center
Martinez, California

William J. Casarella, M.D.
Professor of Clinical Radiology
College of Physicians and Surgeons
Columbia University
Director, Cardiovascular Radiology
Presbyterian Hospital
New York, New York

David B. Case, M.D.
Associate Professor of Medicine
Cornell University Medical College
The New York Hospital
New York, New York

Gwen C. Cho, M.D.
Clinical Instructor in Anesthesiology
Baylor College of Medicine
The Methodist Hospital
Houston, Texas

Julius Conn, Jr., M.D.
Professor of Surgery
Northwestern University Medical School
Chicago, Illinois

E. Stanley Crawford, M.D.
Professor of Surgery
Baylor College of Medicine
The Methodist Hospital
Houston, Texas

Richard H. Dean, M.D.
Associate Professor of Surgery
Head, Division of Vascular Surgery
Vanderbilt University School of Medicine
Nashville, Tennessee

Ralph G. DePalma, M.D.
Professor of Surgery
Case Western Reserve University School of Medicine
Cleveland, Ohio

Allan R. Downs, M.D., F.R.C.S.(C), F.A.C.S.
Professor and Head
Department of Surgery
University of Manitoba Faculty of Medicine
Winnipeg, Manitoba

William S. Dye, M.D.
Professor of Surgery
Rush Medical College
Chicago, Illinois

William R. Flinn, M.D.
Fellow in Peripheral Vascular Surgery
Northwestern University Medical School
Chicago, Illinois

H. Edward Garrett, M.D.
Professor and Chairman
Department of Thoracic and Cardiovascular Surgery
University of Tennessee Center for the Health Sciences
Memphis, Tennessee

R. M. Greenhalgh, M.A., M. Chir., F.R.C.S.
Senior Lecturer in Surgery
Honorary Consultant Surgeon
Charing Cross Hospital Medical School
London, England

Sidney P. Haid, M.D.
Associate in Surgery
Northwestern University Medical School
Chicago, Illinois

Ronald D. Harris, M.D.
Assistant Professor of Radiology
University of California School of Medicine
San Diego, California

B. Heyden, M.D.
Department of Surgery
University of Ulm
Ulm, West Germany

James A. Hunter, M.D.
Professor of Surgery
Rush Medical College
Chicago, Illinois

John H. Isch, M.D.
Chief, Section of Cardiovascular-Thoracic Surgery
St. Vincent Hospital
Assistant Clinical Professor of Surgery
Indiana University School of Medicine
Indianapolis, Indiana

Hushang Javid, M.D.
Professor of Surgery
Rush Medical College
Chicago, Illinois

Norris D. Johnson, M.D.
Fellow in Peripheral Vascular Surgery
Northwestern University Medical School
Chicago, Illinois

Ormand C. Julian, M.D.
Professor of Cardiovascular-Thoracic Surgery (Emeritus)
Rush Medical School
Chicago, Illinois

Kalish Kedia, M.D.
Associate Professor of Urology
Case Western Reserve University School of Medicine
Cleveland, Ohio

Leonard H. Kleinman, M.D.
Assistant Instructor in Surgery
Medical College of Wisconsin
Milwaukee, Wisconsin

Thomas W. Kornmesser, M.D.
Associate in Surgery
Northwestern University Medical School
Chicago, Illinois

John H. Laragh, M.D.
Master Professor of Medicine
Director, Cardiovascular Center
Chief, Cardiovascular Division
Cornell University Medical College
The New York Hospital
New York, New York

George R. Leopold, M.D.
Professor of Radiology
University of California School of Medicine
San Diego, California

Michael Lesch, M.D.
Professor of Medicine and Chief
Cardiology Section
Northwestern University Medical School
Chicago, Illinois

Leonardo T. Lim, M.D.
Assistant Professor and Chief
Section of Vascular Surgery
University of Illinois Abraham Lincoln School of Medicine
Chicago, Illinois

Fred N. Littooy, M.D.
Assistant Professor of Surgery
Loyola University Medical Center
Associate Director, Peripheral Vascular Surgery
Hines Veterans Administration Hospital
Hines, Illinois

Lawrence L. Michaelis, M.D.
Associate Professor of Surgery and Chief
Division of Cardiothoracic Surgery
Northwestern University Medical School
Chicago, Illinois

John M. Moran, M.D.
Associate Professor of Surgery
Northwestern University Medical School
Chicago, Illinois

Hassan Najafi, M.D.
Professor and Chairman
Department of Cardiovascular-Thoracic Surgery
Rush Medical College
Chicago, Illinois

Harvey L. Neiman, M.D.
Associate Professor of Radiology
Chief, Angiography and Sectional Imaging
Northwestern University Medical School
Chicago, Illinois

Lester Persky, M.D.
Professor of Urology
Case Western Reserve University School of Medicine
Cleveland, Ohio

Luis A. Queral, M.D.
Assistant Professor of Surgery
University of Maryland School of Medicine
Baltimore, Maryland

Arthur J. Roberts, M.D.
Assistant Professor of Surgery
Northwestern University Medical School
Chicago, Illinois

John O. F. Roehm, Jr., M.D.
Clinical Associate Professor of Radiology
Baylor College of Medicine
The Methodist Hospital
Houston, Texas

David C. Sabiston, Jr., M.D.
James B. Duke Professor and Chairman
Department of Surgery
Duke University Medical Center
Durham, North Carolina

John H. Sanders, Jr., M.D.
Assistant Professor of Surgery
Northwestern University Medical School
Chicago, Illinois

Donald E. Schwarten, M.D.
Head, Cardiovascular Laboratory
St. Vincent Hospital and Health Care Center
Indianapolis, Indiana

H. William Scott, Jr., M.D.
Professor and Chairman
Department of Surgery
Vanderbilt University School of Medicine
Nashville, Tennessee

James C. Stanley, M.D.
Associate Professor of Surgery
Head, Division of Peripheral Vascular Surgery
University of Michigan Medical School
Ann Arbor, Michigan

Jesse E. Thompson, M.D.
Clinical Professor of Surgery
University of Texas Southwestern Medical School
Attending Surgeon
Baylor University Medical Center
Dallas, Texas

Jonathan B. Towne, M.D.
Associate Professor of Surgery
Medical College of Wisconsin
Milwaukee, Wisconsin

Otto H. Trippel, M.D.
Clinical Professor of Surgery
Northwestern University Medical School
Chicago, Illinois

Frank J. Veith, M.D.
Professor of Surgery and Chief
Division of Vascular Surgery
Albert Einstein College of Medicine
Montefiore Hospital
New York, New York

J. F. Vollmar, M.D.
Professor of Surgery
University of Ulm
Ulm, West Germany

Leonard Wade, M.S.
Research Assistant
Department of Anesthesiology
Northwestern University Medical School
Chicago, Illinois

Walter M. Whitehouse, Jr., M.D.
Assistant Professor of Surgery
University of Michigan Medical School
Ann Arbor, Michigan

Carolyn J. Wilkinson, M.D.
Assistant Professor of Anesthesiology
Northwestern University Medical School
Chicago, Illinois

Introduction

Surgery of the aorta forms the central core of peripheral vascular surgery. This volume recognizes that fact and concentrates on currently available information regarding surgical treatment of this organ system. There are many ways to solve the problems that arise in aortic surgery. This book is extensive in offering between two covers the best ways of achieving these solutions.

While this volume is the product of a symposium which brought together recognized authorities in vascular surgery, it differs from most symposium volumes in that the text does not consist of the verbal presentations given at the meeting; instead, it is a collection of manuscripts prepared by the authors for formal publication. Such a multi-author text inevitably contains duplications. This potential weakness is, however, countered with the strength of multiple viewpoints presented in authoritative fashion.

Chicago as a city was important in the development of vascular surgery, not only because of the work of Guthrie and Carrel at the turn of the century, but also because of the contributions of Ormand Julian whose many pioneering efforts included resecting an abdominal aortic aneurysm within weeks of the time that DuBost was doing this same work in Paris. In this volume, Dr. Julian describes the early days of vascular surgery in Chicago, mentioning his important and influential presentation before the American Surgical Association on direct surgery of artherosclerosis.

Because patients with aortic lesions almost routinely present with cardiac lesions as well, an important section of this book on assessment of cardiac risk and management of cardiac problems during aortic cross-clamping provides useful information. The former, by Michael Lesch, a recognized young cardiologist at Northwestern University, and the latter, by the team of a cardiac surgeon, Dr. Arthur Roberts, and an experienced cardiac anesthesiologist, Dr. Carolyn Wilkinson, document cardiac performance during surgery and challenge some outstanding dogma in this field.

Imaging techniques in aortic evaluation are very well described by the San Diego group led by Eugene Bernstein, and by the Northwestern interventional radiologist, Dr. Harvey Neiman.

Because of the gradual separation of peripheral vascular surgery from cardiothoracic surgery, thoracic aneurysms are increasingly the province of peripheral vascular surgeons. As an experienced surgeon and student of cardiac surgery, peripheral vascular surgery, and the physiology of pulmonary embolism, Dr. David Sabiston is in a unique position to describe the management of aneurysms of the thoracic aorta. His section in this volume is particularly lucid and informative.

Frequently, surgery of the thoracic aorta involves the use of bypass techniques and other forms of organ protection. These are thoroughly discussed in the section by Lawrence Michaelis and Arthur Roberts of Northwestern. While traumatic disruption of the thoracic aorta is usually the province of trauma centers, such lesions may come to any general hospital and may require urgent care by the most experienced surgeon on the staff. John Moran's description of the diagnosis and operative treatment of this lesion is complete and authoritative.

Thoracoabdominal aneurysms of the aorta are rare. Even experienced vascular centers have accumulated little experience with these lesions. No one in the world has contributed so much to an understanding of the surgery of these lesions as Stanley Crawford. His chapter on the management of these lesions represents the definitive statement on the problem and shows the way for other surgeons so that the mortality of this type of surgery can be reduced to an acceptable level.

Management of dissecting aneurysms of the aorta can be medical or surgical. The choice between these is not clear to all peripheral vascular surgeons, but Dr. John Sanders's presentation on this subject provides the information necessary to allow an intelligent choice between the two modalities of care.

Dr. Roger Greenhalgh has become increasingly well known in this country because of his contributions to peripheral vascular surgery and to the understanding of lipoprotein abnormalities in patients with atherosclerosis. His contribution on the small aorta syndrome briefly summarizes all that is known about this condition.

In Chicago, Hassan Najafi has assumed the leadership of a group founded by Ormand Julian, and their experience with occlusive lesions of the aortic arch is massive. Najafi's summary of management of these cases is totally authoritative and clear.

While Jesse Thompson has an international reputation for care of carotid artery lesions, he carries a local reputation in Dallas for superlative surgery of abdominal aortic aneurysms. His technique for resection of abdominal aortic aneurysms and the results achieved by him are carefully elucidated in his chapter.

Ruptured abdominal aortic aneurysms remain a challenge to the vascular surgeon. Garrett and Anderson have presented a very scholarly approach, summarizing extant literature on the subject and adding their own personal touches as suggestions for the care of patients with these dangerous lesions. Similarly, Julius Conn presents an authoritative and complete discussion of the various forms of colon ischemia that follow aortic surgery, and he explains how these can be avoided.

Jorge Vollmar stands in a preeminent position among vascular surgeons in Europe. His publications in this country have been well respected because of their scientific analysis of huge experience. His description of reconstructive surgery of the aortoiliac segment reflects his approach and is an important part of this volume.

Although Leriche described changes in sexual function during development of aortic lesions, only recently have vascular surgeons taken an investigative approach to these problems. The experience in vascular measurements at Northwestern University by Queral and the experience with nerve sparing operations at Case Western Reserve University by De Palma are well described in their chapters. At the time of this symposium, these chapters consolidate the best thinking on this subject.

Nonanatomic vascular reconstructions were pioneered in this country by Blaisdell, in whose chapter are presented various alternatives to direct surgery for aortoiliac disease. He is joined in this chapter by a Northwestern surgical trainee, Stanley Carson, who is making his mark as a peripheral vascular surgeon in California.

The Cook County Hospital in Chicago is well known for its care of vascular trauma. Responsibility for such care has come upon Dr. Leonardo Lim, who summarizes his large experience with aorto-vena caval injury in a clear chapter on this subject.

Acute thrombotic occlusion of the abdominal aorta becomes a surgical problem only occasionally. When it does, such lesions present at inconvenient times, and decisions must be made swiftly so that proper care can be administered. Thomas Kornmesser has summarized the experience of his group with such lesions, pointing out guidelines for care as well as results to be achieved.

Visceral branches of the aorta are important to vascular surgeons. Nowhere would a discussion of renovascular hypertension be complete without the contribution by Dr. John Laragh. His clarity of thought is well illustrated by a chapter contributing to the understanding of the renin system in renovascular hypertension.

The anatomic curiosity of fibromuscular dysplasia has fascinated physicians and surgeons alike. Dr. James Stanley's morphologic studies have contributed useful knowledge in this area, and these are beautifully illustrated in his chapter.

The Vanderbilt University group of vascular surgeons has accumulated massive experience in surgical care of renovascular hypertension. Their work has set the standard for other practicing surgeons. Dr. Richard Dean has a thorough grasp of the knowledge gained in the Vanderbilt experience and summarizes this completely in his presentation.

In the future, some surgery of the renal artery axis will become obsolete because of transluminal dilatation techniques. Among the earliest to employ these techniques in this country was the St. Vincent's Hospital group in Indianapolis. Dr. John Isch, a cardiovascular surgeon, both summarizes the group's experience with renal artery dilation and shows illustrative cases that go far to explain the indications for this technique. Dr. William Casarella supplements Isch's information with a description of renal artery dilatation techniques, adding as well a knowledge of iliac artery dilation.

Other important visceral branches of the aorta include those to the intestines. Scott Boley has been a student of the physiology of mesenteric blood flow and has contributed greatly to knowledge of the pathophysiology produced by occlusive lesions. His chapter on the subject is most informative.

Surgery of acute visceral artery occlusions has become clarified by acceptance of precise diagnosis. Such precision in diagnosis is described in Bergan's chapter on acute mesenteric ischemia, in which he discusses problems arising from surgery of acute mesenteric infarction.

Acute occlusion of the renal artery creates an interesting problem for vascular surgeons. Fortunately, there is now sufficient information about this lesion that Dr. Jonathan Towne has been able to summarize both these data and his own point of view to present a very rational approach to the problem.

The Ann Arbor group's interest in pathology of arterial lesions is again demonstrated in Stanley's and Whitehouse's contribution on aneurysms of the splanchnic and renal arteries. This is supplemented by a very sensible and well-delineated approach to surgery of these lesions.

Inevitably, patients with aortic graft sepsis gravitate to major vascular centers. Because of this, Frank Veith has been able to accumulate some experience with the problem, just as Victor Bernhard has amassed experience with aortoenteric fistulas. These problems and their solutions are discussed by both authors in their respective chapters. Such lesions may represent failure of an entire aortic graft, but it is also true that single graft limb occlusions develop after aortic bifurcation grafting. The problems of such unilateral occlusions are described by Allan Downs whose solutions provide guideposts for care of such lesions.

Abdominal and other subisthmic aortic coarctations are rare enough that few centers have accumulated much experience with them. Nevertheless, Richard

Dean's description of these lesions and their management at Vanderbilt summarizes all available information on this subject very well.

Norris Johnson's scholarly summation of the knowledge about spinal cord ischemia in abdominal aortic surgery is authoritative and complete.

Finally, stretching complications of aortic grafts as studied by Roger Greenhalgh, and management of arteriovenous fistulas of the aortic territory as described by Fred Littooy, complete this volume, providing ancillary information that will be of great value.

As can be seen from an inspection of the table of contents, a glance at the academic credentials of the contributors, and a random view of the pages of this volume, the book goes far to achieve its object. It provides authoritative information both about aortic surgery and about surgery of the branches of the aorta. As such, it illustrates the character of aortic surgery in 1979, defines the limits of such surgery as peripheral vascular surgery enters the 1980's, and points out problems for clinical and basic science research for the next decade of peripheral vascular surgical care.

John J. Bergan, M.D.
James S. T. Yao, M.D., Ph.D.

Basic Considerations

Ormand C. Julian, M.D., Ph.D.
William S. Dye, M.D.
Hushang Javid, M.D., Ph.D.

Chicago and Its Contribution to Aortic Surgery

Some mention of what must be called the ancient history of arterial surgery is appropriate insofar as it is descriptive of the background against which present day arterial, and especially aortic, surgery came into being. Until surprisingly recently, surgical methods were directed only toward the management, not even to say the repair, of traumatic lesions of the vessels [12]. Boiling oil and the red hot iron were the methods used until some unknown genius applied the first ligature. The ligature was mentioned by Celsus in the ninth century, but was brought into practical use – but not general use – by Pare (1507-1590). Actual repair of a fresh arterial wound was accomplished, probably for the first time, by Hallowell at Newcastle-on-Tyne on June 15, 1759. He passed a hare-lip pin through the adjacent edges of a brachial artery laceration which he had accidentally made. He then tied a ligature about the protruding ends of the pin, closing the wound.

By 1901 much scholarship, but little technique, had been brought to bear on the field of trauma of arteries. Pulsating hematoma and arteriovenous fistula were described as such. The terms contusion and laceration were accurately used. According to C. C. Guthrie, Dorfler reported in 1900 that only nine cases of arterial repair had been reported to be successful up until that date. Guthrie also found in the literature available to him that Stich, a German surgeon, had collected something over a hundred successful repairs in the year 1910. The reliability of these statistics is questionable, since little is known of the stimulus to report cases or the accuracy of the authors mentioned.

The experimental work of Carrell, some of which was done in Chicago during 1910-12, led him to develop practical techniques of blood vessel suture and anastomosis. At first he complicated the work by insisting that the intima of an artery must not be included in the suture.

The assistance of the Medical Library of Eisenhower Medical Center, Rancho Mirage, California (Mrs. Jean Atkinson, Chief Librarian) is gratefully acknowledged.

Guthrie and Carrell contributed the concept of fine sutures and demonstrated arterial suture, using both over-and-over sutures and an everting mattress suture. It is remarkable that the field of reconstructive arterial surgery in man did not start at that time. If the Parisian surgeon Delbet [8] had succeeded in his remarkable case in 1907, it is possible that even direct repair of arteriosclerotic lesions would have started 60 years earlier than it did. Delbet's patient was a 74-year-old man whose right leg was gangrenous and whose left leg was threatened by a large femoropopliteal aneurysm. Delbet transplanted the femoral artery of the gangrenous leg in replacement of the resected aneurysm of the other. He reported that the "chalky" character of the vessels defied his attempt to make secure anastomoses. The attempt is a first, however.

In 1945, one of the most active vascular surgical services in the country was that headed by Geza deTakats at the Hines V.A. Hospital just west of Chicago. When I joined this service in 1946, not many World War II injuries were present as yet. Our armamentarium in the treatment of the numerous patients with arteriosclerotic lesions and Buerger's disease was rest, well-supervised foot care, 1½ ounces of good bourbon twice daily, sympathectomy, and amputation. The intense and attractive personality of Dr. deTakats, perhaps aided by the bourbon, accounted for the large size of the service. It could be noted that the census fell in the summer and increased in the cold weather.

Lumbar sympathectomy was generously applied, almost to the point of becoming incidental to the work-up. From 1946 the vascular surgeons were allowed to invade the Radiology Department at Hines and arteriograms were done. It became apparent that the segmental nature of arteriosclerosis described by LeRiche [22] to occur at the aortic bifurcation also occurred in the femoral system [23]. The femoral arteriograms were read with particular attention to the presence of collateral vessels which would be caused to dilate with a sympathectomy. The x-rays also were a guide as we began to test a LeRiche idea that excision of the most involved arteriosclerotic segment in the femoral artery would remove a source of afferent vasoconstrictor impulses and add to the effectiveness of lumbar sympathectomy.

The first of the femoral grafts was done in 1951 in a patient whose planned procedure was lumbar sympathectomy plus excision of the segment of the superficial femoral artery shown in the arteriogram to be occluded. The adjacent superficial femoral vein intruded on the field, and Dr. Dye and I removed a piece of it, reversed it, and sutured it in place of the resected obstructed artery. The immediate appearance of the iatrogenic aneurysm alarmed us a bit, but it was left in place and functioned for a period of follow-up of nine years, including several arteriograms. From that day, our outlook on the treatment of arteriosclerosis changed and we went on a constant search for arteriosclerosis of segmental nature. The features that characterize segmental occlusion became evident. In April of 1952, Dye and I, joined by Olwin and Jordan [15], presented this work before the American Surgical Society, including 18 cases of femoral reconstruction with a maximum of 11 months follow-up. In closing the discussion of that paper, we stole the opportunity to report a resection and homologous graft replacement of the aortic bifurcation in a man with LeRiche syndrome which had been done only two weeks before the meeting. I believe that in this instance we stole the march on Michael DeBakey, although this never happened again.

At the time of the presentation, we were not aware of the 1948 report in Europe of dos Santos [9], who had "disobstructed" the aortic bifurcation, or the 1949 report of Bazy on the femoral [1]. Neither did we know of the report in *Presse Medicale* of 1951 in which Oudot [24, 25] described resection and graft of a bifurcation. We were aware of the thromboendarterectomy which had been performed by Jack Wylie and reported in 1951 [28]. Wylie had been impressed by the thin character left in the wall of the aorta and had strengthened it by the application of fascia lata. The mass of work since that time has shown this hazard to be essentially nil, but the work was an example of tremendous ingenuity. Our technical background was, of course, the resections and grafts done in the femoral area. Our intellectual background was Robert Gross's [13] use of arterial homografts in resection of difficult coarctations in children. We had also listened to Conrad Lam [21] report resection of the descending thoracic aorta for aneurysm with graft replacement. His case ended in a most unfortunate infection, but experimental work he had done encouraged further trials.

The following year, 1953, we presented another paper [16] on arterial resection and graft at the American Surgical Society, including the resections of abdominal aneurysms, as well as obstructed aortas and further femoral surgery. By this time, DeBakey and Cooley [7] were well started on their large series of bifurcation grafts which was to become the most oustanding of all in this area.

At this point, I think it may be interesting to consider the backgrounds of the surgeons who embarked early on programs of reconstructive arterial surgery – some of them also going into cardiac surgery. This was the early period of cardiovascular surgery, 1948-1952. The American Board of Thoracic Surgery was being developed from a recommendation of the American Association for Thoracic Surgery passed by its Board of Governors in May of 1947. General surgeons were doing the embolectomies, the repairs of arterial trauma, and the sympathectomies. Thoracic surgeons were concerned with lung disease, diseases of the pleura, and the esophagus. The only common complicated arterial procedure was coarctation repair, and this was done mostly by surgeons working in children's hospitals. The only exception to this classification is Geza deTakats. He had been a general surgeon doing routine hernia and intraabdominal work in Chicago, but he had a particular technical competence in varicose vein surgery and an appreciation for the need of careful attention to treatment of peripheral arterial emboli. Some years before I became associated with him at Hines Hospital, he had confined his work to arterial and venous surgery. Therefore, at the time under consideration, Geza deTakats was without doubt the only specialized vascular surgeon in the Chicago area; probably there were few like him in the world. No one was trained in aortic surgery and every step had to be carried out by each surgeon for the first time for himself. Each had to learn the technique of anastomosing a graft to a diseased segment of artery, whether aorta or femoral artery. It is true that most availed themselves of some significant opportunity to carry out these procedures in experimental animals, but the pathology made a difference.

The first experiences of the authors in abdominal aortic resection illustrate the meaning of a lack of training and experience. For many of the first cases, resection of an abdominal aortic aneurysm was exactly that, a complete resection. We were reluctant to clamp the aorta above the lesion for the prolonged period of dissection about the aneurysm wall. Therefore, always fighting the blood pressure within the lesion, we moved it back and forth as we did tedious ligation of the lumbar arteries and tedious, as well as hazardous, separation of the plane between the aneurysm and the adjacent vena cava. It was a happy morning when an aneurysm could be resected without accidentally entering the vena cava at least once. It was Javid who finally made the inspirational leap to the fact that the posterior wall of the aneurysm could be left in place. Thereafter, the lesion was simply opened after proximal clamping and its contents evacuated. The lumbar branches were easily suture-ligated from within and the whole procedure was tremendously simplified.

The first group of trainees to be present while this work was going on didn't have to make these advances and their residents after them were able to take most of them for granted.

In spite of the fact that many of the surgeons in this early period of arterial surgery also took on repairable cardiac valve lesions, the certification process of the Board of Thoracic Surgery seemed unimportant.

Of the authors of this paper, the first to earn the certificate of the Thoracic Board was Hushang Javid, who went through this process in a normal sequential manner. Through certain kindnesses by the then sitting Board, Julian was examined and passed in 1967, 23 years after being accredited by the American Board of Surgery. The Thoracic Board offered examination to a number of such anomalous surgeons that year. These included William Glenn; Charles Hufnagle, who had made great contributions to cardiovascular surgery; and perhaps five other surgeons who had been operating on the heart and great vessels within the chest for years without sanction of the Board. Egbert Fell, an outstanding thoracic and pediatric surgeon, never sought accreditation by the Board, although Milton Weinberg, his closest associate for years, went through the General and Thoracic Boards in routine fashion. Starzl, who was prominent in the earlier Northwestern group, is an accredited thoracic surgeon, while Bergan, who has done prodigious work on the visceral branches of the aorta, is not. Otto Tripple, prominent as a vascular surgeon in our Chicago group, is qualified as a general surgeon officially, but is most familiar with the contents of the chest. The stimulus for fragmentation which produced the American Board of Thoracic Surgery is again present, this time directed toward the establishment of a Board of Vascular Surgery, or perhaps of Cardiovascular Surgery.

There is no better example of the dissociation of accomplishment from the name given the field of enterprise than that of surgical treatment of thoracic aortic disease. Chicago had the leadership for a time in aortic surgery while it was confined to the abdomen. DeBakey, with Cooley in Texas and Bahnson in Pittsburgh, took away from us any semblance of leadership. In the early 1950's a number of reports appeared of resection and graft of the thoracic aorta for aneurysms below the origin of the left subclavian artery. We in Chicago participated in this area and followed DeBakey in his unfortunate technique of doing a re-entry operation for dissecting aneurysms originating in the thoracic area before the need for resection and graft for this lesion was appreciated.

In this field it became apparent that the surgeons' backgrounds in terms of field of training were unimportant. Thoracic aortic surgery was therefore fragmented in Chicago between Potts at the Children's Memorial, who saw no aneurysms, the general surgeons in metamorphosis toward thoracic cardiovascular surgery, and the established lung and bronchi surgeons who took no interest in the matter. Among the first to be trained in both disciplines again is one of our authors, who took leadership in developing some of the more difficult aspects of aneurysm and dissecting aneurysm therapy.

Resection of the proximal aorta and its upper visceral branches followed complete development of the means by which the pump-oxygenator could be applied. Such operations continue today to present individual unique problems not conducive to the development of routine procedures.

Early success with aortic bifurcation surgery brought quite another problem to Chicago. The grafts used in all of the earlier cases were homologous bifurcations taken under sterile conditions at autopsy. Most of these autopsies were actually carried out in the operating room and the graft was delivered in fresh state from one operating room to another for implantation. That this was a tenuous supply can be appreciated in terms of a Peoria police captain whose aneurysm was causing him pain and its potential danger causing him anxiety [20]. He told us that if we did not get him a graft soon, he would go out and shoot his own. We responded to his blackmail by moving him well up on the list.

The supply problem was solved for us by the Chicago Heart Association which financed an artery bank under the direction of Egbert Fell and Milton Weinberg. The bank was located in the Hektoen Building across from Cook County Hospital. The aortic bifurcation could be taken from any autopsy as a specimen and sent to the Bank, where it was sterilized and then freeze-dried. The grafts arrived in the operating room in a flame-sealed test tube, the outer surface of which could be reliably sterilized. The stiff, chalky, lyophilized artery was restored to normal consistency when it was rehydrated in saline at the operating table. More than a hundred of these specimens were used before the era of the arterial prosthesis began.

Chicago made a contribution in the field of prosthetic arterial grafts [17, 18] through the ingenuity of a fabric engineer in a weaving plant owned by a patient of one of our surgeons. Titus Haffa of Chicago at that time had control of the plant, and his engineer, William Liebig, devised a method of duplicate weaving on a jacquard loom which produced two flat layers of dacron cloth connected by a selvedge along any line fed into the design. Straight tubes and bifurcations of all sizes were made. These replaced the homemade prostheses we had made by stitching together of dacron cloth on an ordinary sewing machine. The plant, long disposed of by Mr. Haffa, has continued in the prosthesis business – producing crimped grafts as well – and is now well known to many as Meadox Medicals. The flat grafts were rigid and difficult to use, but filled a need for a time.

The flexible crimped dacron prostheses proved to be as easily used as homologous bifurcations for implantation as bypasses instead of end-to-end replacements. This improvement in technique over the method of resection and graft of the LeRiche bifurcation resulted in much time saved. As was the case with many of the improvements of method, this important detail came into being in various centers during a short period of time and no one has claimed particular credit for its origination.

Many of the Chicago vascular surgeons have been interested in reparative surgery of the visceral branches of the aorta. The manner in which stenosis and occlusion of these vessels produce the characteristic syndromes of brain, heart, gastrointestinal tract, and kidney ischemia is in itself fascinating. Leadership in Chicago in the area of renovascular hypertension with the variety of techniques available to correct the arterial lesions was taken by the Northwestern surgeons who followed the 1954 work of Freeman [11] and Castillo [6]. Tripple [27], O'Connor, Starzl [26], and Bergan [4] have made many contributions. The Northwestern center participated in a national multicenter study of the problem of renovascular hypertension and the effectiveness of renal artery surgery and nephrectomy.

Javid [14] and Dye did the earliest work in Chicago in the surgical treatment of cerebrovascular insufficiency. They pointed out the significance of lesions at the carotid bifurcation which had the x-ray appearance of being ulcerated [10]. This added an important indication for surgical intervention designed to remove the hazardous thrombi usually found lodged in the ulcer and repair the artery.

Bergan [2], Tripple [5], and others described in 1969 the essentials of a syndrome accompanying mesenteric artery stenosis. They presented an understanding of the position and amount of interference in the superior and inferior mesenteric arteries required to produce the clinical picture. Earlier, in 1964, Bergan [3] had pointed out the hyperkalemia which can be produced when the intestinal tract is revascularized.

Finally, in 1957 [19], at the University of Illinois laboratory we ignored a spectacular chance to develop in its entirety the operation of aorto-coronary bypass as it is so widely used today. We implanted arterial autografts between the base of the aorta in dogs and various levels of the circumflex or anterior descending coronary arteries. The animal results were excellent and almost as free of danger as the technique is now in clinical use. Postautopsy arteriograms showed wide patency. The conclusion was that such surgery was feasible, but was probably not available for the management of human coronary arteriosclerosis because of the *known* diffuse nature of the disease.

REFERENCES

1. Bazy L, Hugier J, Reboul H, et al: Technique des endarterectomies pour arterites obliterantes chroniques des membres inferieurs des iliaques et de l'aorte abdominale inferieure. J. Chir. 65:196, 1949
2. Bergan JJ, Dry L, Conn J Jr, et al: Intestinal ischemic syndromes. Ann. Surg. 169:120, 1969
3. Bergan JJ, Gilliland V, Troop C, et al: Hyperkalemia following intestinal revascularization. JAMA 187:17, 1964
4. Bergan JJ, O'Connor VJ Jr: Renovascular hypertension. Am. J. Surg. 109:262, 1965
5. Bergan JJ, Tripple OH: Management of juxtarenal aortic occlusions. Arch. Surg. 87:230, 1963
6. Castillo PA, Barrera F: Human hypertension due to thrombotic occlusion of both renal arteries: Report of a case cured by surgical removal of the thrombus. Am. Heart J. 56:769, 1958
7. DeBakey ME, Creech O, Cooley DA: Occlusive disease of the aorta and its treatment by resection and homograft replacement. Ann. Surg. 140:290, 1954
8. Delbet P: Chirurgee Arterielle et Veineuse. Les Modernes Acquisitions. Paris, J. B. Bailliere et Fils, 1906
9. Dos Santos JC: Sur las desobstruction des thromboses arterielles anciennes. Mem. Acad. Chir. 73:409, 1948
10. Julian OC, Dye WS, Javid H, et al: Ulcerative lesions of the carotid bifurcation. Arch. Surg. 86:803, 1963
11. Freeman NE, Leeds FH, Elliott WG, et al: Thromboendarterectomy for hypertension due to renal artery occlusion. JAMA 156:1077, 1954
12. Garre C: Über Gefassnaht, Rostocher Aertzteverein. Dtsch. Z. Chir. 82: 287-294, 1906
13. Gross RE, Hurwitt ES, Bill AH Jr, et al: Preliminary observations on the use of human arterial grafts in the treatment of certain cardiovascular defects. N. Engl. J. Med. 239:578, 1948
14. Javid H, Julian OC: Surgical management of internal carotid occlusion. Heart Bull. 11:84, 1962
15. Julian OC, Dye WS, Olwwn J, et al: Direct surgery of arteriosclerosis. Ann. Surg. 136:459, 1952

16. Julian OC, Grove WJ, Dye WS, et al: Direct surgery of arteriosclerosis: Resection of the abdominal aorta with homologous aortic graft replacement. Ann. Surg. 138:387, 1953
17. Julian OC, Deterling RA, Su HD, et al: Dacron tube and bifurcation prostheses produced to specification: Experimental and clinical use. Surgery 41:50, 1957
18. Julian OC, Lopez-Belio M, Deterling RA, et al: Dacron tube and bifurcation produced to specification: II. Continued clinical use and the addition of microcrimping. Arch. Surg. 78:260, 1959
19. Julian OC, Lopez-Belio M, Morehead D, et al: Direct surgical procedures on the coronary arteries: Experimental studies. J. Thoracic Surg. 34:654, 1957
20. Julian OC: Chicago and the treatment of abdominal aortic aneurysm: Proc. Inst. Med. Chicago 30:24, 1974
21. Lam CR, Aram HH: Resection of the descending thoracic aorta for aneurysm: A report of the use of a homograft in a case and an experimental study. Ann. Surg. 134:743, 1951
22. LeRiche R: Des obliterationes arterielles hautes comme des insuffisances. Bull. Soc. Chir. Paris 29:1404, 1923
23. LeRiche R: De las resection du carrefour aortoiliaque avec double sympathectomie lombaire pour thrombose arteritique de l'aorte. Pr. Med. 48:601, 1940
24. Oudot J: La greffe vasculaire dans les thromboses du carrefour aortique. Pr. Med. 59:234, 1951
25. Oudot J, Beaconsfield P: Thrombosis of the aortic bifurcation treated by resection and homograft replacement. Arch. Surg. 66:365, 1953
26. Starzl TE, Trippel OH: Reno-mesentero-aorto-iliac thromboendarterectomy in patient with malignant hypertension. Surgery 46:556, 1959
27. Trippel OH, Bergan JJ, Simon NM, et al: Bilateral simultaneous renal endarterectomy. Arch. Surg. 88:818, 1964
28. Wylie EJ, Kerr E, Davies O: Experiments and clinical experience with use of fascia lata applied as a graft to major arteries after thromboendarterectomy and aneurysmorrhaphy. Surg. Gynecol. Obstet. 93:257, 1951

Evaluation of the Patient for Aortic Surgery

Michael Lesch, M.D.

Assessment of Cardiac Status in the Patient Requiring Aortic Surgery

In pragmatic terms the assessment of cardiac function in patients requiring surgical treatment for the sequelae and complications of aortic atherogenesis requires development of a data base which allows the cardiologist to answer the following general questions: In the patient with no known heart disease, what is the likelihood of occult heart disease? If occult disease is thought probable or the patient has a definite history of cardiac disease, what is (are) the specific cardiac diagnosis (diagnoses)? To what degree is cardiac function compromised? Is cardiac function compromised to such a degree as to warrant cancellation or postponement of aortic surgery? Traditionally these questions have been approached by utilizing the clinical parameters of history and physical examination supplemented primarily by the chest roentgenogram and electrocardiogram. When further information is needed, localization and quantification of the disease has usually been obtained by cardiac catheterization and/or intracardiac angiography.

Due to the obvious drawbacks attendant to these latter invasive procedures, clinicians have been disinclined to utilize the catheterization laboratory for routine preoperative evaluation. In view of the known limitations of diagnostic accuracy of the stethoscope, electrocardiogram, and chest roentgenogram, the advanced age of the average patient with atherosclerosis, and the increased prevalence of heart disease of all types in this population, one can only surmise that many such patients have frequently entered the operating room either inaccurately or incompletely evaluated insofar as cardiac disease and functional capacity is concerned.

Recently developed techniques for noninvasive assessment of cardiac function have significantly reduced the cardiologist's reliance upon the catheterization laboratory and have concurrently improved the quality of care available to cardiac patients with severe aortic atherogenesis which requires operative therapy. Moreover, cardiac catheterization and particularly coronary angiography can be more efficiently utilized when patients are screened in the noninvasive laboratory.

Although congenital heart disease and other less common forms of heart disease cannot be ruled out a priori in the population group under discussion, the most common and pressing issues in the cardiologic evaluation of these patients usually relates to the following specific questions:

1. Does the patient have coronary artery disease?
2. Does the patient have valvular heart disease?
3. What is the status of left ventricular function?
4. Should corrective cardiac surgery (valve replacement, coronary artery bypass graft, or ventricular aneurysmectomy) be contemplated prior to abdominal or thoracic aortic surgery?

In this chapter techniques of particular value in answering these particular questions will be reviewed and guidelines for their use proposed.

ECHOCARDIOGRAPHY

General Considerations

Echocardiography involves the application of reflected ultrasound – i.e., sound waves of frequency far above the normally audible range – to the evaluation of the heart. Pulsed ultrasound waves in the frequency range of 1.60 to 3.50 MHz are emitted from a transducer probe that also acts as a receiver for reflected waves. Since ultrasound is reflected at interfaces having different acoustic impedances, internal structures of the heart possessing different impedances – such as myocardium, atrial and ventricular chambers, and valves – can be readily imaged. There are two basic techniques of echocardiography currently in clinical use: M-mode and cross-sectional. The M-mode (time-motion) technique utilizes a single beam of ultrasound beginning at the chest wall and traversing identifiable cardiac structures at various depths. The reflected ultrasound waves ("echoes") are displayed on an oscilloscope (in proportion to the depth of the tissues from which they are reflected) on the vertical axis, as a function of time on the horizontal axis. Structures are identified by the intensity and motion of the reflected echoes, as well as by the characteristic anatomic relationships of the various structures to each other. The transducer is usually placed in the second to fourth intercostal spaces to the left of the sternum and a "sweep" performed from the region of the ventricles to the aortic root-left atrial interface [4, 10] (Figs. 1 and 2).

Cross-sectional echocardiography is an attempt to provide a two-dimensional image rather than the single dimension (over time) afforded by the M-mode

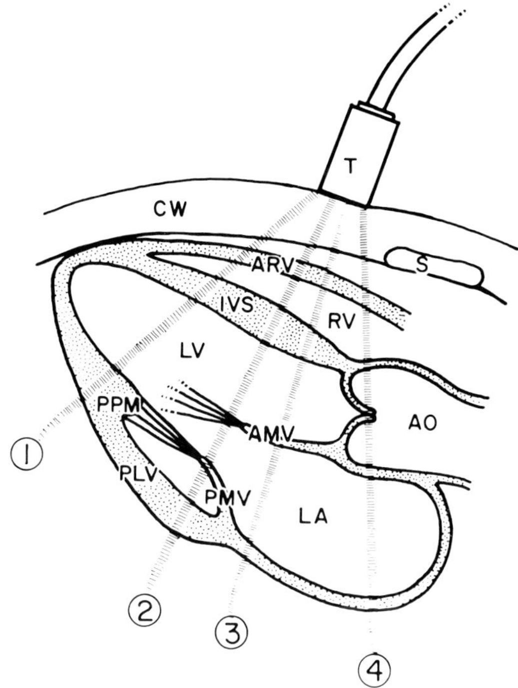

Fig. 1. Diagrammatic representation of the heart in longitudinal section depicting the structures through which the ultrasound beam passes as it is directed from the apex toward the base of the heart. The numbers (1-4) refer to standard positions for recording the M-mode echocardiogram (see Fig. 2). CW = chest wall, T = transducer, S = sternum, ARV = anterior right ventricular wall, RV = right ventricular cavity, IVS = interventricular septum, LV = left ventricle, PPM = posterior papillary muscle, PLV = posterior left ventricular wall, AMV = anterior mitral valve, PMV = posterior mitral valve, Ao = aorta, LA = left atrium. [From Feigenbaum H: Clinical applications of echocardiography. Prog. Cardiovasc. Dis. 14:531, 1972. By permission of the author and Grune & Stratton, Inc.]

technique. Various methods have been developed to produce a continuous (real-time) oscilloscopic display of cardiac function in up to a 90° arc (sector). The two most popular cross-sectional methods are the mechanical and the electronic sector scanners. In mechanical sector scanners, a single ultrasound crystal is rocked through a 30°-90° sector on the chest wall, with simultaneous oscilloscopic display of echoes from each position in the arc. In electronic (or "phased array") sector scanners, a small multicrystal transducer is held stationary on the chest wall while the echo beam is swept back and forth electronically

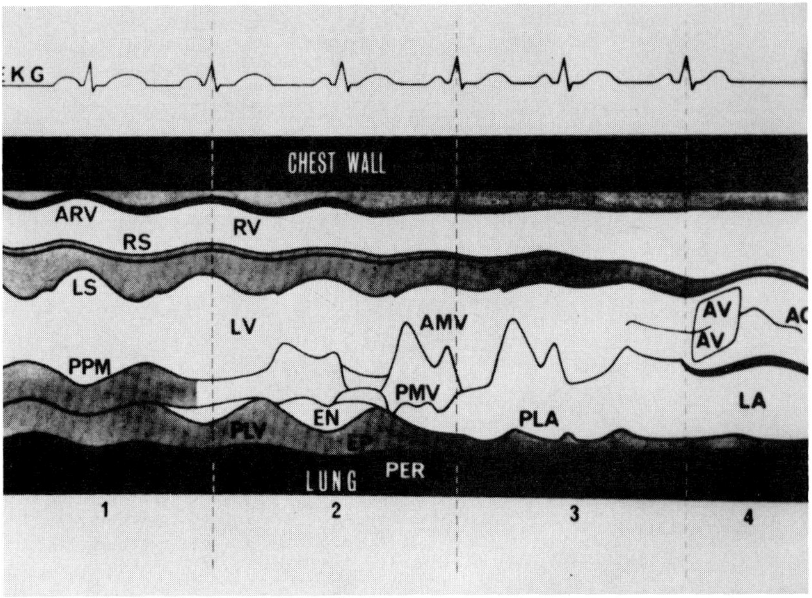

Fig. 2. Diagrammatic representation of the M-mode echocardiogram as the transducer is directed from the cardiac apex (position 11) to the base (position 4). The areas between the dotted lines correspond to the transducer positions as depicted in Fig. 1. EN = endocardium of the left ventricle, EP = epicardium of the left ventricle, PER = pericardium, PLA = posterior left atrial wall. Other symbols are those used for Fig. 1. [From Feigenbaum H: Clinical applications of echocardiography. Prog. Cardiovasc. Dis. 14:531, 1972. By permission of the author and Grune & Stratton, Inc.]

over an arc of up to 90° [2]. Sweeps are generally performed in longitudinal and cross-sectional views, allowing for visualization of most areas of the heart (Fig. 3).

Assessment of Left Ventricular Function by Echocardiography

In the absence of localized disorders of left ventricular function such as seen in coronary artery disease, echocardiographic measurements have been shown to correlate with left ventricular volume and ejection fraction as determined angiographically [4, 12]. While left ventricular ejection fraction does not perfectly characterize the functional state of this chamber, this measurement is accepted as providing an overall assessment of pump performance. The ejection fraction, defined as the ratio of ventricular stroke volume to end-diastolic volume, is thought a more sensitive measurement of myocardial contractile state than cardiac output or end-diastolic pressure and has been successfully used in the evaluation of numerous cardiac disorders. As such, the ability to obtain this value by a noninvasive technique represents a significant development.

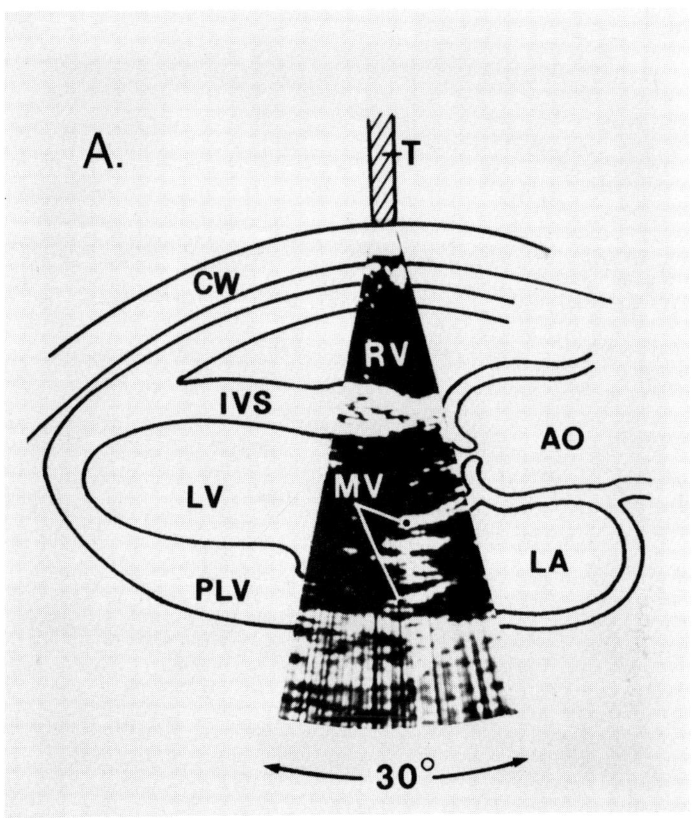

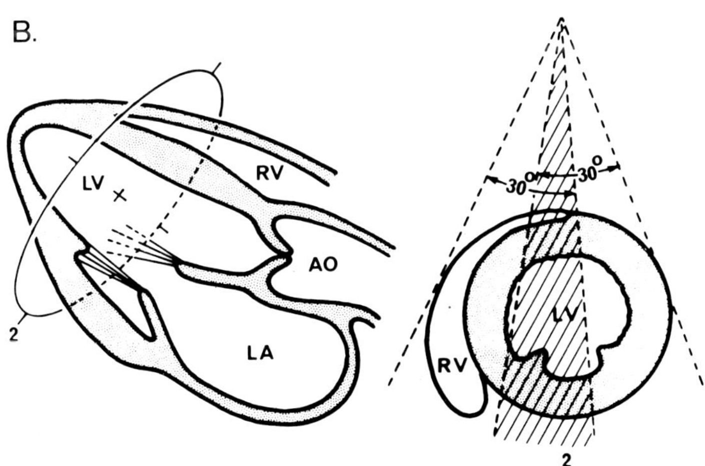

Fig. 3. Two-dimensional echocardiography. [Abbreviations are those used in Fig. 1]. (A) Diagrammatic representation of the heart in longitudinal section with photography of actual 30° sector view of heart. (B) Diagrammatic representation of heart as viewed in cross-section by two dimensional echocardiography. [Part B from Feigenbaum H: Echocardiography, (ed. 2). Philadelphia, Lea & Febiger, 1976. By permission of the author and Lea & Febiger.]

The approach to volume determination by echocardiography relies on the assumption that the left ventricle is a uniformly contracting prolate ellipsoid and that its volume in systole and diastole approximates the cube of the left ventricular transverse dimension in systole and diastole, respectively. Left ventricular transverse dimensions are measured from the left ventricular septal surface to the endocardium of the posterior left ventricular wall (Fig. 2). Left ventricular ejection fraction, it follows, equals

$$\frac{LVTD_D{}^3 - LVTD_S{}^3}{LVTD_D{}^3}$$

where $LVTD_S$ and $LVTD_D$ are left ventricular transverse dimension in systole and diastole, respectively [12]. Stroke volume is obtained by multiplying left ventricular ejection fraction by $LVTD_D$, and left ventricular (or cardiac) output is approximated by multiplying stroke volume by the heart rate (determined from the ECG recorded with the echocardiogram). Conditions such as coronary artery disease, by giving rise to segmental zones of ischemia, scarring, and abnormal contractility, invalidate the above geometric assumptions regarding calculation of left ventricular volume. Conversely, however, echocardiographic demonstration of assymetric thickening of any left ventricular wall during systole is strong evidence towards the diagnosis of coronary artery disease.

Assessment of Mitral Valvular Disease by Echocardiography

Mitral stenosis. M-mode echocardiography may add additional information in determining the presence and relative severity of mitral stenosis in patients in whom the physical examination is not conclusive. Figure 4A is an echocardiogram showing a normal mitral valve. Note that in diastole the anterior leaflet of the mitral valve exhibits an "M-shaped" pattern, whereas the posterior leaflet exhibits a "W" shape. The two leaflets separate relatively widely and abruptly, reflecting normal transmitral flow during ventricular filling. After partial closure during middiastole, the leaflets move apart again during atrial systole (at ventricular end-diastole). During ventricular systole, the anterior and posterior leaflets are seen to approximate and remain together in a neutral position or to move slightly anteriorly. In mitral stenosis, M-mode echocardiography usually reveals a number of characteristic findings (Fig. 4B). There are dense echoes from the mitral leaflets reflecting fibrosis and/or calcification. There is a diminished opening excursion and a diminished rate of early diastolic closure (decreased E-F slope) of the anterior leaflet [4, 10]. Because of fusion of the mitral leaflets, the posterior leaflet moves in parallel fashion to the anterior leaflet in 90% of cases. Although the degrees of diminution of mitral early diastolic closure rate (E-F slope) and of maximal diastolic leaflet separation have been roughly correlated with the severity of mitral stenosis, cross-sectional echocardiography has proved to be a distinctly more accurate means of assessing mitral orifice size. Henry et al. [5] have shown that cross-sectional echocardiographic measurements of mitral orifice area correlate well with mitral orifice size measured at surgery.

Mitral valve prolapse. Echocardiography has been useful in making a presumptive diagnosis of mitral valve prolapse (Barlow's syndrome) in patients with or without a midsystolic click and/or late systolic murmur. Mitral valve prolapse has been found to be an extremely common entity in otherwise normal women of childbearing age, its incidence variously estimated at from 6% to 28% [6, 13]. This condition is generally benign, but may be associated with symptoms of chest pain, palpitations, and, rarely, with sudden death – presumably related to ventricular dysrhythmia. Antibiotic prophylaxis against subacute bacterial endocarditis is recommended in individuals with this condition at the time of dental, urologic, and other surgical procedures.

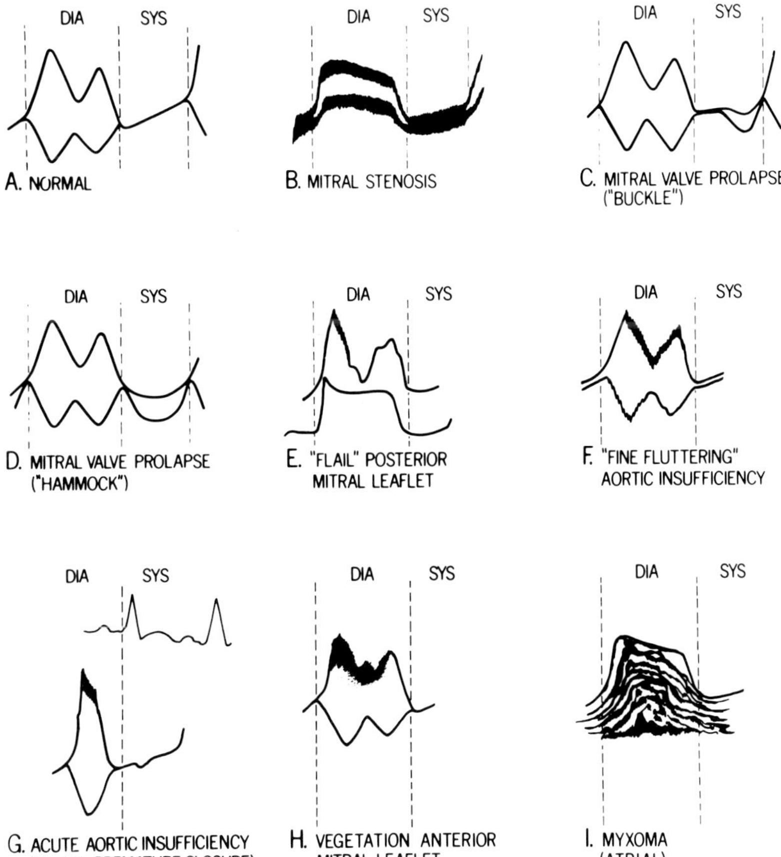

Fig. 4. Composite diagrammatic representation of mitral valve echocardiogram seen in various normal and abnormal states.

There have been two major M-mode echocardiographic patterns reported in patients with mitral valve prolapse [6]. Figure 4C demonstrates a late systolic posterior "buckling" of the mitral leaflets. Figure 4D depicts a pansystolic posterior movement of the mitral leaflets ("hammock" pattern), which may be also produced as an artifact of improper angulation of the transducer on the chest wall.

Mitral regurgitation. Echocardiography does not provide specific findings in mitral regurgitation not related to mitral valve prolapse, ruptured chordae, or calcified mitral annulus. Nonetheless, the presence of a dilated left atrium and left ventricle when associated with increased excursion of the mitral leaflets and exaggeration of normal left ventricular contractility is consistent with the diagnosis of mitral regurgitation [10].

Assessment of Aortic Valve, Root, and Outflow Tract Disease by Echocardiography

Aortic stenosis. The M-mode examination of the aortic valve may normally reveal a parallelogram or boxlike motion of two cusps within the aortic root during systole (Fig. 5A). The third (or left coronary) cusp is not usually visualized because it moves roughly perpendicular to the ultrasound beam. In aortic stenosis, the degree of opening of the aortic box is diminished. In addition, the finding of dense linear echoes within the aortic root suggests fibrosis or calcification of the valve apparatus and favors the presence of aortic stenosis [4, 10] (Fig. 5B). However, it is difficult to determine the severity of aortic stenosis from the M-mode examination of the aortic valve. Although the ratio of left ventricular wall thickness to left ventricular internal dimension is a helpful index of severity of stenosis, two-dimensional echocardiography has proved more useful in separating the degree of aortic obstruction into mild, moderate, and severe [15].

Bicuspid aortic valve. The presence of so-called "eccentric closure" of the aortic valve leaflets in diastole (Fig. 5C) has been associated with a bicuspid aortic valve – although the finding is neither entirely specific nor sensitive [7]. A bicuspid aortic valve has been estimated to be present in 1%-2% of otherwise normal individuals. It may be associated with a systolic ejection sound, and may or may not result in calcific aortic stenosis, aortic insufficiency, and/or subacute bacterial endocarditis.

Aortic insufficiency. The most common (although not universal) echocardiographic finding in aortic insufficiency of any severity and etiology is "fine fluttering" (high-frequency vibration) of the anterior (and occasionally, posterior) mitral leaflet in diastole (Fig. 4F). In acute aortic insufficiency, premature coaptation of the anterior and posterior mitral leaflets (Fig. 4G) indicates severe

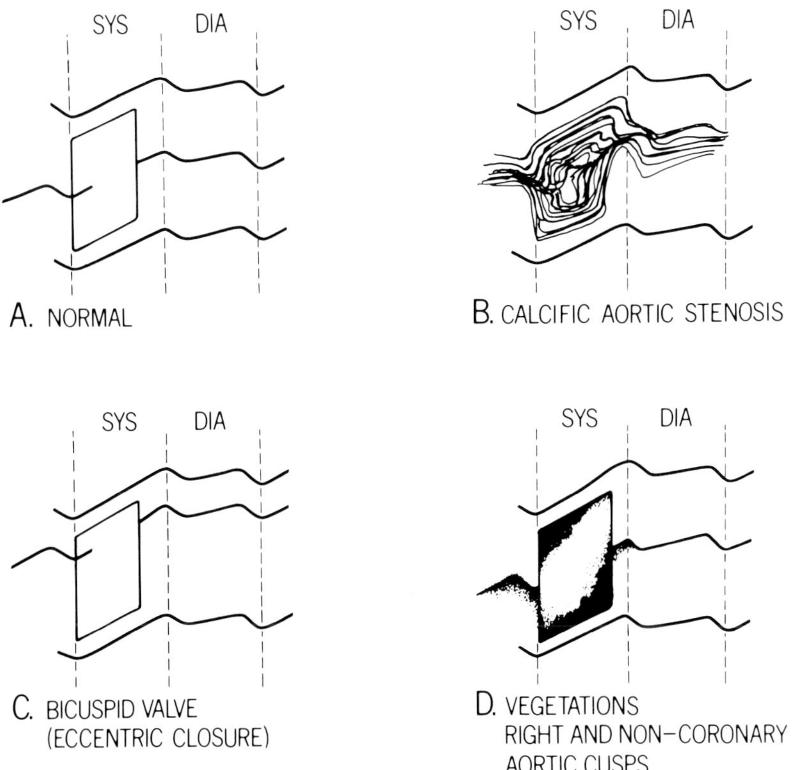

Fig. 5. Composite diagrammatic representation of aortic valve echocardiograms seen in various normal and abnormal states (see text).

regurgitation, generally acute. Left ventricular dilatation [2] and a subnormal left ventricular ejection fraction [1] are felt to reflect severe, long-standing aortic insufficiency.

Marfan's syndrome. Echocardiography may be helpful in the evaluation of patients with the uncommon Marfan syndrome. In particular, the presence of aortic insufficiency and mitral valve prolapse, with redundant (or flail) mitral or aortic leaflets, may be detected by the M-mode technique. In one small series of patients with Marfan's syndrome, there was a 91% incidence of mitral valve prolapse and a 60% incidence of aortic root dilatation [9]. Furthermore, the detection of aortic root dissection is also possible in selected cases by M-mode and cross-sectional methods. There have been, however, some difficulties – including false-positive studies – reported with the M-mode technique [8].

Idiopathic hypertrophic subaortic stenosis. A number of abnormalities of the M-mode echocardiogram have been defined in idiopathic hypertrophic subaortic stenosis (IHSS). The spectrum of IHSS begins with asymmetric septal hypertrophy (ASH), in which the septum is thicker than the left ventricular (LV) posterior free wall by a ratio of at least 1.3 to 1 (Fig. 6A). The presence, in addition, of systolic anterior motion (SAM) (Fig. 6B) of the anterior mitral leaflet is usually associated with a subvalvular gradient at rest [4, 10].

Aortic root dissection. Aortic dissection which extends into the aortic root causes the intima to separate from the external layers of the aortic wall, resulting in an increase in aortic wall width. The echocardiographic correlate of this anatomical situation is an increase of the aortic wall dimensions at the root. Unfortunately, this finding has neither sufficient sensitivity nor specificity to render the M-mode echocardiogram of great value in this condition. However, when the diagnosis of aortic dissection has been established by angiography or CAT scanning, serial echocardiographic examination can aid in the detection of developing aortic insufficiency or pericardial tamponade.

RADIONUCLIDE EVALUATION OF CARDIAC FUNCTION

The past decade has witnessed the development of numerous scanning techniques which permit noninvasive diagnosis and physiologic assessment of cardiac disease [9]. Three techniques are of particular value in the patient population under discussion and are reviewed.

Determination of Left Ventricular Ejection Fraction and Wall Motion Analysis

Two radionuclide techniques are available for the determination of left ventricular ejection fraction [1]. Both utilize external monitoring of the cardiac blood pool with a gamma camera, but, in the "first pass" technique the initial transit of radioactive tracer is monitored, whereas in the "equilibrium" method images are obtained only after the isotope has equilibrated within the blood pool.

In the first pass technique, counts over the left ventricle are measured with a gamma camera as the intravenously injected bolus traverses the central circulation. The number of counts emanating from the left ventricle is proportional to the quantity of isotope in the ventricle and this is, in turn, related to the volume of the ventricle. Thus a plot of radioactivity in the ventricle versus time, during the first minute after injection, reveals cyclical fluctuations in count rate that reflect alterations of ventricular volume during successive cardiac cycles – the frequency of these fluctuations being related to heart rate. The "peak" of each cycle represents the counts in the ventricle at end-diastole (i.e., greatest ventricular volume), and the subsequent "valley" corresponds to the activity in the ventricle at end-systole (i.e., smallest ventricular volume). Five to ten such peaks

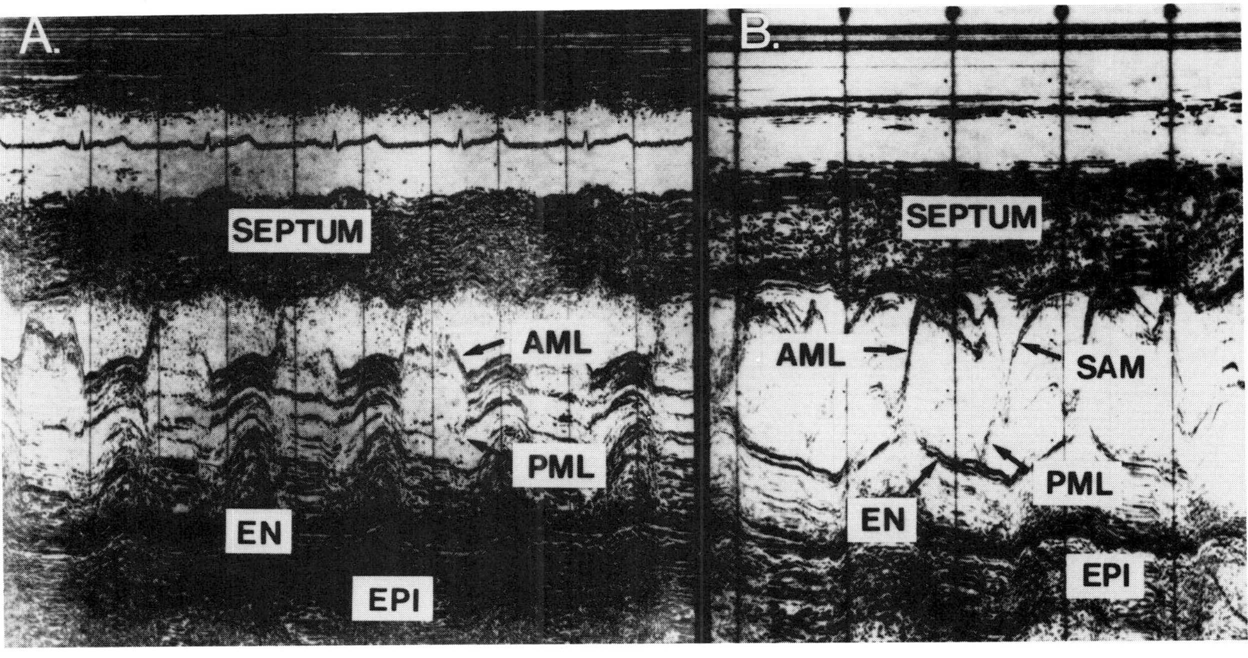

Fig. 6. Echocardiographic spectrum of asymmetric septal hypertrophy (ASH). (A) Nonobstructive ASH, in which the septum is thicker than the left ventricular posterior wall by a ratio of greater than 1.3 to 1. (B) Obstructive ASH (idiopathic hypertrophic subaortic stenosis, IHSS), in which systolic anterior motion of the anterior mitral leaflet (SAM) is also present and reflects a subaortic gradient. Abbreviations are those used in Fig. 2.

and valleys can be identified following a single bolus injection. The difference in number of counts in each successive peak and valley is proportional to the volume change in the ventricle in that cycle and represents stroke volume. When related to the number of counts at end-diastole, this difference gives a measure of ejection fraction.

In the equilibrium method, the tracer is first allowed to equilibrate within the blood pool. Gamma scintillation images of the cardiac silhouette are then constructed by gating the gamma camera to the ECG, since the counts generated during a single cardiac cycle are insufficient to create a scintillation image. For example, the gamma camera can be gated to count for 0.06 sec at the peak of the QRS complex (end-diastole) and for 0.06 sec on the downslope of the T wave (end-systole). The camera is "off" for all other portions of the cardiac cycle, and the data gathered in each successive cycle are stored with computer methodology until enough end-systolic and end-diastolic counts have been accumulated to generate images of the ventricle at these times. With increasing sophistication of the computer and the gating mechanism, the cardiac cycle may be divided into 20 or 30 equal time periods and images developed for each. In effect, this produces a scintillation angiogram with 10-20 frames per cycle and allows for calculation of ejection fraction in a manner analagous to that used in the catheterization laboratory with routine contrast angiography. An obvious advantage of the "equilibrium" technique is that an actual "angiogram" is generated and estimates of wall motion dysfunction can be obtained (Fig. 7). For example, a globally diseased ventricle with poor overall contractile function and low ejection fraction could be distinguished from a ventricle with a depressed ejection fraction due to a large apical aneurysm but with good contractile function in the nondiseased segments of myocardium. Similarly, an area of transmural infarction will appear as a hypokinetic or akinetic segment of an otherwise normally contracting ventricular silhouette.

Myocardial Perfusion Scanning

In this procedure, a radiolabeled monovalent cation (potassium-43, rubidium-81, cesium-129, and, more recently, thallium-201) is injected intravenously either at rest or during exercise testing. The initial distribution of these tracers within the heart is related to both coronary blood flow and myocardial Na^+-K^+ATPase, but the major determinant is coronary flow, and thus images obtained with these nuclides index myocardial perfusion. Although a variety of factors which modify this relation – e.g., high flow states, digitalis, insulin – have been identified, regional distribution of these tracers is sufficiently related to regional flow so as to be of clinical utility [14].

Due to certain unfavorable features of potassium-43 (e.g., short half-life), perfusion imaging was not widespread prior to the development of thallium-201. The relatively long half-life of this nuclide (74 hours), its favorable energy spectrum, dosimetry, and high cardiac and low hepatic extraction have allowed

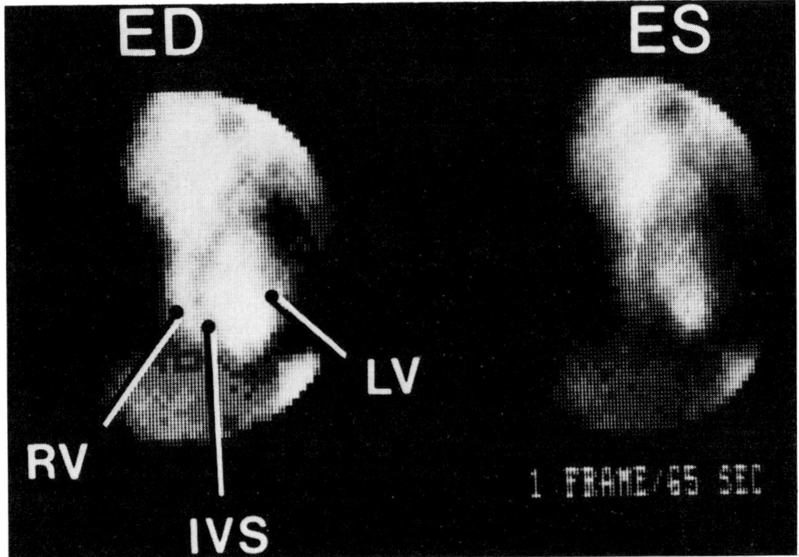

Fig. 7. Radionuclide angiogram at "equilibrium" is shown in the left anterior oblique projection at end-diastole (ED) and end-systole (ES). The left ventricular wall motion is normal during systole. LV = left ventricle, RV = right ventricle, and IVS = interventricular septum.

perfusion scanning to be utilized at all institutions possessing nuclear capability [2, 17, 18].

In the normal heart, thallium distribution is relatively uniform throughout the cardiac silhouette. Areas of transmural infarction can thus be diagnosed if regions of total or near total absence of tracer are found (i.e., a "cold spot"). The relatively high accuracy (greater than 80%) of this technique for the retrospective diagnosis of transmural myocardial infarction has been fully documented [11]. As noted above, gated blood pool scanning is frequently utilized to confirm this diagnosis by matching perfusion defects on thallium scans to areas of dyskinetic wall motion. The accuracy of thallium scanning for the retrospective diagnosis of nontransmural myocardial infarction is considerably less than that with transmural infarction, but recent improvements in data processing of the thallium image suggest the technique will be of some value in this condition also [11].

Most centers now utilize perfusion scanning in conjunction with exercise stress testing. When injected at the time of peak exercise in patients with exercise-induced myocardial ischemia, areas of transient ischemia are identified as zones of decreased tracer uptake not found when the examination is performed at rest. Due to the decreased exercise capability of patients with claudication and the inadvisability of maximally exercising a patient with a large abdominal aneurysm, exercise-perfusion testing is not practical in the group of patients discussed in this symposium.

Myocardial Infarction Imaging

Various nuclides which concentrate in acutely infarcted myocardium are now available. Technetium-99m pyrophosphate is the nuclide most widely used at present [16]. These agents are thought to bind to calcium stores, sulfhydryl groups, or denatured protein sites not available to the tracer in normal myocardium or scar and which are present only transiently (1-13 days) during the process of acute infarction. Operationally the heart is imaged 1-3 hours after injection of the tracer to allow for clearance of the blood pool. Most episodes of acute transmural infarction (greater than 95%) are detected with this technique, while a lower sensitivity and specificity has been reported with nontransmural infarction. Following transmural infarction a positive scan is usually obtainable for up to 13 days. Conditions reported to yield false-positive scans include ventricular aneurysm, cardiac calcification, and cardiac necrosis due to trauma or electrical current.

REFERENCES

1. Ashburn WL, Schelbert HR, Verba JW: Left ventricular ejection fraction – A review of several radionuclide angiographic approaches using the scintillation camera. Prog. Cardiovasc. Dis. 20:267, 1978
2. Bradley-Moore PR, Lebowitz E, Greene MW, et al: Thallium for medical use. II. Biologic behavior. J. Nucl. Med. 16:156, 1975
3. Brown OR, Demots H, Kloster FE, et al: Aortic root dilatation and mitral valve prolapse in Marfan's syndrome: An echocardiographic study. Circulation 52:651, 1975
4. Feigenbaum H: Echocardiography (ed 2). Philadelphia, Lea & Febiger, 1976
5. Henry WL, Griffith JM, Michaelis LL, et al: Measurement of mitral orifice area in patients with mitral valve disease by real-time, two dimensional echocardiography. Circulation 51:827, 1975
6. Markiewicz W, Stoner J, London E, et al: Mitral valve prolapse in one hundred presumably healthy young females. Circulation 53:464, 1976
7. Nanda NC, Gramiak R, Manning J, et al: Echocardiographic recognition of the congenital bicuspid aortic valve. Circulation 49:870, 1974
8. Nanda NC, Gramiak R, Shah PM: Diagnosis of aortic root dissection by echocardiography. Circulation 48:506, 1973
9. Nuclear medicine. Prog. Cardiovasc. Dis. 20 (Nos. 1-4), 1977-78
10. Parisi AF, Two DE, Felix WR, et al: Noninvasive cardiac diagnosis. N. Engl. J. Med. 296:316, 368, 427, 1977
11. Pitt B, Strauss HW: Myocardial imaging in the noninvasive evaluation of patients with suspected ischemic heart disease. Am. J. Cardiol. 37:797, 1976
12. Pombo JF, Troy BL, Russell RO Jr: Left ventricular volumes and ejection fraction by echocardiography. Circulation 43:480, 1971

13. Procacci PM, Savran SV, Schreiter SL, et al: Prevalence of clinical mitral valve prolapse in 1169 young women. N. Engl. J. Med. 294:1086, 1976
14. Schelbert HR, Ashburn WL, Chauncey DM, et al: Comparative myocardial uptake of intravenously administered radionuclides. J. Nucl. Med. 15:1092, 1974
15. Weyman AE, Feigenbaum H, Dillon JC, et al: Cross-sectional echocardiography in assessing the severity of valvular aortic stenosis. Circulation 52:828, 1975
16. Wynne J, Holman BL, Lesch M: Myocardial scintigraphy by infarct avid radio tracers. Prog. Cardiovasc. Dis. 20:242, 1978
17. Zaret BL: Myocardial imaging with radioactive potassium and its analogs. Prog. Cardiovasc. Dis. 20:81, 1977
18. Zaret BL, Martin ND, Flamm MD: Myocardial imaging for the noninvasive evaluation of regional perfusion at rest and after exercise, in Strauss HW, Pitt B, James AE (eds): Cardiovascular Nuclear Medicine. St. Louis, C. V. Mosby, 1974, pp 35-51

Carolyn J. Wilkinson, M.D., Arthur J. Roberts, M.D.
Leonard Wade, M.S., John J. Bergan, M.D.
James S. T. Yao, M.D., Ph.D.

Hemodynamic Measurements During Aortic Cross-Clamping

Aortic surgery is well established as treatment of abdominal aortic aneurysm and aortoiliac occlusive disease. With improvement of operative and anesthetic techniques, hospital mortality for elective abdominal aortic surgery has dropped below 5% in most reported series [14, 18, 31]. Despite this accomplishment, myocardial infarction still accounts for over 50% of the postoperative deaths [14, 28, 31].

The hemodynamic effects of aortic cross-clamping on the lower extremities are well known [16, 28]. Myocardial effects of abdominal aortic cross-clamping, however, received little attention until 1968, when Perry [26] reported decreased cardiac output in dogs and variable hemodynamic changes in patients undergoing abdominal aortic surgery.

Since most patients who have aortic atherosclerotic disease have a high incidence of atherosclerotic heart disease [12, 14, 29, 31], the major question is to what extent aortic cross-clamping influences myocardial performance. Secondly, is aortic cross-clamping detrimental to the myocardium in the perioperative period?

Recently, a number of studies have documented hemodynamic changes during aortic cross-clamping. Despite these reports, confusion still exists concerning the magnitude of these changes and their significance in determining operative morbidity and mortality. Furthermore, the influence of various forms of anesthetic agents on cardiac output and hemodynamic parameters during aortic clamping is unclear. Finally, indications for routine use of the Swan-Ganz catheter in aortic surgery have not yet been clarified.

The present study was undertaken to determine the hemodynamic and electrocardiographic changes which occurred during abdominal aortic cross-clamping to ascertain whether these changes could be prevented during halothane anesthesia supplemented with nitroglycerin.

EFFECTS OF AORTIC CROSS-CLAMPING

The effects of aortic cross-clamping on lower extremity blood flow and in other organs have been of interest to vascular surgeons. In addition to producing changes in hemodynamic parameters, cross-clamping of the aorta also causes changes in renal blood flow [13] and affects the release of renin [4]. After aortic declamping, severe hypotension has been observed and various mechanisms have been offered to explain this so-called "declamping phenomenon." Observations in patients undergoing resection of ruptured aortic aneurysm have shown a washout acidosis immediately following declamping [22]. This has been shown to be detrimental to cardiac performance.

It seems that of all the events which follow declamping, the cardiac manifestations appear to be most important. These have received much attention because of recent developments in intraoperative monitoring devices.

Table 1 summarizes reports by investigators interested in hemodynamic parameters during and following aortic clamping. The consistent finding in each study was the lack of change in heart rate after clamping. As expected, there was an increase of systolic pressure and peripheral resistance [2, 3, 15, 24, 30], together with a decrease of cardiac index during cross-clamping. However, three studies reported the absence of significant changes in these measurements [1, 9, 10]. Altogether, these changes in hemodynamic parameters have been proposed to affect the tolerance of patients with severe coronary artery disease to the stress of infrarenal aortic cross-clamping.

Hemodynamic Studies

At the Northwestern University McGaw Medical Center, 11 patients, 10 males and 1 female, ranging in age from 48 to 71 years, were studied. There were four patients with aortic aneurysms, and seven had aortoiliac occlusive disease. All patients underwent aortic bypass grafting procedures.

Preoperative evaluation. The multifactorial index of cardiac risk suggested by Goldman et al. [17] (Table 2) was used to screen these patients. According to these authors, cardiac risk index greater than 13 is considered poor risk. The cardiac risk indices for our patients were as follows: seven patients, 3 points; three patients, 8 points; one patient, 13 points. No patient had a cardiac risk index greater than 13 points, although a history of hypertension was present in eight patients, old myocardial infarction in three patients, history of congestive heart failure in one patient, and stable angina in one patient.

In order to assess serial changes in left ventricular function, all patients had their ejection fractions (EF) determined by radionuclide equilibrium gated blood pool (GBP) studies. This radiopharmaceutical technique has been shown to correlate well with contrast ventriculography [8], and it allows a noninvasive assessment of left ventricular performance which is highly reproducible [32]. The GBP study was done 24 hours prior to and after surgery.

Table 1
Hemodynamic Effects of Aortic Cross-Clamping

AUTHORS	PATIENTS	TYPE OF ANESTHESIA	HR	SAP	SVR	CI	CVP	PCWP	LVSWI
Moloche et al 1977	9 AAA 9 Leriches	N_2O-Fentanyl-Droperidol	OΔ	↑ 13%	↑ 37%	↓ 18%	OΔ	—	OΔ
Dunn et al 1977	13 AAA 14 AID	"Balanced" anesthesia or Halothane	—	↑	↑	↓	—	—	—
Silverstein 1976	15 AAA	Morphine and Halothane	OΔ	↑ 17%	↑ 36%	↓	OΔ	OΔ	—
Asicitopolou 1978	10 AID	N_2O-Fentanyl-Droperidol	OΔ	OΔ	—	OΔ	OΔ	—	—
Carroll et al 1976	12 AAA 2 AFB	(5) N_2O-Narcotic Tranquilizer (9) Halothane	OΔ	OΔ	OΔ	OΔ	OΔ	↑ (2)	OΔ
Bush et al 1977	22 AAA	(10) Halothane or Ethrane (12) N_2O Narcotic Tranquilizer	—	OΔ	—	OΔ	—	OΔ	↑
Attia et al 1976	5 AAA No CAD	N_2O Morphine	OΔ	↑	↑ 33%	↓	↓	↓	—
	10 AAA Severe CAD		OΔ	↑	—	—	↑	↑	—
Kouchoukos et al 1979	8 Descending Thoracic TAA	Halothane	OΔ	↑	—	↓ 29%	↑ 56%	↑ 90%	OΔ
Peterson et al 1978	6 Dogs	Dialurethane	—	↑	↑	↓	—	—	—
	6 Dogs NTG		—	↓	↓	OΔ			

HR - Heart Rate
SAP - Systolic Arterial Pressure
SVR - Systemic Vascular Resistance
CI - Cardiac Index
CVP - Central Venous Pressure
PCWP - Pulmonary Capillary Wedge Pressure
LVSWI - Left Ventricular Stroke Work Index
AAA - Abdominal Aortic Aneurysm
AID - Aorto Iliac Disease
CAD - Coronary Artery Disease
NTG - Nitroglycerin
TAA - Thoracic Aortic Aneurysm

Table 2
Computation of Cardiac Risk Index

Criteria*	Multivariate Discriminant-Function Coefficient	"Points"
1 History:		
(a) Age >70 yr	0.191	5
(b) MI in previous 6 mo	0.384	10
2 Physical examination:		
(a) S_3 gallop or JVD	0.451	11
(b) Important VAS	0.119	3
3 Electrocardiogram:		
(a) Rhythm other than sinus or PAC's on last preoperative ECG	0.283	7
(b) >5 PVC's/min documented at any time before operation	0.278	7
4 General status:		
Po_2<60 or Pco_2>50 mm Hg, K<3.0 or HCO_3<20 meq/liter, BUN>50 or Cr>3.0 mg/dl, abnormal SGOT, signs of chronic liver disease or patient bed ridden from noncardiac causes	0.132	3
5 Operation:		
(a) Intraperitoneal, intrathoracic or aortic operation	0.123	3
(b) Emergency operation	0.167	4
Total possible		53 points

*MI denotes myocardial infarction, JVD jugular-vein distention, VAS valvular aortic stenosis, PAC's premature atrial contractions, ECG electrocardiogram, PVC's premature ventricular contractions, Po_2 partial pressure of oxygen, Pco_2 partial pressure of carbon dioxide, K potassium, HCO_3 bicarbonate, BUN blood urea nitrogen, Cr creatinine, & SGOT serum glutamic oxalacetic transaminase.

Reproduced with permission of author and publisher from Goldman, et al: Multifactorial index of cardiac risk in noncardiac surgical procedures. N. Engl. J. Med. 297:845, 1977.

Intraoperative Studies

All patients were premedicated with morphine 10 mg and atropine 0.4 mg. Prior to induction of anesthesia, a standard 12-lead ECG was obtained and recorded on a chart recorder (Marquette Mac-cart machine). Increments of 5 mg Valium were given for sedation during insertion of (1) a No. 7 Fr. Swan-Ganz pulmonary artery catheter for measurement of central venous pressure (CVP), pulmonary artery pressure ($\overline{\text{PAP}}$), and pulmonary capillary wedge pressure (PCWP) and (2) a No. 20 Teflon catheter for systolic radial artery pressure

(SAP). Pressures were recorded continuously on a Tektronix 414 recorder. Heart rate (HR) was determined by the electrocardiogram. Cardiac outputs (CO) were measured in triplicate by the thermodilution method using a computer (Edwards output computer Model 9520) [34].

Cardiac index (CI) was calculated by dividing cardiac output by body surface area (BSA) and stroke index (SI) by dividing CI by heart rate. Left ventricular stroke work index (LVSWI) was calculated from the $\overline{AP}$, PCWP, and SI using

$$LVSWI\ (g \cdot m/m^2) = \frac{1.36\ (\overline{AP} - PCWP)}{100} \times SI$$

Systemic vascular resistance (SVR) (dynes · sec/cm^{-5}) was calculated by

$$SVR = \frac{\overline{AP} - \overline{CVP}}{CO} \times 80$$

Rate pressure product was calculated by multiplying SAP by HR.

Baseline hemodynamic measurements of HR, SAP, AP, PAP, PSWP, CVP, and CO were taken before and after induction of anesthesia 5 min before as well as 5 and 30 min after infrarenal clamping of the abdominal aorta. A 12-lead ECG was taken with each set of hemodynamic measurements.

Anesthesia was induced with sodium thiopental 3-5 mg/kg. Endotracheal intubation was facilitated with succinylcholine 1.0 mg/kg and anesthesia maintained with inspired concentrations with 50% nitrous oxide and halothane 0.5%-1.5%. Muscle relaxation was provided by pancuronium bromide following tracheal intubation.

Intravenous nitroglycerin in increments of 60 μg or by continuous infusion was given prior to and during induction and intubation when the rate pressure product was over 15,000 or the systolic blood pressure was over 160 mm Hg. Throughout the operation, special attention was paid to keeping the rate pressure product below 12,000, either by increasing the concentration of halothane or increasing the dose of nitroglycerin being infused. Ventilation was controlled mechanically with a total gas flow of 5 liters per minute, arterial oxygen tension was maintained above 100 torr, and arterial carbon dioxide tension between 35 and 40 torr. No other drugs were administered. All patients received 100 ml/hr 5% dextrose in lactated Ringer's solution 12 hours prior to surgery and 10 to 15 ml/kg/hr prior to aortic clamping.

Hemodynamic data obtained 5 min before and after aortic cross-clamping were analyzed by Student's *t* test for paired data. All values were expressed as mean and standard deviation of the mean.

RESULTS

Table 3 and Fig. 1 summarize hemodynamic parameters taken during the preoperative, preincision, 5 min preclamp, 5 min postclamp, and 30 min postclamping periods. Although there was an increase in HR between the preoperative and 5 min postclamp determinations ($p<0.025$) and a decrease between the preoperative and 5 min postclamp $\overline{AP}$ ($p<0.025$), there were no statistical

Table 3
Hemodynamic Effects of Aortic Cross-Clamping During Halothane Anesthesia With Nitroglycerin Supplement in Patients ($N = 11$)

	Pre-Op	Pre Incision	5 Min. Pre Clamp	5 Min. Post Clamp	30 Min. Post Clamp	5 Min. Post Declamp	30 Min. Post Declamp
H.R.	65.9 ± 11.85	73.0 ± 27.55	81.4 ± 16.32	82.4 ± 17.91	79.0 ± 15.61	80.4 ± 15.22	77.5 ± 16.42
R.P.P.	10054 ± 1660	9925 ± 2408	10158 ± 2873	9912 ± 2574	9652 ± 1516	10653 ± 2255	10048 ± 1532
S.A.P.	152.5 ± 19.09	124.1 ± 26.05	125.18 + 28.40	120.36 + 17.52	122.5 ± 12.98	132.3 ± 13.88	130.9 ± 11.20
$\overline{\text{A.P.}}$	98.5 ± 7.19	89.7 ± 16.99	87.9 ± 20.19	85.0 ± 14.48	84.1 ± 11.17	90.5 ± 15.21	88.54 ± 11.76
$\overline{\text{P.A.P.}}$	20.1 ± 5.59	19.7 ± 5.08	17.9 ± 5.5	17.9 ± 5.65	15.1 ± 5.51	18.2 ± 4.62	18.0 ± 4.86
P.C.W.P.	14.3 ± 5.38	14.9 ± 4.28	13.3 ± 4.90	11.9 ± 4.46	11.6 ± 4.14	12.7 ± 5.12	11.7 ± 5.12
C.V.P.	9.5 ± 4.43	10.7 ± 4.00	9.4 ± 5.35	8.4 ± 3.83	7.9 ± 3.98	8.0 ± 3.00	8.4 ± 3.91
C.O.	5.43 ± 1.69	5.11 ± 9.35	5.50 ± 1.39	5.11 ± 1.49	4.50 ± .91	5.17 ± 1.19	4.86 ± 1.21
S.V.R.	1530 ± 715	1283 ± 390	1181 ± 399	1268 ± 365	1401 ± 395	1353 ± 440	1413 ± 435
C.I.	2.8 ± .94	2.62 ± .46	2.81 ± .16	2.64 ± .72	2.29 ± .47	2.64 ± .56	2.49 ± .61
L.V.S.W.I.	41.36 ± 19.48	31.48 ± 10.08	32.26 ± 9.71	29.78 ± 8.20	25.76 ± 5.84	32.90 ± 11.11	33.86 ± 6.33

$\overline{\text{AP}}$ – Mean Arterial Pressure
CI – Cardiac Index
CO – Cardiac Output
CVP – Cental Venous Pressure
HR Heart Rate
LVSWI – Left Ventricular Stroke Work Index
$\overline{\text{PAP}}$ – Mean Pulmonary Artery Pressure
PCWP – Pulmonary Capillary Wedge Pressure
RPP – Rate Pressure Product
SAP – Systolic Arterial Pressure
SVR – Systemic Vascular Resistance

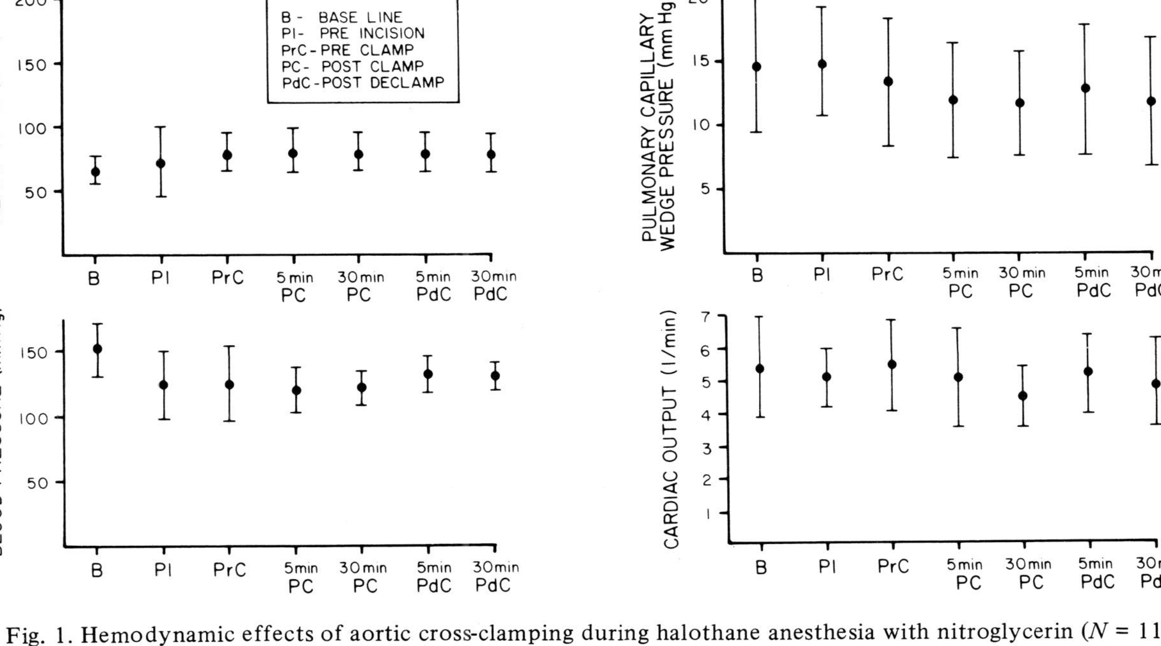

Fig. 1. Hemodynamic effects of aortic cross-clamping during halothane anesthesia with nitroglycerin ($N = 11$).

differences between any of the 5 min preclamp and 5 min postclamp hemodynamic measurements. In addition, there were no significant differences between the highest and lowest RPP, PCWP, CVP, and CO. Similarly, there were no ventricular arrhythmias or significant ST-segment depressions (⩾1 mm) seen in the 12-lead electrocardiograms during any of the above periods. Analysis of preoperative and 24 hour postoperative ejection fractions determined by radionuclide gated blood pool studies also showed no changes (preoperative EF 54.91 ± 6.32, 24 hour postoperative EF 51.45 ± 7.89 [$p>0.05$]) (Fig. 2).

DISCUSSION

Goldman et al. [17] identified nine independent significant correlates of life-threatening and fatal cardiac complications. The multifactorial index (with a maximum of 53 points) is an estimate of cardiac risk independent of surgical risk. Patients with scores over 13 warrant extensive preoperative medical evaluation, and those with scores over 26 should have only life-saving surgical procedures performed. In 1001 patients studied, preoperative evidence of congestive heart failure, recent myocardial infarction (less than 6 months), frequent premature ventricular contraction (greater than five per minute), rhythms other than sinus or premature arterial contractions, and age over 70 years were

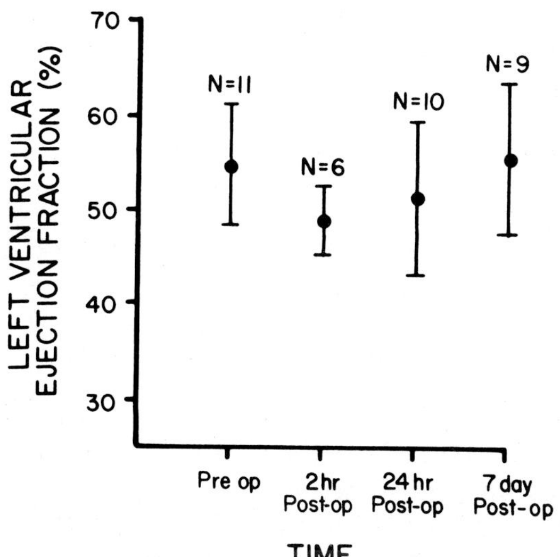

Fig. 2. Ventricular ejection fractions determined by radionuclide gated blood pool studies.

associated with significant increased cardiac risk, while the old myocardial infarction, bundle branch block, hypertension, stable angina, and nonspecific ST- and T-wave changes were not useful in assessing risk. None of our patients had an index greater than 13.

Myocardial ischemia occurs when there is an imbalance between myocardial oxygen supply and demand, and it is predominantly subendocardial [6]. The major determinants of myocardial oxygen demand, which may change markedly under the influence of various surgical and anesthetic techniques, are (1) ventricular wall tension, reflected by systolic arterial pressure (afterload) and ventricular volume (preload), (2) heart rate, and (3) myocardial contractility [7]. Testing the significance of these determinants, McDonald et al. [23] showed the best indicator of myocardial oxygen demand was peak developed tension multiplied by heart rate. Recently, it has been shown that rate pressure product (RPP), i.e., heart rate times systolic arterial pressure, correlates well with MVO_2, and ischemic electrocardiographic changes are more common when RPP exceeds 15,000-20,000 [25, 33].

Systemic arterial pressure, cardiac output, and ventricular filling pressure are used to reflect myocardial function. In a patient with normal ventricular function, however, cardiac output is far more dependent on the effects of peripheral factors on ventricular preload and afterload than on central factors such as the contractile state of the myocardium [6]. Only recently have the effects of afterload been considered significant in left ventricular failure.

In the study of cardiac function, several authors have advocated the use of the Swan-Ganz catheter to monitor PCWP, since CVP may not reflect left ventricular filling pressure [2, 9, 30]. An elevated PCWP may precipitate subendocardial ischemia and reflect left ventricular dysfunction, but the cause may be factors such as hypervolemia, depressed contractility secondary to changes in anesthetic agents, or hypertension. In order to elucidate the cause of myocardial ischemia, a study of MVO_2 is necessary, and RPP is a simple clinical measurement which may be used as an indicator of MVO_2 in the perioperative period. Using a rise in PCWP to predict ischemia is of little benefit to the patient if, at the same time, the RPP is allowed to exceed 15,000-20,000. In one patient reported by Attia [2], electrocardiographic ST-segment depression was seen when the systolic pressure was over 200 mm Hg and the RPP exceeded 20,000.

In the present study, there were no significant changes seen in cardiac output, cardiac index, left ventricular stroke index, or systemic ventricular resistance before and after aortic cross-clamping. Central venous pressure, pulmonary artery pressure, and pulmonary capillary wedge pressure were found to change insignificantly after clamping. In addition, increased myocardial oxygen consumption, as reflected by rate pressure product exceeding 15,000, was not seen. Correspondingly, there was no myocardial ischemia demonstrated by the electrocardiographic monitoring. Furthermore, both hemodynamic parameters and indices of myocardial oxygen consumption were unchanged during and after aortic cross-clamping, indicating no adverse myocardial effects. Our study differs from others in that all patients had strict control of rate pressure product before and during aortic clamping and had normal preoperative left ventricular ejection fractions by radionuclide angiograms.

Hemodynamic changes during aortic cross-clamping have been studied in a total of 140 patients, including the 11 cited here. A rise in systolic arterial pressure and systemic vascular resistance and a decrease in CI have been reported frequently. In all these patients, only one postoperative myocardial infarction was reported [15]. No episodes of pulmonary edema were reported. During infrarenal cross-clamping, five patients had marked elevations in PCWP, four of whom had ST-segment depression on the electrocardiogram. The ST-segment depression reverted to normal with nitroprusside infusion in three of these patients. Two of the patients who developed ischemic electrocardiographic changes had documented severe coronary artery disease. They were anesthetized with morphine and nitrous oxide and had marked rise in blood pressure and heart rate when the aorta was clamped. Despite the reports of myocardial ischemic changes, no study showed aortic cross-clamping alone to cause myocardial infarction. Our results support other observations that detrimental hemodynamic effects causing myocardial infarction due solely to aortic cross-clamping are rare.

The anesthetic agent influences hemodynamic parameters measured during aortic clamping. Most of the current knowledge of cardiovascular physiology and pharmacology is based on findings in anesthetized animals. Unfortunately, some investigators have assumed that the type of anesthesia within a given experiment does not alter the conclusions derived from the experiment, but it is well known that anesthetics and adjuvants do have direct and indirect effects upon the heart and circulation and anesthetic techniques must be considered in any analysis of results. For example, half of the patients summarized in Table 1 had either a narcotic or halothane anesthesia [9, 10, 15, 30]. In half the studies, nitroprusside was an adjuvant [2, 10, 21, 30]. Some patients received combinations of halothane and morphine [30]. No study compared different anesthetic techniques and their influence on myocardial parameters during aortic clamping.

Since many patients with abdominal aortic disease have arteriosclerotic heart disease, an anesthetic technique which improves the balance between myocardial oxygen and demand is desirable. Although no studies are available in patients with coronary artery disease undergoing noncardiac surgical procedures. Kistner et al. [20] compared the effects of halothane and morphine on MVO_2 during coronary artery revascularization in patients without severe ventricular dysfunction. Fewer signs of ischemia occurred in the prebypass period when halothane rather than morphine was used in combination with nitrous oxide. Ischemia changes and increase in RPP were noted in the patients anesthetized with morphine despite the fact that nitroprusside was used to minimize hypertension often seen in these patients. In the nonfailing canine heart, halothane decreased the severity of experimentally produced myocardial ischemia, suggesting that it influences the relationship between myocardial oxygen supply and demand in a favorable way when coronary blood flow is limited [5].

Besides anesthetic agents, the use of pharmacologic agents to control hypertension during the anesthetic period also may play a role in myocardial performance. While both nitroprusside and nitroglycerin can control hypertension and decrease oxygen demand, nitroglycerin has been shown to improve ischemic changes on the electrocardiogram during myocardial infarction [9] and coronary artery bypass [19] more often than nitroprusside. Nitroglycerin is thought primarily to dilate large coronary conductance vessels, increase collateral blood flow, and redistribute blood to subendocardial areas. Nitroprusside may dilate arterioles in normal areas of the heart by shunting blood from ischemic to nonischemic areas [11]. Peterson et al. [27] reported that infusion of nitroglycerin produced a 44% increase in cardiac index during aortic cross-clamping in animals with depressed myocardial function. The judicious use of nitroglycerin to control systolic pressure when it exceeded 160 mm Hg in the present study may account for the absence of electrocardiographic evidence of ischemia and subsequent infarction. Although the present study series is small, it appears that perioperative control of hypertension with nitroglycerin may decrease myocardial ischemia in patients undergoing abdominal aortic surgery.

One of the central questions in the management of patients undergoing aortic surgery is the role of perioperative hemodynamic monitoring. Other studies [2, 30] have stressed the importance of using Swan-Ganz catheterization to monitor PCWP and prevent electrocardiographic changes during aortic cross-clamping. In the present series, these changes did not occur.

CONCLUSIONS

Data from a number of investigations have shown an increased systolic blood pressure, peripheral vascular resistance, and decreased cardiac index during infrarenal aortic cross-clamping. Despite the propensity for these changes, they can be mitigated by strict attention to the rate pressure product during halothane anesthesia with nitroglycerin as an adjuvant.

Our data do not indicate that aortic cross-clamping precipitates myocardial ischemia in patients with normal preoperative ventricular function. Monitoring the PCWP may be a helpful guide to fluid management in patients with left ventricular dysfunction, but it is not essential in patients with good ventricular function. It remains to be seen whether patients with multifactorial cardiac risk factors of more than 13 may show myocardial ischemic changes. Further study is necessary to identify patients who need hemodynamic monitoring with the Swan-Ganz catheter during abdominal aortic surgery. Previous studies have not classified patients in sufficient detail as to cardiac risk. Therefore serious doubt is raised about the need for a Swan-Ganz catheter during surgery in patients with normal preoperative ventricular function.

REFERENCES

1. Askitopolou H, Young CA, Morgan M, et al: Some cardiopulmonary effects of infrarenal clamping of the abdominal aorta. Anaesth. Intensive Care 6:44, 1978
2. Attia RK, Murphy J, Snider M, et al: Myocardial ischemia due to infrarenal aortic cross-clamping during aortic surgery in patients with severe coronary artery disease. Circulation 53:961, 1976
3. Au A, Evans D, Crago R, et al: Blood pressure effects of lower abdominal aortic surgery with particular reference to the use of morphine and droperidol in modifying the responses. Can. Anesth. Soc. J. 24:293, 1977
4. Berkowitz HD, Shetty S: Renin release and renal cortical ischemia following aortic cross-clamping. Arch. Surg. 109:612, 1974
5. Bland HL, Lowenstein E: Halothane induced decrease in experimental myocardial ischemia in the non-failing canine heart. Anesthesiology 45:287, 1976
6. Braunwald E: On the difference between the heart's output and its contractile state. An analysis of different muscle models. Circulation 43:171, 1971
7. Braunwald E: The determinants of myocardial oxygen consumption. Physiologist 12:65, 1969
8. Burow RP, Strauss HW, Singleton R, et al: Analysis of left ventricular function from multiple gated acquisition cardiac blood pool imaging. Comparison to contrast angiography. Circulation 56:1024, 1977
9. Bush HL, LoGerfo FW, Weisel RD, et al: Assessment of myocardial performance and optimal volume loading during elective abdominal aortic aneurysm resection. Arch. Surg. 112:1301, 1977
10. Carroll M, Laravuso B, Schaube JF: Left ventricular function during aortic surgery. Arch. Surg. 111:740, 1976
11. Chiariello M, Gold M, Leinbach R: Comparison between the effects of nitroglycerin and nitroprusside on ischemic injury during myocardial infarction. Circulation 54:766, 1976
12. Cooperman M, Pflug B, Martin EW, et al: Cardiovascular risk factors in patients with peripheral vascular disease. Surgery 84:505, 1978
13. Cronenwett J, Lindenauer SM: Distribution of intrarenal blood flow following aortic clamping and declamping. J. Surg. Res. 22:469, 1977
14. DeBakey ME, Crawford ES, Cooley DA, et al: Aneurysms of abdominal aorta. Analysis of results of graft replacement therapy one to 11 years after operation. Ann. Surg. 160:622, 1964
15. Dunn E, Prager L, Fry W, et al: The effect of abdominal aortic cross-clamping on myocardial function. J. Surg. Res. 22:463, 1977
16. Fry WJ, Keitzer WE, Kraft RO, et al: Prevention of hypotension due to aortic release. Surg. Gynecol. Obstet. 116:301, 1963
17. Goldman L, Caldera L, Nussbaum S, et al: Multifactorial index of cardiac risk in noncardiac surgical procedures. N. Engl. J. Med. 297:845, 1977

18. Hicks GL, Eastland MW, DeWeese JA, et al: Survival improvement following aortic aneurysm resection. Ann. Surg. 181:863, 1975
19. Kaplan JA, Jones EL: Vasodilator therapy during coronary artery surgery: Comparison of nitroglycerin and nitroprusside. J. Thorac. Cardiovasc. Surg. 77:301, 1979
20. Kistner JR, Miller ED Jr, Lake C, et al: Indices of myocardial oxygenation during coronary artery revascularization in man with morphine versus halothane anesthesia. Anesthesiology 50:324, 1979
21. Kouchoukos N, Lell WA, Karp B, et al: Hemodynamic effects of aortic clamping and decompression with a temporary shunt for resection of the descending thoracic aorta. Surgery 85:25, 1979
22. Mansberger AR, Cos EF, Flotle CT, et al: "Washout" acidosis following resection of aortic aneurysms. Clinical metabolic study of reactive hyperemia and effect of Dextran on excess lactate and pH. Ann. Surg. 163:778, 1966
23. McDonald RH, McDonald RR, Cingolani HE: Measurement of myocardial developed tension and its relation to oxygen consumption. Am. J. Physiol. 211:667, 1966
24. Meloche R, Pottecher T, Audet J, et al: Haemodynamic changes due to clamping of the abdominal aorta. Can. Anaesth. Soc. J. 24:20, 1977
25. Nelson RR, Gobel FL, Jorgensen CR, et al: Hemodynamic predictors of myocardial oxygen consumption during static and dynamic exercise. Circulation 50:1179, 1974
26. Perry MO: Hemodynamics of temporary abdominal aortic occlusion. Ann. Surg. 168:193, 1968
27. Peterson A, Brant D, Kirsh MM: Nitroglycerin infusion during infrarenal aortic cross-clamping in dogs: An experimental study. Surgery 84:216, 1978
28. Proven JL, Fraenkel GL, Austen WG: Metabolic and hemodynamic changes after temporary aortic occlusion in dogs. Surg. Gynecol. Obstet. 123:1417, 1966
29. Sabawala PB, Strong MJ, Keat A: Surgery of the aorta and its branches. Anesthesiology 33:229, 1970
30. Silverstein PR, Caldera DL, Cullen DJ, et al: Avoiding hemodynamic consequences of aortic cross-clamping and unclamping. Anesthesiology 50:462, 1979
31. Thompson JE, Hollier LH, Patman RD: Surgical management of abdominal aortic aneurysms: Factors influencing mortality and morbidity – A 20 year experience. Ann. Surg. 181:654, 1975
32. Wackers FJT, Berger HJ, Johnstone DE, et al: Multiple gated cardiac blood pool imaging for left ventricular ejection fraction: Validation of the technique and assessment of variability. Am. J. Cardiol. 43:1159, 1979
33. Wilkinson PL, Moyders JR, Ports T, et al: Rate pressure product and myocardial oxygen consumption during surgery for coronary artery bypass. Scientific Abstract Presented at the American Heart Association Meeting, Nov. 1979
34. Weisel RD, Berger RL, Hechtman HB: Measurement of cardiac output by thermodilution. N. Engl. J. Med. 292:682, 1975

Eugene F. Bernstein, M.D., Ph.D.
Ronald D. Harris, M.D.
George R. Leopold, M.D.

Ultrasound and CT Scanning in the Noninvasive Evaluation of Abdominal Aortic Aneurysms

Aneurysm of the abdominal aorta is a common and dangerous manifestation of diffuse atherosclerosis. The incidence of this lesion increases after the sixth decade of life and it has therefore become progressively more important in our aging society. The presence of an abdominal aortic aneurysm is most commonly first identified by the patient, who becomes aware of midabdominal discomfort and a palpable pulsatile abdominal mass. In about one-fourth of the cases, however, the lesion is entirely asymptomatic and detected on routine physical examination, by abdominal X-ray, ultrasound, or CT exam, at laparatomy for some other indication, or at postmortem examination.

It is important to accurately confirm a clinical diagnosis of aneurysm which may be made on the basis of physical examination or plain X-ray films alone, since a few patients operated upon on the basis of such limited diagnostic studies prove to have other lesions responsible for these findings, including a calcified tortuous aorta, overlying retroperitoneal masses, or other visceral masses superimposed upon a normal abdominal aortic pulsation. For these reasons, to avoid unnecessary surgery, independent objective confirmation of the diagnosis is appropriate.

The availability of more detailed information concerning the size and configuration of the aneurysm increases the data base available to the physician who must decide upon an operative or nonoperative course. Both noninvasive techniques of ultrasonic imaging and computerized tomography have proven extremely useful in this regard, and are now being widely applied to the management of such patients.

Angiography, both of the conventional contrast and newer isotope types [6], has also been advocated in the diagnosis and characterization of abdominal aortic aneurysms. Conventional contrast angiography is clearly invasive, requires hospitalization, has a small but definite complication rate, and is quite expensive. All angiographic studies define only the inner lumen of the aneurysm, which may provide grossly inaccurate data regarding size. For this reason, it is our feeling that aortography should not be performed as a diagnostic procedure, but rather as a preoperative investigation, once surgery has been definitely decided upon, to further delineate the anatomy of the paraaneurysmal structures, with particular emphasis on renal artery involvement or stenosis, multiple renal arteries, visceral artery lesions (including SMA and hypogastric involvement and the possibility of colonic ischemia), and other vascular anomalies. In our view, therefore, angiography is a complementary procedure to ultrasound or CT scanning. The latter are best for confirming the diagnosis and defining aneurysm size and configuration, while angiography provides additional useful and valuable preoperative information.

THE PLAIN X-RAY

Both AP and lateral views of the abdomen may show calcification in the wall of an abdominal aneurysm and therefore be diagnostic of its presence and indicative of its size. However, only 55%-85% of patients with abdominal aneurysms have such calcification [18]. Further, in the AP view, the right wall of the aneurysm generally overlies the vertebral column and therefore does not always permit an accurate estimate of the transverse diameter of the lesion. In addition, such films may not reveal that the calcified left aortic wall is simply a portion of a tortuous aorta and not an aneurysmal one. In contrast, the lateral abdominal X-ray is clearly diagnostic when positive and does provide a reasonably accurate estimate of aneurysm size. Unfortunately, particularly in the smaller aneurysms where size is more critical in evaluating the need for surgery, calcification is often absent.

THE ROLE OF ULTRASOUND AND CT SCANNING

In view of the limitations of the physical examination and conventional radiographs and the fact that both aortography and radionuclide aortic scans document only the lumen size and do not indicate the thickness of laminated clot and atheromatous material, other noninvasive and accurate means of diagnosis and sizing of abdominal aneurysms are important. Both ultrasound and CT scanning fulfill these requirements and permit routine documentation of the presence or absence of an abdominal aneurysm, an accurate depiction of its configuration and location, and good estimates of aneurysm size.

Until 1977, grey-scale echography was the most reliable tool for the evaluation and detection of abdominal aortic aneurysms. However, computed tomographic body scanning also has been recognized as a valuable radiographic diagnostic tool.

The applications of computed tomography are quite similar to echography in the investigation of the aorta in both normal and pathologic states. The two methods are similarly accurate in identifying those patients with an aneurysm and properly diagnosing those in whom clinical suspicion of aneurysm is raised but who prove to have aortic ectasia and tortuosity, an overlying abdominal mass, or a normal aorta in an asthenic person. Both techniques are safe, fast, noninvasive, and can be easily performed on an outpatient basis without discomfort to the patient. The fine detail obtained by these imaging modalities also provides added information about other structures important to the surgeon at the time of operation. These include the position and state of the renal vessels, vena cava, and associated vascular anomalies such as retroaortic or circumaortic renal veins. Details of the technical requirements for obtaining high quality studies with both of these modalities, and of the relative differences in information obtained by the two techniques, form the basis of this chapter.

ULTRASOUND TECHNIQUES

The use of a reflected beam of ultrasound to identify and characterize clinical pathology has been developed during the past two decades. In 1961, Donald and Brown first demonstrated an intraabdominal aortic aneurysm with ultrasound. Further development of this methodology has involved the use of the A-mode, B-mode scan, B-mode real-time, and M-mode ultrasound modalities. In each of these techniques a crystal is oscillated by electrical energy, producing sound at frequencies exceeding 2 million cycles/second, with each burst of ultrasound lasting approximately 1 microsecond. This ultrasonic beam is directed at the tissues to be studied and is reflected when it contacts any change in tissue density or tissue interface with a different acoustic impedance. The reflected waves then may be displayed on an oscilloscopic screen in a variety of ways.

In the A-mode presentation the reflected echoes are demonstrated as vertical deflections from a horizontal baseline, which represents the time for the echo to travel to the target and return to the receiver. Knowing the velocity of sound in human tissues permits accurately converting this time delay into a depth scale in the direction of the sound beam. A stronger echo will produce a greater deflection, or amplitude of echo, on this horizontal time (or depth) base tracing. Such echo strength is dependent on the nature of the reflecting interface, with more marked acoustic mismatching, or impedance, from more markedly different tissues. Accordingly, the A mode permits the precise measurement of the depth of various tissue planes in a straight line from the transducer through the body. It is a one-dimensional determination that is highly accurate (Fig. 1).

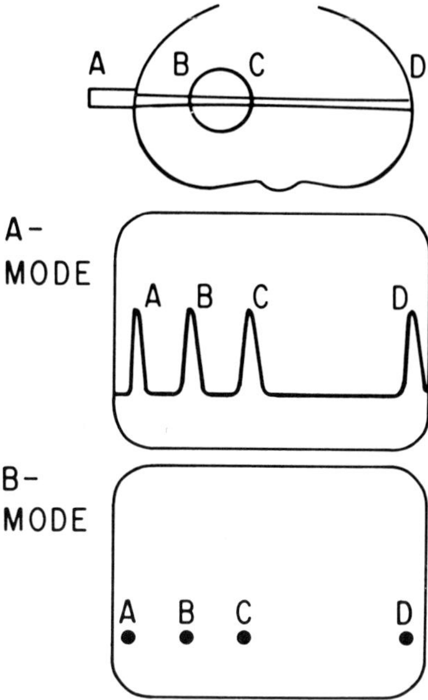

Fig. 1. Scheme of A-mode echography, which represents each reflecting surface as a spike on the oscilloscope, the height of which is proportional to the acoustic density difference between the two materials at the interface. In the B-mode each such interface between different layers is represented as a dot, the brightness of which is proportional to the density difference. It is comparable to looking down onto the top of the A-mode spikes. Each of these techniques provides a one-dimensional output of the distance between layers traversed by the sound beam. [From Bernstein EF: Ultrasound techniques in the diagnosis and evaluation of abdominal aortic aneurysms, in Bernstein EF (ed): Noninvasive Diagnostic Techniques in Vascular Disease. St. Louis, C. V. Mosby, 1978.]

By moving the transducer in a plane of section and representing echoes on the oscilloscope in accordance with the transducer position, a two-dimensional impression of the interior of the body may be obtained by what is referred to as B-mode scanning, or ultrasonic scanning (Fig. 2). This procedure usually involves the manual movement of a single transducer to fill in the picture of a particular body section [11, 12, 25, 26, 34].

Early efforts with ultrasound in the diagnosis of abdominal aortic aneurysms involved the use of both the A and B modes by Goldberg and Segal in 1966 [13,

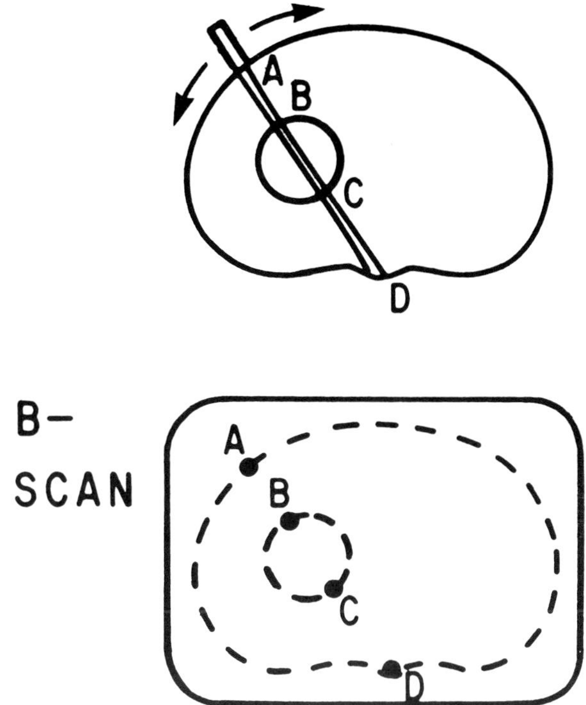

Fig. 2. B scan is obtained by rotating the B-mode transducer to obtain many B-mode reflections and storing them on an oscilloscope screen. This permits building up a detailed two-dimensional image in any plane or section. [From Bernstein EF: Ultrasound techniques in the diagnosis and evaluation of abdominal aortic aneurysms, in Bernstein EF (ed): Noninvasive Diagnostic Techniques in Vascular Disease. St. Louis, C. V. Mosby, 1978.]

39]. In a subsequent study Evans first utilized B scanning to demonstrate the value of the cross-sectional technique in two planes to obtain a three-dimensional picture of the aneurysm [10]. In 1970, Leopold pointed out the advantages of combining the A-mode and B-scan techniques, utilizing the B scan to identify and characterize the shape of the aneurysm, particularly in the longitudinal echogram, with follow-up identification of the maximum diameters in both AP and transverse planes with the A-mode technique (Figs. 3-8) [27]. The accuracy in sizing aneurysms using the combined technique approached 3 mm. Our current experience with this approach exceeds 400 cases at the University of California, San Diego, and we have increasingly more confidence in the sensitivity and accuracy of the method [5, 28, 29].

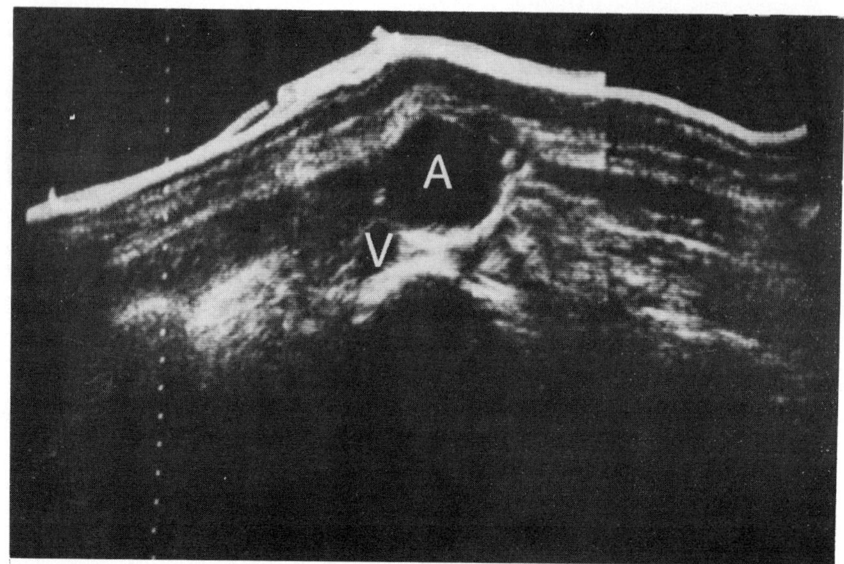

Fig. 3. B-scan echogram in transverse plane demonstrating an abdominal aortic aneurysm (A) and the inferior vena cava (V). [From Bernstein EF: Ultrasound techniques in the diagnosis and evaluation of abdominal aortic aneurysms, in Bernstein EF (ed): Noninvasive Diagnostic Techniques in Vascular Disease. St. Louis, C. V. Mosby, 1978.]

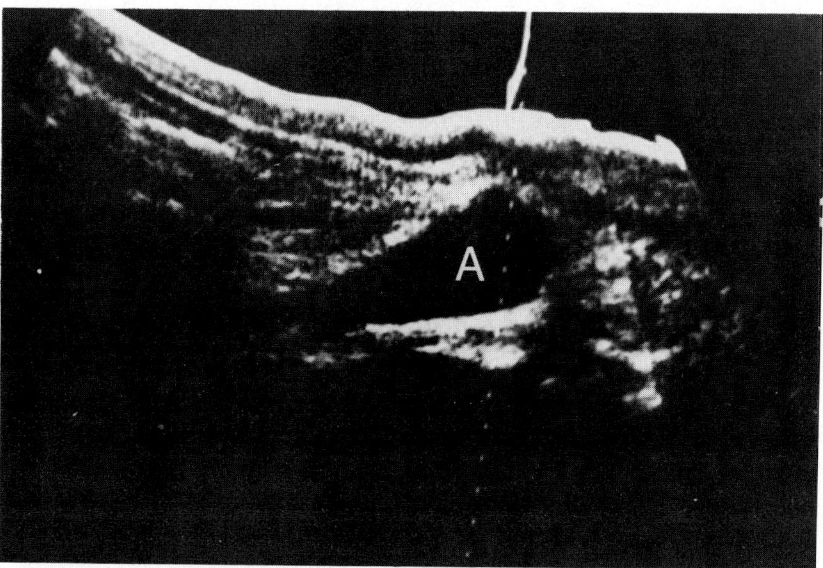

Fig. 4. Sagittal plane B-scan echo through an abdominal aortic aneurysm (A) with sizing scale. [From Bernstein EF: Ultrasound techniques in the diagnosis and evaluation of abdominal aortic aneurysms, in Bernstein EF (ed): Noninvasive Diagnostic Techniques in Vascular Disease. St. Louis, C. V. Mosby, 1978.]

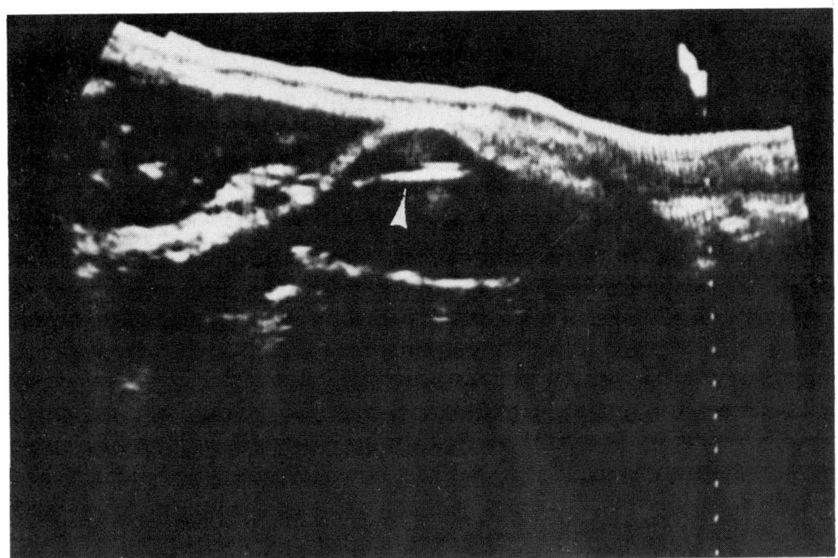

Fig. 5. Sagittal plane demonstration of a large abdominal aortic aneurysm with a thrombus (arrow) within the lumen. [From Bernstein EF: Ultrasound techniques in the diagnosis and evaluation of abdominal aortic aneurysms, in Bernstein EF (ed): Noninvasive Diagnostic Techniques in Vascular Disease. St. Louis, C. V. Mosby, 1978.]

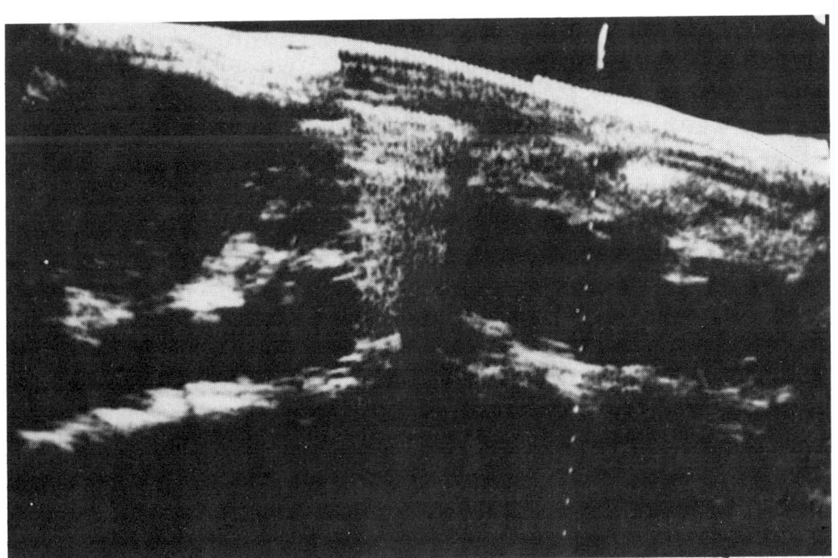

Fig. 6. Sagittal plane through a large and tortuous abdominal aortic aneurysm, which leaves the plane of the echogram in the center of the study as it extends to the patient's left beyond the plane of the examination. [From Bernstein EF: Ultrasound techniques in the diagnosis and evaluation of abdominal aortic aneurysms, in Bernstein EF (ed): Noninvasive Diagnostic Techniques in Vascular Disease. St. Louis, C. V. Mosby, 1978.]

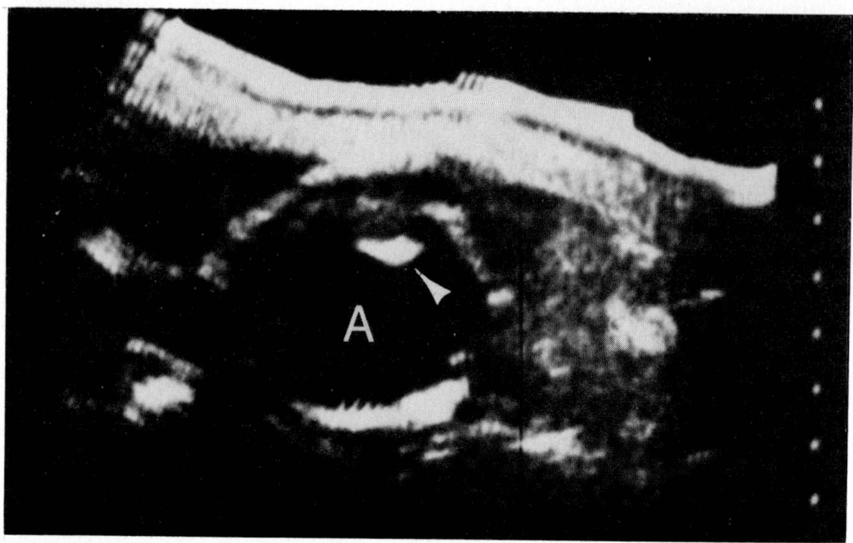

Fig. 7. Transverse B scan of an abdominal aneurysm (A) with a thrombus (arrow) of varying acoustic density in the anterior portion of the lumen. [From Bernstein EF: Ultrasound techniques in the diagnosis and evaluation of abdominal aortic aneurysms, in Bernstein EF (ed): Noninvasive Diagnostic Techniques in Vascular Disease. St. Louis, C. V. Mosby, 1978.]

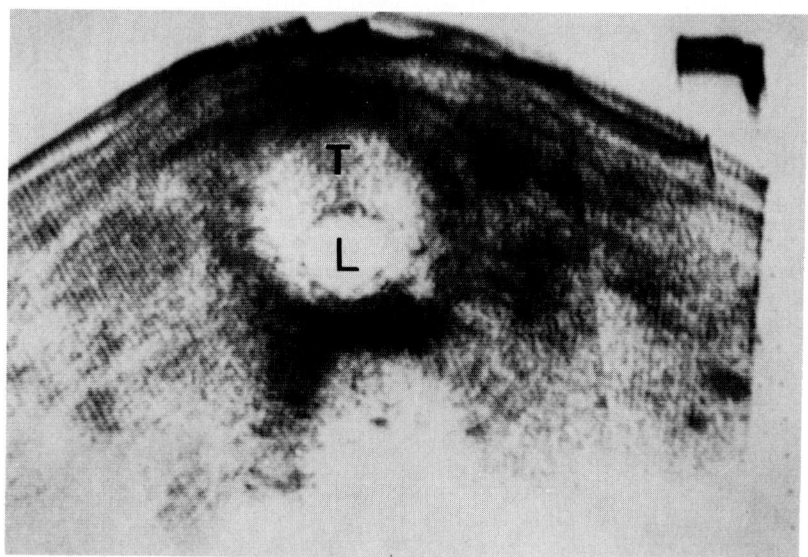

Fig. 8. Transverse section of a large abdominal aneurysm, in which the intraluminal thrombus (T) is circumferential and the lumen (L) is of normal size. Such a lesion might well appear normal on aortography. [From Bernstein EF: Ultrasound techniques in the diagnosis and evaluation of abdominal aortic aneurysms, in Bernstein EF (ed): Noninvasive Diagnostic Techniques in Vascular Disease. St. Louis, C. V. Mosby, 1978.]

Accuracy of B-Mode Ultrasound

Earlier studies of abdominal aneurysms with ultrasound, involving both A- and B-mode investigations to obtain three-dimensional data and accurate sizing, demonstrated the ability of the technique to adequately visualize such lesions in a routine manner. The first published correlation of the diagnostic capability of ultrasound with surgery, in 1971, indicated that B-scanning accurately diagnosed 79 of 80 cases of abdominal aneurysms with one false positive result in a patient with a paraaortic lymph node enlargement [35]. More recently, a study of the sizing accuracy of B-mode ultrasound by Maloney and associates measured the AP and transverse diameter of the abdominal aortic aneurysm at surgery in 47 patients, in comparison with AP and lateral X-rays and B-mode ultrasound images [30]. In only 72% of these patients was the lateral X-ray suggestive of the diagnosis, and size measurements were possible in only 55% of the cases. On the other hand, B-mode ultrasound accurately made the diagnosis and permitted size measurements in each instance. In both the AP and transverse planes, the ultrasonic estimates of size averaged within 4 mm of the surgical measurement. In those patients in whom measurements could be obtained from the plain X-ray films, there was an average of 8.7 mm of variance in the AP dimension and 15 mm in the transverse plane, which had to be evaluated from the AP X-ray. On the basis of this study, it is clear that ultrasound not only is a better diagnostic technique than the plain X-ray, with little or no likelihood of false negative or positive reports, but also is more precise in sizing abdominal aortic aneurysms in both the AP and transverse dimension. A similar study was recently published from the Cleveland Clinic, comparing physical examination, the lateral abdominal X-ray, and B-mode ultrasound with operative measurements in 53 cases. Physical examination overestimated the aneurysm size by an average of 1 cm, as did the lateral X-ray [24]. The B-mode ultrasound measurements were identical with the operative measurements in 34% of the patients and within 0.5 cm in 75%. The mean diameter of the aneurysms measured by ultrasound was within 2 mm of that measured directly at operation.

Finally, the reproducibility of B-mode ultrasound measurements has been demonstrated in our own experience in which over 100 patients have been followed rather than operated upon because they represented poor-risk patients with small asymptomatic lesions [2-4]. These patients have had repeated studies, some over periods up to 6 years. Studies performed at 3 month intervals rarely vary by more than 2 or 3 mm, and produce such consistent data that growth rates can be accurately defined, as indicated in the next section.

ABDOMINAL ANEURYSM GROWTH RATES

In a group of poor-risk patients with asymptomatic abdominal aortic aneurysms measuring less than 6 cm in largest transverse diameter, a policy of continued observations with sequential A- and B-mode echo scans at 3 month intervals initially provided data concerning small aneurysm growth rate in 49 patients. The mean aneurysm growth rate was 0.4 cm a year in those patients observed for at least one year. However, in 10 patients there was no evidence of growth over periods of observation extending to 42 months, whereas in others there was sudden, unexpected, and rapid growth within a very short period of time, often without the development of symptoms. The growth of small aneurysms was not correlated with patient age or blood pressure.

This growth rate information appears valuable in evaluating the risk of elective surgery in a poor-risk patient with an asymptomatic abdominal aneurysm measuring less than 6 cm. It suggests that the average aneurysm takes 7.5 years to grow from 3 to 6 cm and permits weighing the mortality of elective surgery in a given case against the known likelihood of rupture at a particular aneurysm size. It has been our policy to observe such high-risk patients until the aneurysm reaches a size of 6 cm or symptoms develop. In contrast, in good-risk patients early elective surgery is indicated for aneurysms of any size.

This data has recently been updated to include a total of 117 patients followed for 181 patient years (Table 1). In those cases followed 12 months or longer, the available data remain quite consistent with our previous study, although the growth rates are somewhat less than the previously reported figure of 0.4 cm/year. As indicated in Table 1, those aneurysms diagnosed between 3 and 5.9 cm in diameter appear to grow at rates between 0.23 and 0.28 cm/year, based on 159 patient years of observation. Those few aneurysms which have been studied at sizes larger than 6 cm indicate a definitely increased growth rate, as would be expected by the law of LaPlace.

CT OPERATING PRINCIPLES

The patient is placed on a couch which passes through an aperture in the scanner gantry. Around the aperture is an array of highly sensitive X-ray detectors which are in precise alignment with the X-ray tube, or single detectors that rotate. The X-ray beam is tightly collimated into a shape that matches the configuration of the detectors. As the beam passes through the anatomic

Table 1
Abdominal Aortic Aneurysm Growth (Cases Followed >12 Months)

Size at Diagnosis (cm)	Points	Months	Growth (cm/yr)
3 - 3.9	23	715	0.23
4 - 4.9	25	646	0.27
5 - 5.9	22	512	0.28
Totals	70	1873*	—

*156 patient years.

structures, the intensity of the beam is altered by tissue absorption in the beam's path. The detectors convert this information into electrical signals which are precisely digitized for each sampling interval or until the scan is completed. The patient is then repositioned and another scan begun. A complex series of computer calculations defines the precise X-ray absorption value for each specific pixel point within the scanned section. These digital values are stored on a magnetic tape and represent a mathematical picture of the patient's anatomy. The data are then available for video display and can be manipulated for optimal evaluation and reproduction. The newest generation of scanners complete a scan in 2-5 sec and have a skin surface radiation dose of as low as 0.1-0.45 rads per section, depending on the manufacturer.

CT TECHNIQUES

The approach should be tailored to each individual patient, depending on the particular problem. In the case of an aortic aneurysm, different techniques can be utilized. One method is to palpate the maximal part of the abdominal mass and then scan 3 cm above and 3 cm below this point [1, 38] at 2 cm intervals. The patient is then given intravenous radiographic contrast material either by a bolus injection of 50-100 cc of a high iodine content substance (Renografin 76 or Conray 400), or by an infusion of 300 cc 25%-30% of a meglumine diatrizoate solution. The scans are then repeated following the contrast injection [21-23].

Another technique is to scan from the xyphoid to below the umbilicus at 2 cm intervals to gain information about other intraabdominal organs, the proximal aorta, and the iliac arteries. Contrast material is then administered and the scans repeated, occasionally overlapping at 1 cm intervals to gain information about the renal and visceral vessels. The renal status can also be determined after the administration of contrast material, particularly to identify problems of excretion and possible obstruction. If necessary, a primary contrast exam may be performed, especially in an emergency situation. After the contrast material is injected, the aorta itself, the aortic lumen, and thrombus within the aneurysm is clearly defined. The procedure without, and then with, contrast takes about 60 minutes. A contrast scan alone takes 30-40 minutes to complete.

EVALUATION OF ANEURYSMS BY CT

In the early experience with CT, scans were done without i.v. contrast material; although aneurysms could be recognized, the wall of the aorta was indistinguishable from the lumen unless the wall was calcified. Thrombi were indistinguishable from the blood in the lumen. The time involved in obtaining these early scans was 4 minutes and the radiation dose approximated 8 rads to the skin [1].

With the newer scanners, especially with the 2 second scan time, the aortic diameter is easily measured even if not calcified and the measurements correlate well with those obtained at surgery [8, 14, 19]. Vertebral body erosions associated with aneurysms are easily identified and aneurysms may be distinguished from other intraabdominal masses or hematomas. CT is also helpful in distinguishing an aneurysm from tortuosity when an aneurysm is suspected by other radiographic or clinical examinations. Additional information gained by CT includes the variation in aortic position from its usual location anterior and slightly to the left of the vertebral bodies. With increasing tortuosity or dilatation, it frequently swings considerably to the right (Fig. 9). Commonly, aneurysms of the iliac arteries are also encountered (Fig. 10) as well as dilatation of the proximal aorta.

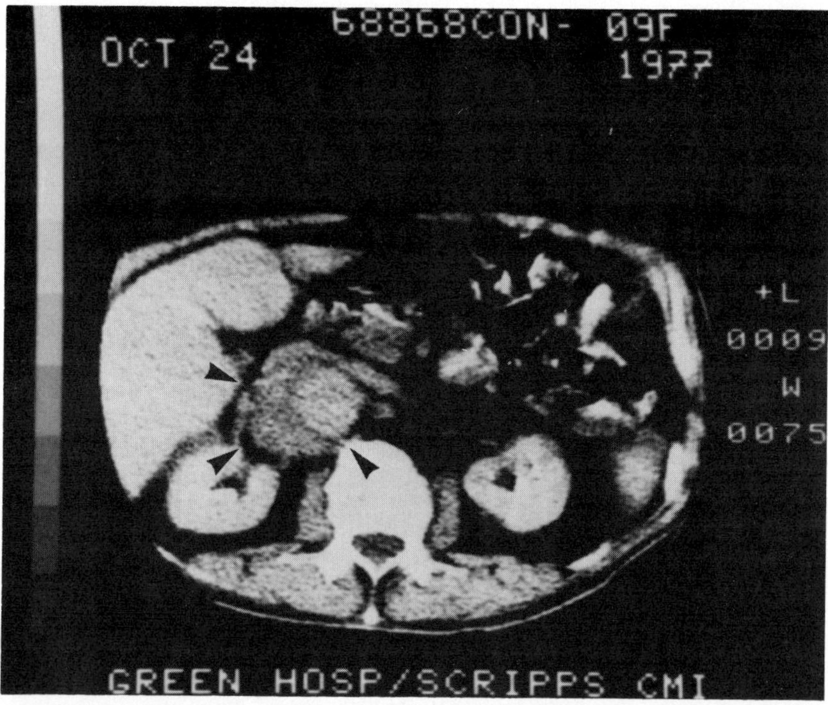

Fig. 9. This contrast enhanced computerized tomographic scan demonstrates the amount of tortuosity which can occur in a dilated aorta. Here the aorta is seen far to the right (arrowheads). The inferior vena cava is sitting on top of the aorta with the renal veins stretched to gain access to it. CT scans are read with the patient's right on the viewer's left, as if looking up at the section from the patient's feet.

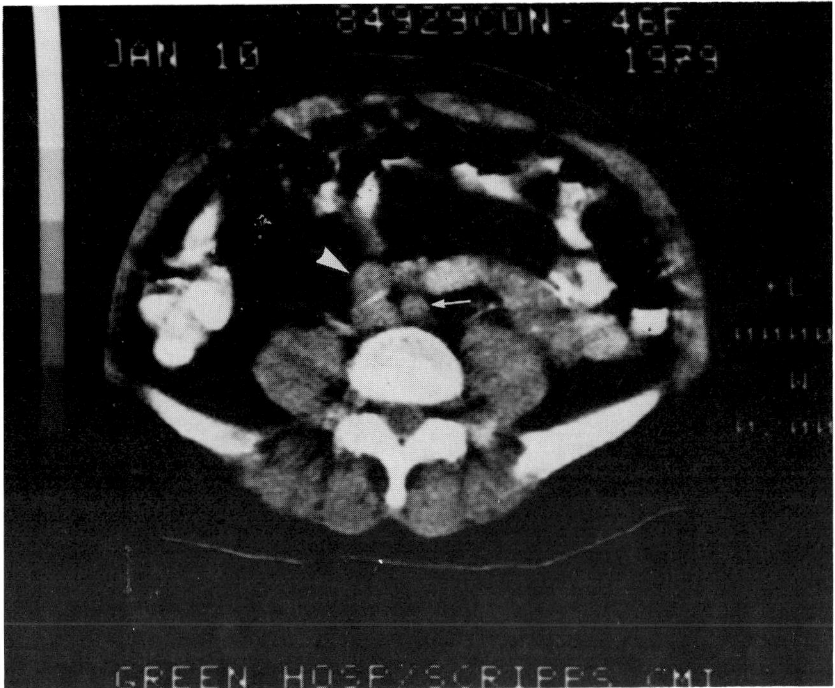

Fig. 10. This scan obtained below the aortic bifurcation shows an aneurysm of the right common iliac artery (arrowhead) next to a normal left side (small arrow).

Of particular interest was the observation that CT may be diagnostic when ultrasound is not effective because of patient obesity, barium retention, or excessive intestinal gas. Obese patients are easily scanned because the fat acts as a contrast against which the soft tissues stand out (Fig. 11). Gas also does not interfere with the CT scans, especially if the patient is given an intravenous injection of 1 mg glucagon to inhibit bowel motility. Barium may produce some artifacts but does not significantly grade the scans. One very important source of CT artifacts is the presence of metallic surgical clips, since small detailed areas are obscured by streaks from the metal.

Size estimates of the aneurysms have been quite accurate on CT when correlated with findings at surgery [15, 17]. They do not vary more than 4 mm, and in a series of 23 patients the measurements were identical in 17 cases.

One of the great advances in CT scanning has occurred with the use of intravenous radiographic contrast material (RCM). Exams with RCM have allowed detailed evaluation of the lumen size and the position and amount of thrombus present in all patients studied. The different phases of clot formation can be sharply defined regardless of the degree of organization [8, 17]. Newer

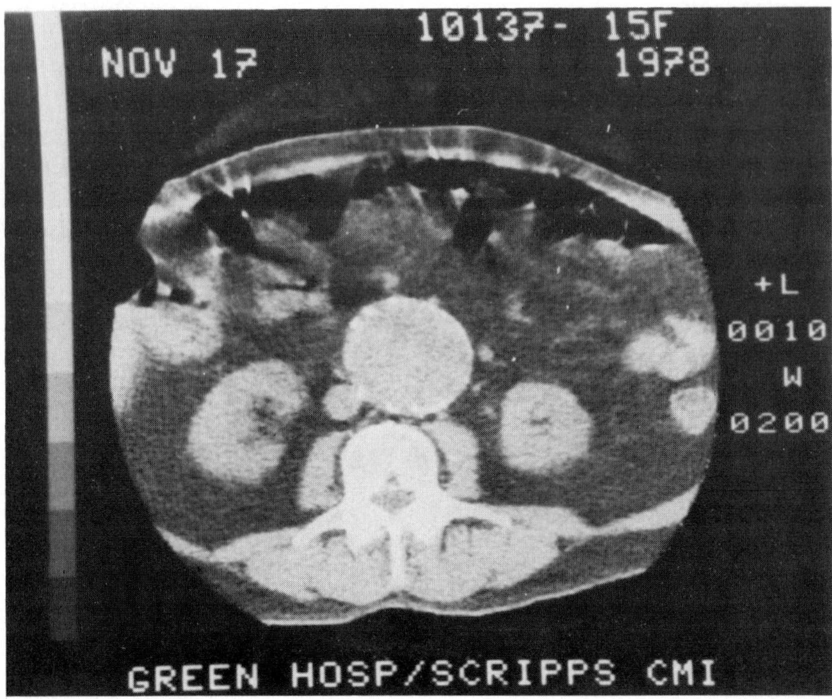

Fig. 11. A scan from a patient with a large amount of body fat shows how the fat acts as a contrast substance against which the organs stand out. Here the aneurysm dwarfs the inferior vena cava.

clot close to the lumen is less dense than the older clot close to the outer wall, as confirmed by serial sectioning of pathologic specimens [17]. In most cases the majority of thrombus lies anterior to the lumen, which is in turn located symmetrically somewhat posterior to the center (Fig. 12). The clot can also be further evaluated after contrast enhancement. Clot liquefication or clot dissection can be identified by the presence of an eccentric lumen, often with a tail of contrast seen close to the lateral wall (Fig. 13). This indicates a dehisence of the clot [17]. A clot dissection can also be recognized by contrast material appearing around the edge of the clot [38] (Fig. 14). This preoperative clot identification may help the surgeon prevent distal emboli at surgery.

The preoperative visualization of the inferior vena cava position in relation to the aorta and the state of the visceral vessels, such as the celiac, superior mesenteric, and renal arteries, also can be ascertained. Aneurysmal dilatation of the iliac arteries is easily determined, especially following contrast enhancement (Fig. 10), and is better seen by CT than by echography. This is important preoperative information when assessing the surgical risk and potential technical operative difficulties [16, 17].

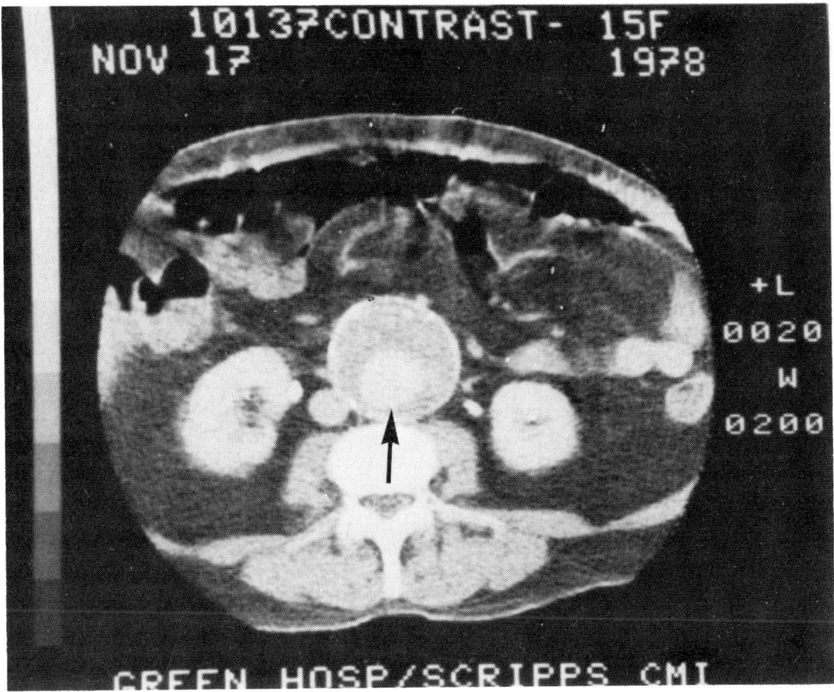

Fig. 12. Following intravenous contrast material, the lumen of the aorta is seen to enhance with flowing blood (arrow). The thrombus is easily differentiated and is typically located anterior and lateral to the lumen.

Although not a common problem in abdominal aortic aneurysms, dissections of the aortic wall have been seen on CT scans as a separation of the wall and development of two lumens (Fig. 15). After contrast material injection, a determination can be made as to whether both lumens are carrying flowing blood or if one lumen is thrombosed [23].

Retroperitoneal hematomas secondary to leaking or rupturing aneurysms can be quickly assessed by CT especially with contrast enhanced scans. Extravascular blood is a high density substance, which disrupts the normal anatomic configurations in the retroperitoneum on the scans (Fig. 16A) [8, 16, 17]. After RCM, the clot takes a characteristic lower density than surrounding structures, which normally "blush" with the contrast (Fig. 16B). The hematoma may also have some rim enhancement (Fig. 16B) because of an inflammatory response around the hematoma to the presence of the blood. These findings are considerably better seen on CT than echo [8].

A new and important role for CT has been the postoperative evaluation of patients undergoing aneurysmectomy. Repeat scans can follow the resolution of

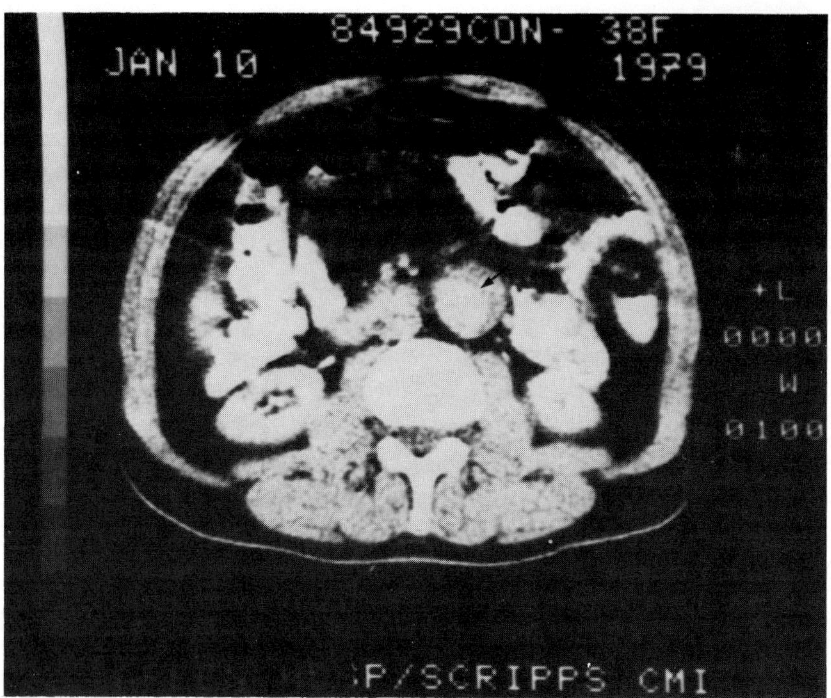

Fig. 13. In this contrast enhanced scan the lumen is eccentric (arrow), suggesting clot dissection.

periprosthetic hematomas. Both aortoprosthesis disruption and false-aneurysm formation have been diagnosed by CT scans which can be done rapidly in emergency situations. There is no need to prepare the bowel in those patients who often have an attendant paralytic ileus which would render echo ineffective. It also may be possible to distinguish between early postoperative changes from those changes due to infection. One of the early signs is the loss of periaortic fat [19]. An exceptional diagnostic finding, however, has been the identification of pockets of gas due to pyogenic organisms (Fig. 17), which are usually multiple and characteristically located posterior to the lumen. RCM enhancement demonstrates that these gas pockets are indeed extraluminal [20]. In distinction, gas can be found in normal patients up to 10 days after surgery, but the gas is seen anteriorly and is usually a single collection compared to the posteriorly located multiple gas bubbles of an abscess [20]. Inflammatory rim enhancement around a postgraft abscess after contrast injection is also a sign of infection (Figs. 18A and 18B).

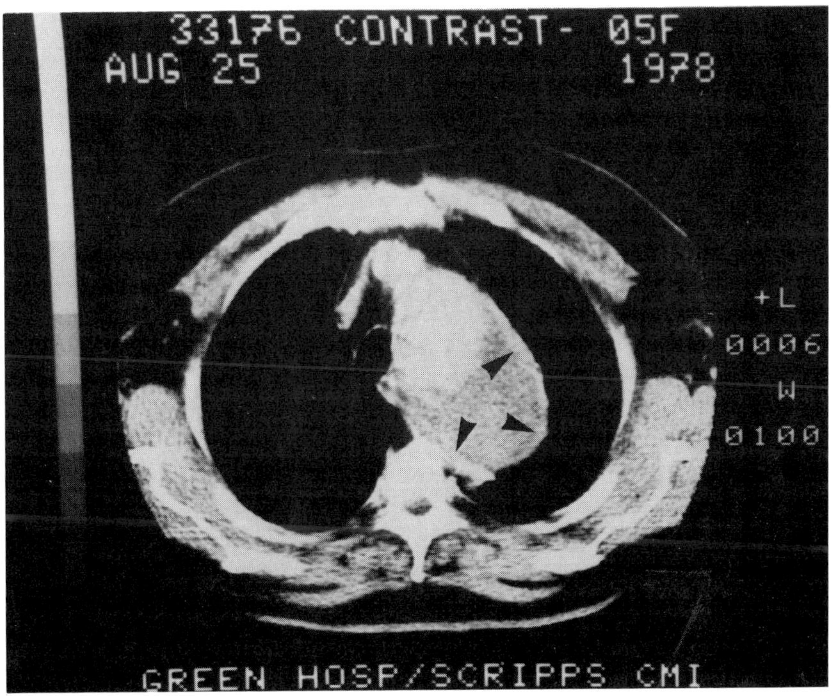

Fig. 14. In this patient contrast material is seen around the edge of the thrombus just beneath the wall of the aorta (arrowheads). This is a sign of clot liquefication and dehisence.

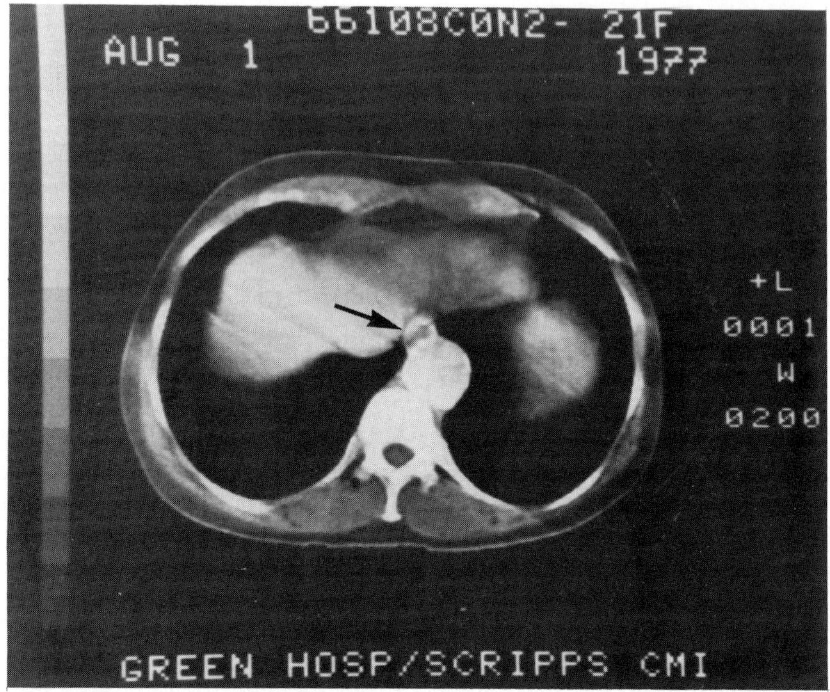

Fig. 15. Following an aortic dissection the two lumens are separated by a calcific rim. The larger, true lumen contains contrast enhanced flowing blood. The smaller, false lumen (arrow) does not enhance, indicating it is thrombosed.

Fig. 16. A retroperitoneal hematoma surrounds a leaking aortic prosthesis. (A) The high density blood obscures the normal anatomic configurations of the aorta and anterior psoas muscle margins. Vertebral body erosions are also noted (arrowheads). The bleeding was due to an aortoprosthetic graft disruption. (B) Contrast enhancement clearly delineates the aortic lumen and the limits of the periprosthetic hematoma (white arrows).

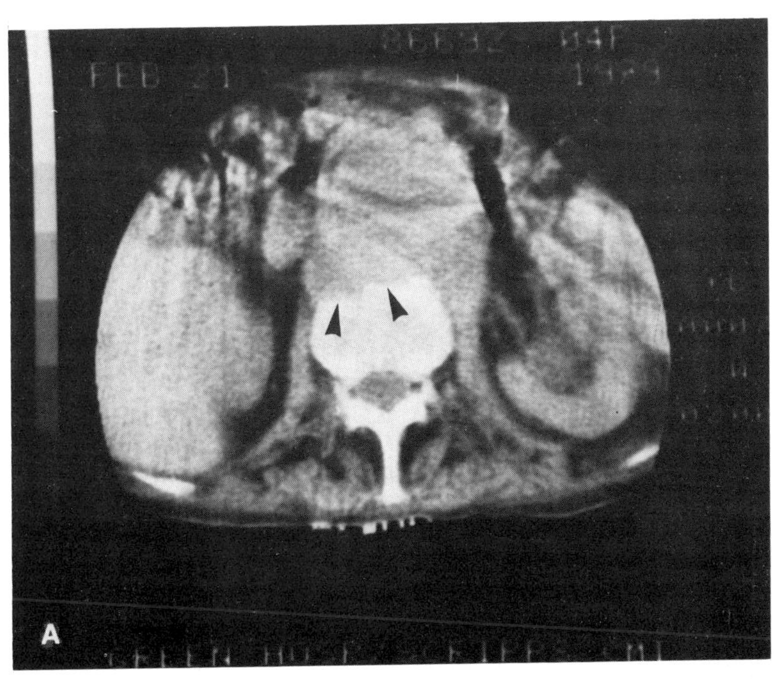
FEB 21
A

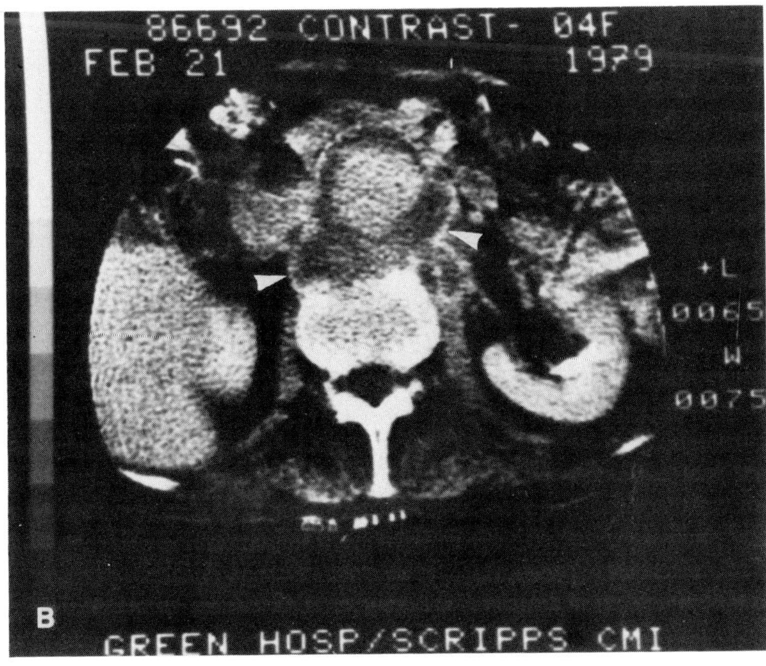
86692 CONTRAST- 04F
FEB 21
1979
+L
0065
W
0075
B
GREEN HOSP/SCRIPPS CMI

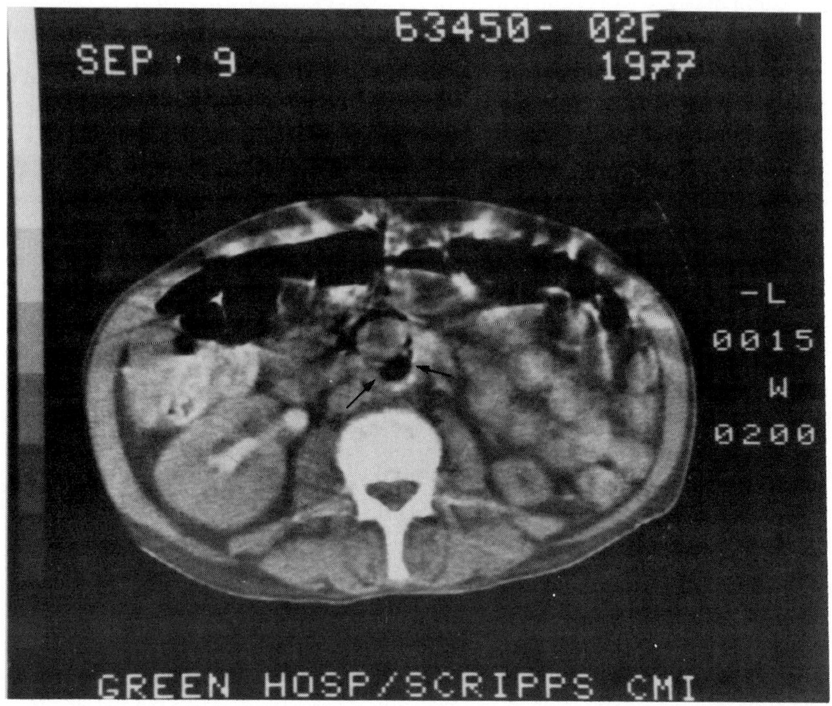

Fig. 17. This patient became febrile after aortic graft surgery. The scan shows collections of gas, which appears as a black area posterior to the lumen of the aorta (arrows). These gas pockets are felt to be pathognomonic for a pyogenic infection.

Fig. 18. This patient became febrile shortly after his aneurysm was resected and the aortic wall wrapped over the graft. (A) Scan done without contrast material shows inhomogeneous soft tissue densities below the graft bifurcation (arrowheads). (B) The postcontrast scan in this patient demonstrates rim enhancement of the wrapped aortic graft (arrowheads). The rim enhancement is also seen with infection, and an abscess was found at this site.

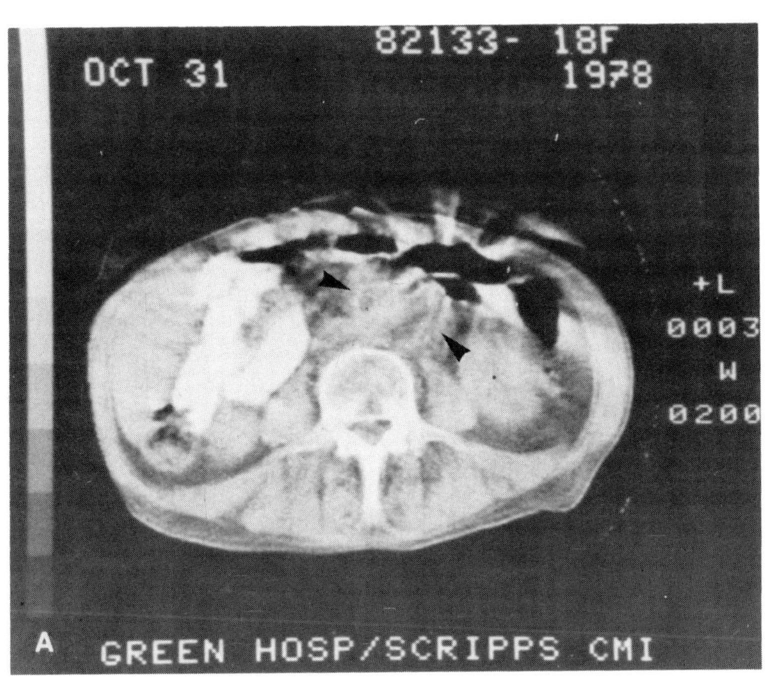
82133- 18F
OCT 31
1978
+L
0003
W
0200
A
GREEN HOSP/SCRIPPS CMI

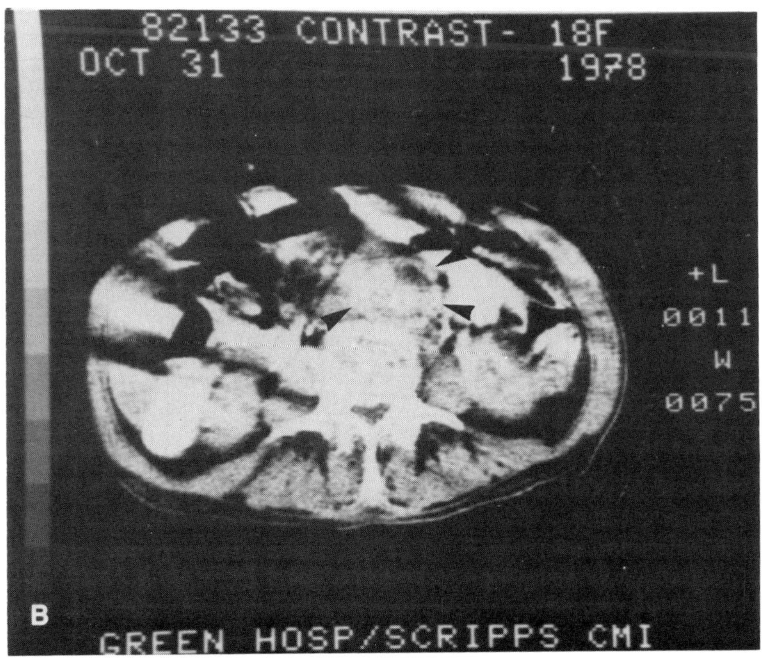
82133 CONTRAST- 18F
OCT 31
1978
+L
0011
W
0075
B
GREEN HOSP/SCRIPPS CMI

COMPARATIVE ANALYSIS OF ULTRASOUND AND CT SCANNING

Echography has been shown to be quite accurate in diagnosing 98.8%-100% of abdominal aneurysms [7, 35, 41] and generally correlates within 3 mm of the findings at surgery (Table 2) [29]. However, in some hands, the results have not been as reliable. One study found a consistent underestimation of size in up to 20% of patients by B-mode scans [7], and another series [32, 33] found that the size underestimation ranged from 1.3 to 3.0 cm. These errors may be due to an increased wall thickness with old organized thrombus, leading to difficulty in acoustically separating the aortic wall from surrounding tissue. In a recent series [17] of 27 patients, the ultrasound findings were identical to those at surgery in 3 patients but underestimated aneurysmal size from 2 to 16 mm in the other 24 patients. Wider discrepancies were present in obese patients or where there was heavy thrombus deposited in the walls of the aneurysm. Whether such variations in data are due to differences in equipment, its application, or skill in interpretation remains unknown at this time.

Table 2
Comparison of Ultrasound and Computerized Tomography in the Diagnosis and Assessment of Abdominal Aortic Aneurysms

	Ultrasound	Computerized Tomography
Examining modality	High frequency sound (1-20 mHz)	X-ray
Radiation dose (skin surface)/slice	None	0.1-2 R
Time for examination	10-60 min	30-60 min
Cost of examination	$75-$150	$75-$300
Dependence upon technician skill	Great	Modest
Dependence upon interpretive skill	Great	Straightforward
Limitations	Intestinal gas, obesity. Cannot distinguish clot from flowing blood.	Motion. Only cross-section images generally available now. Metallic clips distort image.
Accuracy in aneurysm diagnosis	Excellent	Excellent
Accuracy in aneurysm size estimates	± 3 mm	Not fully documented but probably ± 3 mm

Ultrasound frequently can detect the presence of thrombus within an aneurysm, although the various phases of clot organization may not be as accurately distinguished as with CT. The clinical importance of these distinctions remain uncertain at this time, however.

The presence of large amounts of interfering intestinal gas (in at least 15% of patients) is a problem for ultrasound. The worst cases occur in patients with paralytic bowel ileus. However, the presence of an abdominal aneurysm usually pushes aside the overlapping bowel, so that the diagnosis can still be made in most instances. Radiodense contrasts in the bowel, such as barium, also serve as an obstacle to ultrasound, but usually do not interfere with aneurysm diagnosis. Finally, in some obese patients, the body size is too great to permit adequate penetration of the sound beam for an accurate anatomic examination [36].

On the positive side, echo has at least two major advantages over CT in being able to scan in a longitudinal plane and that the energy used is nonionizing. In a comparison between the two techniques in 20 patients, Raskin et al. [37] felt that ultrasound was indeed superior because it was less expensive as well as nonionizing and provided longitudinal scans. They felt echography was as accurate as CT in determining aneurysm size and in revealing intraluminal thrombus. The CT limitation to transverse scanning would increase the likelihood of falsely diagnosing an aneurysm as an ectatic aorta swings transversely. However, whether such errors are common is still not known.

Finally, real-time ultrasonography represents an additional modality for the study of aortic wall motion, which eliminates the need for highly skilled technical specialists and permits the recognition of aortic dissection.

One of the problems with the older CT scanners was the time required for each study. However, with the newer machines, the entire procedure can be accomplished within 30 to 60 minutes, which compares with 10 to 60 minutes for ultrasound examinations.

Radiation dosage has also been a CT drawback, but with the newer scanners, the skin dose has been significantly reduced to 0.1-2 rads per slice [31, 42], and the patient dosage is no greater than that received from a GI series.

The earlier advantage of ultrasound in being able to perform longitudinal scans is rapidly being equalized by newer CT software packages which allow both longitudinal and coronal reconstruction images of the abdomen, but these are available in less than 1% of the installations in this country at the present time.

Metallic hemostatic surgical clips produce serious CT image artifacts, especially when they are located adjacent to moving structures such as a pulsatile aorta. Because of their dependence on postoperative CT scans, most neurosurgeons have ceased using such clips for hemostasis, and vascular surgeons may find a similar tactic useful if the frequent postoperative use of CT scanning becomes progressively more valuable.

REFERENCES

1. Axelbaum SP, Schellinger D, Gomes MN, et al: Computed tomographic evaluation of aortic aneurysms. Am. J. Roentgenol. 127:75-78, 1976
2. Bernstein EF: Considerations in the management of poor-risk patients with small asymptomatic abdominal aortic aneurysms, in Varco RL, Delaney JP (eds): Controversy in Surgery. Philadelphia, W. B. Saunders, 1976
3. Bernstein EF, Dilley RB, Goldberger LE, et al: Growth rates of small abdominal aortic aneurysms. Surgery 80:765, 1976
4. Bernstein EF: The natural history of abdominal aortic aneurysms, in Delaney JB, Najarian JS (eds): Vascular Surgery. Miami, Symposia Specialists, 1978
5. Bernstein EF: Ultrasound techniques in the diagnosis and evaluation of abdominal aortic aneurysms, in: Non-Invasive Diagnostic Techniques in Vascular Disease. St. Louis, C. V. Mosby, 1978, pp 330-338
6. Birnholtz JC: Alternatives in the diagnosis of abdominal aortic aneurysm: Combined use of isotope aortography and ultrasonography. Am. J. Roentgenol. Radium Ther. Nucl. Med. 118:809, 1973
7. Brewster DC, Darling C, Raines JK: Assessment of abdominal aortic aneurysm size. Cardiovasc. Surg. 1976 [Suppl II]; Circulation 56:164-169, 1977
8. Carter BL, Wechsler RJ: Computed tomography of the retroperitoneum and abdominal wall. Semin. Roentgenol. 13:201, 211, 1978
9. Donald L, Brown TG: Demonstration of tissue interfaces within the body by ultrasonic echo sounding. Br. J. Radiol. 34:539, 1961
10. Evans GC, Lehman JS, Segal BL, et al: Echo-aortography. Am. J. Cardiol. 19:91, 1967
11. Goldberg BB: Suprasternal aortosonography. JAMA 215:245, 1971
12. Goldberg BB, Lehman JS: Aortosonography: Ultrasound measurement of the abdominal and thoracic aorta. Arch. Surg. 100:652, 1970
13. Goldberg BB, Ostrum BJ, Isard HJ: Ultrasonic aortography. JAMA 198:119, 1966
14. Gomes MN: CT scanning in the diagnosis of abdominal aortic aneurysms. Computed Tomography 1:51-61, 1977
15. Gomes MN, Schellinger D, Hufnagel CA: Abdominal aortic aneurysms and CT scanning. Symposium on Total Body Computerized Tomography, Heidelberg, Sept. 29-Oct. 1, 1977
16. Gomes MN, Hufnagel CA: The use of CT scanning in the evaluation of aneurysms of the abdominal aorta. International Cardiovascular Society, Los Angeles, June 1978
17. Gomes MN, Hakkal HG, Schellinger D: Ultrasonography and CT scanning: A comparative study of abdominal aortic aneurysms. Computerized Tomography 2:99-110, 1978
18. Gore I, Hirst AJ: Arteriosclerotic aneurysms of the abdominal aorta: A review. Prog. Cardiovasc. Dis. 16:113, 1973
19. Haaga J, Reich NE: Computed Tomography of Abdominal Abnormalities. St. Louis, C. V. Mosby, 1978, pp. 163-169

20. Haaga JR, Baldwin GN, Reich NE, et al: CT detection of infected synthetic grafts: Preliminary report of a new sign. Am. J. Roentgenol. 131:317-320, 1978
21. Harris RD, Hougen ML: Early diagnosis of tuberculous thoracic aortic aneurysm by computerized axial tomography. Computerized Tomography 2:49-54, 1978
22. Harris RD, Seat SG: Value of computerized tomography in evaluation of kidney. Urology 12:729-732, 1978
23. Harris RD, Usselman JA, Vint VC, et al: Computerized tomography of aneurysms of the thoracic aorta. Computerized Tomography (in press)
24. Hertzer NR, Beven EG: Ultrasound measurement and elective aneurysmectomy. JAMA 240:1966, 1978
25. Holm HH, Kvist KJ, Mortensen T, et al: Ultrasonic diagnosis of arterial aneurysms. Scand. J. Thorac. Cardiovasc. Surg. 2:140, 1968
26. Lautela E, Tahti E: Echoaortography in abdominal aortic aneurysm. Ann. Chir. Gynaecol. Fenn. 57:506, 1968
27. Leopold GR: Ultrasonic abdominal aortography. Radiology 96:9, 1970
28. Leopold GR: Gray scale ultrasonic angiography of the upper abdomen. Radiology 117:665, 1975
29. Leopold GR, Goldberger LE, Bernstein EF: Ultrasonic detection and evaluation of abdominal aortic aneurysms. Surgery 72:939, 1972
30. Maloney JD, Pairolero PC, Smith BF Jr, et al: Ultrasound evaluation of abdominal aortic aneurysms. Circulation 56 [Suppl II]:1180, 1977
31. Margulis AR, Boyd DP, Korobkin MT: Advantages and disadvantages of rotary body CT scanners. Symposium on Total Body Computerized Tomography, Heidelberg, Sept. 29-Oct. 1, 1977
32. McGregor JC, Pollock JG, Anton HC: The value of ultrasonography in the diagnosis of abdominal aortic aneurysm. Scot. Med. J. 20:133-137, 1975
33. McGregor JC, Pollock JG, Anton HC: The diagnosis and assessment of abdominal aortic aneurysms by ultrasonography. Ann. R. Coll. Surg. Engl. 58 (5):388, 1976
34. Mulder DS, Winsberg F, Cole CM, et al: Ultrasonic "B" scanning of abdominal aneurysms. Ann. Thorac. Surg. 16:361, 1973
35. Nusbaum JW, Freimanis AK, Thomford NR: Echography in the diagnosis of abdominal aortic aneurysm. Arch. Surg. 102:385, 1971
36. Pederson R, Schellinger D, Hakkal H, et al: CT in the evaluation of abdominal aortic aneurysms. International Symposium and Course on Computed Tomography, Miami Beach, March 1978
37. Raskin MM, Cunningham JB: Comparison of computed tomography and ultrasound for abdominal aortic aneurysms: A preliminary study. J. Comput. Tomogr. 2:21-23, 1978
38. Schellinger D: CT of abdominal aortic aneurysms. Society of Computerized Tomography Post-Graduate Course, San Diego, Feb. 24-Mar. 1, 1979
39. Segal BL, Likoff W, Asperger Z, et al: Ultrasound diagnosis of an abdominal aortic aneurysm. Am. J. Cardiol. 17:101, 1966
40. Wheeler WE, Beachley MC, Ranniger K: Angiography and ultrasonography. Am. J. Roentgenol. Radium Ther. Nucl. Med. 126:95, 1976

41. Winsberg F, Cole-Beuglet C, Mulder DS: Continuous ultrasound "B"-scanning of abdominal aortic aneurysms. Am. J. Roentgenol. 121:626, 1974
42. Zaklad H: Low dose in computerized tomography. Abstracts, Symposium on Total Body Computerized Tomography, Heidelberg, Sept. 29-Oct. 1, 1977

Harvey L. Neiman, M.D.

Combined Imaging Techniques in Vascular Radiology

Multiple imaging techniques are available which allow complete evaluation of the arterial system. Plain radiography is the most limited of these; it shows only mural calcification. Angiography, in contrast, has been the mainstay of vascular imaging for the past two decades, although radionuclide techniques have been helpful occasionally. With the introduction of computed body tomography and diagnostic ultrasound, the choice of the most appropriate imaging technique has become somewhat perplexing. Also, with the increase in number of imaging techniques, there have been marked advances in older, solidly established techniques such as angiography. Lately, comparison studies have been carried out [18, 28] to provide guidelines as to the best imaging modality for a particular clinical problem. This presentation addresses itself to the current state of the art imaging for the aorta and its body branches and describes associated advances, particularly transcatheter interventional angioplasty.

THORACIC AORTA

Plain radiography of the chest is of limited usefulness in diagnosis of thoracic aortic aneurysms, aortic dissection, and suspected aortic trauma. The changes demonstrated are usually nonspecific and suggestive only when correlated with the clinical findings. Kirsh et al. [16] found, for example, that in patients with traumatic rupture of the thoracic aorta, the plain films demonstrated widening of the superior mediastinal shadow, abnormality of the aortic contour, loss of sharpness of the aortic margin, and inferior displacement of the left mainstem bronchus. Less frequently seen was deviation of the trachea to the right, left-sided hemothorax, pneumothorax, and pulmonary contusion. As a constellation of findings, in the clinical setting they offer some specificity. As individual findings, however, these are quite nonspecific. They were frequently seen in control patients who had sustained blunt chest trauma but who were subsequently shown to have an intact thoracic aorta.

The situation in thoracic aortic aneurysms and dissection of the thoracic aorta is analogous. Multiple authors have emphasized the necessity for thoracic aortography in the definitive diagnosis of aortic laceration, dissection, or aneurysm [1, 10, 11, 16, 19]. The point is that arteriography is a relatively safe technique in these cases and most importantly is definitive. The angiographic findings have been previously well described [10, 11, 16].

The negative aspect of angiography is that it is an invasive procedure and requires the skills of a trained angiographer. In particular, the performance of a percutaneous axillary approach is difficult, and this method is helpful in aortic dissection and aortic lacerations.

Recently, computed tomography (CT) has been noted to be helpful in evaluation of the thoracic aorta (Fig. 1). Computed tomography demonstrates the major mediastinal vessels simply and with great clarity [14]. In our initial series of 19 patients, we found that CT scanning vividly demonstrated the presence of aortic dissection and the relationship of the true to the false lumen [24] (Fig. 2). In a series of patients, computed tomography of the chest

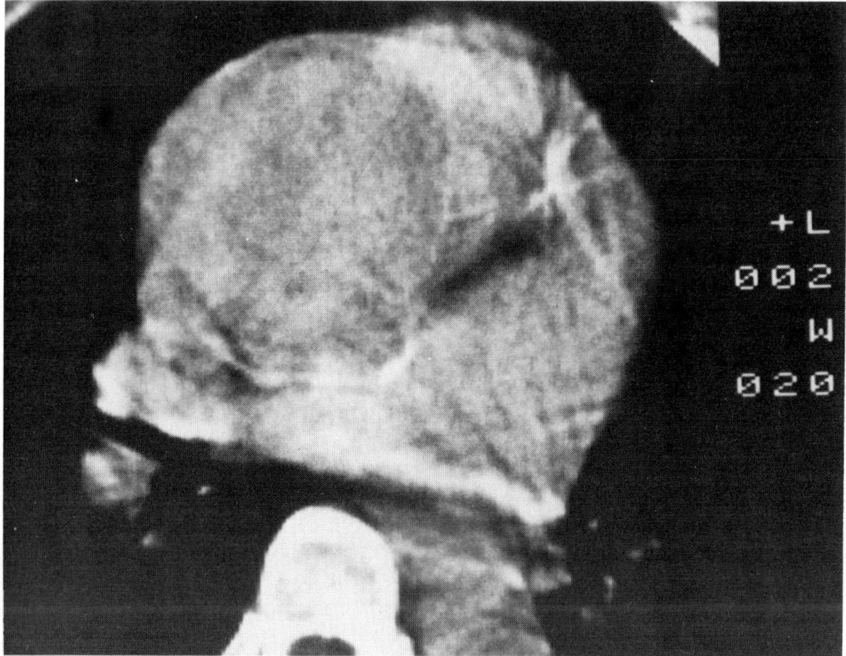

Fig. 1. Large aneurysm involving the ascending thoracic aorta. Note curvilinear calcification in the wall.

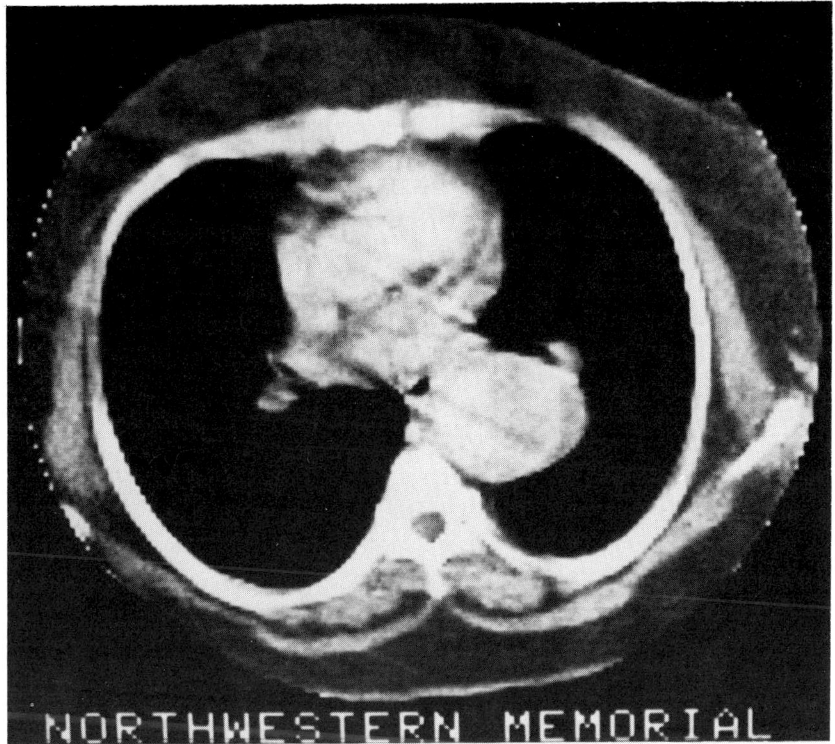

Fig. 2. Type III aortic dissection. Contrast opacified lumen is differentiated from surrounding false lumen.

was performed on 297 patients because plain x-ray films suggested mediastinal disease. Nineteen were suspected of having significant disease of the thoracic aorta. The CT scan was performed using an 18 sec scanner and intravenous infusion of 300 ml of 30% contrast material [23]. In this series, the following conclusions were made: The aorta was readily visualized and an accurate diagnosis ascertained. In cases of thoracic aortic aneurysm, CT was able to determine the size of the aneurysm and the vertical extent. It was able also to define the extent of laminated thrombus and its relation to the patent lumen. The relative size of true lumen and thrombosed segment was measured by CT and arteriography. There was a correlation within 0.5 cm.

Computed tomography easily distinguished an aneurysm from a tortuous aorta, thus obviating the need for arteriography in asymptomatic individuals. Additionally, progression of an aneurysm could be monitored accurately with CT. This allowed outpatient management. Finally, an aneurysm at an aortic graft site could be determined with CT scanning.

Experience has shown that the normal aorta demonstrates sharp margination. The contrast enhanced lumen extends to the margins. The vessel tapers normally and is of expected diameter. In contrast, thoracic dissection demonstrates a widened diameter and a separate false lumen. In two of four patients with ascending aortic dissection, widening of the aorta was seen but CT could not distinguish between the false lumen of dissection and the laminated thrombus of aneurysm. In the other two cases and in four cases with type III dissection, contrast material in the false lumen allowed differentiation between true and false lumen.

The use of CT in the evaluation of potential aortic trauma has been impressive. If aortic rupture is *strongly* suspected, we would recommend angiography as a first procedure. However, many such patients have multiple injuries, thus making CT an attractive alternative. The aorta is clearly seen by this method and fluid or hematoma causing the plain film abnormalities can be identified. If the hematoma is periaortic, angiography must be done to rule out rupture [23].

At Northwestern University, CT scanning is utilized in the stable patient. With present equipment, CT is not able to differentiate dissection from fusiform aneurysm consistently. However, in either situation, it is able to determine the extent of disease and degree of involvement of the abdominal aorta. In the future, use of bolus injection of contrast material and faster scanning times with newer generation equipment will further expand the capabilities of CT in the chest.

ABDOMINAL AORTA

Aortic Aneurysm

In visualization of the abdominal aorta and its branches, plain radiography is of little value except to demonstrate extensive calcification. While oblique and cross-table lateral radiographs are still frequently obtained for diagnosis of abdominal aortic aneurysm, such use should be discouraged. The technique suffers because of the variable amounts of calcification within the wall of an abdominal aneurysm and varying degrees of radiographic magnification. Furthermore, the technique has been superceded by diagnostic ultrasound, which is more accurate (Fig. 3). This procedure is greatly sensitive and is able to diagnose the presence of an aneurysm, its transverse, ventral-dorsal, and cephalocaudad dimensions [18, 28]. Of particular importance is the fact that ultrasound is able also to document the absence of an aneurysm in a patient who is suspected of having aortic widening by clinical examination.

Ultrasound is presently the imaging procedure of choice for diagnosis of abdominal aortic aneurysms and differentiation from other abdominal masses. It is more accurate than clinical examination, plain radiography, aortography, or isotope aortography in the diagnosis of abdominal aortic aneurysms [28]. Hertzer and Beven [15] found that B-mode aortic ultrasonography closely

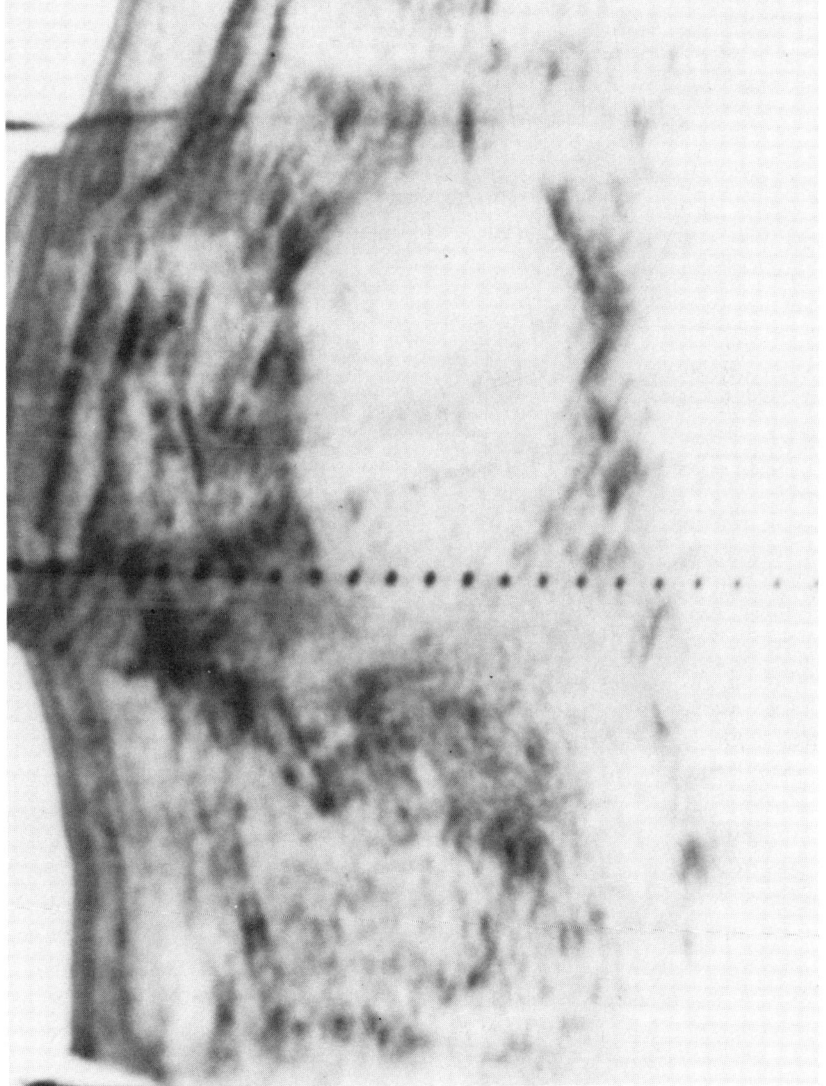

Fig. 3. Saccular abdominal aortic aneurysm.

approximated intraoperative aneurysm measurements. Additionally, ultrasound has the ability to demonstrate that a suspected abdominal aortic aneurysm may in reality relate to a retroperitoneal or intraperitoneal malignancy or retroperitoneal fibrosis [8, 17]. Finally, ultrasound is able to differentiate total cross-sectional diameter from residual lumen and to document the amount of thrombus filling the lumen (Fig. 4).

Diagnostic ultrasound also has been shown to be useful in the followup observation of abdominal aortic aneurysms. Since it is highly accurate in measuring an aneurysm, enlargement with time can be noted and appropriate surgical management carried out or withheld as indicated.

Although ultrasound can frequently detect extension of an aneurysm into the iliac artery, at the present time it is unable to assess accurately extension of the aneurysm into the renal arteries or other branches of the aorta (Fig. 5). It is for this reason that angiography remains uniquely useful for preoperative evaluation of a patient who is a candidate for elective abdominal aortic aneurysmectomy. Biplane aortography allows for assessment of (1) proximal extent of the aneurysm with respect to the renal arteries, (2) extension into the renal arteries, (3) the size of the suprarenal segment of the abdominal aorta, (4) distal extension of the aneurysm into the iliac and femoral arteries, (5) presence of other frequently associated aneurysms, i.e., popliteal artery, and (6) the mesenteric blood supply, particularly the status of the blood supply to the left side of the colon. Finally, angiography may occasionally be helpful in evaluating a ruptured abdominal aortic aneurysm. Generally, this is true in cases which are clinically silent and in which the situation allows for an elective study [9].

Computed body tomography is also able to image abdominal aneurysms, to assess the cross-sectional diameter, and to differentiate residual lumen from overall aneurysm diameter. It has the same limitations as ultrasound in terms of staging the aneurysm with respect to extent. At the present time, there is no advantage of CT over ultrasound in the diagnosis of abdominal aortic aneurysms. Actually, there are several disadvantages, including the need for intravenous injection of iodinated contrast material and the additional cost of the procedure.

RENOVASCULAR HYPERTENSION

Radiologic evaluation plays a central role in surgical management of the patient with renovascular hypertension. The limitations and use of plain films and intravenous urography in the evaluation of the hypertensive patient have been well documented previously. Data from the Cooperative Study of Renovascular Hypertension are particularly useful in this regard [4].

Both diagnostic ultrasound and computed body tomography may occasionally demonstrate a renal artery aneurysm. The present techniques offer little in assessing the presence of renal artery stenosis, however.

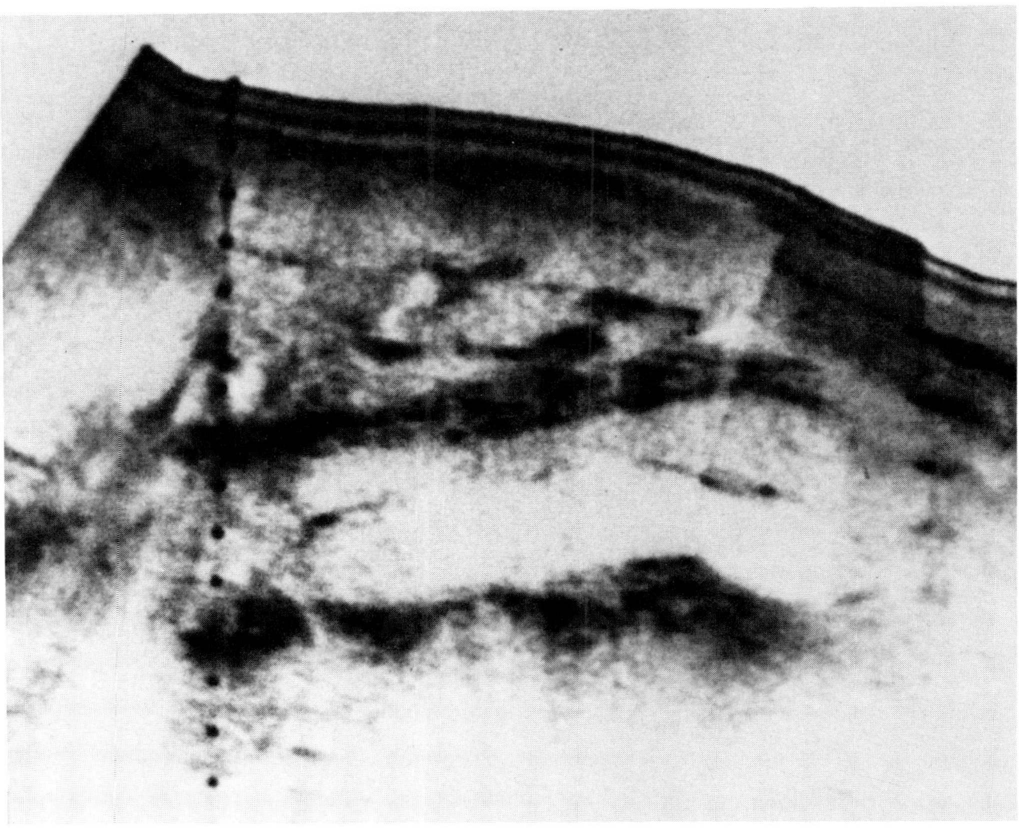

Fig. 4. Extensive aneurysm of abdominal aorta with an echogenic band of thrombus along the ventral surface.

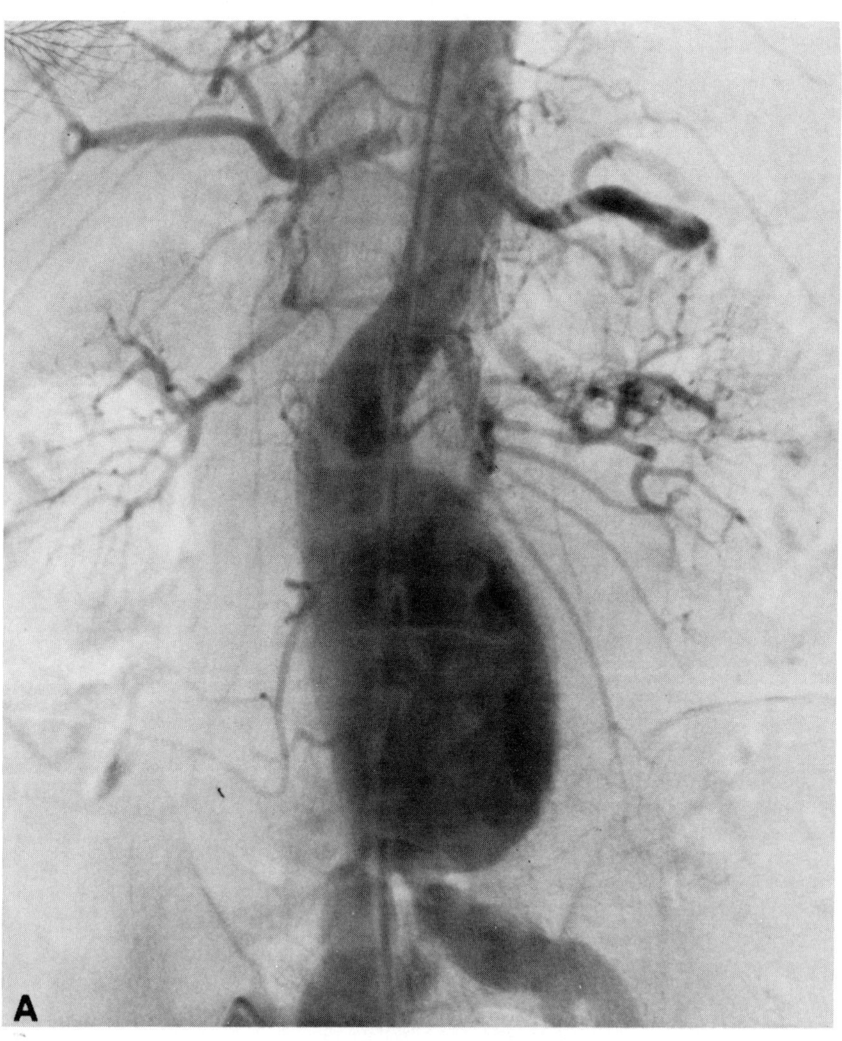
A

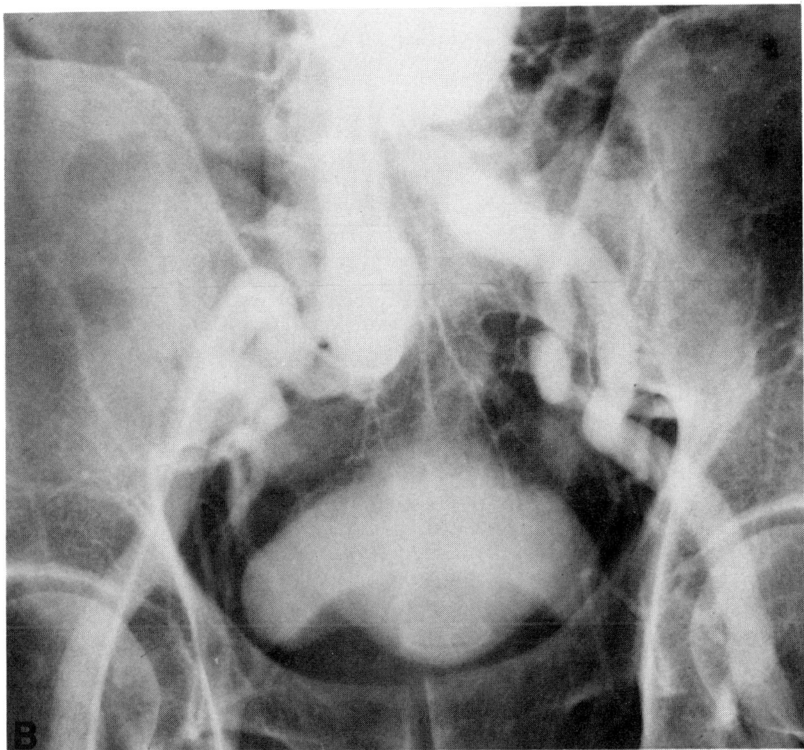

Fig. 5A (left) and B. Aortogram demonstrating aneurysm with extent into common iliac arteries bilaterally.

Of particular moment is the necessity of deciding which patients are candidates for hypertensive evaluation by radiographic screening techniques, i.e., intravenous urography and radionuclide renography. It is our feeling as well as that of others [7] that the need for a specific diagnosis of renovascular hypertension exists only in those individuals who are potential operative or radiologic intervention candidates. These are individuals who are young and might require a lifetime of medical management or are older and poorly controlled on medical management. These indications may change somewhat as additional experience is gained with percutaneous transluminal angioplasty for renal artery stenosis [13, 25].

The angiographic workup for renovascular hypertension includes aortography (Fig. 6), followed by bilateral selective renal arteriography. The latter should be routinely performed except in patients with a high grade stenosis of definite hemodynamic significance involving the ostium of a renal artery. At Northwestern University, magnification filming is utilized routinely for the selective studies using a grid biased 0.3 mm spot x-ray tube.

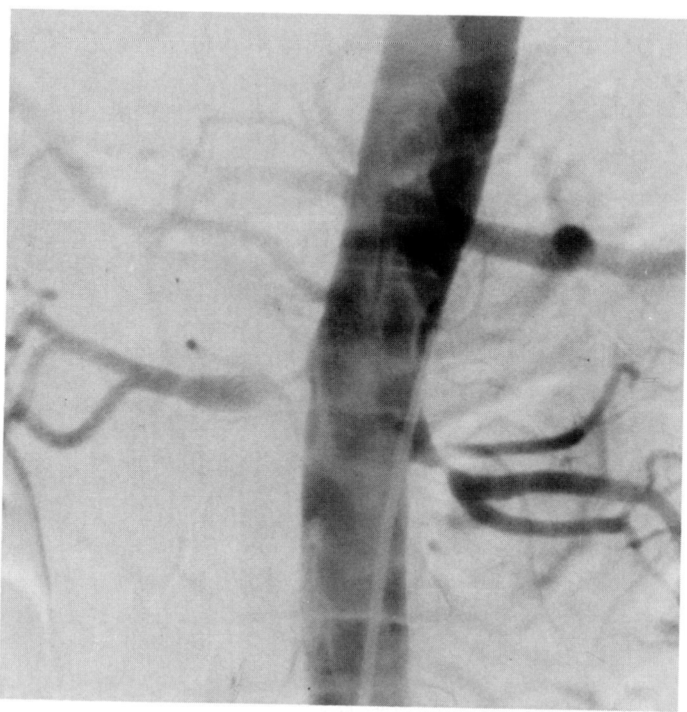

Fig. 6. Bilateral high-grade renal artery stenosis of atherosclerotic etiology.

The results of the Cooperative Study of Renovascular Hypertension confirm the sensitivity of angiography in detecting renal artery stenoses [5]. The presence of false-negative results is exceedingly rare. Additionally, arteriography offers a great deal of specificity about particular lesions. Arteriography is able to classify the etiology of the lesion as atherosclerotic, which is found in the majority of cases, fibromuscular dysplasia, and, occasionally, uncommon entities such as aneurysm, trauma, embolism, neurofibromatosis, and arteriovenous fistula [7]. Arteriography also is specific with respect to localization of the disease process, i.e., bilateral, unilateral, or segmental. Finally, arteriography is able to define the extent of the disease process within the involved kidney.

It is important that differentiation be made between an arteriographically demonstrated renal artery stenosis as an incidental finding in a hypertensive patient and one in whom the stenosis is etiologically significant, i.e., differentiating renovascular disease from renovascular hypertension. Renal vein renin ratios are widely utilized to evaluate the functional importance of a renal artery stenosis. It has been noted, however, that while lateralizing renin data are highly predictive of operative benefit, nonlateralizing data do not necessarily indicate potential operative failure [20]. In unilateral disease as well, the renin ratio may incorrectly indicate the hemodynamic significance. Multiple reasons exist for this situation, including sampling errors, patient positioning, and dietary and assay errors.

As an adjunct, therefore, to renal vein renin assay much work has been done attempting to correlate the angiographic appearance of renal artery stenosis with hemodynamic significance [3, 6]. Only two angiographic signs have proven reliable in this setting: (1) A stenosis greater than 75%, usually indicating a cross-sectional diameter under 1.5 mm. This is useful in evaluation of athero-sclerotic narrowing but is of less value in patients with the medial fibroplasia with aneurysms type of fibromuscular dysplasia. (2) Demonstration of collateral circulation bridging the site of stenosis (Fig. 7). The collateral circulation arises

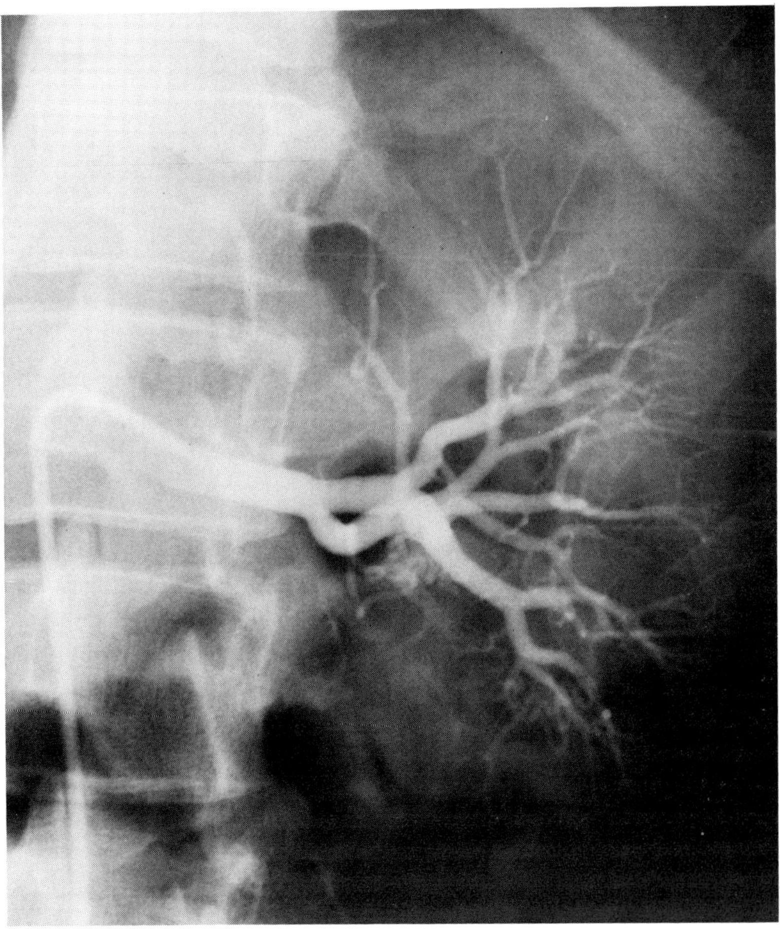

Fig. 7A. Early arterial phase of selective left renal arteriogram demonstrating prominent renal sinus collateral vessels and a missing interlobar artery to the lower pole.

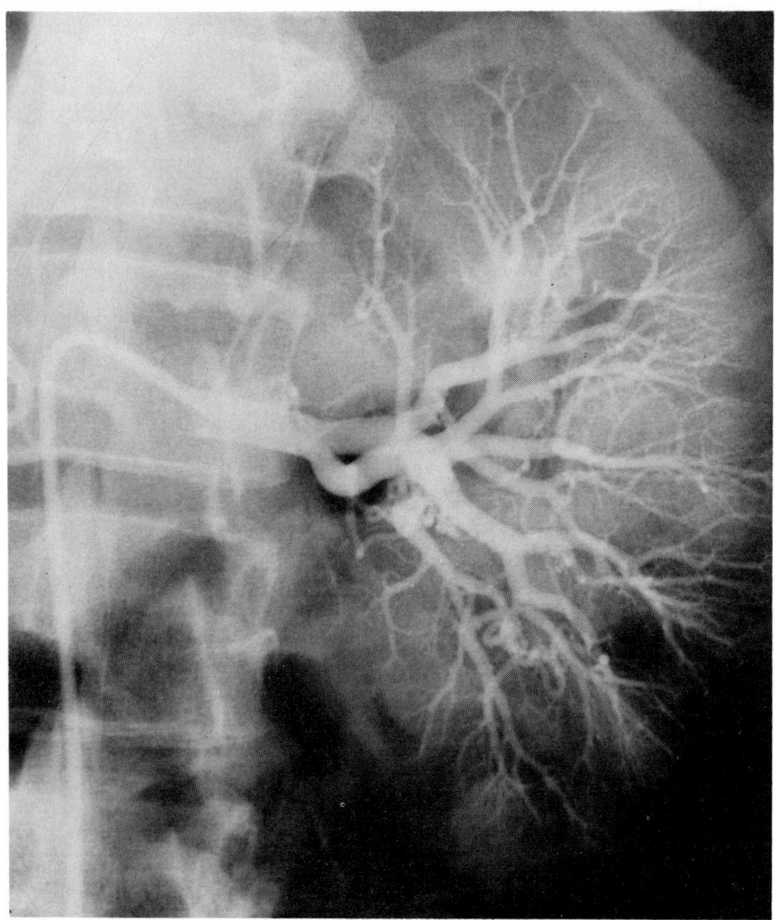

Fig. 7B. Late arterial phase demonstrating opacification of lower pole interlobar artery, filling via collaterals.

from several groups of arteries: the renal capsular complex, ureteral, lumbar, adrenal, renal-pelvic, gonadal, and arteries of the renal sinus in individuals with segmental disease. These potential collateral arteries are usually seen on a good quality selective magnification renal arteriogram. Bookstein and co-workers noted that the direction of flow in these nonparenchymal renal artery branches is normally antegrade (away from the renal artery) [6]. In a small number of normal individuals these extrarenal arterial branches are not seen even with optimal radiographic techniques.

In a renal artery stenosis which is not hemodynamically significant the nonparenchymal branches are visualized as in a normal individual (antegrade flow). However, in a hemodynamically significant stenosis, those nonparen-

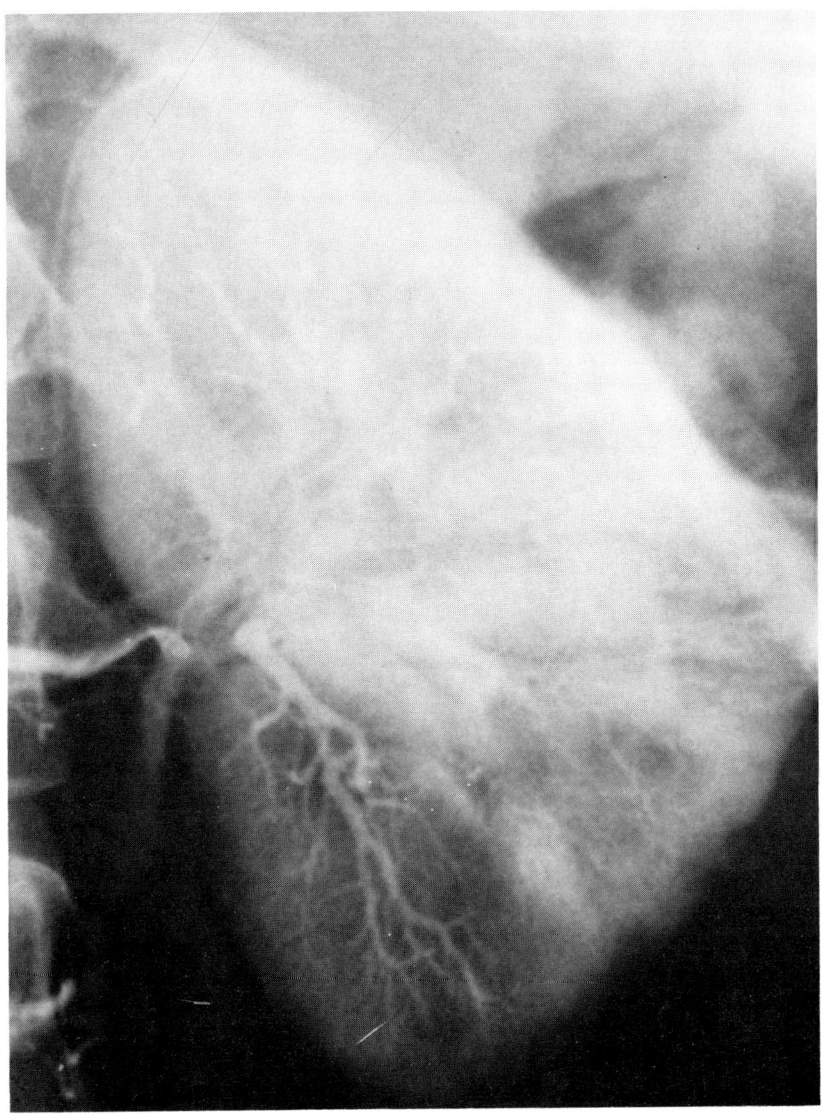

Fig. 7C. Nephrographic phase demonstrating delayed washout of the occluded segmental branch.

chymal renal artery branches arising distal to the stenosis function as collateral vessels and carry blood in a retrograde direction into the renal artery. Thus on a selective renal arteriogram this collateral flow may be noted as a flow defect within the main renal artery or an interlobar artery. Alternatively, it may be manifested as nonvisualization of nonparenchymal branches. In order to differentiate the latter situation from the individual with a "normally naked" renal artery 3-4 g epinephrine is injected into the renal artery, followed immediately by a repeat selective injection of contrast material. In this situation, if the stenosis is hemodynamically significant, the increase in the peripheral arterial resistance of the renal bed allows contrast to enter the previously nonvisualized nonparenchymal branches, demonstrating that in a steady state they are present and carry blood in a retrograde fashion.

If nonparenchymal branches are not seen even after epinephrine, this substantiates the fact that it is most likely a "normal naked" renal artery.

Further manipulation with vasodilator drugs is also occasionally useful and has been discussed at length elsewhere [6].

In the patient who is postrenal artery bypass, angiography accurately demonstrates graft patency or occlusion [12, 27] (Fig. 8). To date, there has been very little work concerning the use of ultrasound or CT in monitoring grafts.

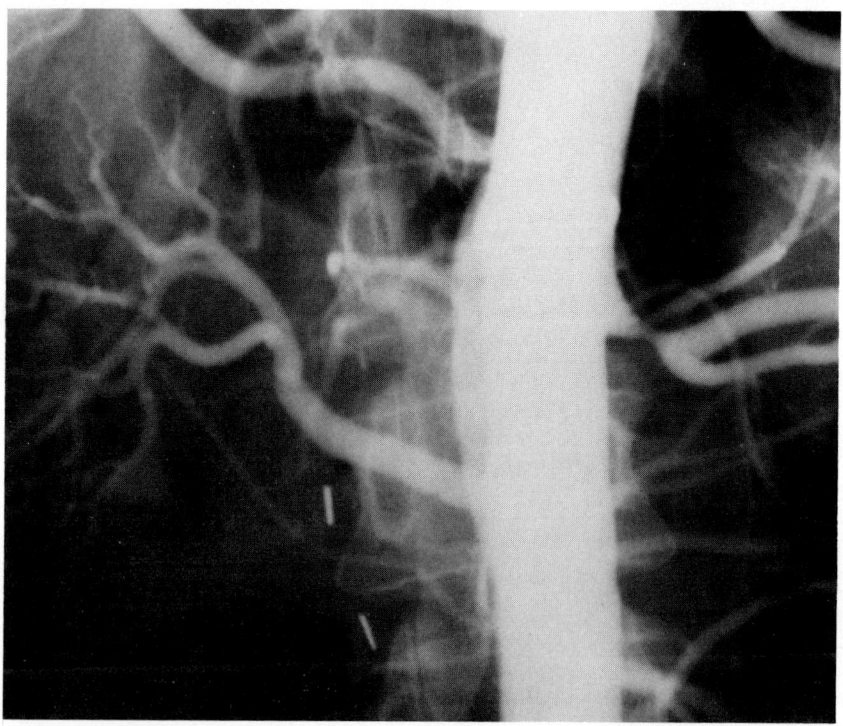

Fig. 8. Same patient as Fig. 6, demonstrating patent graft.

Recently, percutaneous transluminal angioplasty of renal artery stenoses (Fig. 9) has received attention [13, 25]. Initial experience with the procedure has been favorable, as manifested by (1) improvement in control of hypertension and (2) pre- and postangioplasty pressure gradients, arteriography, renal plasma flow, and renins. However, large series and long term results have as yet not been reported.

MESENTERIC ISCHEMIA

Although on occasion aneurysm of the celiac and superior mesenteric arteries has been demonstrated by ultrasound, imaging of these vessels is for the most part the province of arteriography. Much has been written concerning the angiographic workup of acute and chronic mesenteric ischemia [2, 22]. There is no question that cross-table lateral aortography can demonstrate occlusive dis-

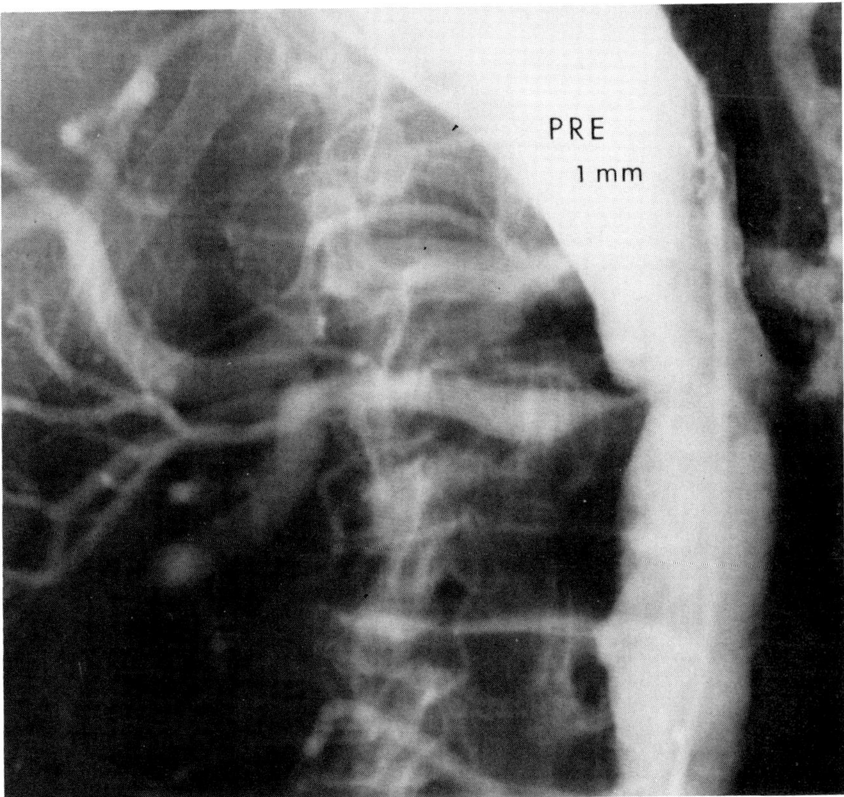

Fig. 9A. High-grade renal artery stenosis. Lateralizing selective renal vein renin to the right side.

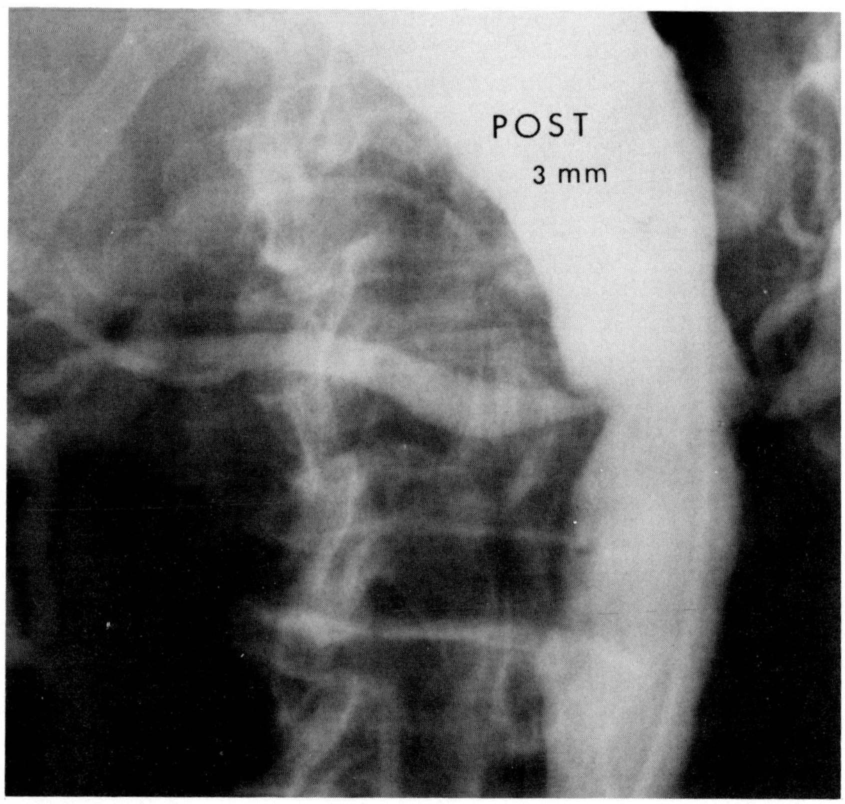

Fig. 9B. Posttransluminal angioplasty with marked decrease in elevated blood pressure.

ease at the origin of the celiac superior mesenteric and inferior mesenteric arteries. There is difficulty, however, in correlating these findings with the clinical syndrome of abdominal angina. Stenosis of one or more of the visceral vessels is frequently seen in asymptomatic individuals. Why some patients are symptomatic while others with identical findings are not is unclear. Similarly, lateral aortography can demonstrate the findings of the median arcuate ligament compression syndrome. There is a characteristic concave impression on the cephalic surface of the celiac artery which is accentuated by expiration. In spite of angiographic findings the existence of a clinical syndrome is also controversial [21].

In contradistinction, selective arteriography plays an important role in the management of the patient with acute mesenteric ischemia (Figs. 10 and 11).

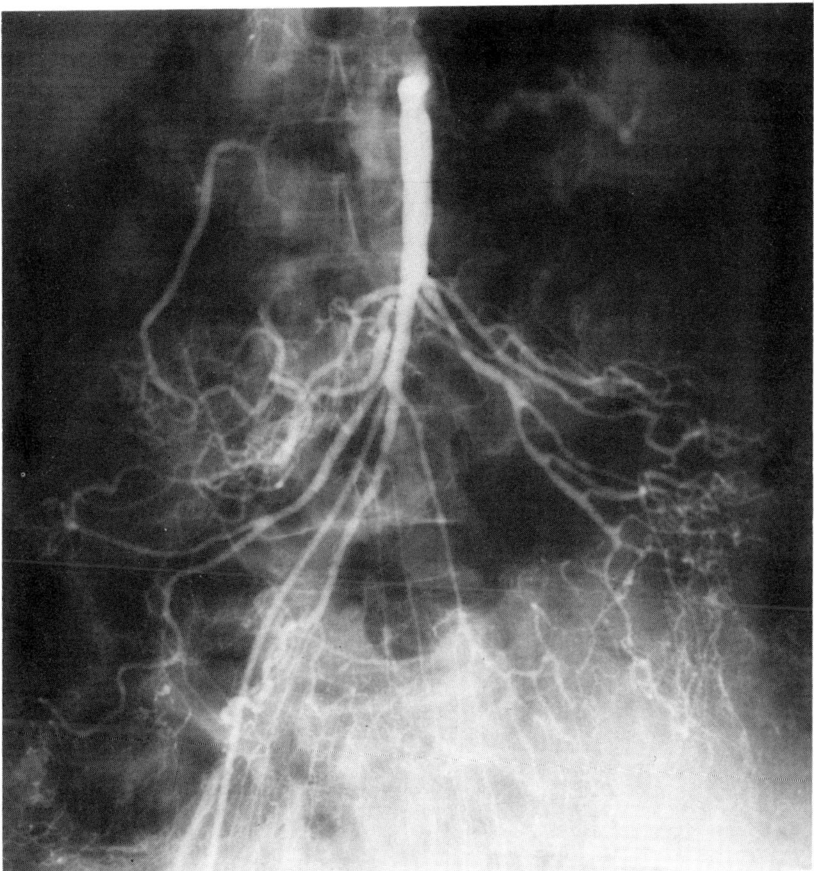

Fig. 10. Seventy-eight year old woman with abdominal pain and rectal bleeding. Note complete occlusion of a proximal jejunal artery at its origin. Decrease in caliber of vessels secondary to nonocclusive ischemia.

Emboli to the mesenteric circulation can be demonstrated during the acute episode. Similarly, changes of nonocclusive mesenteric ischemia in patients with hypovolemic shock or digitalis toxicity are noted as an intense vasoconstriction of the mesenteric arteries.

The use of interventional angiography – superior mesenteric artery infusion of papaverine – has been suggested as a treatment for nonocclusive mesenteric ischemia [26]. An additional interventional angiographic technique, transluminal angioplasty, may be of value in chronic mesenteric ischemia for dilatation of proximal atherosclerotic lesions.

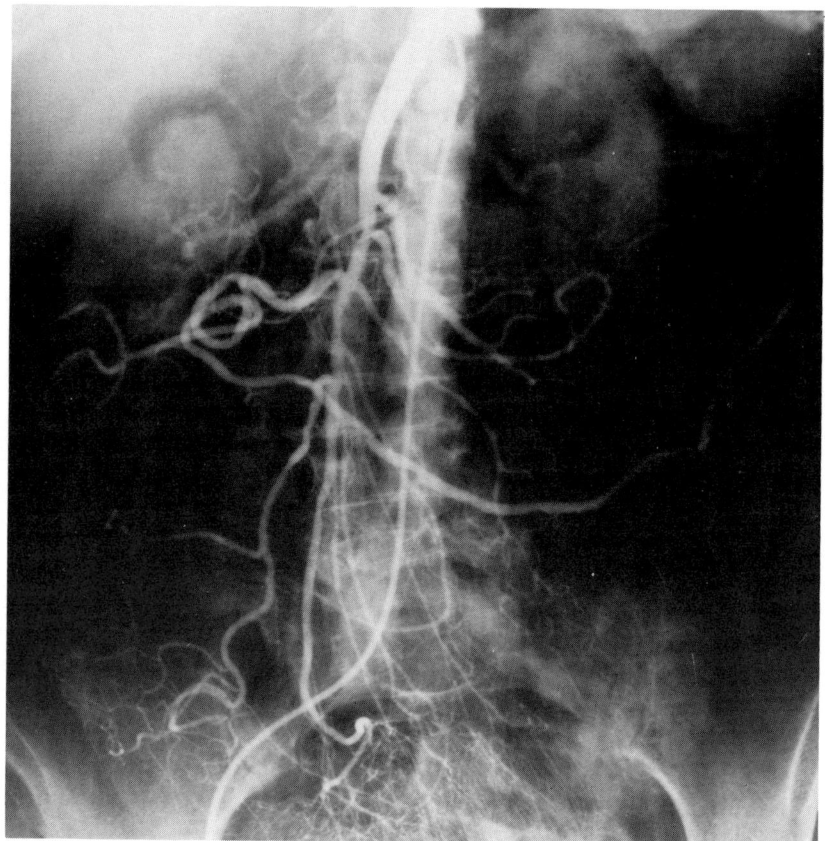

Fig. 11. Acute mesenteric ischemia secondary to hypovolemic shock. Note threadlike visceral branches.

REFERENCES

1. Ambros JA, Rothberg M, Lefleur RS, et al: Unsuspected aortic dissection: The chronic "healed" dissection. Am. J. Roentgenol. 131:221, 1979
2. Boley SJ, Krieger H, Schultz L, et al: Experimental aspects of peripheral vascular occlusion of the intestine. Surg. Gynecol. Obstet. 121:789, 1965
3. Bookstein JJ: Appraisal of arteriography in estimating the hemodynamic significance of renal artery stenosis. Invest. Radiol. 1:284, 1966
4. Bookstein JJ, Abrams HL, Buenger RE, et al: Radiologic aspects of renovascular hypertension. The role of urography in unilateral renovascular disease. JAMA 220:1225, 1972
5. Bookstein JJ, Abrams HL, Buenger RE, et al: Radiologic aspects of renovascular hypertension. Appraisal of arteriography. JAMA 221:368, 1972

6. Bookstein JJ, Ernst CB: Vasodilatory and vasoconstrictive pharmacoangiographic manipulation of renal collateral flow. Radiology 108:55, 1973
7. Bookstein JJ, Walter JF: The role of abdominal radiography in hypertension secondary to renal or adrenal disease. Med. Clin. North Am. 59:169, 1975
8. Bowie JD, Bernstein JR: Retroperitoneal fibrosis: Ultrasound findings and case report. J. Clin. Ultrasound 4:435, 1976
9. Chisolm AG, Sprayregen S: Angiographic manifestations of ruptured abdominal aortic aneurysms. Am. J. Roentgenol. 127:769, 1976
10. Dinsmore RE, Wilkerson JT, Buckley MJ: Dissecting aneurysm of the aorta. Radiology 105:567, 1972
11. Earnst F, Muhm JR, Sheedy PF: Roentgenographic findings in thoracic aortic dissection. Mayo Clin. Proc. 54:43, 1979
12. Ekelung L, Gerlock J, Goncharenko V, et al: Angiographic findings following surgical treatment for renovascular hypertension. Radiology 126:345, 1978
13. Gruntzig A, Vetter W, Meier B, et al: Treatment of renovascular hypertension with percutaneous transluminal dilatation of a renal artery stenosis. Lancet 1:801, 1978
14. Heitzman ER, Goldwin RL, Proto AV: Radiological analysis of the mediastinum utilizing computed tomography. Radiol. Clin. North Am. 15:309, 1977
15. Hertzler NR, Beven EG: Ultrasound aortic measurement and elective aneurysmectomy. JAMA 240:1966, 1978
16. Kirsh MM, Crane JD, Kahn DR, et al: Roentgenographic evaluation of traumatic rupture of the aorta. Surg. Gynecol. Obstet. 131:900, 1970
17. Lee TG, Henderson SC: Ultrasonic aortography: Unexpected findings. Am. J. Roentgenol. 128:273, 1977
18. Leopold G: Ultrasonic abdominal aortography. Radiology 96:9, 1970
19. Marsh DG, Sturm JT: Traumatic aortic rupture: Roentgenographic indications for angiography. Ann. Thorac. Surg. 21:337, 1976
20. Maxwell MH, Marks LS, Lupu AN, et al: Predictive value of renin determinations in renal artery stenosis. JAMA 238:2617, 1977
21. Reuter SR: Accentuation of celiac compression by the median arcuate ligament of the diaphragm during deep expiration. Radiology 98:561, 1971
22. Reuter SR, Kanter IE, Redman HC: Angiography in reversible colonic ischemia. Radiology 97:371, 1970
23. Sanders JH, Malave S, Neiman HL, et al: Thoracic aortic imaging without angiography. (Submitted for publication)
24. Sanders JH, Neiman HL, Malave SR, et al: The use of computerized axial tomography in the diagnosis of surgical diseases of the thoracic aorta. Proc. Inst. Med. Chicago 32:133, 1979
25. Schwarton D: Percutaneous transluminal angioplasty of the renal artery. Presented at Annual Meeting, Radiologic Society of North America, Dec. 1978

26. Siegelman SS, Sprayregen S, Boley SJ: Angiographic diagnosis of mesenteric arterial vasoconstriction. Radiology 112:553, 1974
27. Stanley JC, Fry WJ: Surgical treatment of renovascular hypertension. Arch. Surg. 112:1291, 1977
28. Wheeler WE, Beachley MC, Ranniger K: Angiography and ultrasonography: A comparative study of abdominal aortic aneurysms. Am. J. Roentgenol. 126:95, 1976

Surgery of the Thoracic and Abdominal Aorta

David C. Sabiston, Jr., M.D.

Management of Aneurysms of the Thoracic Aorta

Aneurysms involving the ascending, transverse, and descending thoracic aorta most frequently result from atherosclerosis, with a smaller number being caused by other disorders. Unless surgical therapy is undertaken, the majority of these aneurysms ultimately produce either seriously disabling complications or death. In selected patients, especially with dissecting aneurysms of the thoracic aorta, pharmacologic therapy directed toward a reduction in cardiac contractility and in the lowering of systemic blood pressure may be indicated. Fortunately, in the recent past surgical therapy has become sufficiently safe and successful so that this approach is now associated with a low operative morbidity and mortality.

ETIOLOGY

Formerly, most aneurysms of the thoracic aorta were due to syphilis, but atherosclerosis is currently the most common etiology. The descending thoracic aorta is the most frequent site of atherosclerotic aneurysms, followed in order by aneurysms of the ascending aorta and of the transverse arch. These lesions are considerably more common in males and are most often fusiform, but may also be saccular. *Congenital* aneurysms, especially in the ascending aorta, including the sinuses of Valsalva, are well recognized and may be associated with aortic valvular insufficiency. In addition, another cause of thoracic aneurysms, particularly in the ascending aorta, is *cystic medial necrosis*, often associated with other stigmata of Marfan's disease. *Trauma* is also a well recognized and relatively frequent cause, especially deceleration injuries such as occur in automobile accidents. The force of the impact produces a tear in the aorta near the site of fixation at the ductus arteriosus. Thus such lesions most frequently occur in the proximal thoracic aorta just distal to the origin of the subclavian artery. Rarely, *bacterial infection* may be an etiologic cause producing a mycotic aneurysm in the thoracic aorta.

In addition to etiology, aneurysms of the thoracic aorta are classified on an *anatomical* basis. This is especially helpful in relationship to surgical management. Anatomic types include (1) aneurysms of the *ascending* aorta, which may extend into the proximal portions of the innominate artery and the left carotid artery, (2) aneurysms of the *transverse arch* of the aorta, which again may involve the innominate, left carotid, and left subclavian, and (3) aneurysms of the *descending* thoracic aorta. In some instances, a combination of these is present indicating more extensive involvement and the necessity for a more involved surgical procedure.

CLINICAL MANIFESTATIONS

Many thoracic aneurysms are *asymptomatic* and are first discovered on a routine chest film. When symptoms are present, they are most often the result of pressure on surrounding structures. Thus pain is the most common symptom and may be located substernally or posteriorly along the spinal column. The pain may be chronic, and increasing pain is an ominous sign, especially if quite severe and suggests impending rupture. With escalation in pain, enlargement of the aneurysm is often noted, and again such manifestations indicate threatened rupture. If the aneurysm produces pressure on the trachea or main bronchi, respiratory insufficiency is apt to ensue. Similarly, esophageal compression may produce dysphagia (Fig. 1). Hoarseness may follow pressure on the recurrent laryngeal nerve. Neurological symptoms from cerebrovascular insufficiency can occur either by compression of the innominate or carotid vessels in the mediastinum or as a result of the passage of emboli from the aneurysmal sac into the cerebral circulation. If free rupture of the aneurysm into the pleural cavity occurs, the loss of blood is usually massive, producing shock and often death. The aneurysm may also rupture into the lung, with massive hemoptysis, or into the esophagus, with exsanguinating hematemesis. If the rupture occurs into the pericardium, severe cardiac decompensation due to cardiac tamponade usually follows. If the dissection compromises blood supply to the spinal cord, neurologic impairment of the lower body and extremities ensues.

ESTABLISHING THE DIAGNOSIS

In current practice, most thoracic aneurysms are first tentatively diagnosed on the basis of the chest film and then confirmed by angiography (Fig. 2). Arteriography is of considerable aid in determination of the size and extent of the aneurysm together with identification of associated lesions such as aortic valve insufficiency. Moreover, if the aneurysm is of the dissecting type, the reentry point may be identified on the films. The distal circulation, especially that to the brain, kidneys, viscera, and lower extremities, is of much importance both in diagnosis and in the planning of effective therapy. Serial roentgenograms often show progressive enlargement, another salient point in selection of the appropriate form of treatment (Fig. 3). It is particularly important to identify the origin at the major branches of the aorta, and in the presence of a dissecting aneurysm to determine whether the origin of the dissection is from the *true* or *false* lumen of the aorta.

In most patients with thoracic aortic aneurysms, resection of the aneurysm and replacement by a plastic graft is the most appropriate form of treatment. In those with *dissecting aneurysms*, pharmacologic management is often the preferred *initial* approach and is directed toward achieving stabilization of the patient. Subsequently a surgical procedure may be performed electively should it be indicated. Some patients with thoracic aortic aneurysms have severe associated disease which may contraindicate operation on the basis of excessive risk. However, with improving techniques, the vast majority of patients with these lesions are amenable to surgical therapy with an acceptable morbidity and mortality.

MEDICAL MANAGEMENT OF DISSECTING ANEURYSMS

Dissecting aneurysms of the thoracic aorta are classified according to their anatomic site and the extent of dissection. The type I dissecting aneurysm begins in the ascending aorta and extends distally to a varying point in the transverse arch or descending aorta. In a type II dissection, the dissection is limited to the ascending aorta and usually occurs as a chronic lesion. Type III is a dissecting aneurysm originating distal to the origin of the left subclavian artery and extending for varying distances into the thoracic aorta and at times into the abdominal aorta and its branches.

The natural history of dissecting aneurysms of the aorta is dismal, a fact which is well recognized. In a large collected series with acute dissecting aneurysms without treatment, only 20% were alive at the end of one month, 7% at the end of one year, and 5% at two years [4]. The immediate mortality began to change rather dramatically with the introduction of appropriately selected pharmacologic therapy. The initiating factor in these aneurysms is an intimal tear, most often arising in the ascending aorta and progressing distally. Once the dissection has occurred, systemic arterial pressure is then present within the arterial wall and the dissection is apt to extend. The dissection can be slowed or arrested by a reduction in the force of ventricular contraction (reduction in the pulse wave of dp/dt_{max}) as initiated by contraction of the left ventricle.

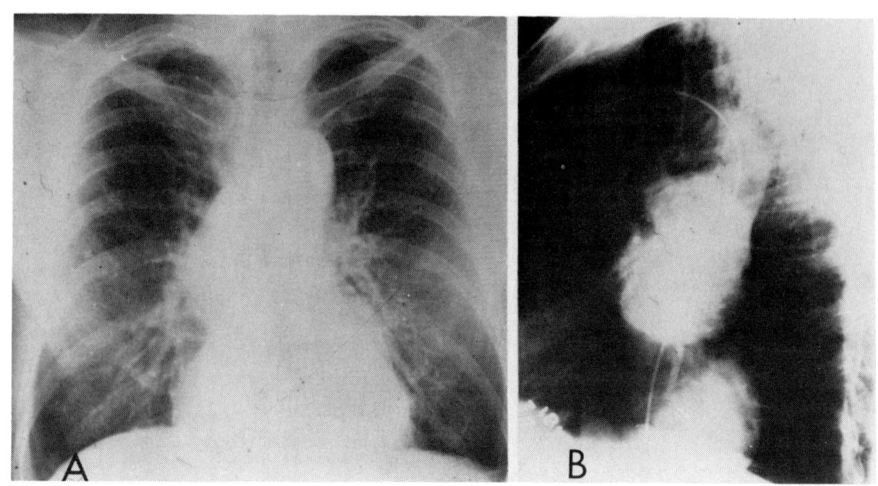
A
B

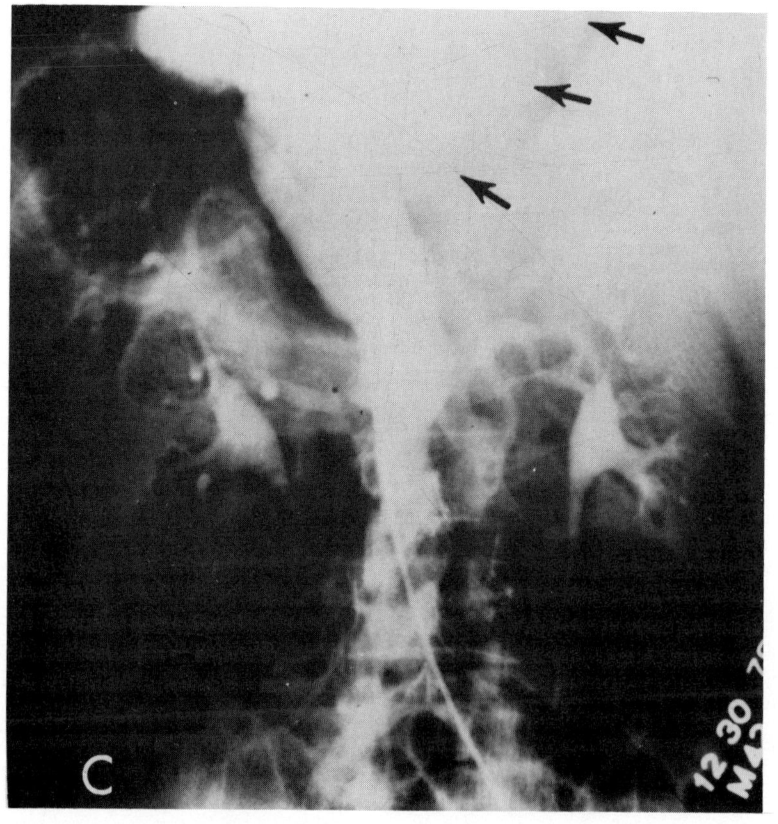
C

The patient with an acute dissecting aneurysm should be placed in a special care unit and carefully monitored with intraarterial blood pressure, serial chest films, and urinary output as measured by an indwelling urinary catheter. Since approximately 90% of such patients will be either hypertensive or have a history of hypertension, such findings are usually indicative of the appropriate diagnosis when accompanied by severe chest, back, or abdominal pain and signs of cardiovascular collapse. The presence of a diastolic murmur may indicate aortic valvular insufficiency.

Pharmacologic therapy is usually the preferred initial therapy in patients with acute dissecting aneurysms. This is particularly true of type III dissections and in patients who are considered poor surgical risks. A number of agents are effective, including *sodium nitroprusside* which is currently the most useful and the one most often selected for primary use. This agent selectively relaxes smooth muscle in the arterial wall and rapidly lowers blood pressure and peripheral resistance. Moreover, it reduces the contractility of the heart by decreasing preload (venous return) and therefore reduces cardiac output. It has the advantage of being effective immediately, and similarly its effect can be terminated rapidly if necessary. The indications for definitive surgical repair include type I and type II aneurysms in which there is a dissecting hematoma or evidence of impending rupture. Moreover, aortic valve insufficiency secondary to a dissecting aneurysm should be considered as indication for operation. If the dissecting hematoma continues to enlarge, especially if associated with severe pain, operation usually becomes necessary. Moreover, blood in the pericardium or pleural space, the inability to relieve and control the pain, or systemic blood pressure which is unyielding to pharmacologic therapy each constitutes indication for operation.

Propranolol is also useful since it specifically blocks beta adrenergic stimulation and exerts its effect on the end-organ receptors in the blood vessels and on the ventricular myocardium directly. The *thiazides* are important for their effect

---

Fig. 1. (A) Chest roentgenogram of 50-year-old man who complained of increasing difficulty with swallowing, revealing posterior mediastinal mass with compression of esophagus. (B and C) Arteriogram showing large aneurysm (arrows) extending from subclavian to celiac axis. Excision and grafting of aneurysm was performed through left-sided lateral thoracotomy using a Carlen double-lumen endotracheal tube. Chest was entered through bed of fifth rib and second incision made at seventh interspace, splitting diaphragm. Heparinized shunt was inserted in the ascending aorta to femoral artery. Patient tolerated the procedure without difficulty. Six months following operation, he ambulates without difficulty, with only slight weakness noted in left leg. [From Wolfe WG, Kleinman LH, Wechsler AS, et al: Heparin-coated shunts for lesions of the descending thoracic aorta. Experimental and clinical observations. Arch. Surg. 112:1481, 1977. Copyright 1977, American Medical Association.]

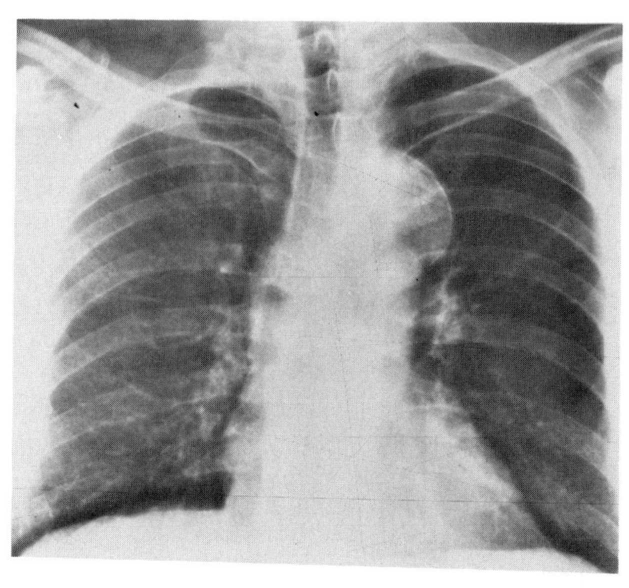

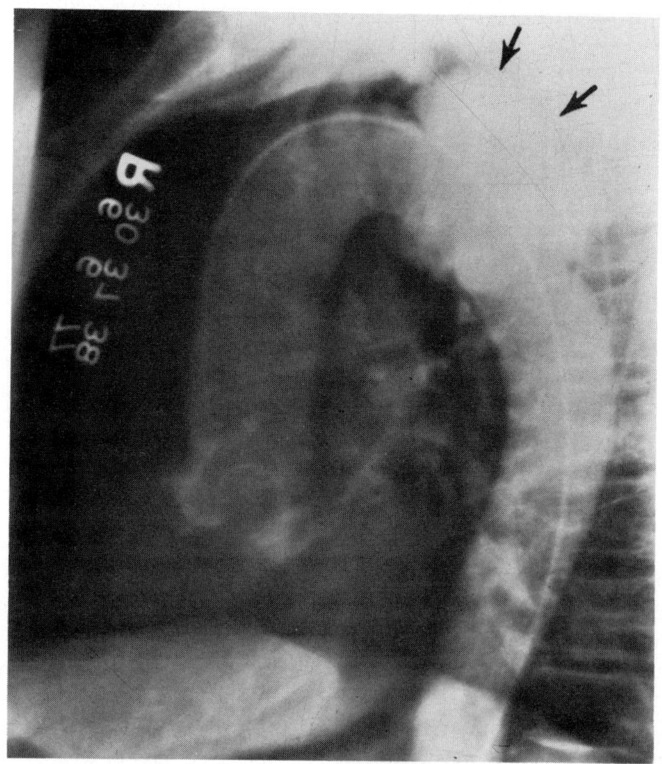

in decreasing tubular reabsorption of chloride and sodium and, with fluid volume depletion, in decreasing the blood pressure. *Reserpine* has also been used, since it depletes catecholamines from the tissue stores and causes a decrease in myocardial contractility. *Guanethidine* and *trimethaphan* may also be useful. Using this approach, most patients will survive and may be treated with drug therapy alone, or undergo an operative procedure at a time of selection.

SURGICAL MANAGEMENT

Aneurysms of the Ascending Aorta

The most proximal aneurysms of the ascending aorta are those involving the *sinuses of Valsalva.* There are two forms: (1) congenital aneurysms resulting from a lack of attachment of the aortic media to the annulus fibrosus, and (2) sinus aneurysms in association with aneurysms of the ascending aorta, usually due to cystic medial necrosis, which also involve the aortic sinuses and in addition may involve the aortic valve and coronary orifices. The congenital aneurysms most often involve the right coronary sinus, next frequently the noncoronary sinus, and very uncommonly the left sinus [1]. These lesions may be asymptomatic for prolonged periods, and the first evidence of their presence may follow rupture of the aneurysm into a cardiac chamber. The most common site of rupture is into the right ventricle, followed by the right atrium, the left atrium, and the pericardium. Males are more commonly involved, by a ratio of five to one.

For congenital lesions, operation is advisable unless the aneurysm is quite small and asymptomatic. Should rupture of the aneurysm of the sinus of Valsalva into a heart chamber occur, surgical management becomes mandatory. If the rupture is into the right atrium, the fistula may be exposed through the right atrium employing cardiopulmonary bypass. Exposure is usually easily achieved, since the aneurysmal sac herniates into the right atrium and can be

---

Fig. 2. Top and bottom, roentgenograms of 57-year-old man seen for evaluation of inguinal hernia. Chest x-ray film revealed calcified mass that, on arteriogram, proved to be aneurysm (arrows). Past history included account of reasonably severe automobile accident in 1949, at which time he had multiple fractures, although he did not specifically recall chest injury. Resection and grafting of aneurysm using heparinized shunt from subclavian artery to femoral artery were performed, chest being entered through resected bed of fourth rib. Carlen's endotracheal tube was used to permit collapse of left lung. Recovery was uneventful. [From Wolfe WG, Kleinman LH, Wechsler AS, et al: Heparin-coated shunts for lesions of the descending thoracic aorta. Experimental and clinical observations. Arch. Surg. 112:1481, 1977. Copyright 1977, American Medical Association.]

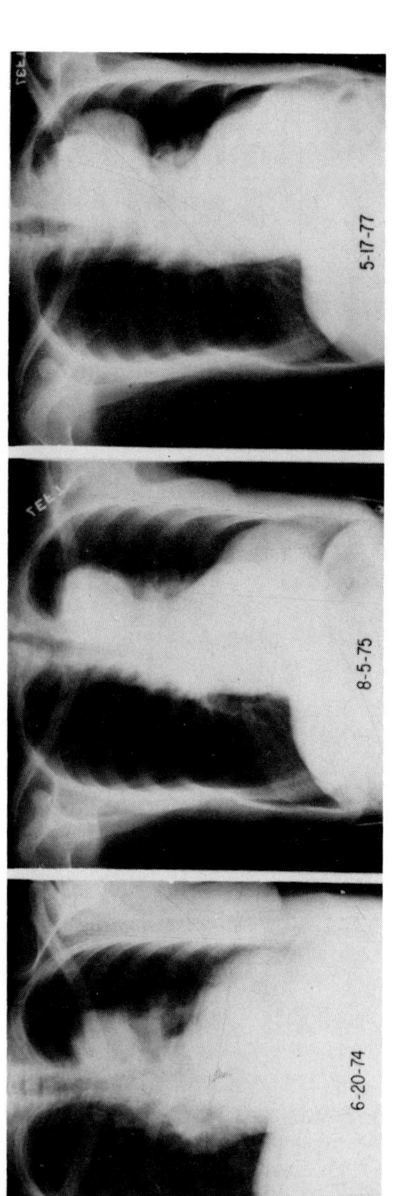
5-17-77
8-5-75
6-20-74

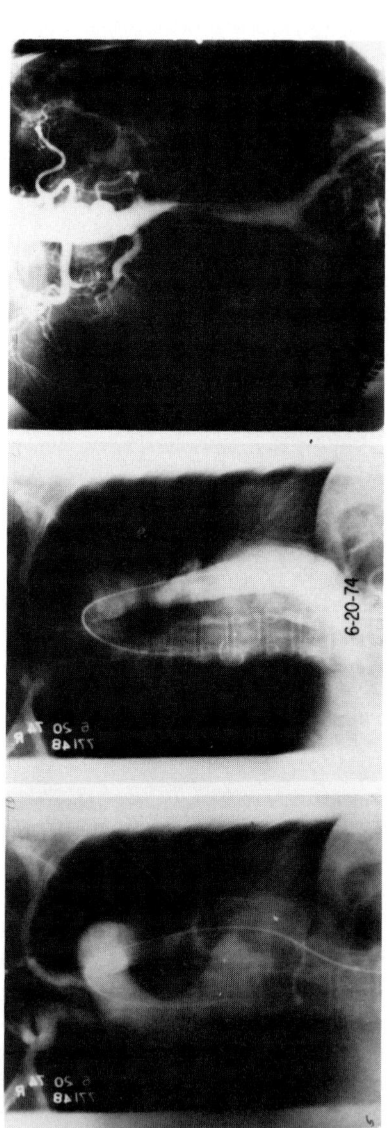
6-20-74

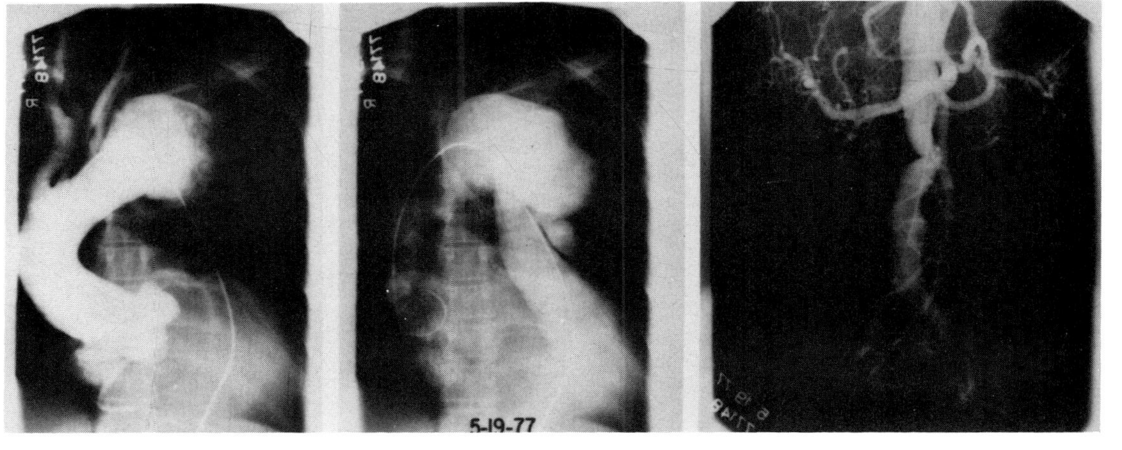

Fig. 3. Roentgenograms of 61-year-old woman known to have had type III dissecting aneurysm that had been managed medically. During previous two years, aneurysm showed progressive enlargement, and patient had recent onset of back and chest pain. Arteriogram revealed large dissection of descending thoracic aorta. Through left-sided lateral thoracotomy with previously placed Carlen's endotracheal tube, heparinized shunt was positioned from left ventricle to femoral artery. Graft was placed from subclavian artery to descending thoracic aorta. Postoperative course was uneventful. [From Wolfe WG, Kleinman LH, Wechsler AS, et al: Heparin-coated shunts for lesions of the descending thoracic aorta. Experimental and clinical observations. Arch. Surg. 112:1481, 1977. Copyright 1977, American Medical Association.]

easily closed. For more involved aneurysms, with or without rupture, open aortotomy with a combined exposure of both the cardiac chamber and the aorta may be necessary. The standard technique of closure of a fistula between the sinus of Valsalva and the right atrium is shown in Fig. 4.

In those instances in which the sinus of Valsalva aneurysm is a part of a more extensive procedure involving the ascending aorta, it is generally preferable to replace the aorta with a woven Dacron graft as well as the insertion of a prosthetic aortic valve. Both the right and left coronary arteries usually require reimplantation into the prosthesis. In such a procedure, all of the diseased tissue is removed and the likelihood of a good long-term result is improved. The operative technique is shown in Fig. 5.

For aneurysms involving the ascending aorta without extension into the sinuses of Valsalva, a median sternotomy is performed, and after dissection of the distal branches of the aorta for control, the patient is placed on extracorporeal circulation with venous catheters in the right atrium and the arterial catheter in the common femoral artery. Cold arrest of the heart with potassium cardioplegia is very useful, especially if the aortic valve requires replacement.

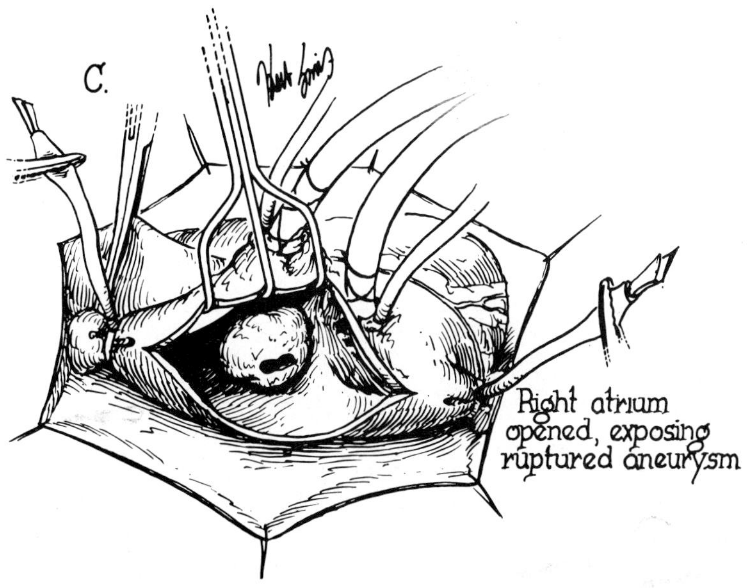

Fig. 4. Demonstration of sinus of Valsalva aneurysm with a fistula to the right atrium. A right atriotomy has been made. Following excision of the fistula, the opening into the atrium is closed directly with sutures. [From DeBakey ME, Dietrich EB, Liddicoat JE, et al: Abnormalities of the sinuses of Valsalva. Experience with 35 patients. J. Thorac. Cardiovasc. Surg. 54:312, 1967.]

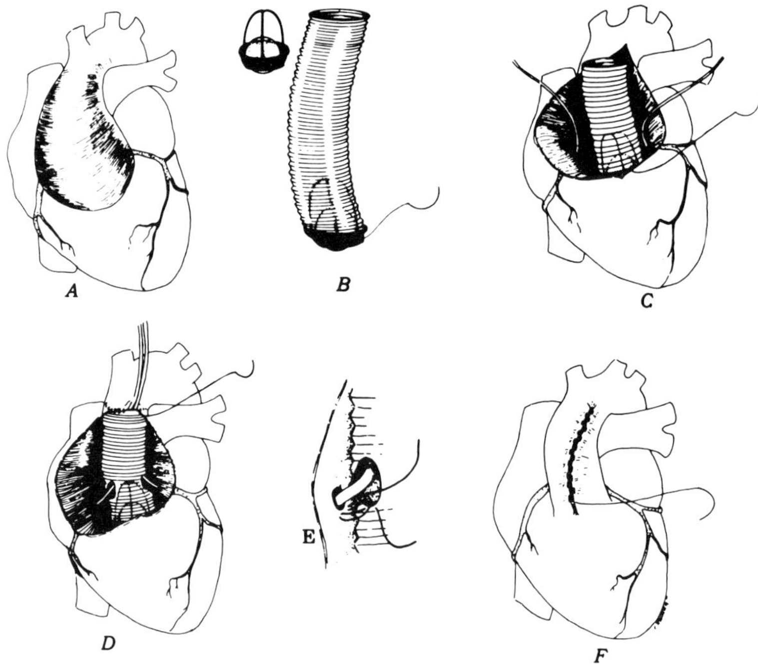

Fig. 5. When ascending aortic aneurysms involve the aortic sinuses (A), the coronary orifices, and the aortic valve, the technique demonstrated has proved safe and effective. (B) Valve prosthesis sutured to a woven graft. (C) Bypass is started, the ascending aorta is opened longitudinally, and the valve is inserted in the aortic annulus with interrupted sutures. (D) Holes are cut in the graft opposite the coronary orifices. (E) The distal anastomosis is completed and the aneurysmal sac is closed around the graft. [From Edwards WS, Kerr AR: A safer technique for replacement of the entire ascending aorta and aortic valve. J. Thorac. Cardiovasc. Surg. 59:837, 1970.]

The aneurysm is then opened and a preclotted Dacron graft then inserted end-to-end. If the proximal portions of the large vessels are involved, these can be appropriately corrected with bypass shunts placed distally. The distal anastomosis is first performed and the proximal suture line is then accomplished. Prior to completion of the proximal anastomosis, the caval tourniquets are released to allow the heart to fill and the entrapped air to escape. A needle is then placed close to the proximal anastomosis for removal of any residual air. The remaining aneurysmal wall may then be used to reinforce the prosthetic graft by closure over the prosthesis. The technique involved in excision of a fusiform aneurysm of the ascending aorta without involvement of the aortic valve is shown in Fig. 6.

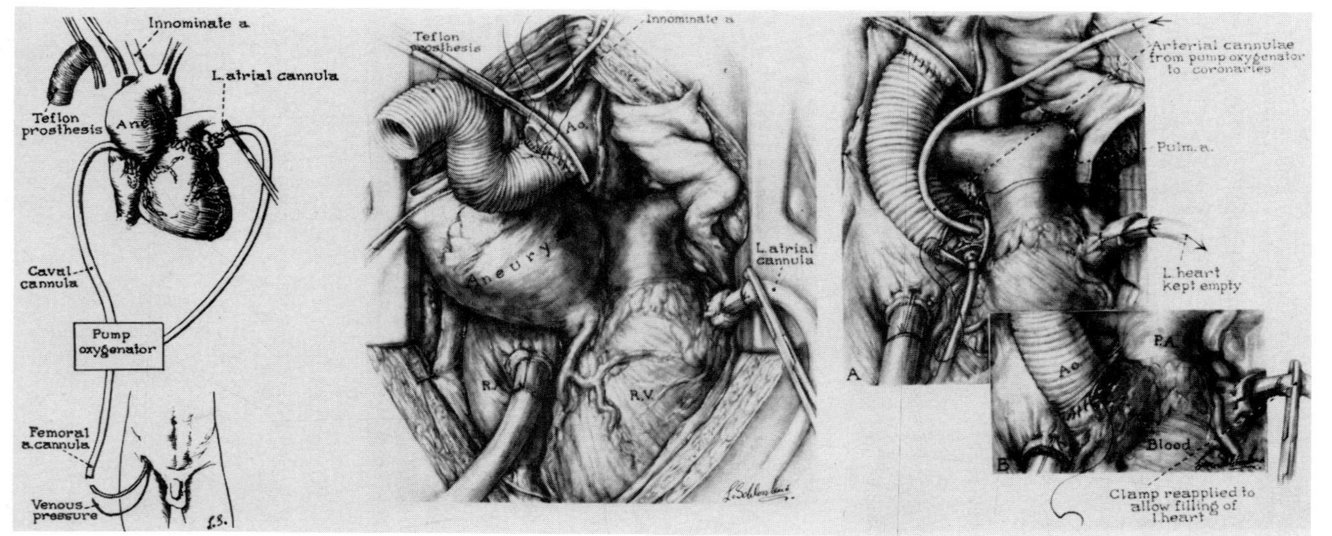

Fig. 6. Excision of fusiform aneurysm of the ascending aorta. (A) Plan of bypass. (B) While the distal anastomosis is made, venous blood is not completely removed from the right atrium and the left atrial suction is used only to prevent excessive pressure in the aneurysm. The coronary circulation is thus maintained intact. (C) After the aneurysm is excised, all blood is aspirated from both sides of the heart while the proximal anastomosis is completed. When the proximal aorta is opened, the coronary arteries should be perfused. [From Bahnson HT, Spencer FC: Excision of aneurysm of the ascending aorta with prosthetic replacement during cardiopulmonary bypass. Ann. Surg. 151:879, 1960. Reproduced by permission of the J. B. Lippincott Company.]

Aneurysms of the Transverse Arch

For lesions involving the transverse arch, a median sternotomy provides good exposure. Preparation is made for cardiopulmonary bypass similar to that for lesions of the ascending aorta. The right and left axillary and left common carotid arteries are then cannulated in addition to the femoral artery. The operative procedure employed for aneurysms of the transverse aortic arch is shown in Fig. 7. After opening the proximal aorta, the heart is protected by infusion of cold potassium solution at 4°C (Fig. 7B). Ice slush is used to maintain cardiac arrest, and separate perfusion of the innominate and left carotid arteries can be achieved by lines from the pump (Fig. 7C). An excised segment of the wall of the aneurysm including the orifices of the innominate, left carotid, and left subclavian arteries may then be sutured to the prosthetic graft.

Aneurysms of the Descending Thoracic Aorta

Aneurysms involving the descending thoracic aorta are most often the result of atherosclerosis, aortic dissection, or those which follow deceleration injuries with a serious aortic tear at the ductus arteriosus. These lesions can be quite effectively managed by one of several techniques including (1) use of a flexible heparin sodium-coated shunt from the proximal aorta (or subclavian artery) or the left ventricular apex to the femoral artery, (2) use of partial cardiopulmonary bypass from the femoral vein to femoral artery, (3) partial extracorporeal circulation with pumping from the left atrium to the femoral artery (oxygenator not required), and (4) simple occlusion of the proximal and distal aorta and rapid excision of the aneurysm without provision for distal arterial circulation.

While all of these methods have been employed successfully, our own preference is generally for the use of the flexible heparin-bonded shunt lined with cationic surfactant tridodecylmethylammonium. We believe this shunt has provided safe clinical conduct of the operation with a lower mortality than that associated with extracorporeal pumping techniques. The primary advantage of this method is the elimination of heparin for systemic anticoagulation. Moreover, it avoids the hypertension which may occur during simple cross-clamping of the aorta. Thus when the lesion is amenable this method is preferable, a choice selected by a number of others [2, 3, 5]. Our experiences in a group of patients with this technique have previously been reported [7], and in this approach a left lateral thoracotomy is used. The patient is intubated with a Carlen catheter for separate inflation of the right and left lung, and the groin is prepared for insertion of the heparin-bonded shunt. The chest is entered through the bed of the resected fourth or fifth rib, and if the aneurysm is an extensive one, a lower incision can be made if needed through the seventh or eighth interspace to facilitate performance of the distal anastomosis. If the left sub-

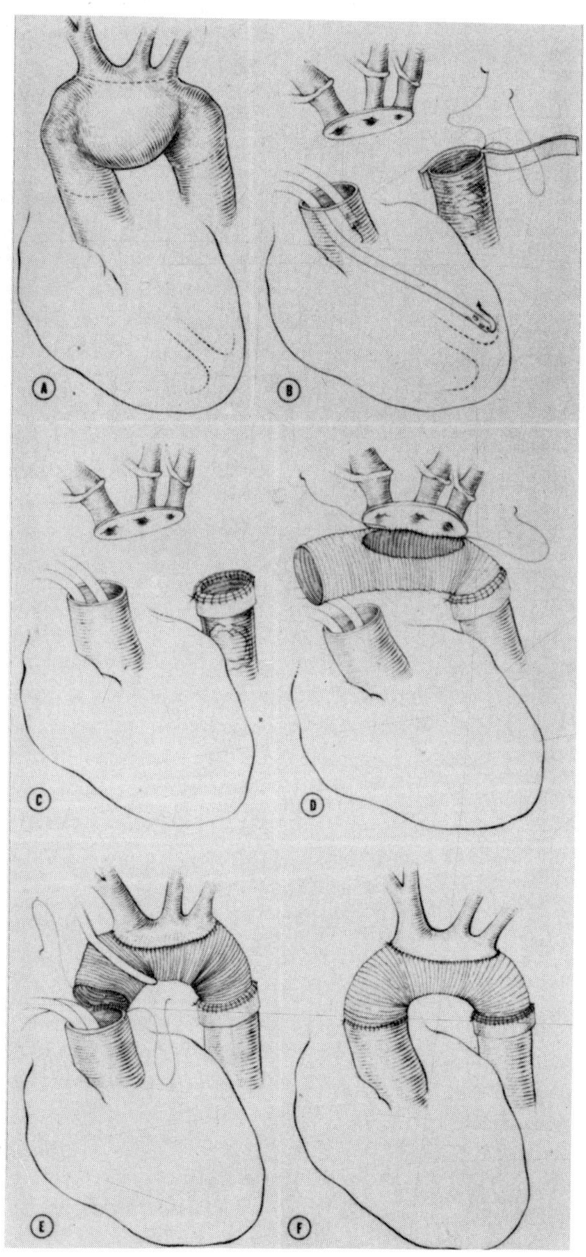
A
B
C
D
E
F

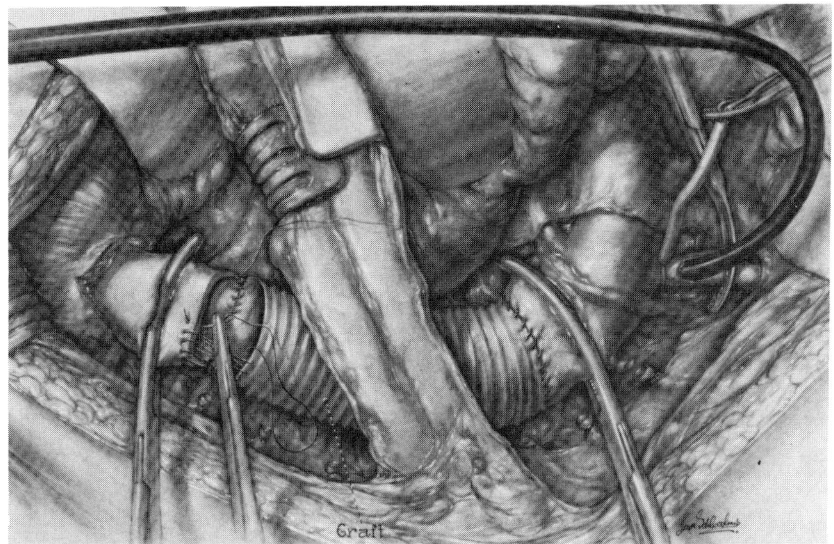

Fig. 8. Placement of the prosthetic graft with the heparinized shunt in position. [From Valiathan MS, Weldon CS, Bender HW Jr, et al: Resection of aneurysms of the descending thoracic aorta using a GBH-coated shunt bypass. J. Surg. Res. 8:197, 1968.]

clavian artery is suitable, it is used for placement of the proximal end of the shunt. If not, the proximal end of the catheter may be inserted through either a purse-string suture into the ascending aorta or in the left ventricular apex. After the distal end of the catheter is placed into the femoral artery, the aorta is clamped above and below the aneurysm. The aneurysm is then opened and the Dacron graft is inserted end-to-end, preserving sufficient aneurysmal wall to encircle the prosthesis for reinforcement after completion of the anastomoses. This technique is shown in Fig. 8 [6].

Fig. 7. Operative procedure for aortic aneurysm involving the transverse arch. (A) Lines of transection of aorta leaving cuff for great vessels. (B) The myocardium is protected by infusion of potassium cardioplegic solution at 4°C with ice slush to maintain the temperature at this level throughout the procedure. (C) The innominate, left carotid, and left subclavian arteries may be separately perfused by cannulae from cardiopulmonary bypass passed into these vessels while the anastomoses of the graft are being made. The body temperature should be lowered to 5°-28°C. (D) Anastomosis of cuff of great vessels to graft. (E) Perfusion of aortic arch and great vessels resumed during suture of graft to ascending aorta. (F) Completed graft in place. [From Griepp RB, Stinson EB, Hollingsworth JF, et al: Prosthetic replacement of the aortic arch. J. Thorac. Cardiovasc. Surg. 70:1051, 1975.]

While some have advocated simple proximal and distal cross-clamping and rapid insertion of the graft without a shunt, it is our view that the spinal cord and kidneys can best be protected by the use of a shunt. Moreover, this is also preferable to the use of extracorporeal circulation, since the latter requires systemic heparinization, which can lead to difficult bleeding problems in these patients. Our experimental results concerning the effects of insertion of a heparin-bonded shunt into the left ventricle (as opposed to insertion into the ascending aorta or subclavian artery) have shown the left ventricular route results in an increase in left ventricular pressure during left ventricle-femoral artery shunting compared with aorta-femoral artery shunting (Figs. 9 and 10). In addition, the *shunt flow* is always greater when the shunt is placed between the aorta (or subclavian artery) than when from the left ventricle. Therefore if the choice exists the evidence suggests that insertion of the shunt distal to the aortic valve is preferable. If anatomic or pathologic reasons preclude the use of either the aortic or subclavian sites for the proximal catheter, the left ventricle can be used as source for the shunt blood.

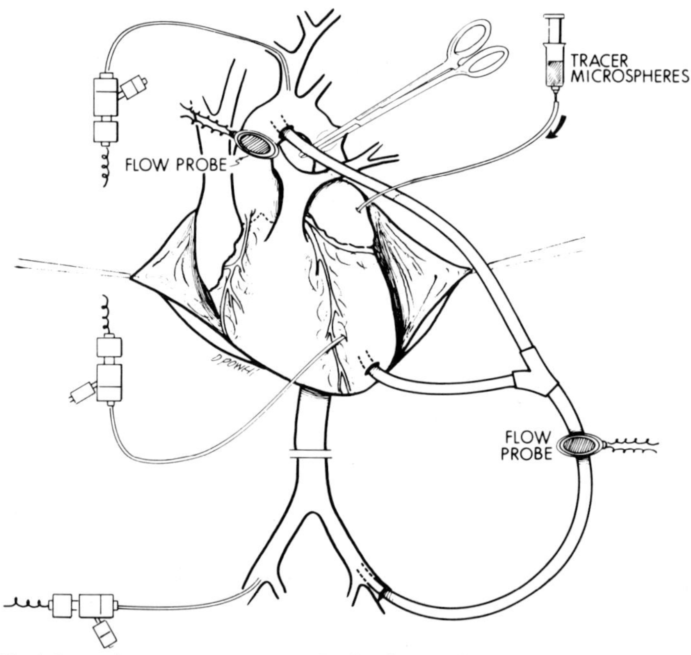

Fig. 9. Model used to compare ventricular-femoral artery shunts with aorta-femoral artery shunts. Tracer microspheres were injected into left atrium. Y conduit was large enough to prevent restriction of blood flow. [From Wolfe WG, Kleinman LH, Wechsler AS, et al: Heparin-coated shunts for lesions of the descending thoracic aorta. Experimental and clinical observations. Arch. Surg. 112:1481, 1977. Copyright 1977, American Medical Association.]

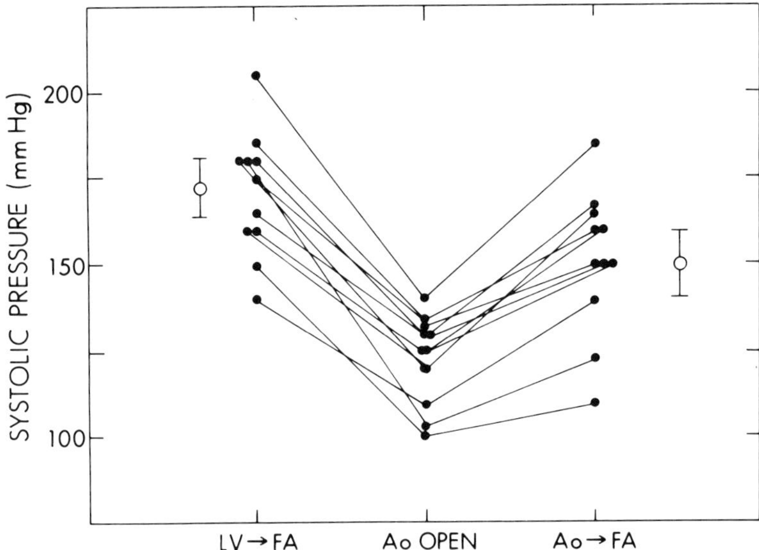

Fig. 10. Effect on left ventricular (LV) pressure of shunting from left ventricle to femoral artery (FA), compared with aorta (Ao) to femoral artery. Neither shunting from left ventricle nor ascending aorta to femoral artery during cross-clamping of proximal descending aorta is fully effective in decompressing left ventricle. However, shunting from aorta appears more effective in decompressing ventricle, probably because of greater shunt flow during diastole. When left ventricular shunting was used, there was only insignificant aortic insufficiency. Coronary blood flow increased in proportion to increased left ventricular systolic pressure and was therefore greater when shunting was from left ventricle to femoral artery. [From Wolfe WG, Kleinman LH, Wechsler AS, et al: Heparin-coated shunts for lesions of the descending thoracic aorta. Experimental and clinical observations. Arch. Surg. 112:1481, 1977. Copyright 1977, American Medical Association.]

REFERENCES

1. Chapman DW, Beazley HL, Peterson PK, et al: Annulo-aortic ectasia with cystic medial necrosis. Am. J. Cardiol. 16:679, 1965
2. Connors JP, Ferguson TB, Roper CL, et al: The use of TDMAC-heparin shunt in replacement of the descending thoracic aorta. Ann. Surg. 181:735, 1975
3. Donahoo JS, Brawley RK, Gott VL: The heparin-coated vascular shunt for thoracic aortic and great vessel procedures: A ten-year experience. Ann. Thorac. Surg. 23:507, 1977
4. Hirst AE Jr, Johns VJ Jr, Kime SW Jr: Dissecting aneurysm of the aorta: A review of 505 cases. Medicine (Baltimore) 37:217, 1958
5. Lawrence GH, Hessel EA, Sauvage LR, et al: Results of the use of the TDMAC-heparin shunt in the surgery of aneurysms of the descending thoracic aorta. J. Thorac. Cardiovasc. Surg. 73:393, 1977

6. Valiathan MS, Weldon CS, Bender HW Jr, et al: Resection of aneurysms of the descending thoracic aorta using a GBH-coated shunt bypass. J. Surg. Res. 8:197, 1968
7. Wolfe WG, Kleinman LH, Wechsler AS, et al: Heparin-coated shunts for lesions of the descending thoracic aorta. Experimental and clinical observations. Arch. Surg. 112:1481, 1977

Arthur J. Roberts, M.D.
Lawrence L. Michaelis, M.D.

The Use of Bypass Techniques and Other Forms of Organ Protection During Thoracic Aortic Cross-Clamping

The increasing frequency of penetrating and nonpenetrating injuries to the thoracic aorta, the development of improved diagnostic techniques, and refinements in the perioperative management of aortic pathology have made operations involving the thoracic aorta more common in surgical practice. While the mortality rate from aortic tears is high [31] and the natural history of thoracic aortic aneurysms has shown that they usually become progressively larger [7] and related complications are common [24], recent advancements in surgical technique and anesthetic management have been associated with a marked decrease in operative mortality. The purpose of this report is to review the development and significance of bypass techniques and other methods of organ preservation during thoracic aortic surgery.

Although operative management of aortic injuries varies according to the site of aortic pathology, direct repair of aortic disease usually requires cross-clamping of the aorta and interruption of distal blood flow. Consequently, proximal blood pressure rises and distal blood pressure falls. The kidneys [46] and the spinal cord [10] are especially vulnerable to even brief periods of ischemia, and temporary aortic occlusion for the repair of an aortic rupture or the excision of a thoracic aortic aneurysm has occasionally resulted in paraplegia [8]. In addition, marked hypertension may develop in the proximal aorta with the subsequent development of left ventricular failure [36]. Some surgeons believe that if accomplished in a short time the thoracic aortic cross-clamping is well tolerated and that special techniques to prevent subsequent hemodynamic changes are unnecessary [19]. Others believe that an anesthetic agent or drug-induced hypotension may be beneficial to reduce proximal hypertension [20, 58]. Finally, some surgeons have advocated the use of bypass techniques to provide protection from the adverse hemodynamic effects of aortic cross-clamping, which they feel may lead to temporary or permanent organ dysfunction.

SURGERY OF THE ASCENDING AORTA

The most common diseases requiring surgery of the ascending aorta are ascending aortic aneurysms and types I and II dissecting hematomas. Regardless of the etiology of ascending aortic disease, the aorta is usually cross-clamped proximal to the innominate artery, total cardiopulmonary bypass is instituted, and some form of sanguinous or asanguinous intracoronary perfusate is usually employed (Fig. 1). In addition, most surgeons favor the use of some form of left ventricular vent to avoid left ventricular distension during bypass. As early as 1960, Bahnson and Spencer [5] described a technique where cardiopulmonary bypass was used and intermittent left atrial suction employed to enable the resection of an ascending aortic aneurysm. More recently, considerable attention has been directed to improving the techniques of myocardial preservation during surgery requiring cross-clamping of the ascending aorta. At the present time, the

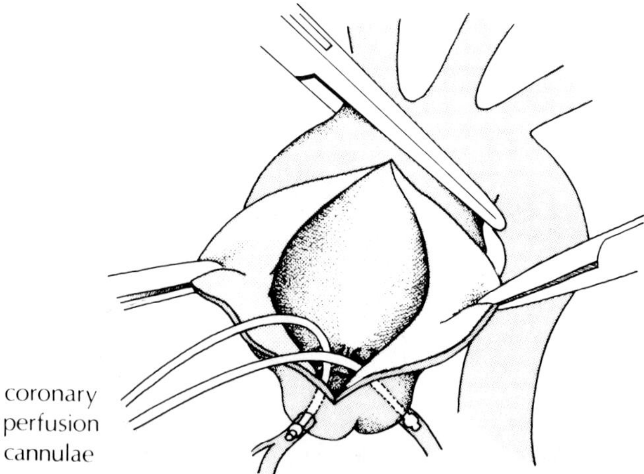

Fig. 1. Technique of myocardial preservation with ascending aortic cross-clamping and the left ventricle is vented. Selective coronary perfusion may be continuous or intermittent and the perfusate may contain blood, hypothermic cardioplegia, or blood cardioplegia. In addition, topical hypothermia may be added.

following measures are considered important during global myocardial ischemia (Table 1). The left ventricular subendocardial muscle is the most susceptible region of the left ventricle to ischemia [35]. This portion of the ventricle receives its blood and oxygen supply only during diastole, since intramyocardial vessels are squeezed shut during systole. Furthermore, subendocardial muscle is in greatest jeopardy in patients with either ventricular hypertrophy or coronary artery disease, conditions which are common in patients with hypertension and aortic dissection or chronic arteriosclerotic aortic aneurysms [12]. Buckberg et al. [11] have been instrumental in defining the importance of perioperative physiological events which occur during cardiopulmonary bypass and information gained from his and other experiments have helped to determine optimal procedures for use in the protection of the ischemic myocardium.

At the present time, the best method of myocardial protection during aortic clamping is uncertain. Behrendt and associates [6] have presented evidence that hypothermic (4°C) potassium (25 mEq/L) cardioplegia provides better immediate myocardial contractility in patients following coronary artery bypass surgery than does ischemic arrest. He also showed that continuous coronary perfusion resulted in protection equivalent to that observed in the cardioplegic group. Furthermore, Conti and Kirkland [17] also studied patients undergoing coronary artery surgery and showed no marked differences in electrocardiographic, hemodynamic, or myocardial-specific enzymatic findings bhtween hypothermic and potassium hypothermic groups. Kuchoukos et al. [39] have reported that systemic hypothermia combined with profound (4°C) topical hypothermia without cardioplegia can be used for combined ascending aortic aneurysm resection and aortic valve replacement with excellent clinical results. Most recently, Follette and Buckberg [28] have used a technique combining blood perfusion and intermittent potassium cardioplegia with encouraging results during ascending aortic cross-clamping. Although the surgical literature is

Table 1
Myocardial Protection Techniques

General
1. Maintain adequate coronary perfusion pressure
2. Use hypothermia (topical, perfusion, intracavitary, systemic)
3. Avoid prolonged ventricular fibrillation
4. Avoid hypotension or hypertension
5. Avoid severe tachycardia or bradycardia
6. Avoid marked hemodilution

Specific Alternatives
1. Multidose potassium crystalloid cardioplegia
2. Multidose blood cardioplegia
3. Continuous coronary perfusion
4. Topical hypothermia

filled with reports concerning the relative efficacy of various forms of myocardial preservation, Ebert [27] states that the large number of solutions and components used in various forms of myocardial protection make it difficult to prove one method superior to others. Furthermore, none of the specialized measures may be as important as the techniques of their application, and thus the safe period of cardiac arrest probably varies with each surgeon.

SURGERY OF THE AORTIC ARCH

Aneurysms of the aortic arch, particularly those involving the transverse arch, have long been considered the most serious form of this disease because excisional therapy in this area is associated with greater technical difficulties and more hazardous consequences, since blood flow to the brain may be compromised.

If the proximal portion of the ascending aorta is uninvolved by aneurysm, bypass can be accomplished by the use of a temporary system of grafts providing circulation to the brain and to the lower part of the aorta while the thoracic aorta is clamped as described by DeBakey et al. [22] (Fig. 2). In addition, the early work of Muller et al. [47] was useful in describing a method of progressive insertion of an ascending aortic graft which protected cerebral blood flow during insertion. Recent modifications of these earlier techniques have had relatively limited clinical trial and include a combination of temporary, permanent, or combined external shunts using woven Dacron tube grafts described by Chu et al. [13] (Fig. 3) or a prefabricated multibranched shunt described by Verdant et al. [55]. Each of the above techniques is performed with systemic heparinization to prevent clot formation and to allow safe autotransfusion if needed.

Fusiform aneurysms of the transverse aortic arch have most commonly been treated by instituting cardiopulmonary bypass from the venae cavae to the femoral artery, followed by selective extracorporeal perfusion of the cerebral and coronary circulations [22] (Fig. 4). Pearce et al. [50] devised a method of perfusing all vessels feeding the circle of Willis as well as the rest of the body during cardiopulmonary bypass utilizing peripheral cannulations and thereby leaving the operative field uncluttered. More recently, Griepp et al. [33] have reported the use of profound hypothermia and circulatory arrest in the successful repair of aortic arch aneurysms (Fig. 5). The basis for the clinical use of hypothermic circulatory arrest was found in experimental data showing that systemic hypothermia at 15°-20°C gave significant protection to the central nervous system in dogs, when the circulation is arrested for 30-60 min [59]. At the present time, however, clinical experience has shown that unexpected neurological complications have occurred with the use of hypothermic circulatory arrest and that postoperative bleeding, pulmonary insufficiency, and poor wound healing are also unsolved problems [13, 49].

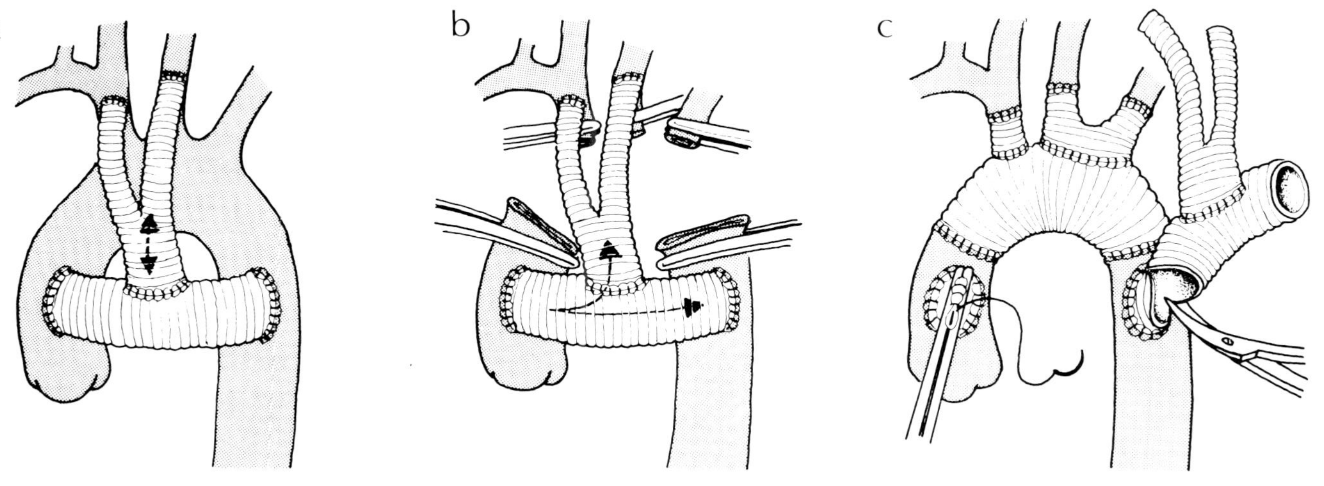

Fig. 2. Sequence of maneuvers used in the placement of temporary grafts during aortic arch replacement. After the temporary grafts are performed using partial occluding clamps (A), the aneurysm is resected (B) and the permanent graft is sewn in place (C). Finally the temporary graft is excised and the ends oversewn.

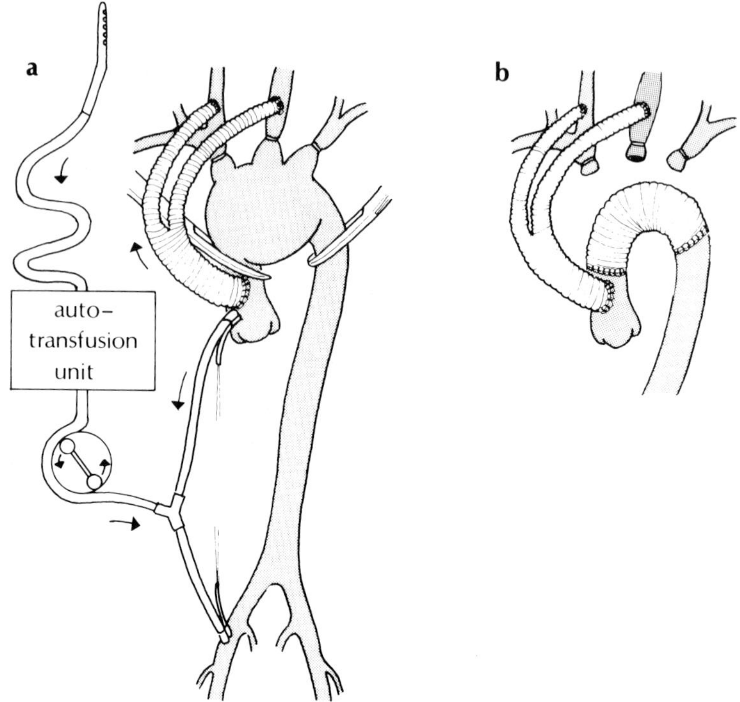

Fig. 3. Modification of earlier bypass techniques used in aortic arch replacement includes the use of Dacron tube grafts to provide a bypass route for cerebral blood flow and replacement of the aortic arch with a second woven graft. Systemic heparin is given and an autotransfusion unit is used to preserve autologous blood.

SURGERY OF THE DESCENDING THORACIC AORTA

The descending thoracic aorta just distal to the left subclavian artery is the site of acute aortic disruptions in the majority of trauma cases, and arteriosclerotic aneurysms are occasionally observed originating in this region.

Some of the earliest resections of aneurysms of the descending thoracic aorta were carried out with either a temporary internal plastic shunt described by Johnson et al. [37] or a temporary external shunt described by Stranahan et al. [52]. Systemic hypothermia was also used in 1953 with full recovery despite 62 min of aortic occlusion [23].

Partial left heart bypass from left atrium to femoral artery popularized by Cooley [18] and Gerbode [29] has more recently been used for acute and chronic descending aortic aneurysms (Fig. 6). Utilizing this technique, one may cross-clamp the aorta proximal to the region of injury while maintaining distal flow to the spinal cord and kidneys. Occasional problems have arisen with this

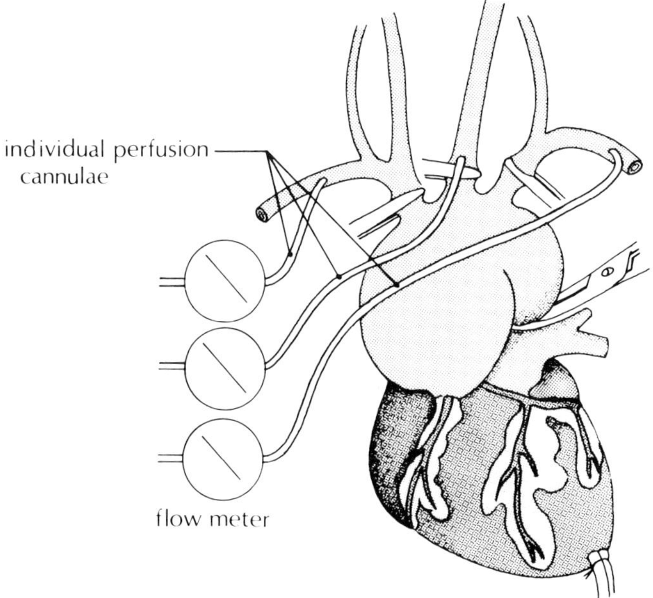

Fig. 4. Another method used to replace the aortic arch includes the utilization of cardiopulmonary bypass and left ventricular decompression in combination with separate perfusion cannulae inserted into the branches of the aortic arch. Individual flowmeters are employed so that careful regulation of cerebral blood flow is obtained. In addition, coronary perfusion may also be added if desired.

technique because of a small or fragile left atrium or when extensive mediastinal hematoma makes exposure in this area difficult and hazardous. Another technique commonly employed in descending thoracic aortic lesions involves the use of femoral vein to femoral artery partial bypass with the use of a pump oxygenator and systemic heparin [21] (Fig. 7). This procedure keeps perfusion lines away from the main operative field and partial bypass may be instituted at any time if sudden hemorrhage should occur. Left atrial or femoral vein to femoral artery bypass flows of 20-30 cc per minute per kilogram of body weight have appeared to provide protection to the spinal cord and kidneys [21, 46]. In addition, some surgeons have advocated that direct intraarterial pressure measurement distal to the site of aortic cross-clamping offers useful information and that maintenance of a distal mean pressure of at least 60 mm Hg provides added security against ischemic damage [15].

More recently, the use of heparin-bonded plastic tubing, which eliminates the need for systemic heparinization, has become increasingly popular [53]. Gott et al. [30] first reported bonding graphite and benzalkonium to heparin

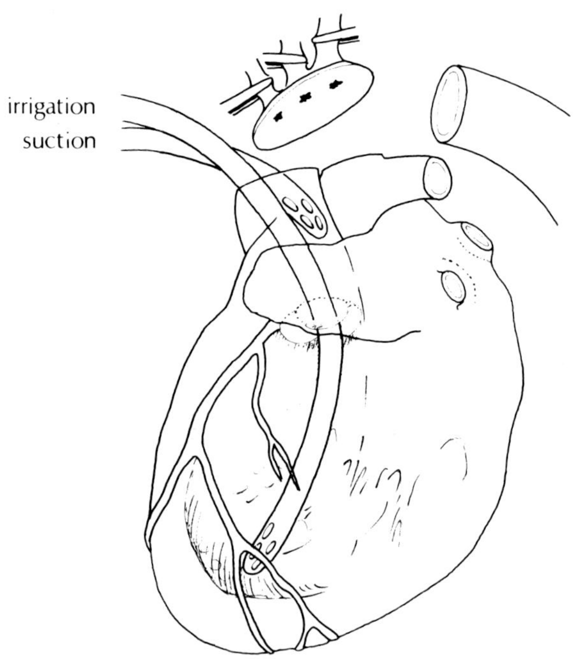

Fig. 5. Technique of profound hypothermia and circulatory arrest during aortic arch replacement. Total cardiopulmonary bypass is instituted and topical hypothermia (4° C) is used to cool the endocardium (irrigation line), while left ventricular distension is controlled by an aortic root vent (suction line). Additionally, epicardial cooling can be achieved by pouring cold Ringer's lactate solution on the surface of the heart.

with excellent thromboresistant properties. Grode et al. [34] produced an improved heparinized surface with the use of tridodecylmethylammonium chloride (TDMAC-heparin). The use of a heparinized shunt bypass without systemic anticoagulation simplifies operations on the thoracic aorta and decreases the likelihood of bleeding complications. The advantage of eliminating the need for systemic heparinization becomes even more important in the trauma patient with coincidental abdominal or cranial injuries when increased bleeding in those areas could lead to serious consequences. The TDMAC-heparin bypass can be inserted proximally into the ascending aorta (Fig. 8) or the apex of the left ventricle (Fig. 9). Earlier use of the subclavian artery for proximal cannulation has generally been abandoned because of its role as a source of collateral blood supply. Technical considerations and relative ease of exposure of the heart or ascending aorta during operation may favor one proximal cannulation site over the other. Distal cannulation may be performed in the descending

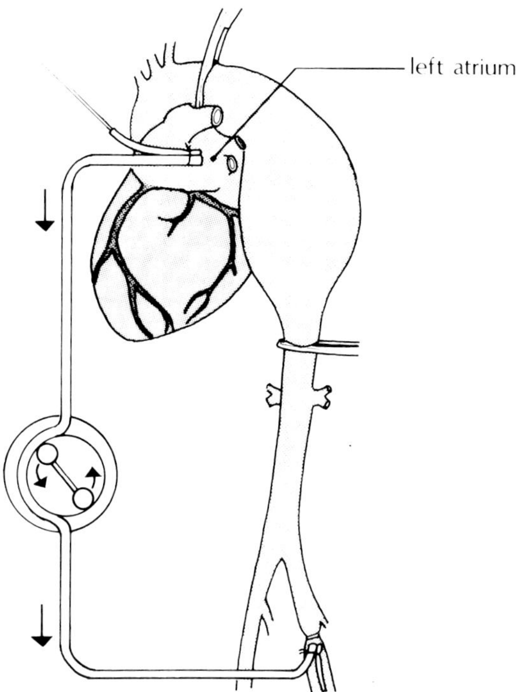

Fig. 6. Partial left heart bypass from left atrium to femoral or iliac artery employed in descending thoracic aortic operations. A standard roller pump is used and systemic heparinization is necessary.

thoracic aorta, iliac, or femoral arteries. This technique is not without difficulties, however, as air emboli have been reported [57], bleeding complications observed [48], and the incidence of paraplegia, although small, not significantly reduced as compared to that noted using other techniques [19]. Wakabayashi and associates [56] have recently described and successfully employed a bypass technique using nonthrombogenic polyurethane-polyvinyl-graphite (PPG) tubing, cannulas, and a roller pump without an oxygenator or systemic heparin. This technique has been used with either femoral vein to femoral artery bypass [45] or left atrial to femoral artery bypass [16] during thoracic aortic cross-clamping. Peripheral cannulation of the femoral vein and artery is very easily performed, but 100% oxygen must be delivered to raise the oxygen content of the venous blood, and a large-bore venous cannula should be passed up to the level of the right atrium in order to obtain mixed venous blood in sufficient quantity to prevent cardiac distention and to maintain adequate oxygenation in the distal aorta [45] (Fig. 10). An additional technique which has been used in conjunction with either thoracic aortic bypass or unprotected

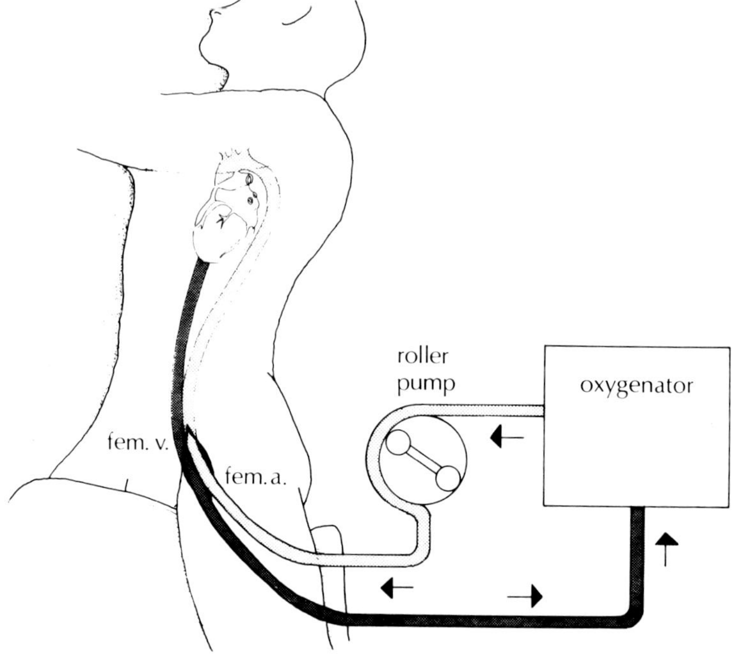

Fig. 7. Partial cardiopulmonary bypass with femoral artery-to-femoral vein perfusion system. A standard roller pump and an oxygenator are used with this method and systemic heparin is mandatory.

aortic cross-clamping has been the use of a Carlens or Robertshaw endotracheal tube [38]. The use of such double-lumen endotracheal tubes allows deflation of the left lung facilitating retraction and decreasing dissection necessary for proper exposure of the thoracic aorta. When this anesthetic adjunct is used and systemic heparin is avoided, pulmonary hemorrhage is decreased and pulmonary complications appear to be fewer postoperatively [38, 57]. An added benefit of the double lumen tube is the prevention of aspiration of secretions or blood into the dependent lung when the patient is in the lateral decubitus position.

THORACIC AORTIC CROSS-CLAMPING WITHOUT BYPASS

Crawford et al. [19] have reported a large and successful series of operations on patients with thoracic aneurysms using a simplified technique involving proximal and distal aortic cross-clamping, minimal dissection, and a rapid suture technique aimed at preventing disruption of collateral circulation to the spinal cord and avoidance of intraoperative hypotension. The incidence of spinal cord injury in his series using aortic cross-clamping without bypass approximates the

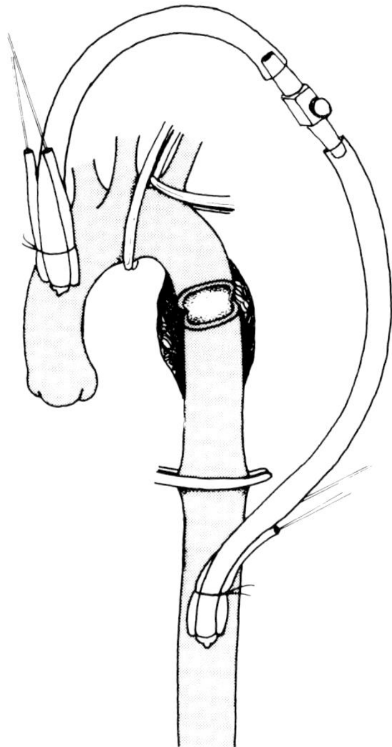

Fig. 8. Temporary partial bypass from ascending to descending aorta used in repair of descending thoracic aortic injury. Systemic heparin is not used and heparin-bonded shunt is preferred bypass conduit.

incidence of spinal cord damage found with other techniques utilizing a bypass system to maintain distal blood flow [2, 10].

Although 30-45 min of normothermic descending aortic cross-clamping is accepted as the upper limit of safety [8, 19], it has been tolerated for periods of over an hour; yet severe neurological damage has resulted from periods of occlusion as short as 18 min [4]. Systemic hypotension or the operative division of intercostal arteries have been identified as important factors in the development of spinal cord injury related to aortic cross-clamping [14]. The major problem confronting the vascular surgeon is that the arteria magna (anterior spinal artery) cannot be readily identified preoperatively and its origin is extremely variable, arising from a segment varying between the eighth thoracic and fourth lumbar vertebrae [1, 4, 10]. Furthermore, the anterior spinal artery is rarely, if ever, a continuous vessel and there may be no vascular communications between the cervical, thoracic, and lumbar sections. Consequently, the placement of the aortic cross-clamp or the occlusion of an intercostal artery may be harmless in one patient but may be extremely perilous in another. Kirklin et

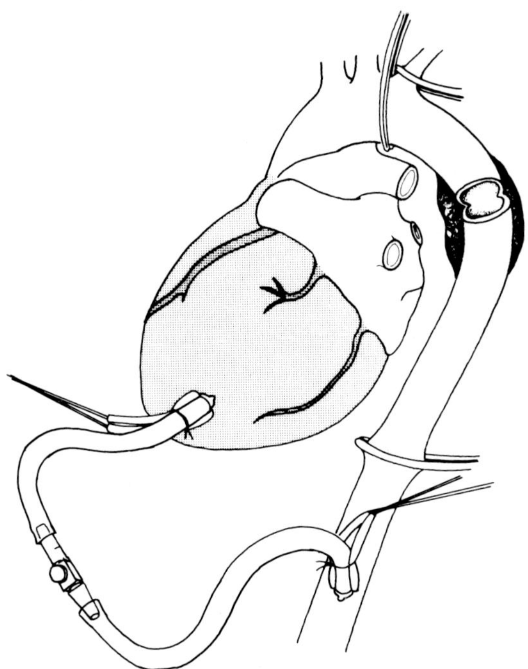

Fig. 9. Partial bypass conduit from left ventricular apex to descending thoracic aorta is used as an alternate cannulation technique in operations involving the descending thoracic aorta. The TDMAC-heparin bypass material is most frequently employed in this procedure and systemic heparin is not needed.

al. [2] and Brewer and colleagues [10] report that their clinical experience supports that of Crawford, and they conclude that in properly trained personnel closed traumatic injuries of the upper descending thoracic aorta should be managed by simply cross-clamping the aorta, thereby decreasing operating time, cross-clamp time, and the need for blood administration, all of which tend to minimize complications. On the other hand, Gott et al. [26] suggest that the shunt method gives surgeons who are less experienced with problems of the descending thoracic aorta an increased safe period of cross-clamping in which to perform the aortic resection and anastomosis. Furthermore, Brewer [9] notes that a surgeon will fare better when there is litigation regarding paraplegia if he has employed an accepted method to protect the spinal cord.

The occurrence of acute tubular necrosis has been a relatively uncommon but persistent problem after thoracic aortic operations. DeBakey et al. [25] have found that the incidence of this complication (approximately 2%) is similar whether a bypass technic or unprotected aortic clamping is employed. Although

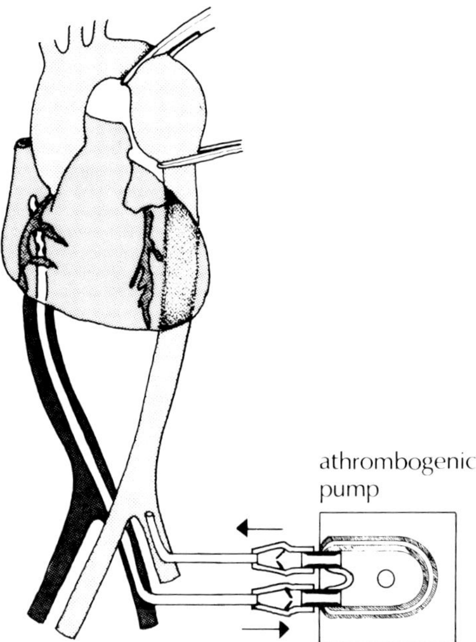

Fig. 10. Partial cardiopulmonary bypass utilizing non-thrombogenic polyurethane-polyvinyl-graphite tubing and a specially constructed roller pump described by Wakabayashi. This system requires neither an oxygenator nor systemic heparin.

some surgeons feel that pretreatment with mannitol, lasix, and/or corticosteroids prior to aortic occlusion is beneficial in protecting the ischemic kidney [42, 54], clinical trials proving the advantage of such pharmacological therapy in thoracic aortic surgery have not been performed. Similarly, the use of sodium bicarbonate to counteract the lactic acid which is released into the systemic circulation during aortic cross-clamping and following declamping has been shown experimentally to be useful against the formation of tissue acidosis [42], but the clinical use of this agent has not been widely employed.

PHARMACOLOGIC TREATMENT OF HYPERTENSION ASSOCIATED WITH THORACIC AORTIC ANEURYSMS

Wheat et al. [62] in 1965 first popularized the pharmacological treatment of acute dissecting aneurysms of the aorta. A more recent report documenting this experience in 50 patients admitted to two different hospitals over a 5 year period showed an immediate hospital survival rate of 86%, with 84% of patients initially discharged still alivc at 1 year [60]. Intensive drug therapy has been used to decrease the cardiac impulse (dp/dt_{max}) and to lower the mean blood pressure. Trimethaphan camsylate was initially used to acutely decrease blood pressure, but more recently sodium nitroprusside has been used with increasing frequency [32]. Advantages of intravenous nitroprusside include a rapid onset and a rapid cessation of action and a relative refractoriness to tachyphylaxis, as was seen with trimethaphan. However, nitroprusside may not reliably decrease dp/dt_{max}; thus simultaneous use of small doses of propranolol may offer additional benefits in the treatment of hypertension associated with thoracic aneurysms. Furthermore, the increased reflex sympathetic activity which occurs secondary to nitroprusside-induced peripheral vasodilation may be blocked by the additional use of reserpine, Aldomet, or propranolol. Presently, specific use of aggressive antihypertensive therapy appears indicated in the initial therapy of hypertension associated with all forms of acute aortic injury, as a temporary measure to allow stabilization during treatment of associated organ damage in patients with multiple traumatic injuries [51], and as primary therapy for type III dissecting aneurysms [61].

PHYSIOLOGICAL STUDIES DURING DESCENDING THORACIC AORTIC OCCLUSION

Experimental hemodynamic studies by Hug and Taber [36] in 1969 revealed that significant elevation in left ventricular systolic and end-diastolic pressures were observed in normal dogs following occlusion of the aorta distal to the left subclavian artery. In addition, marked elevation of mean left atrial pressure from 25 to 45 mm Hg sometimes occurred with the appearance of large V waves indicative of acute mitral regurgitation. The V waves persisted in eight of ten dogs for 30 min following a 30 min period of occlusion, despite return of the atrial and ventricular pressures to normal levels, suggesting persistent impairment of cardiac function. Shumacker et al. [43] studied the effects of thoracic aortic cross-clamping on kidney and spinal cord integrity and observed that a brachial artery to femoral artery bypass in dogs prevented paraplegia and elevation of BUN following thoracic aortic cross-clamping. Wechsler et al. [57] analyzed the cardiac effects of ventriculofemoral and ascending aortic to femoral bypass by comparing paired observations in dogs and found using flow probes and trace microspheres as well as conventional pressure recordings that greater decompression of the left ventricle and less demand on myocardial blood flow was observed when the ascending aorta was the proximal site for decompression during thoracic aortic cross-clamping.

In a clinical study involving ten patients with severe coronary artery disease who had occlusion of the infrarenal aorta for resection of abdominal aortic aneurysms, significant increases in pulmonary arterial, pulmonary capillary wedge, and mean arterial pressures occurred [3]. Three of these patients who showed the greatest increases in pulmonary capillary wedge pressure developed electrocardiographic evidence of myocardial ischemia which was reversed in two of the three patients by preload and afterload reduction by sodium nitroprusside. In addition, Wilkinson, Roberts, et al. in this volume have shown that intravenous nitroglycerin can prevent elevations in pulmonary capillary wedge pressure and electrocardiographic evidence for myocardial ischemia in patients undergoing infrarenal aortic cross-clamping (see page 27). Kouchoukos et al. [40] assessed the effects of clamping of the proximal thoracic aorta and subsequent decompression with a temporary shunt in eight patients undergoing descending thoracic aortic aneurysm resection. They found that a significant decrease in left ventricular performance associated with an increase in pulmonary capillary wedge pressure and a decrease in cardiac index resulted from thoracic aortic clamping and that these deleterious effects were almost completely reversed by the use of a temporary shunt. In addition, Crawford [20] has observed that peripheral vasodilator type of anesthetics such as Innovar and Sublimaze and intraoperative regulation of peripheral resistance with nitroprusside provides pharmacologic control of adverse hemodynamic responses to cross-clamping of the thoracic aorta.

Further investigations are necessary to accurately delineate the relative efficacy of various methods employed to protect organs rendered ischemic during thoracic aortic cross-clamping. Although operative mortality from this condition has decreased in recent years, further advances must await a better definition of the pathophysiology of thoracic aortic disease and a more critical analysis of physiologic responses noted during the use of various techniques used to protect the circulation during thoracic aortic cross-clamping.

REFERENCES

1. Adams HD, van Geertruyden HH: Neurologic complications of aortic surgery. Ann. Surg. 144:574, 1956
2. Appelbaum A, Karp RB, Kirklin JW: Surgical treatment for closed thoracic aortic injuries. J. Thorac. Cardiovasc. Surg. 71:458, 1976
3. Attia RR, Murphy JD, Snider M, et al: Myocardial ischemia due to infrarenal aortic cross-clamping during aortic surgery in patients with severe coronary artery disease. Circulation 53:961, 1976
4. Bahnson HT: Thoracic aneurysms, in Sabiston DC Jr, Spencer FC (eds): Gibbon's Surgery of the Chest (ed 3). Philadelphia, W. B. Saunders, 1976
5. Bahnson HT, Spencer FC: Excision of aneurysm of the ascending aorta with prosthetic replacement during cardiopulmonary bypass. Ann. Surg. 151:879, 1960
6. Behrendt DM, Kirsh MM, Jochim KE, et al: Effects of cardioplegic solution on human contractile element velocity. Ann. Thorac. Surg. 26:499, 1978

7. Bennett DE, Cherry JK: The natural history of traumatic aneurysms of the aorta. Surgery 61:516, 1967
8. Blaisdell FW, Cooley DA: The mechanism of paraplegia after temporary thoracic aortic occlusion and its relationship to spinal fluid pressure. Surgery 51:351, 1962
9. Brewer LA III, as discussed by Lawrence GH, Hessel EA, Sauvage LR, et al: Results of the use of the TDMAC-heparin shunt in the surgery of aneurysms of the descending thoracic aorta. J. Thorac. Cardiovasc. Surg. 73:393, 1977
10. Brewer LA, Fosburg RG, Mulder GA, et al: Spinal cord complications following surgery for coarctation of the aorta. J. Thorac. Cardiovasc. Surg. 64:368, 1972
11. Buckberg GD: Left ventricular subendocardial necrosis. Ann. Thorac. Surg. 24:379, 1977
12. Ching CC, Hughes RK: Arteriosclerotic aneurysms of the thoracic aorta: Late state of a diffuse disease. Am. J. Surg. 114:853, 1967
13. Chu S-H, Lee Y-T, Lien W-P, et al: Resection of aneurysm of the aortic arch without cardiopulmonary bypass. J. Thorac. Cardiovasc. Surg. 74:928, 1977
14. Clatworthy HW, Sako Y, Chisholm TC, et al: Thoracic aortic coarctation. Surgery 28:245, 1950
15. Connolly JE, Kountz SL, Boyd RJ: Left heart bypass: Experimental and clinical observations on its regulation with particular reference to maintenance of maximal renal blood flow. J. Thorac. Cardiovasc. Surg. 44:577, 1962
16. Connolly JE, Wakabayashi A, German JC, et al: Clinical experience with pulsatile left heart bypass without anticoagulation for thoracic aneurysms. J. Thorac. Cardiovasc. Surg. 62:568, 1971
17. Conti VR, Bertranou EG, Blackstone EH, et al: Cold cardioplegia versus hypothermia for myocardial protection. J. Thorac. Cardiovasc. Surg. 76:577, 1978
18. Cooley DA, DeBakey ME, Morris GC Jr: Controlled extracorporeal circulation in surgical treatment of aortic aneurysm. Ann. Surg. 146:473, 1957
19. Crawford ES, Rubio PA: Reappraisal of adjuncts to avoid ischemia in the treatment of aneurysms of descending thoracic aorta. J. Thorac. Cardiovasc. Surg. 66:693, 1973
20. Crawford ES, as discussed by Kouchoukos NT, Lell WA, Karp RB, et al: Hemodynamic effects of aortic clamping and decompression with a temporary shunt for resection of the descending thoracic aorta. Surgery 85:25, 1979
21. Symbas PN: Trauma to the Heart and Great Vessels. New York, Grune & Stratton, 1978
22. DeBakey ME, Beall AC Jr, Cooley DA, et al: Resection and graft replacement of aneurysms involving the transverse arch of the aorta. Surg. Clin. North Am. 46:1057, 1966
23. DeBakey ME, Cooley DA: Successful resection of aneurysm of distal aortic arch and replacement of graft. JAMA 155:1398, 1954

24. DeBakey ME, Cooley DA, Crawford ES, et al: Aneurysms of the thoracic aorta: Analysis of 179 patients treated by resection. J. Thorac. Cardiovasc. Surg. 36:393, 1958
25. DeBakey ME, McCollum CH, Graham JM: Surgical treatment of aneurysms of the descending thoracic aorta: Long term results in 500 patients. J. Cardiovasc. Surg. 19:571, 1978
26. Donahoo JS, Brawley RK, Gott VL: The heparin-coated vascular shunt for thoracic aortic and great vessel procedures: A ten-year experience. Ann. Thorac. Surg. 23:507, 1977
27. Ebert PA (ed): Aspects of myocardial protection. Ann. Thorac. Surg. 26:495, 1978
28. Follette DM, Mulder DG, Maloney JV, et al: Advantages of blood cardioplegia over continuous coronary perfusion or intermittent ischemia: Experimental and clinical study. J. Thorac. Cardiovasc. Surg. 76:604, 1978
29. Gerbode F, Braimbridge M, Osborn JJ, et al: Traumatic thoracic aneurysms: Treatment by resection and grafting with the use of an extracorporeal bypass. Surgery 42:975, 1957
30. Gott VL, Whiffen JD, Dutton RC: Heparin bonding on colloidal graphite surfaces. Science 142:1297, 1963
31. Greendyke RM: Traumatic rupture of aorta – Special reference to automobile accidents. JAMA 195:119, 1966
32. Greenfell RF: Treatment of hypertensive crisis. Chest 59:212, 1971
33. Griepp RB, Stinson EB, Hollingsworth JF, et al: Prosthetic replacement of the aortic arch. J. Thorac. Cardiovasc. Surg. 70:1051, 1975
34. Grode GA, Anderson SJ, Grotta HM, et al: Nonthrombogenic materials via a simple coating process. Trans. Am. Soc. Artif. Intern. Organs 15:1, 1969
35. Hoffman JI: Determinants and prediction of transmural myocardial perfusion. Circulation 58:381, 1978
36. Hug HR, Taber RE: Bypass flow requirements during thoracic aneurysmectomy with particular attention to the prevention of left heart failure. J. Thorac. Cardiovasc. Surg. 57:203, 1969
37. Johnson J, Kirby CK, Lehr HB: A method of maintaining adequate blood flow through the thoracic aorta while inserting an aorta graft to replace an aortic aneurysm. Surgery 37:54, 1955
38. Kirsh MM, Behrendt DM, Orringer MB, et al: The treatment of acute traumatic rupture of the aorta: A 10-year experience. Ann. Surg. 184:308, 1976
39. Kouchoukos NT, Karp RB, Lell WA: Replacement of the ascending aorta and aortic valve with a composite graft: Results in 25 patients. Ann. Thorac. Surg. 24:140, 1977
40. Kouchoukos NT, Lell WA, Karp RB, et al: Hemodynamic effects of aortic clamping and decompression with a temporary shunt for resection of the descending thoracic aorta. Surgery 85:25, 1979
41. Lawrence GH, Hessel EA, Sauvage LR, et al: Results of the use of the TDMAC-heparin shunt in the surgery of aneurysms of the descending thoracic aorta. J. Thorac. Cardiovasc. Surg. 73:393, 1977
42. Lempert N, Pakdaman P, Stein A, et al: Further studies on enzymatic

histochemical alterations in the renal tubular epithelium of dogs. II. The effect of aortic cross-clamping below the renal arteris. III. The effect of pretreatment with 10% mannitol in peripheral trauma. Ann. Surg. 160:115, 1964

43. Leshnower AC, Shumacker HB Jr: Experimental unassisted right brachial-to-femoral bypass. Arch. Surg. 109:542, 1974
44. Mansberger AR, Cox EF, Flotte CT, et al: "Washout" acidosis following resection of aortic aneurysms: Clinical metabolic study of reactive hyperemia and effect of dextran on excess lactate and pH. Ann. Surg. 163:778, 1966
45. May IA, Ecker RR, Iverson LI: Heparinless femoral venoarterial bypass without an oxygenator for surgery on the descending thoracic aorta. J. Thorac. Cardiovasc. Surg. 73:387, 1977
46. Morris GC Jr, Witt RR, Cooley DA, et al: Alterations in renal hemodynamics during controlled extracorporeal circulation in the surgical treatment of aortic aneurysms. J. Thorac. Cardiovasc. Surg. 34:590, 1957
47. Muller WH, Warren WD, Blanton FS Jr: A method for resection of aortic arch aneurysms. Ann. Surg. 151:225, 1959
48. Murray GF, Young WG Jr: Thoracic aneurysmectomy utilizing direct left ventriculofemoral shunt (TDMAC-heparin) bypass. Ann. Thorac. Surg. 21:26, 1976
49. Nicks R: Aortic arch aneurysm: Resection and replacement: Protection of the nervous system. Thorax 27:239, 1972
50. Pearce CW, Weichert RF, del Real RE: Aneurysms of the aortic arch: Simplified technique for excision and prosthetic replacement. J. Thorac. Cardiovasc. Surg. 58:886, 1969
51. Pezzella TA, Todd EP, Dillon ML, et al: Early diagnosis and individualized treatment of blunt thoracic aortic trauma. Am. Surg. 44:699, November 1978
52. Stranahan A, Alley RD, Sewall WH, et al: Aortic arch resection and grafting for aneurysm employing an external shunt. J. Thorac. Surg. 29:54, 1955
53. Symbas PN, Shedeva JS: Penetrating wounds of the thoracic aorta. Ann. Surg. 171:441, 1970
54. Vasko JS, Raess DH, Williams TE Jr, et al: Nonpenetrating trauma to the thoracic aorta. Surgery 82:400, 1977
55. Verdant A: Technique simplifée de derivation en chirurgie de la crosse aortique. Union Med. Can. 105:941, 1976
56. Wakabayashi A, Nakamura Y, Woolley T, et al: Successful prolonged heparinless venoarterial bypass in sheep. J. Thorac. Cardiovasc. Surg. 71:648, 1976
57. Wechsler AS, Wolfe WG: Heparinless shunting during cross-clamping of the thoracic aorta (Editorial). Ann. Thorac. Surg. 23:497, 1977
58. Wheat MW Jr: Acute dissecting aneurysm of the aorta. Primary Cardiol. Clin. 1:31, 1978
59. White RJ, Donald DE: Selective hypothermic perfusion and circulatory arrest. Arch. Surg. 84:292, 1962
60. Wheat MW Jr, Harris PD, Malm JR, et al: Acute dissecting aneurysms of the aorta. J. Thorac. Cardiovasc. Surg. 58:344, 1969

61. Wheat MW Jr, Palmer RF: Dissecting aneurysms of the aorta, in Sabiston DC Jr, Spencer FC (eds): Gibbon's Surgery of the Chest (ed 3). Philadelphia, W. B. Saunders, 1976, p 913
62. Wheat MW Jr, Palmer RF, Bartley TD, et al: Treatment of dissecting aneurysms of the aorta without surgery. J. Thorac. Cardiovasc. Surg. 50:364, 1965

John M. Moran, M.D.

Traumatic Disruption of the Thoracic Aorta

The voluminous literature of recent years on the subject of disruption of the aorta due to blunt trauma attests to the fact that our highly mobile society produces vehicular accidents which, in turn produces this common and highly lethal syndrome. If diagnosed early and treated aggressively, the result may be significant salvage of otherwise healthy individuals. Blunt trauma to the aorta is seen wherever automobiles go; speeds of 55 miles per hour are more than sufficient to provide opportunities for rapid deceleration. Aortic disruption by knives and bullets is relatively rare (survivors, that is) – except during wartime – and is limited mainly to metropolitan areas. This chapter deals with the results of blunt trauma to the aorta and the considerable diagnostic and therapeutic challenges which it creates.

BACKGROUND

In the 16th century Vesalius first described blunt trauma as a cause of rupture of the aorta, but only in the past 25 years has this become a surgical entity. Widespread appreciation of the problem has been slow in developing. For instance, in his review of 72 autopsy cases in 1947, Strassman [26] was able to state "traumatic rupture of the aorta caused by blunt force injuries is considered to be a rare occurrence." It is of considerable epidemiologic interest that 51 of 72 autopsied cases were the result of automobile accidents and that more pedestrians were afflicted by this injury than drivers or passengers of cars. Currently the most common victims of this type of injury are drivers involved in high-speed accidents with abrupt deceleration by virtue of contact with the steering wheel, the passenger in the "death seat" (front right) colliding with the dashboard, or from landing on the ground after being thrown from the car. More recently in another pathological review, Greendyke [12] encountered 42 deaths from traumatic aortic rupture in 420 autopsies done for accidental death, an incidence of 10%. He found also that approximately one-sixth of all auto accident deaths were due to aortic rupture. Interestingly, in 151 passenger and driver fatalities, the incidence of aortic rupture was 27% among those ejected from the vehicle. Among 102 passengers not ejected from the automobile, the incidence of rupture was only 8.5%. Parmley and associates [20] in yet another autopsy study from the Walter Reed Army Hospital accumulated 296 cases of aortic injury produced by nonpenetrating trauma. In 38% of these cases the aortic rupture was combined with cardiac injury, and 21 (8%) cases had only partial tears of the aorta. At that time (1958), they were able to quote eight reported cases of successfully operated chronic traumatic aneurysms dating from 1953 and in this report added two more successful cases. From these reports it has been estimated that approximately 10% of patients will survive the initial rupture and reach the hospital, thus becoming candidates for surgical repair.

Among those patients reaching the hospital it has been estimated that approximately one-third will die within 6 hours, that two-thirds will die within 10 days, and that 90% will rupture the aorta within 10 weeks if not treated surgically; 5%-10% of patients with significant lacerations of one or more layers of the aorta escape initial diagnosis and develop chronic posttraumatic aneurysm which may or may not eventually come to light.

The concern of the surgeon therefore has become twofold: (1) the establishment of early diagnosis and (2) expeditious and appropriate operative management. The high incidence of multiple injuries in part explains the reason for a missed diagnosis and emergence into the chronic phase by some patients. Head injuries, multiple fractures, abdominal parenchymal, intestinal, and vascular injuries, flail chest, and lung contusion all may contribute to obfuscation of aortic tear, perhaps the most dangerous lesion of all.

Another pitfall that awaits the surgeon is the presence of multiple aortic lacerations. The great majority of lacerations are located in the so called "isthmus" of the aorta in proximity to the ligamentum arteriosum and just beyond the left subclavian artery. This area has been involved in 80%-90% of cases in the comprehensive series and 100% in some surgical reports.

MECHANISMS CAUSING AORTIC DISRUPTION

Because of all the types of blunt trauma and deceleration injury and because of the somewhat complex anatomy, the precise etiology of aortic tears remains to some extent a matter of conjecture. In general, however, there is some agreement that shear/stress at the aortic isthmus is a primary etiologic factor in most deceleration injuries. The descending thoracic aorta becomes a relatively fixed structure, being tethered to the chest wall by intercostal arteries, blanketed by the parietal pleura and dense connective tissue between the aorta and the preaortic fascia. In comparison, the ascending aorta, transverse arch, and great vessels are relatively mobile, so that differences in the rate of deceleration of these two regions of the aorta undoubtedly accounts for some aortic tears. Germane to this theory is the fact that with aortic disruption at the isthmus, intercostal arteries are virtually never torn. In addition, especially with compressive trauma, there is undoubtedly some torsion stress at the aortic isthmus brought about by displacement of the heart into the left chest and an acute bending phenomenon in the area of the isthmus. Again, with acute compression or with vertical deceleration, a "water-hammer" mechanism is the most likely cause for disruption of the aortic valve and for transverse laceration of the ascending aorta.

Oppenheim [18] and Zehnder [31] have gathered data to illustrate the tremendous pressure necessary to disrupt the aorta and have thus laid to rest the earlier theories that a sharply elevated blood pressure was responsible for aortic disruption in blunt trauma. They have found that a healthy aorta can withstand up to 2000 mm Hg pressure before rupturing. Some injuries of the ascending aorta may be attributed to direct compression with or without fracture of the sternum, usually by a sharp blow and enormous impact such as described in the case report of Charles et al. [5].

Regardless of the precise mechanism of the aortic disruption, the reason for any survival whatsoever after injury of such a large vessel is the containment of the blood flow by an intact adventitia supported by pleura and extravasated hematoma. The strongest of the three layers of the aorta is the adventitia, which figures strongly not only in the containment of disruption but also in any aortic repair. Circumferential transection of aortic intima and media is seen more often than partial transections; occasionally the distal intima and media may invaginate into the distal aorta, thus creating the hemodynamics of coarctation (Fig. 1).

Subclavian and/or innominate artery avulsion have been described in conjunction with aortic disruption. Fleming and Green [9] reported that in two of ten aortic disruptions at the isthmus in their acute series, innominate artery avulsion was also found. Similarly, Gunnlaugsson et al. [13] collected 17 cases of avulsion of the innominate artery due to blunt trauma, most often associated with a false aneursym. The mechanism for this is felt to be chest compression together with hyperextension of the cervical spine, thus fixing the innominate artery before compression displaces the heart to the left and caudad, producing sufficient shearing force to avulse the innominate artery.

DIAGNOSIS

Acute Aortic Disruption

Any patient reaching the emergency room with a history of blunt chest injury from an automobile must be considered to have an aortic disruption until reasonably proven otherwise. A very high index of suspicion and the willingness

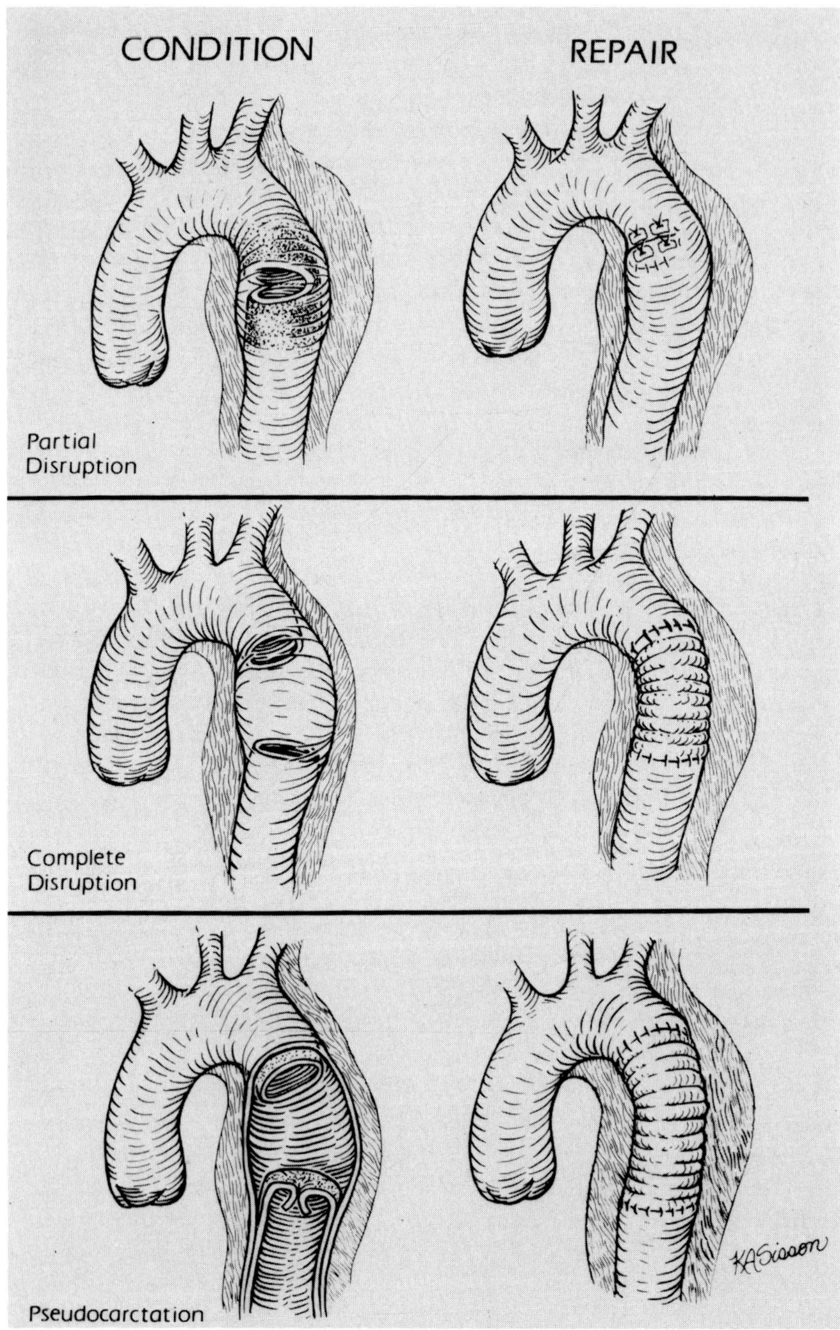

Fig. 1. Degrees of aortic disruption.

to obtain definitive diagnostic studies are the two attitudes which must be present in order to allow optimal salvage in these patients. The usual problem in early diagnosis is the associated injuries which may distract attention from the possibility of aortic rupture. The patient may be unconscious, in pain from extremity fractures, in shock from intraabdominal bleeding, and possibly in respiratory distress from flail chest and lung contusion. The high index of suspicion and the willingness to act definitively to obtain a diagnosis must be based on the awareness that an undetected aortic laceration may be fatal within minutes, hours, or days following admission to the emergency room.

The best screening test is the chest roentgenogram. Mediastinal widening, particularly if progressive on sequential films, subpleural displacement of the left lung from the apex by hematoma, deviation of the trachea to the right as well as deviation of a nasogastric tube to the right, loss of sharpness of the superior aortic contour, and downward displacement of the left bronchus are all signs which may be associated with aortic disruption. If some or all of these findings are present, an early decision must be made by the triage surgeon or the thoracic surgical consultant about the role of angiography in relation to treatment of the associated injuries. Other roentgenographic clues to the types of patients for whom angiography should be considered are those with multiple rib fractures with or without flail, those with sternal fracture, first rib fracture, displaced clavicular fractures, and those with massive hemothorax, particularly with signs of continued bleeding once the hemothorax has been evacuated. Also, patients with pulse deficits in any area, upper body hypertension relative to lower body pressures, or unexplained hypotension must be considered to have aortic rupture until proven otherwise.

Certain symptoms are associated with aortic disruption, but not infrequently patients are surprisingly lacking in symptoms, which, however, may simply be overshadowed by more painful injuries. Chest pain is usually present in conscious patients; in diminishing order of frequency dyspnea, back pain, dysphagia, and hoarseness may be found. The latter two complaints are usually due to tense hematoma about the esophagus and aortic arch, respectively.

Physical findings in addition to the pulse deficits and upper body hypertension mentioned above are a systolic murmur that may be audible over the neck, upper chest, and back, which is caused by turbulencc in the area of tear or occasionally the stenosis of pseudocoarctation due to invaginated intima distally. A few patients with aortic disruption will present with paraplegia. Symbas [28] has listed a triad of signs which he states has a high degree of association with aortic rupture. These are a widened mediastinum, increased blood pressure in the upper body, and decreased blood pressure in the lower body. This view suggests that hypertension associated with rupture at the isthmus is always due to a coarctation effect, but this appears not to be so. In 1951 Rice and Wittstruck [23] first reported the association of acute hypertension with thoracic aortic disruption. In 1965, Laforet [16] documented upper-extremity hypertension in a case of traumatic aortic rupture. He reexamined the previously reported series and encountered 15 instances of significant hypertension associated with this syndrome. He theorized that upper body hypertension was caused by the hematoma under pressure which compressed the false lumen of the rupture. However, Fox and associates [10] carefully reexamined this subject and noted that in the review by Symbas of 204 aortic ruptures, only 37% of the hypertensive patients had pressure differences between the upper and lower extremities. Turney and associates [29] have reviewed 31 consecutive patients having operation for aortic rupture at the University of Maryland and found insignificant pressure differences between upper and lower extremities in those patients that were hypertensive. Lioy and associates [17], working on cats, demonstrated that mechanical stretching of the thoracic aorta without interference to blood flow induces significant rises in arterial blood pressure, heart rate, and maximum rate of rise of ventricle pressure (dp/dt) in vagotomized cats. These responses could be abolished by lidocaine administrated to the aortic adventitia. There is no question that a pseudocoarctation syndrome may occasionally follow aortic disruption, but it is likely that the hypertension following such trauma in most cases is due to reflex phenomena and sympathetic discharge. Gray and Kirsch [11] recently described a new x-ray finding associated with aortic disruption. Separation of a calcified intima from the adventitia, as delineated on chest roentgenogram and confirmed by angiography and surgery, was a sign of aortic disruption at the isthmus.

Angiography remains the mainstay of definitive diagnosis in this condition. There are three important reasons for obtaining angiography [8]: (1) mediastinal hematoma of significant and often impressive degree can come from causes other than aortic disruption, mainly lacerations of small arteries and veins within the mediastinum, (2) there may be multiple tears from the aortic root on through the abdominal aorta, (3) there may often be injury to the great vessels, e.g., innominate artery avulsions, the documentation of which will allow a more reasoned approach by the surgeon.

Although retrograde brachial catheterization has some appeal, it is rarely done in this condition because of the ease of transfemoral angiography in patients who may often be unconscious or uncooperative. Abdominal angiography is thus simplified, and the catheter can be more safely threaded through a complete disruption from below with the use of a soft, J-shaped catheter. The radiologist must be aware of the potential catastrophic complication of excessive manipulation and forceful injection within the area of disruption, and small test injections of contrast material should be made to precede forceful injections of the usual large quantities of dye. Although rarely recorded, an occasional death in the x-ray suite has been caused by injection into the false lumen of a tenuously contained disruption.

Computerized axial tomography (CAT) may find a place in the diagnosis of traumatic aortic disruption. Although we have documented the precision of CAT scan diagnosis in other aortic conditions such as dissection, in which old and recent clot can be clearly distinguished from lumen, we have not yet used it in aortic trauma [24]. A definitive noninvasive study clearly has great appeal in this condition. It is not inconceivable that CAT scan, together with classical roentgenographic and physical findings, may allow contrast angiography to be eliminated in some cases.

It is important to perform careful neurologic evaluation before surgery in order to assess whether or not paraplegia is present so that a better postoperative evaluation can be made. In addition, the presence of paraplegia should be recognized as an indication for prompt operation. In a few instances paraplegia has been reversed with immediate intervention, e.g., the case report of DeMuth [7], who operated without angiography because of an immediate life-threatening situation which included the paraplegia. Repair of the aortic rupture was followed by complete recovery from the paraplegia.

Posttraumatic Aortic Aneurysm

The setting for the development of chronic aortic aneurysm due to disruption is usually the previously mentioned multiple injuries and chest x-ray findings which may have been absent or misinterpreted. Patients may become symptomatic at any stage following injury, often many years later. Alternatively, aortic calcification in the area of the isthmus, with or without obvious signs of descending thoracic aneurysm on the chest roentgenogram, may be found. Fleming and Green [9] have recently reviewed a series of 43 patients and divided them into two groups: an acute group comprised of those operated within the first 90 days following injury, and the chronic group subsequently operated after 90 days. This distinction was based on the previous review of surgery for chronic traumatic aneurysm by Bennett and Cherry [4]. In order to characterize the natural history of emergence of patients into the chronic group, Fleming and Green found that in the acute group, 50% of patients had hemothorax whereas only 12% developed hemothorax if they eventually proved to have chronic traumatic aneurysms. Similarly, 50% in the acute group had major abdominal injuries, whereas none in the chronic group were so afflicted. In the acute group, only 10% had evidence of significant chest wall contusion, whereas in the chronic group 33% had evidence of such contusion. Of 33 chronic patients, only one had been even suspected of aortic injury during the original hospital admission after trauma. Sixty-one percent of chronic aneurysms were found on incidental chest film; calcification of the wall is a common finding if the aneurysm is more than 10 years old. Immobilization of patients with skeletal trauma, who are subject to less frequent chest films of poorer quality, was the usual setting for nondiscovery of this important lesion. In their review of 105 cases of chronic traumatic aneurysm in the French and English literature from 1950 to 1965 from 48 series then in the literature, Bennett and Cherry found that 50% of patients developed symptoms and 21% showed x-ray enlargement as late signs of instability. Such instability was first manifested after 5 years in approximately 55 patients. This was similar to the experience of Fleming and Green, in which 40% of the patients who became unstable developed symptoms after 5 years. Bennett and Cherry noted aortic rupture as late as 27 years following the original injury. Fleming and Green found 13 patients from the English literature who were recorded as having ruptured aneurysms, 6 of them after the 5 year mark. In their review they concluded that the risk of rupture was about 6% in those diagnosed as having posttraumatic aneurysms.

OPERATIVE TREATMENT

The operative approach to aneurysms of the descending aorta in the early 1950s was a logical sequel to the earlier experience with patent ductus and coarctation surgery. The first posttraumatic aneurysm repair, performed in 1953 by Stranahan, Alley, and Sewell [25], was reported in 1955. Passaro and Pace [21] in 1959 reported the first surgical correction of acute aortic disruption, although the operation was actually performed by Klassen [31]. Since then the literature on this subject has expanded almost exponentially, so that diagnostic and therapeutic approaches to this problem have become somewhat standardized and the surgical results reasonably good.

In preparation of the patient for operation, once the diagnosis has been made, carefully individualized judgment must be utilized to place operation for aortic disruption within the context of other injuries. Due to mistaken priorities, fatal disruptions have occurred while rather routine intraabdominal injuries were attended surgically. Obviously, if a patient is exsanguinating from intra-abdominal trauma, repair of the aortic rupture must follow the abdominal exploration. On occasion, it is necessary to operate on a moribund patient in whom angiography is clearly not feasible and in whom there are certain diagnostic features compatible with rupture at the isthmus – e.g., hemothorax with continued bleeding, mediastinal widening, a pleural cap, loss of the left radial pulse, etc. We recently encountered an unusual situation in which surgery without angiography seemed justified.

Case 1. A 64-year-old man, involved in an automobile accident as the driver approximately 10 hours prior, was transferred from another hospital after a fracture of C1 and C2 had been documented, the so-called "hangman's fracture" (Fig. 2). Progressive widening of the upper mediastinum was noted on the chest films. The blood pressure in the left arm was 20 mm Hg lower than on the right, and there was a significant hematoma lowering the apex of the left lung (Fig. 3). The patient was placed in cervical traction by means of Crutchfield tongs. Because of time considerations and the difficulties in moving a patient with a broken neck to the angiographic suite and again to the operating room, it was considered appropriate to simply operate. Left thoracotomy revealed the diagno-

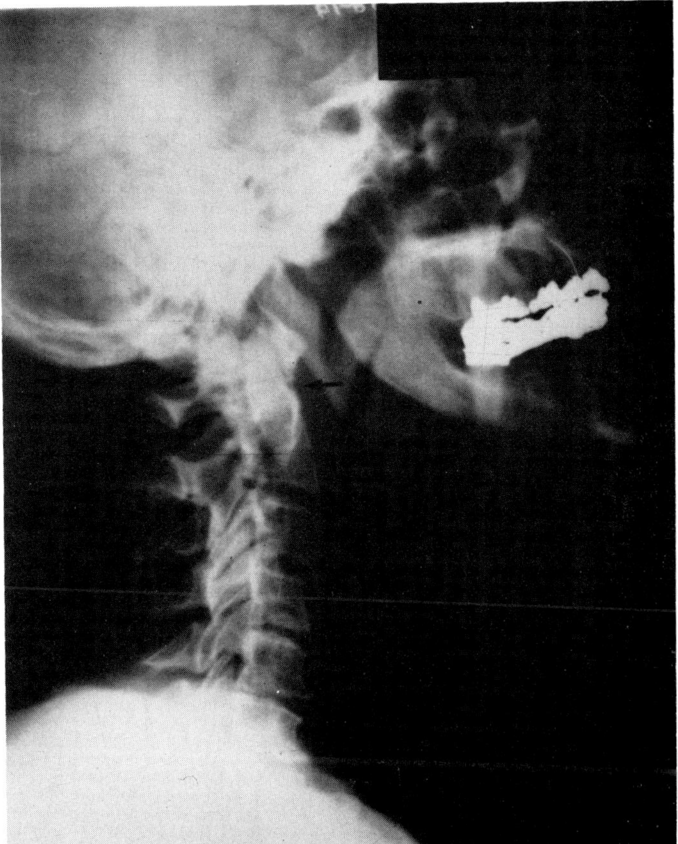

Fig. 2. Case 1. "Hangman's fracture" of C1-C2.

sis to be correct, and after proximal and distal control was achieved and the large hematoma entered, a partial transection of about 75% of the lumen circumference was documented. Secure primary repair was achieved without bypass or shunt during a 24 min period of clamping. Subsequently, the patient did well but unfortunately died 2 weeks later while straining at stool, presumably from a pulmonary embolus. Resuscitation was delayed by the halo and minerva plaster jacket which was used for stabilization of the vertebrae fractures. Permission for autopsy was denied.

An example of successful immediate surgery without angiography in a moribund patient serves to make the point that dogmatism regarding angiographic diagnosis is inappropriate [27].

Case 2. A 34-year-old female victim of an automobile accident presented in hemorrhagic shock, unresponsive to volume replacement, with a grossly widened mediastinum and a distended abdomen. She was transferred immediately to the operating room, where femorofemoral bypass was begun and left thoracotomy

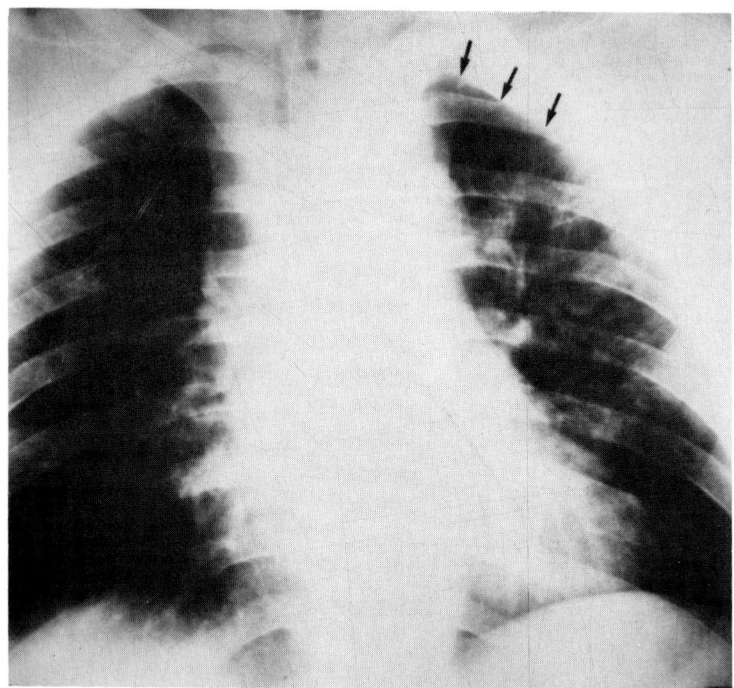

Fig. 3. Case 1. Mediastinal widening, left pleural cap.

performed. Blood was evacuated from the chest; extensive subpleural periaortic hematoma was documented, but there was no further bleeding. The incision was extended across the costal margin into the abdomen, a ruptured spleen was removed, and a laceration of the liver was repaired. Dacron graft interposition was carried out for a typical complete disruption of the aortic isthmus. The patient was discharged 3 weeks later.

The following illustrates a typical "textbook" case of aortic rupture.

Case 3. A 28-year-old driver and single occupant of an automobile had his vehicle struck head-on by another car which crossed the median strip of a divided highway. Upon arrival in the emergency room he was hemodynamically stable without hypertension or pulse deficit, and the only pertinent physical findings were unimpressive bruises of the anterior chest wall and multiple facial lacerations. The chest film revealed mediastinal widening, taking into consideration the portable nature of the film (Fig. 4). There were no limb or apparent intraabdominal injuries. Immediate transfemoral angiography was performed, revealing aortic disruption at the isthmus, with intact arch and great vessels. The patient was transferred directly to the operating room where simultaneous institution of femorofemoral bypass and left thoracotomy were carried out. Abundant subpleural hematoma surrounded the upper descending aorta. It was entered after proximal and distal control were achieved. Complete transection of

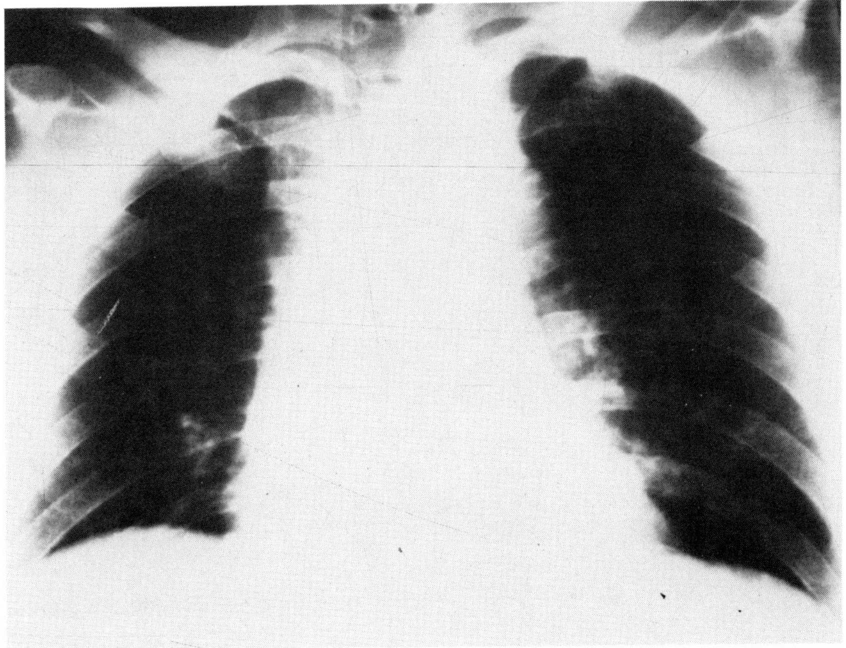

Fig. 4. Case 3. Mediastinal widening, portable film.

the media and intima were found, with intact adventitia. A short woven Dacron graft was interposed, the patient was removed from bypass, and the procedure terminated. He was discharged 10 days later.

During the time between hospital admission and surgery, if the patient is hypertensive, it is clearly desirable to maintain blood pressure control by means of intravenous alpha adrenergic blocking agents or intravenous nitroprusside or nitroglycerine. The experience with a pharmacologic therapy of aortic dissections is entirely germane to the false aneurysm caused by trauma as originally pointed out by Aronstam et al. [3]. This method is currently not widely used, but clearly seems appropriate when hypertension is documented, and probably should be used in most cases, if hemodynamically stable, to keep the systolic blood pressure around 100 mm Hg at most. Although difficult to document, it is likely that some patients who exsanguinate while being prepared for surgery or during angiography, especially with uncontrolled hypertension, might conceivably have been salvaged with pharmacologic control of the blood pressure.

In the rare instance in which disruption of the ascending aorta is documented by angiography, preparation for cardiopulmonary bypass and a midsternotomy approach should be made. Femoral cannulation for the institution of early bypass is entirely appropriate in this setting, and will provide a significant degree of protection and blood salvage during the early phases of operation. Since survival in this situation is extremely rare, there is very little

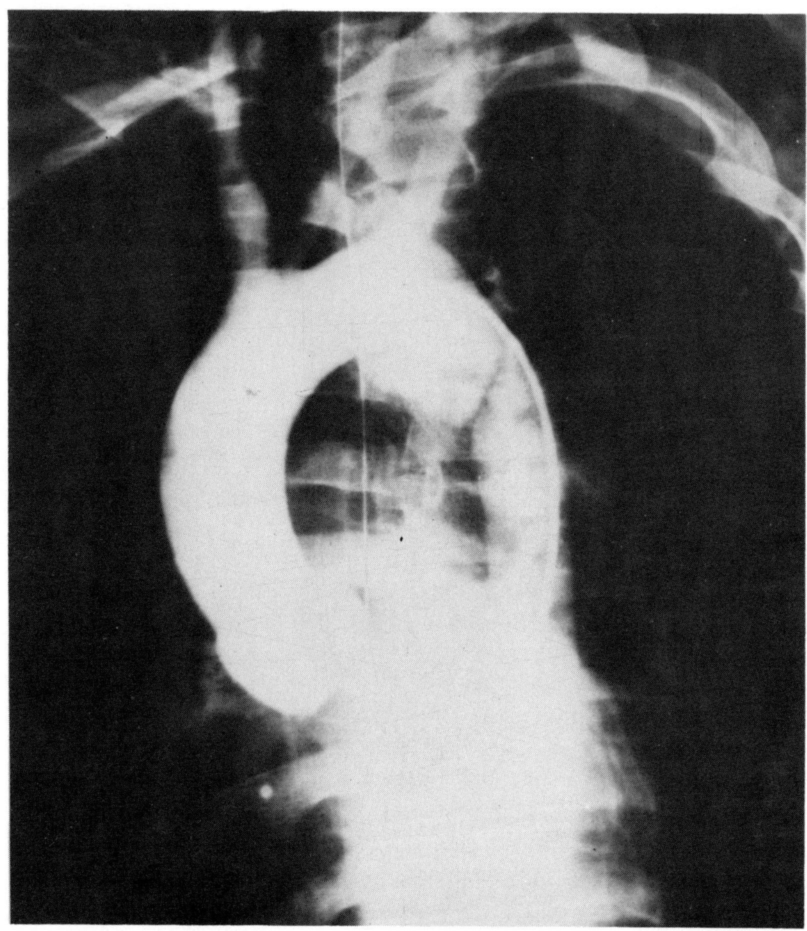

Fig. 5. Aortic disruption at isthmus. Ascending aorta, transverse arch, and great vessels intact.

reported experience with the alternatives of direct repair versus graft interposition. In two cases, Kirsh and Sloan [15] have successfully repaired the ascending aortic tear by direct end to end anastomosis.

When angiography demonstrates the usual disruption at the isthmus, the patient is prepared for left posterolateral thoracotomy through the fourth or fifth interspace. Positioning should allow for femoral cannulation by keeping the left leg straight and the patient laid back slightly to allow easy access to the groin. The initial surgical maneuver, assuming time permits, is to obtain proximal and distal control of the aorta prior to incising the pleura over the hematoma. Proximal control can be gained distal to the left subclavian artery or proximally depending on the extent of the hematoma. Opening the pericardium is advocated by some as a means to safely obtain control proximal to the left subclavian artery. Perhaps a more important reason for opening the pericardium is to assess the possibility of hemorrhage from intrapericardial injury which has occasionally been described.

Primary surgical repair without graft interposition is sometimes appropriate, usually in the setting of an incomplete aortic tear. Even with complete transection of intima and media with some retraction, primary repair has been utilized on occasion for both acute and chronic aneurysms. The great majority of surgeons, however, prefer graft interposition to avoid the mobilization of the aorta necessary for a primary repair.

Until recently it was considered mandatory by nearly all authors that some form of lower body perfusion and upper body decompression be used during aortic cross-clamping for graft interposition. In recent years, stimulated by the report of Crawford et al. [6] a number of authors have, on the basis of considerable experience, advocated simple cross-clamping and repair without any form of bypass or shunt. Sufficient evidence currently exists to suggest that the occasional case of paraplegia attending surgery for this condition is caused by factors other than the presence or absence of lower body perfusion during aortic clamping. By avoiding heparinization attendant to the various forms of bypass, except for tube shunts, hemorrhagic lung, a formidable and occasionally lethal complication, as well as other organ hemorrhage, can thus be avoided. In addition, the operation is invariably more expeditious, better tolerated and associated with less blood loss. At the present time, it is probably advisable for the highly expert and well trained surgical teams to avoid bypass methods if a primary repair or graft interposition can be accomplished within half an hour or so. If more time is necessary, the safer of the bypass methods would appear to be a tube shunt with the use of minimal or no heparinization. Finally, the Carlens tube is a valuable adjunct to surgery for this condition because minimal lung retraction is required, and the incidence of hemorrhagic lung complications is thus greatly reduced.

Today, most patients who can reach the operating room with traumatic aortic disruption should survive. In the reporting of results of operation for acute disruption of the aorta there is a surprising uniformity from the larger series. In the largest series, that of Kirsch et al. [14], in which 43 patients with acute rupture were treated, the overall survival was 70%. The attrition is also quite typical, with five patients dying prior to surgery either in the emergency room, the radiology department, or while waiting for angiography. Six patients with severe abdominal trauma underwent exploration prior to thoracotomy, and five of these six patients died from the aortic rupture. Survival of patients actually undergoing surgery was 76%. The overall survival from other primary treatment centers such as that reported by Allmendinger et al. [1] was 68%, Reul et al. [22], and O'Sullivan et al. 75% [19].

On the other hand, reports emanating from referral centers indicate some degree of selection process. For instance, the report of Fleming and Green records 9 out of 10 survivals in acute rupture and 30 of 33 survivors in chronic aneurysm or 91%. In 25 cases, Appelbaum et al. [2] recorded an 89% success rate for acute rupture and 92% survival in chronic aneurysm surgery. Thus at the present time it appears that 10%-20% of victims of decelerating trauma will reach the hospital alive. About 20% of these will succumb for one reason or another prior to thoracotomy, and the mortality rate from this point on varies from 5% to 10%. For patients who, by the selection process, develop chronic thoracic aortic aneurysms due to trauma, the mortality rate of surgery is 8%-10%. This figure must be kept in mind when one is recommending surgery for chronic aneurysm. In the thorough review of Fleming and Green, only 13 patients in the English literature could be found who ruptured a chronic aneurysm, and from the available literature the risk of rupture appeared to be about 6%. There is little question that a patient who demonstrates enlargement of a posttraumatic aneurysm or one which has clearly become symptomatic should be offered surgery. But for the patient whose small, perhaps calcified aneurysm has been discovered incidentally, if he is truly asymptomatic, careful observation is a reasonable alternative to operation.

REFERENCES

1. Allmendinger P, Low HBC, Takata H, et al: Deceleration injury: Laceration of the thoracic aorta. Am. J. Surg. 133:490-491, 1977
2. Appelbaum A, Karp RB, Kirklin JW: Surgical treatment for closed aortic injuries. J. Thorac. Cardiovasc. Surg. 71:458, 1976
3. Aronstam EM, Gomez AC, O'Connell TJ Jr, et al: Recent surgical and pharmacologic experience with dissecting and traumatic aneurysm. J. Thorac. Cardiovasc. Surg. 59:231, 1970
4. Bennett DE, Cherry JK: The natural history of traumatic aneurysms of the aorta. Surgery 61:516, 1967
5. Charles KP, Davidson KG, Miller H, et al: Traumatic rupture of the ascending aorta and aortic valve following blunt chest trauma. J. Thorac. Cardiovasc. Surg. 73:208, 1977
6. Crawford KS, Rubio PA: Reappraisal of adjuncts to avoid ischemia in the treatment of aneurysms of the descending thoracic aorta. J. Thorac. Cardiovasc. Surg. 66:693, 1973
7. DeMuth WE Jr, Roe H, Hobbie W: Immediate repair of traumatic rupture of thoracic aorta. Arch. Surg. 91:602, 1965
8. Fishbone G, Robbins DI, Osborn DJ, et al: Trauma to the thoracic aorta and great vessels. Radiol. Clin. North Am. 11:543-554, 1973
9. Fleming AW, Green DC: Traumatic aneurysms of the thoracic aorta: Report of 43 patients. Ann. Thorac. Surg. 18:91-101, 1974
10. Fox S, Pierce WS, Waldhausen JA: Acute hypertension: Its significance in traumatic aortic rupture. J. Thorac. Cardiovasc. Surg. 77:622, 1979

11. Gray L, Kirsch M: A new roentgenographic finding in acute traumatic rupture of the aorta. J. Thorac. Cardiovasc. Surg. 70:86, 1975
12. Greendyke RM: Traumatic rupture of aorta: Special reference to automobile accidents. JAMA 195:527, 1966
13. Gunnlaugsson GH, Hallgrimsson JG, Sigurdsson HL, et al: Complete traumatic avulsion of the innominate artery from the aortic arch with a unique mechanism of injury. J. Thorac. Cardiovasc. Surg. 66:235, 1973
14. Kirsh MM, Behrendt DM, Orringer MD, et al: The treatment of acute traumatic rupture of the aorta. Ann. Surg. 184:308-316, 1976
15. Kirsh MM, Sloan J: Blunt Chest Trauma: General Principles of Management. Boston, Little, Brown, 1977
16. Laforet EG: Acute hypertension as a diagnostic clue in traumatic rupture of the thoracic aorta. Am. J. Surg. 110:948, 1965
17. Lioy F, Malliani A, Fagani M, et al: Reflex hemodynamic responses initiated from the thoracic aorta. Circ. Res. 34:78-84, 1974
18. Oppenheim F: Gibt es eine spontanruptur der gesunden aorta und wie kommt sie zustande? Munch. Med. Wochenschr. 65:1234, 1918
19. O'Sullivan MJ Jr, Folkerth TL, Morgan JR, et al: Post-traumatic thoracic aortic aneurysm. Recognition and treatment. Arch. Surg. 105:14, 1972
20. Parmley LF, Mattingly TW, Manion WC, et al: Nonpenetrating traumatic injury of the aorta. Circulation 17:1086, 1958
21. Passaro E Jr, Pace WG: Traumatic rupture of the aorta. Surgery 46:787, 1959
22. Reul GA, Rubio PA, Beal AC: The surgical management of acute injury to the thoracic aorta. J. Thorac. Cardiovasc. Surg. 67:272-281, 1974
23. Rice WG, Wittstruck KP: Acute hypertension and delayed traumatic rupture of the aorta. JAMA 147:915, 1951
24. Sanders JH Jr, Neiman HL, Malave S, et al: The use of computerized axial tomography in the diagnosis of surgical diseases of the thoracic aorta. Proc. Inst. Med. Chicago 32:133, 1979
25. Stranahan A, Alley RD, Sewell WH, et al: Aortic arch resection and grafting for aneurysm employing an external shunt. J. Thorac. Surg. 24:325, 1952
26. Strassman G: Traumatic rupture of the aorta. Am. Heart J. 33:508, 1947
27. Sullivan HJ: Personal communication
28. Symbas PN, Tyras DH, Ware RE, et al: Rupture of the aorta. A diagnostic triad. Ann. Thorac. Surg. 15:405, 1973
29. Turney SZ, Attar S, Ayella R, et al: Traumatic rupture of the aorta. A five-year experience. J. Thorac. Cardiovasc. Surg. 72:727-734, 1973
30. Vasco JS, Raess DH, Williams TE: Non-penetrating trauma to the thoracic aorta. Surgery 82:400-406, 1977
31. Zehnder MA: Delayed post traumatic rupture of the aorta in a young healthy individual after closed chest injury: Mechanical etiological consideration. Angiology 7:252-267, 1956

E. Stanley Crawford, M.D.
Gwen C. Cho, M.D.
John O. F. Roehm, Jr., M.D.

Thoracoabdominal and Abdominal Aortic Aneurysms Involving Celiac Axis, Superior Mesenteric, and Renal Arteries

Extensive aneurysms involving both the thoracic and abdominal aorta or the abdominal aorta from which the visceral arteries arise, like aneurysms located elsewhere, eventually rupture and cause death. Death from rupture has occurred in our experience from 3 to 18 months in all patients referred to us in whom operation was not advised because of risks associated with advanced cardiopulmonary and other disease. Death has also occurred in 5 patients being transferred from other institutions for operation. Death occurred suddenly in 2 patients in the hospital awaiting operation. More unfortunately, death has occurred from rupture of suprarenal aneurysmal segments left in patients in whom larger infrarenal aneurysms were removed. Finally, a significant number of patients successfully treated presented with rupture and hemorrhage, some of whom had been treated elsewhere by wrapping or ligation and bypass. Consequent to these experiences, we conclude that this is a most serious form of disease and that the only effective method of treatment is graft replacement, so well established in the treatment of similar lesions in other locations.

The application of this form of therapy, however, presents the most difficult challenge in the field of arterial and aortic reconstruction owing to the difficulties of exposure, the control of blood loss both during and after operation, the problems of aortic and arterial reconstruction needed for permanent restoration of circulation, the occurrence of paraplegia, and the preservation of multiple organ function – including the heart – during aortic clamping and the kidneys after operation.

A number of operations have been successfully employed in the treatment of these lesions. The first devised was excision and graft replacement with reattachment of visceral arteries either directly to the side of the aortic graft or to branches arising from the aortic graft [6-8]. Temporary shunts and/or hypothermia were used in most of these cases, for it was thought that organ damage would occur during the period of aortic clamping. The second method of treatment was insertion of permanent bypass graft with attachment of visceral arteries to ends of side-arm grafts attached to the aortic graft, attached in sequence starting with the left renal artery to minimize the period of renal ischemia [5]. With the grafts in place and functioning, the aneurysm was either removed, embricated upon itself, or partially wrapped around the graft. We have preferred the graft inclusion technique with reattachment of visceral vessel origin to openings made in the graft [1, 3, 9]. This method requires less dissection and reduces the need for branch grafts with their tendency to kink and obstruct and their association with suture line bleeding. The aneurysmal wall is tightly sutured around the graft at the end of operation. This step both tamponades the entire region of aortic reconstruction and separates the graft from adjacent structures, eliminating the possibility of hemorrhage and erosion into adjacent abdominal and thoracic viscera. The method lends itself to a more rapid operation, obviating the need for shunts, and it is associated with less intraoperative and postoperative blood loss, the most frequent fatal complication associated with the other methods of reconstruction. Consequent to these advantages, the present survival rate, both immediate and long-term, compares favorably with that following treatment of aneurysms located elsewhere; thus reconstruction should be considered in all of these cases. This report is concerned with our experience in the treatment of 108 patients employing the technique during the past 19 years.

CLINICAL MATERIAL

There were 90 males and 18 females in the series whose ages ranged from 23 to 83 years, with the majority being over 60 years of age. The disease was due to arteriosclerosis in most but dissection and cystic medial necrosis were common, the latter being present in the younger patients. The etiology was trauma in 1, syphilis in 2, and infection in 1 patient. The typical Marfan's syndrome was present in 7 patients, all of whom had extensive lesions, dissection in 5, and cystic medial necrosis in 2.

EXTENT OF DISEASE

The extent of aneurysm was variable, ranging from relatively short segments of aorta to total involvement, and for simplicity may be divided into 6 groups depending upon location, extent, and visceral vessel involvement (Table 1). In

Table 1
Results of Treatment of Thoracoabdominal and Abdominal Aortic Aneurysms Involving Celiac, Superior Mesenteric, and Renal Arteries Classified According to Extent of Disease

Group	Involvement	No. Cases	Paraplegia	Survival
I	Thoracic and abdominal aorta without vessels	13	1	12
II	Entire aorta	1	0	0
III	Most descending thoracic and abdominal aorta with vessels	33	8	29
IV	Distal thoracic and abdominal aorta with vessels	24	1	21
V	Abdominal aorta with vessels	22	0	20
VI	Abdominal aorta with renal arteries	15	0	15
	Total	108	10	97

group I were 13 patients in whom the aneurysm extended from the left subclavian artery in the chest down into the abdomen opposite the celiac axis. There was one patient in group II in whom the aneurysm extended from the proximal ascending aorta to the bifurcation of the abdominal aorta. In group III, there were 33 patients in whom the aneurysm involved most of the descending thoracic aorta and most of the abdominal aorta (Figs. 1-3). In group IV, there were 24 patients with involvement of the distal thoracic and most abdominal aorta (Figs. 4 and 5). There were 22 patients in whom the aneurysm involved the entire abdominal aorta (group V), and in 15 (group VI) the aneurysm was primarily infrarenal but involved the aorta up to the origin of the superior mesenteric artery (Figs. 6 and 7). The aneurysms in these cases frequently extended out into the renal arteries. Associated aneurysm either of the descending thoracic aorta or infrarenal abdominal aorta was frequent in patients with the more limited involvement (Fig. 6). In fact, such lesions had been removed previously in a number of cases.

CLINICAL MANIFESTATIONS

All patients in this series were symptomatic. Chest, abdominal, and back pain were frequent. Hoarseness from left recurrent laryngeal nerve paralysis was present in 15% of cases. Most patients had history of enlarging aneurysm. Bone erosion was present in a large number of cases. Rupture into pleural or abdominal cavities, mediastinum, retroperitoneum, or duodenum had occurred

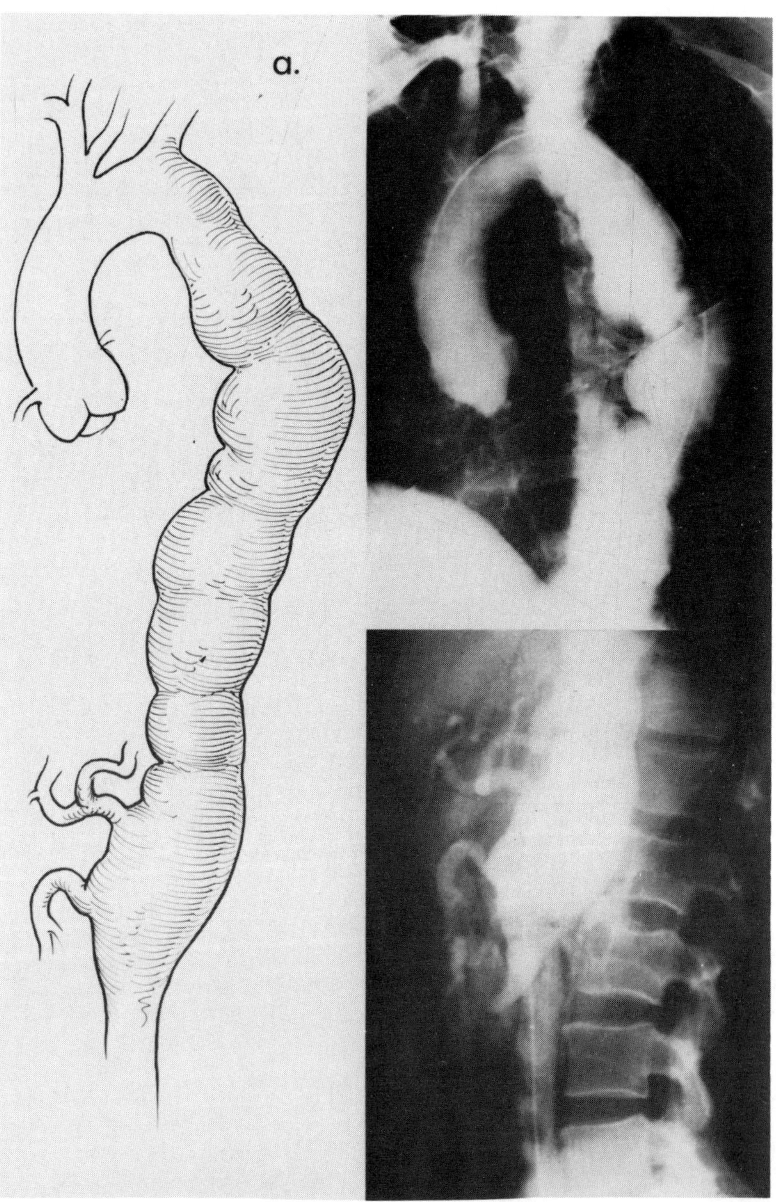

Fig. 1. Treatment in patient with extensive thoracoabdominal aortic aneurysm. (A) Diagram and aortogram made before operation showing location and extent of aneurysm. (B, C) Diagram and aortogram made after operation showing inclusion graft with reattached intercostal and visceral arteries. [From Crawford ES, Snyder DM, Cho GC, et al: Progress in treatment of thoracoabdominal and abdominal aortic aneurysms involving celiac, superior mesenteric, and renal

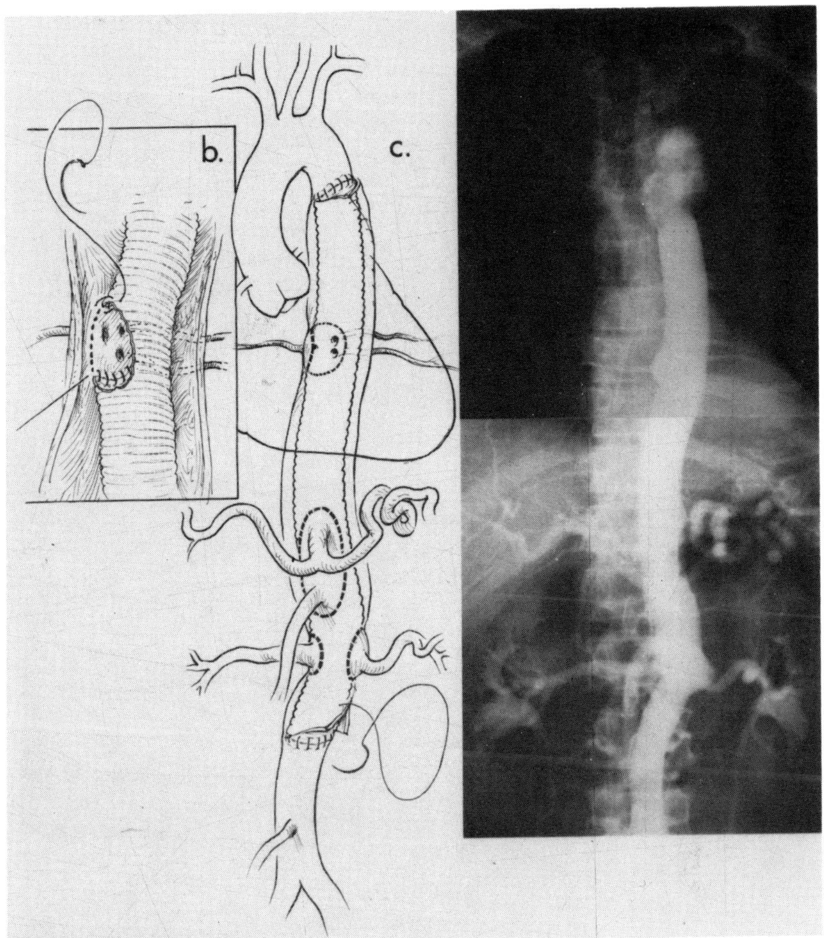

arteries. Ann. Surg. 188:404-422, 1978. Reproduced by permission of the J. B. Lippincott Company.]

in 15 patients. Associated occlusive disease of the mesenteric, renal, and iliac arteries was common, being present in 17% of cases (Fig. 2 and 4). Two patients had been on chronic hemodialysis for over 1 year. A large horseshoe kidney was present in 1 patient, and a kidney had been removed previously in 6 patients (Fig. 5). Some form of heart disease was present in 25%, hypertension in 18%, and chronic fibrotic obstructive pulmonary disease in 22%. Gallstones were present in 5 and peptic ulcers in 8 patients. Previous aortic exploration or some type of reconstruction or reinforcement had been performed in 17 patients. Coronary artery bypass operations had been performed previously in 5 patients, and 2 had had aortic valve replacement. One patient had had a laryngectomy, 1 a lobectomy, 2 had previous leg amputations, 1 was partially paraplegic, and 1 was

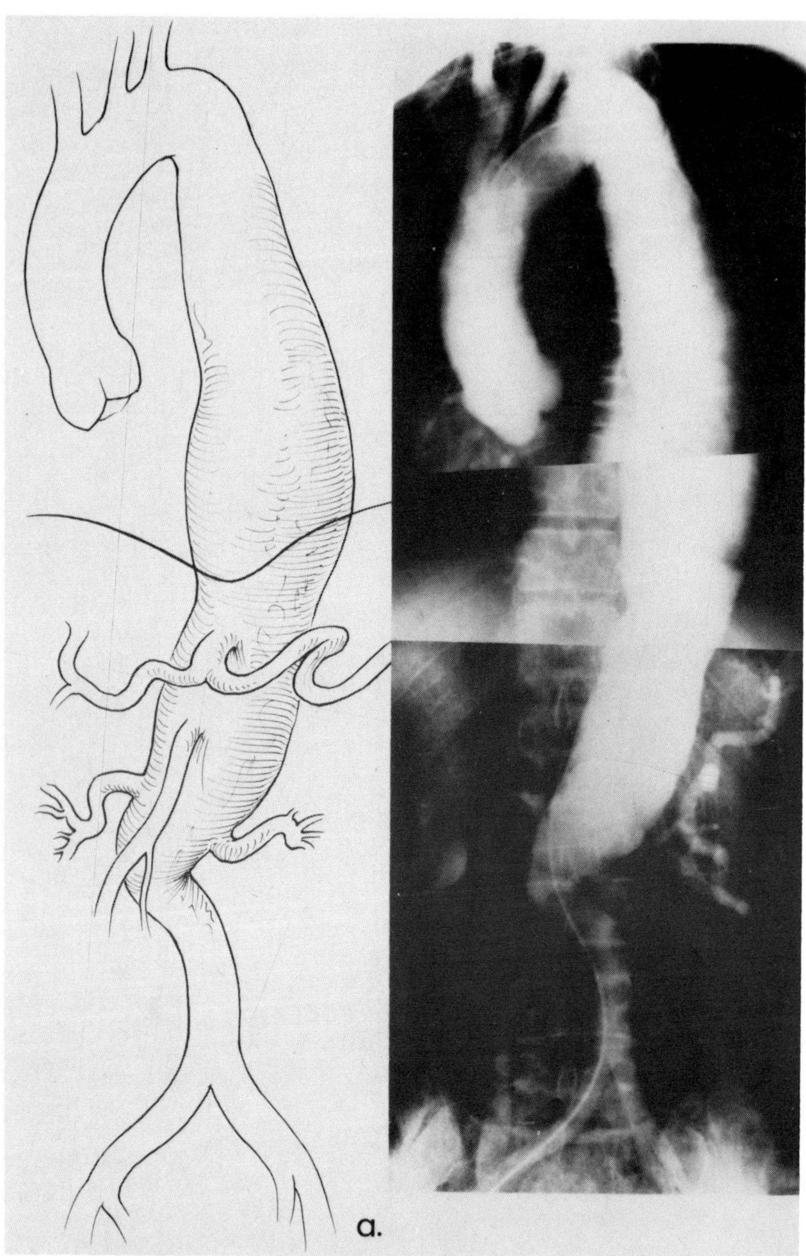

Fig. 2. Illustrations of patient with extensive thoracoabdominal aortic aneurysm involving most of the descending thoracic aorta and the abdominal aorta showing method of reconstruction. (A) Diagram and aortogram before operation showing extent of disease. (B) Diagram and aortogram made after operation showing method of reconstruction including intercostal reattachment and reattachment of superior mesenteric and right renal artery by direct suture and

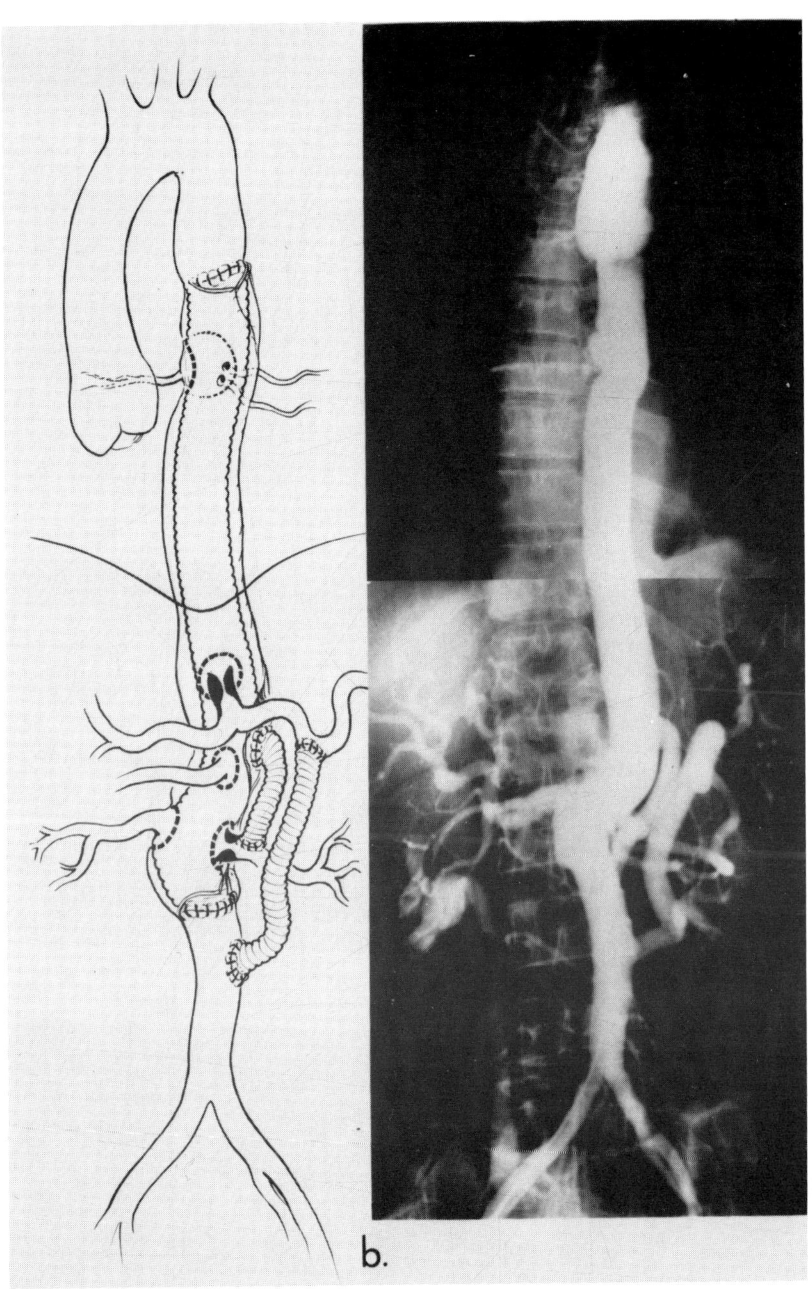

celiac axis and left renal artery reconstruction by graft for associated occlusive disease. [From Crawford ES, Snyder DM, Cho GC, et al: Progress in treatment of thoracoabdominal and abdominal aortic aneurysms involving celiac, superior mesenteric, and renal arteries. Ann. Surg. 188:404-422, 1978. Reproduced by permission of the J. B. Lippincott Company.]

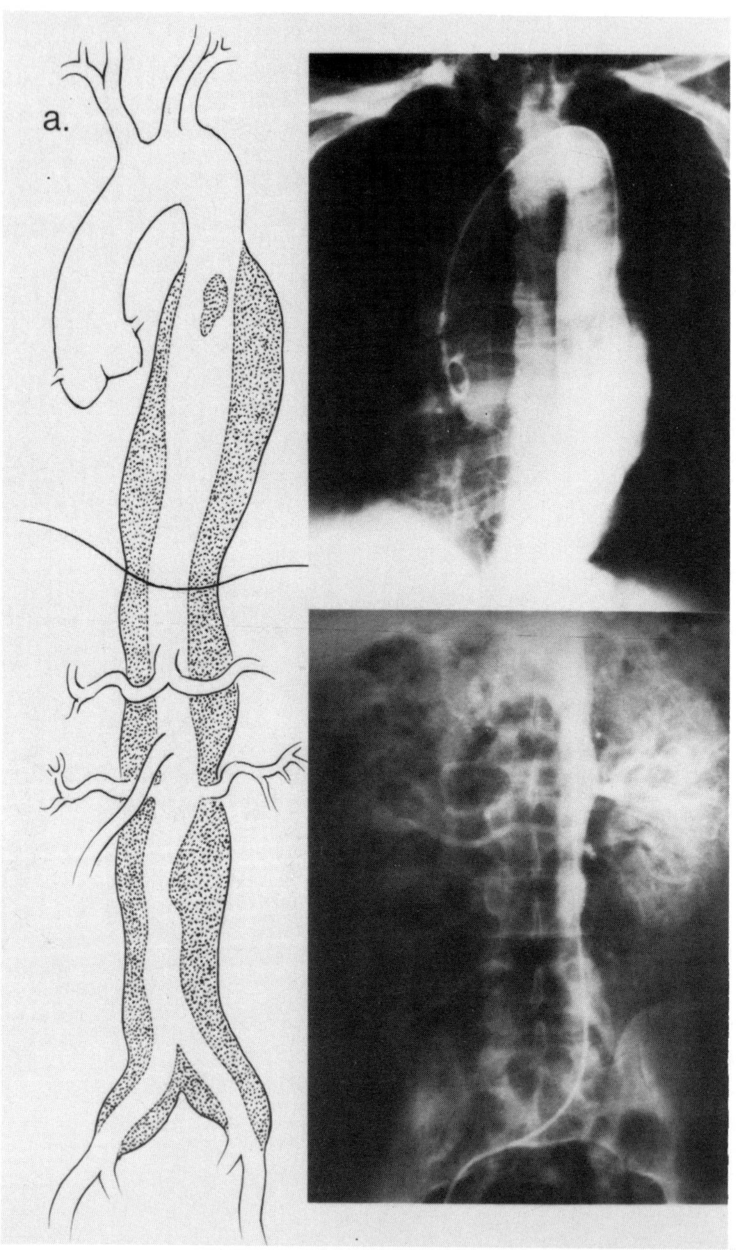

Fig. 3. Illustrations of treatment of patient with chronic dissecting aortic aneurysm diffusely involving the descending thoracic and abdominal aorta. (A) Diagram and aortogram made before operation showing extent of disease. (B) Method of aneurysmal replacement preserving intercostal blood flow and re-

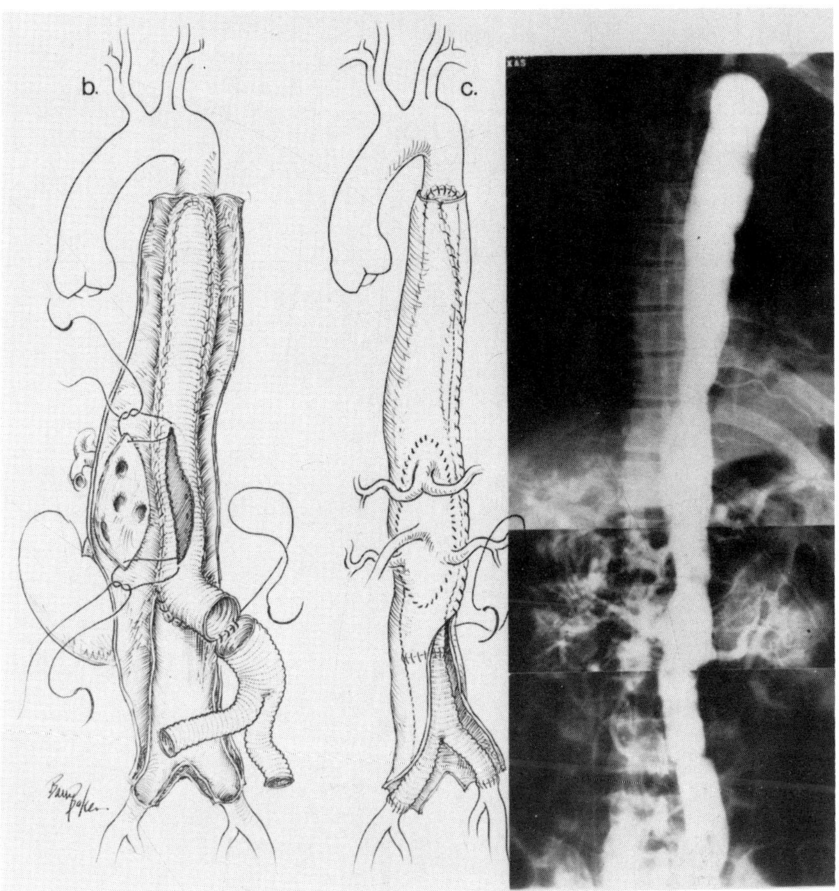

attachment of visceral arteries. (C) Diagram and aortogram made after operation showing reconstruction.

totally deaf. All patients with Marfan's syndrome had deformed sternums and rib cages. Obesity was common except in those with Marfan's syndrome and those over 65 years of age.

TECHNIQUE OF OPERATION

Groups I-V are best exposed through a left thoracoabdominal incision with the patient lying at about 45° on the right side. The abdominal component of the incision may be oblique or midline depending upon the extent of abdominal involvement. Midline incisions provide more exposure for extensive lesions. The abdominal incision is extended across the costal arch posteriolaterally into the

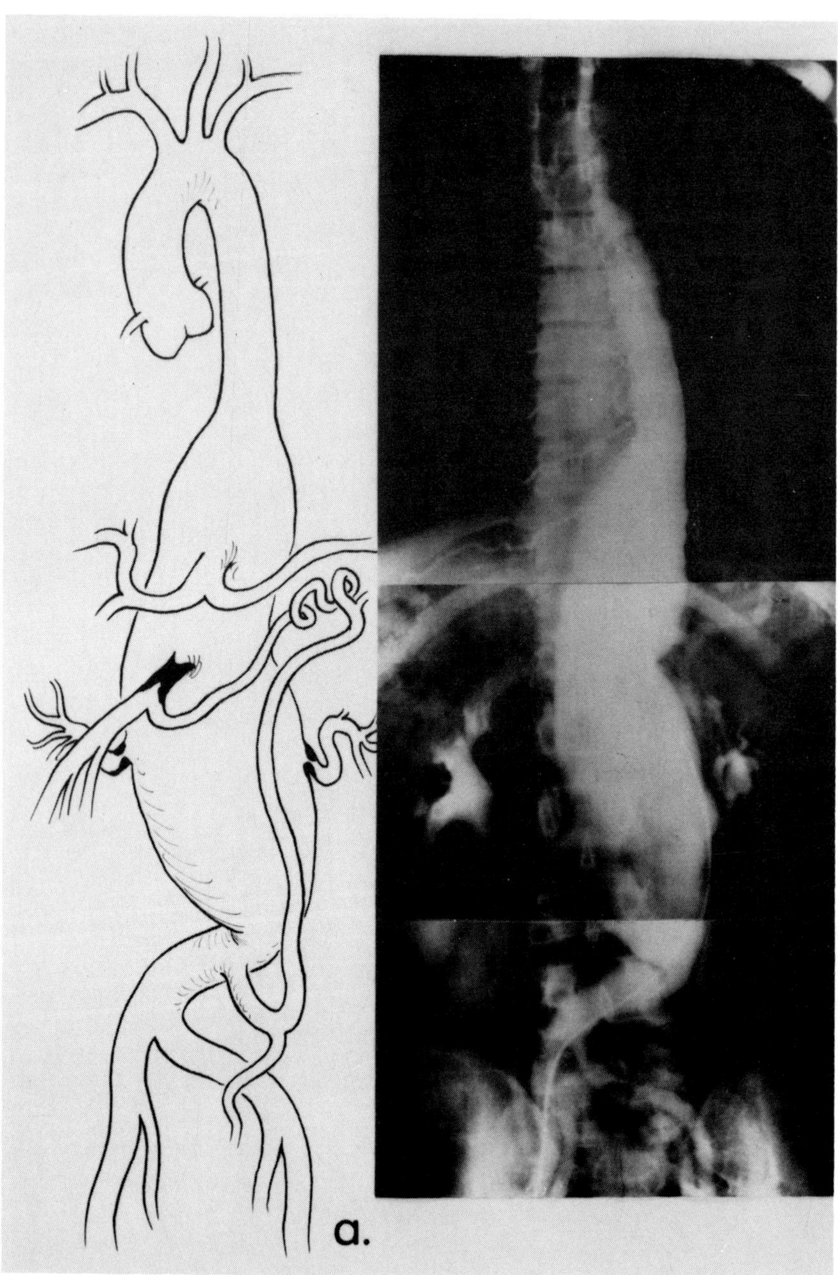

Fig. 4. Illustrations of patient with thoracoabdominal aortic aneurysm with bilateral renal artery occlusion and complete obstruction of the superior mesenteric artery with good collateral circulation and no gastrointestinal symptoms showing treatment by graft inclusion, bilateral renal artery endarterectomy, and preservation of superior mesenteric artery collateral circulation. (A) Diagram and

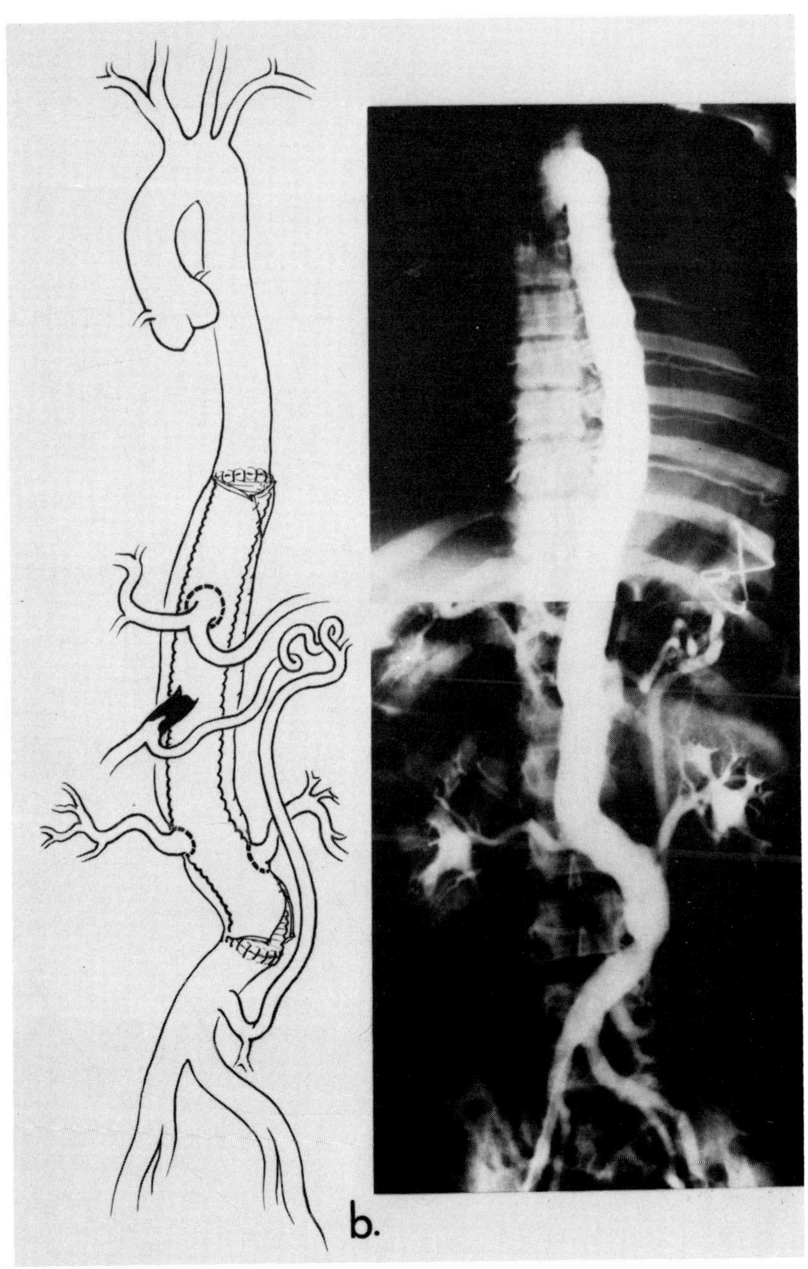

aortogram showing extent of aneurysm and location of obstruction. (B) Diagram and aortogram after operation showing inclusion graft and vessel reattachment with patent renal arteries. [From Crawford ES, Snyder DM, Cho GC, et al: Progress in treatment of thoracoabdominal and abdominal aortic aneurysms involving celiac, superior mesenteric, and renal arteries. Ann. Surg. 188:404-422, 1978. Reproduced by permission of the J. B. Lippincott Company.]

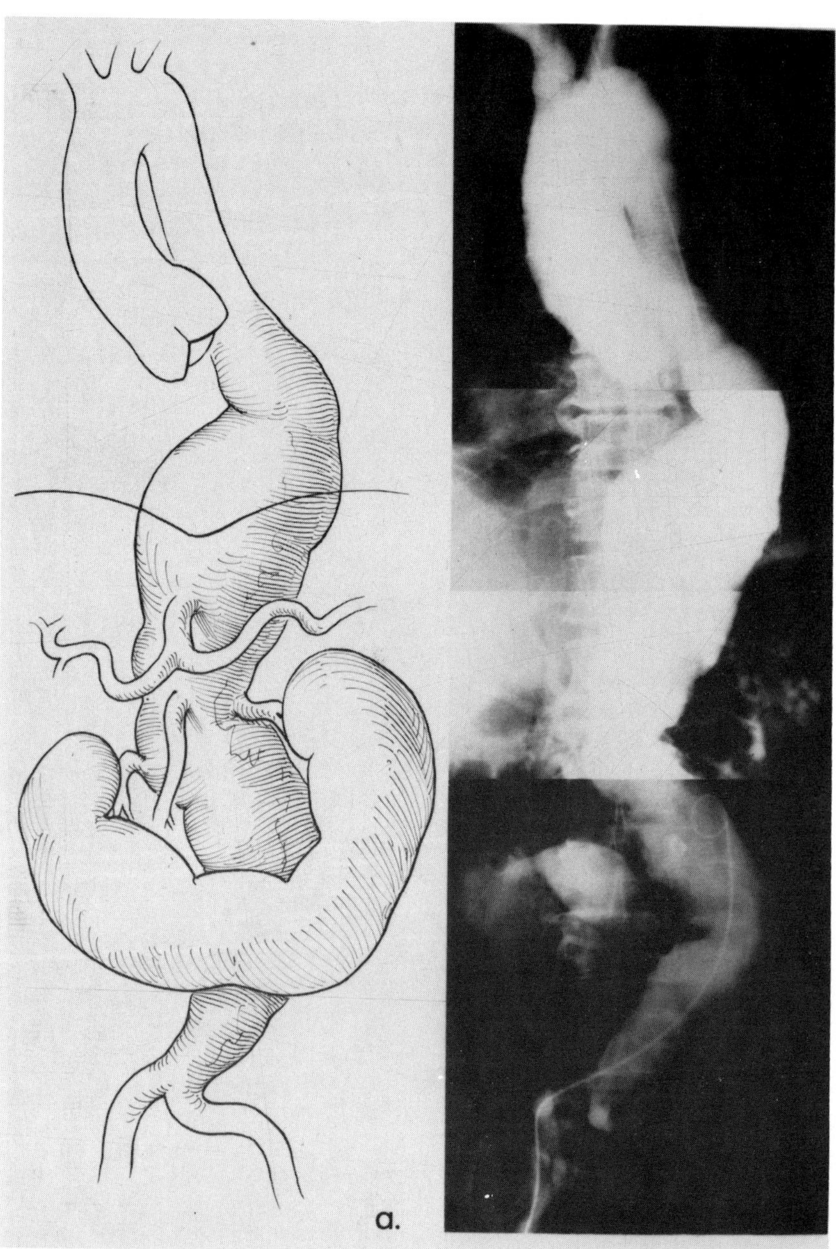

Fig. 5. Illustrations of patient with ruptured thoracoabdominal aortic aneurysm and horseshoe kidney. (A) Diagram and aortogram showing extent of aneurysm and location of abnormal kidney. (B) Diagram and aortogram showing vascular reconstruction in this case. [From Crawford ES, Snyder DM, Cho GC, et al:

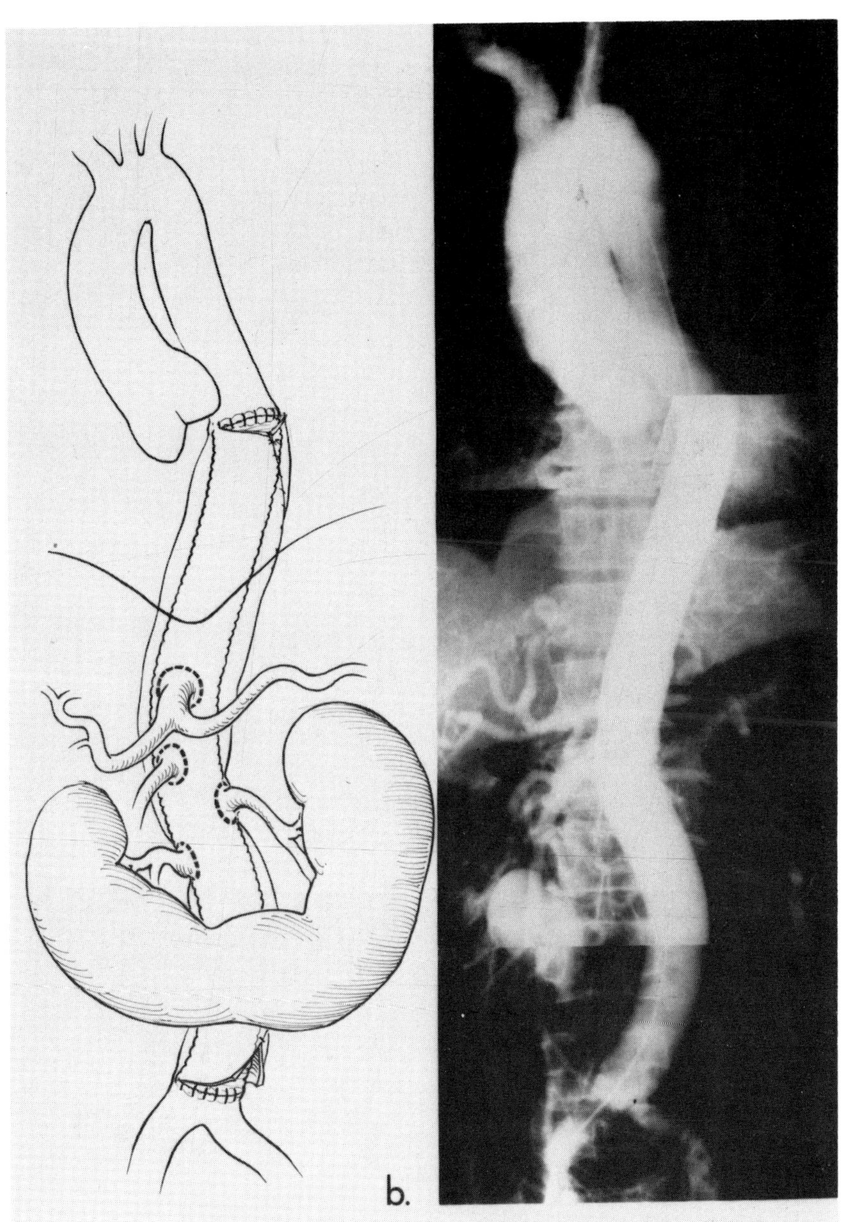

Progress in treatment of thoracoabdominal and abdominal aortic aneurysms involving celiac, superior mesenteric, and renal arteries. Ann. Surg. 188:404-422, 1978. Reproduced by permission of the J. B. Lippincott Company.]

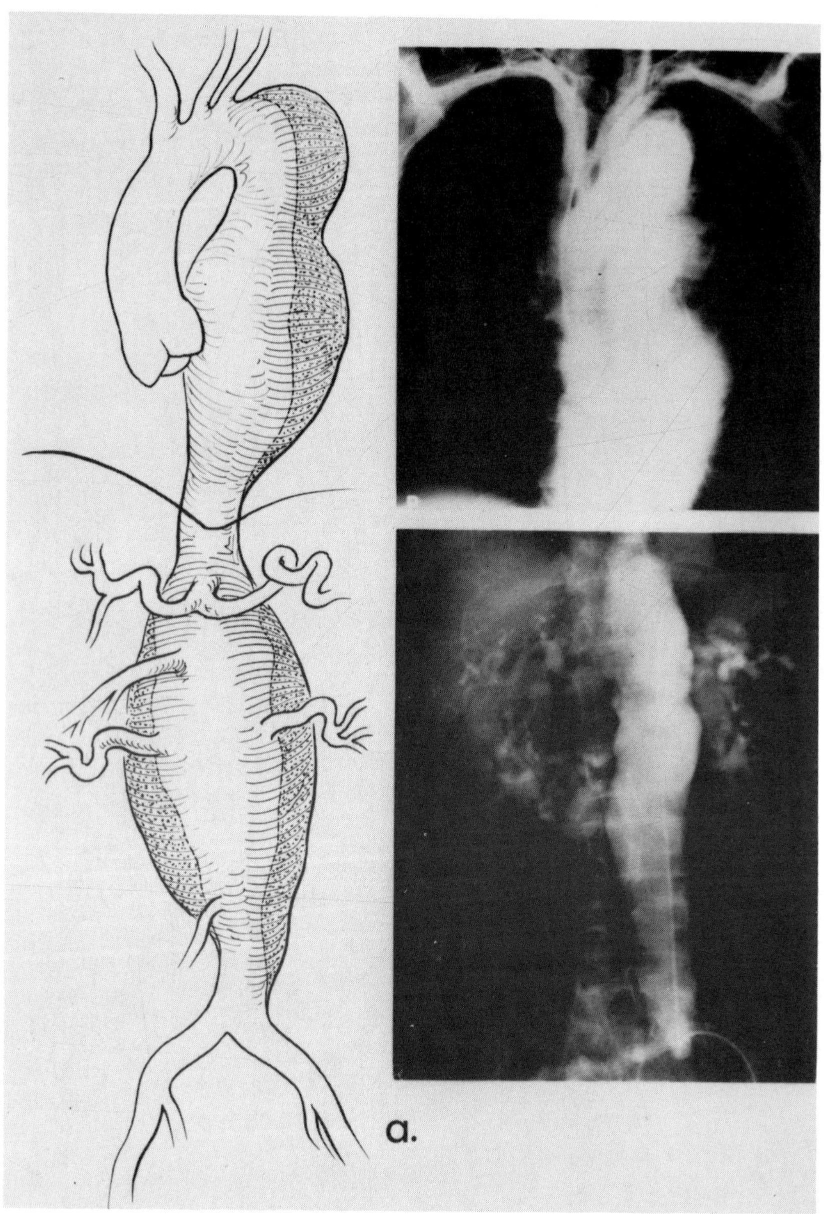

Fig. 6. Illustrations of patient with aneurysm of both the descending thoracic aorta and the entire abdominal aorta. (A) Diagram and aortogram showing extent of disease. (B) Diagram and aortogram showing method of treatment performed in two stages. [From Crawford ES, Snyder DM, Cho GC, et al:

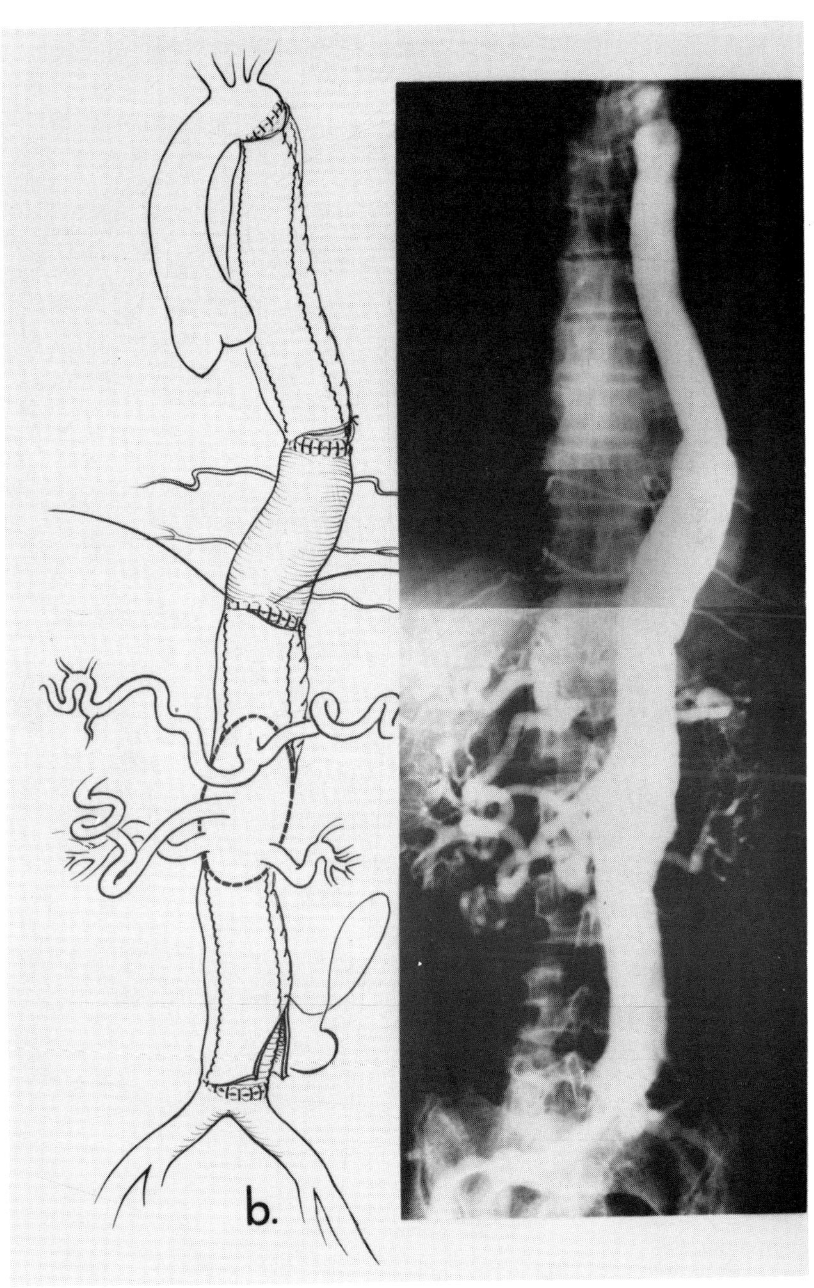

Progress in treatment of thoracoabdominal and abdominal aortic aneurysms involving celiac, superior mesenteric, and renal arteries. Ann. Surg. 188:404-422, 1978. Reproduced by permission of the J. B. Lippincott Company.]

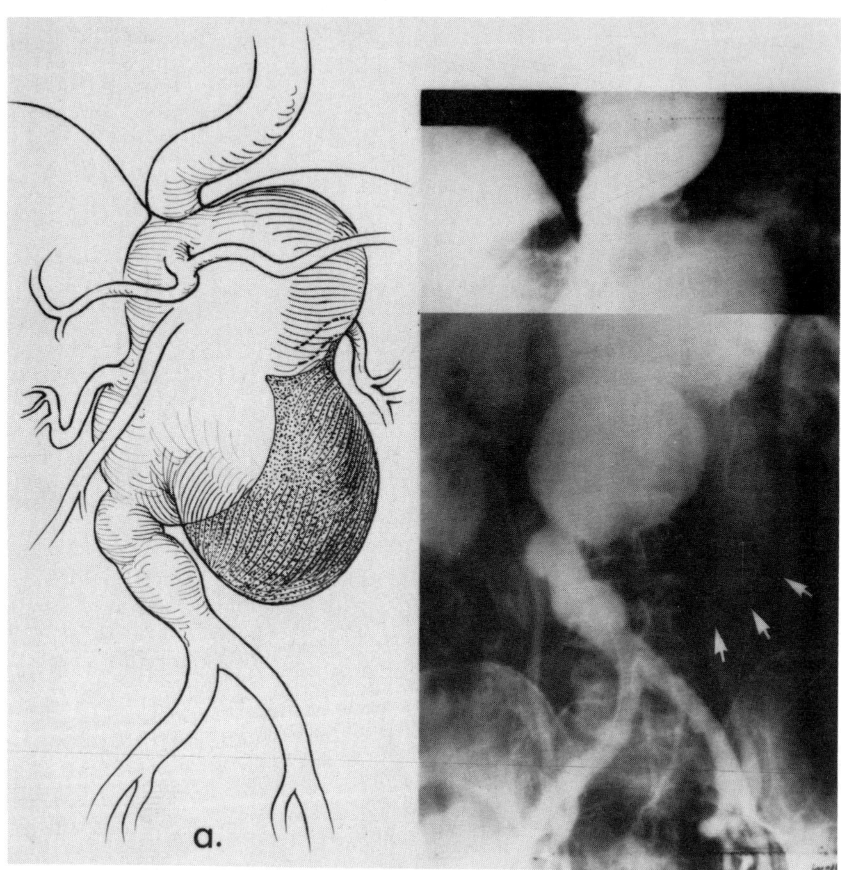

Fig. 7. Illustrations of patient with large abdominal aortic aneurysm involving origins of visceral arteries treated by inclusion graft technique. (A) Diagram and aortogram showing nature and extent of disease. (B) Diagram and aortogram after operation showing successful reconstruction. [From Crawford ES, Snyder DM, Cho GC, et al: Progress in treatment of thoracoabdominal and abdominal aortic aneurysms involving celiac, superior mesenteric, and renal arteries. Ann. Surg. 188:404-422, 1978. Reproduced by permission of the J. B. Lippincott Company.]

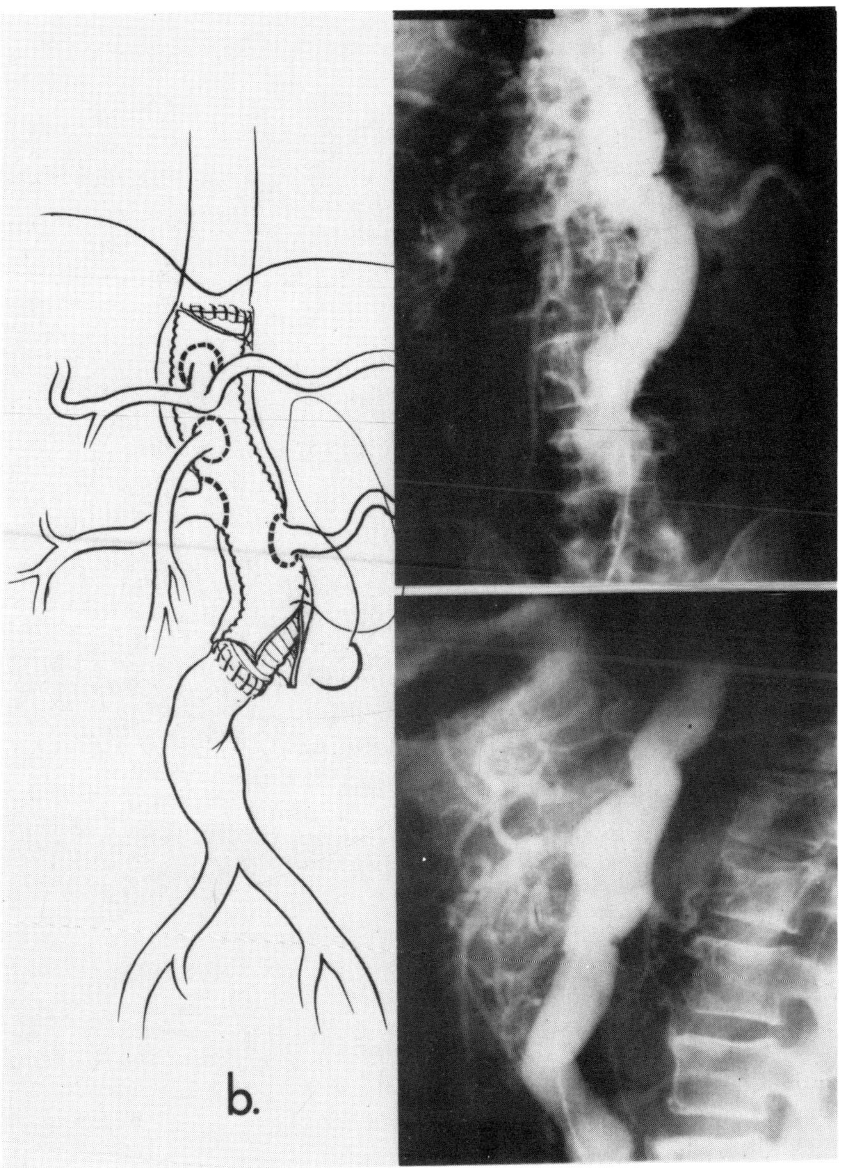
b.

appropriate intercostal space varying from the 9th to the 6th depending upon the proximal extent of aneurysm. The left posteriolateral aspect of the abdominal segment of aneurysm is exposed by retracting the stomach, spleen, tail of pancreas, left kidney, and descending colon upward and to the right [1]. This step of the operation mobilizing the viscera is performed by combining all the steps in mobilizing the left colon to perform left colectomy; mobilizing spleen, tail of pancreas, and stomach for radical cancer operation; or mobilization for extensive abdominal sympathectomy. The diaphragm is incised radically from costal arch to aortic hiatus. To avoid both bleeding and injury to intercostal collateral circulation, the thoracic aneurysm is not mobilized. The aorta proximally and the aorta or iliac arteries distally are minimally mobilized for application of clamps.

The proximal and distal clamps are applied and the aneurysm incised longitudinally using cautery beginning proximally and extending distally through the entire involved segment posteriorly near the spine to avoid injury to the origin of the left renal artery unless intercostal and visceral vessel back bleeding is excessive (Fig. 8). To reduce blood loss in these cases, the incision may be made in stages and back bleeding controlled with balloon catheters. The cut edges of the aneurysm are retracted using heavy stay sutures attached to weights. This maneuver adds significantly to the exposure by retracting the lung and abdominal viscera and by bringing the origins of the visceral vessels into view.

Aortic and arterial reconstruction is then performed by inclusion technique and its application is dependent upon the type and extent of aneurysm and the distance between visceral vessel origins (Fig. 8A) [1, 3]. One end of a woven Dacron tube of appropriate size is sutured to the uninvolved proximal aorta. Intercostal and lumbar arteries are reattached in patients with aneurysms involving most of the thoracic and abdominal aorta (Figs. 1, 3, and 8B). The graft is placed under tension and an oval opening made opposite the pairs of these vessels to be reattached. The edges of the opening made in the graft are sutured around the origins of these vessels. Back bleeding is controlled with balloon catheters until reconstruction is completed. Traction is again applied and oval openings made in the graft opposite the origins of the visceral arteries (Figs. 3, 8, and 9). Separate openings are made in patients when these vessels are spaced more than 2 cm apart and each sutured around the vessel origins. The celiac axis, superior mesenteric, and right renal arteries arise near each other in many cases. This permits reattaching the origins of these vessels to one opening made in the graft or in various combinations (Figs. 3 and 9). The left renal artery is almost always attached to a separate opening, and the graft must be twisted to the right to insure that the renal artery is attached to the left side of graft to prevent kinking and obstruction upon return of viscera into normal position. This may be impossible in some cases, and in others the left renal artery may be involved by aneurysm or distal occlusive disease. Left renal artery reconstruction in these cases is perfomed by using separate Dacron tube graft or by removing the spleen

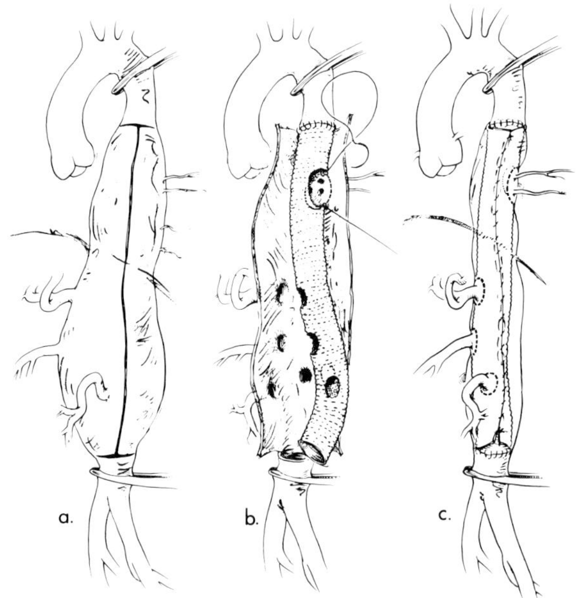

Fig. 8. Diagrams showing graft inclusion and direct vessel reattachment technique as employed in patients with extensive lesions in whom the visceral vessel origins are widely separated. [From Crawford ES, Snyder DM, Cho GC, et al: Progress in treatment of thoracoabdominal and abdominal aortic aneurysms involving celiac, superior mesenteric, and renal arteries. Ann. Surg. 188:404-422, 1978. Reproduced by permission of the J. B. Lippincott Company.]

and performing end-to-end anastomosis between the distal end of splenic artery and the distal uninvolved end of renal artery (Fig. 2). After completing this phase of reconstruction, the graft is evacuated by suction and flushed by temporary removal of proximal aortic clamp. The balloon catheters are removed, the graft clamped distal to renal artery reconstruction, and finally the proximal aortic clamp removed, restoring flow into intercostal and visceral arteries. Reconstruction is then completed by distal anastomosis of the tube graft to distal uninvolved aorta or by bifurcation graft in patients with involvement of the bifurcation either by aneurysm or occlusive disease. Bleeding from suture lines and origins of intercostal and lumbar vessels are thoroughly secured and the aneurysmal wall sutured tightly around the graft and the wound closed in layers.

These same principles are employed in the treatment of chronic dissecting aortic aneurysms; however, variations may be employed to preserve more intercostal arteries. The dissected intimal layer of the false lumen may be trimmed away and this part of aortic circumference replaced by beveling a Dacron tube graft (Fig. 3). This technique preserves the intercostal arteries arising from the

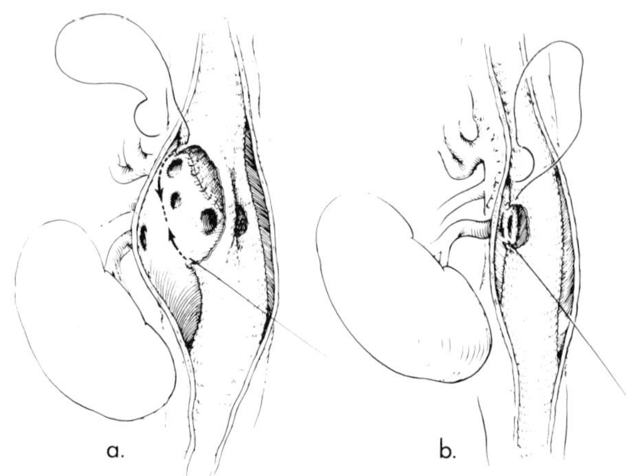

Fig. 9. Diagrams showing variation in visceral vessel reattachment when origins are close together. [From Crawford ES, Snyder DM, Cho GC, et al: Progress in treatment of thoracoabdominal and abdominal aortic aneurysms involving celiac, superior mesenteric, and renal arteries. Ann. Surg. 188:404-422, 1978. Reproduced by permission of the J. B. Lippincott Company.]

undissected circumference of aorta. Distally the reconstruction is accomplished as described above. In 80% of cases the dissection in the abdomen is located on the left side and the left renal artery arises from the false lumen. In 20% of cases the dissection is on the right and the right renal artery arises from the false lumen. The other visceral vessels usually arise from the true lumen; however, this is variable. In any case, the inner septum produced by the dissection is excised and visceral artery reattachment performed as described.

Infrarenal aortic aneurysms that extend to involve the renal arteries are exposed similar to ordinary infrarenal aortic aneurysms except that the aorta is cross-clamped in the aortic hiatus of the diaphragm and the proximal anastomosis made just distal to the origin of the superior mesenteric artery from inside the aneurysm. The renal arteries are reattached as described above unless the aneurysm extends distally into these vessels. Renal artery reconstruction in the latter cases is performed by 8 mm Dacron graft insertion extending from the side of the aortic graft to the distal uninvolved renal artery.

TREATMENT OF ASSOCIATED ARTERIAL LESIONS

Partial occlusive lesions involving the origins of the renal and mesenteric arteries are treated by endarterectomy before reattachment [1, 3]. A circular incision is made in the intimal layer of aorta around the vessel origin, and the tissue plane between inner and outer layer is entered. Dissection is extended within this layer out into involved vessel beyond the obstructing lesion. All intimal fragments are removed and the vessel origin then reattached. Distal obstructing lesions are treated by bypass grafts, and associated visceral vessel aneurysms are repaired either by patch graft or tube grafts (Fig. 2). Most are sacciform in nature and are treated by the former method. Distal occlusive lesions of the aorta and iliac arteries are treated by aortoiliac or aorta-common femoral artery bypass grafts using bifurcation knitted Dacron tubes. Associated diseases such as duodenal ulcer, gallstones, and hiatus hernia are treated by appropriate operation to avoid troublesome postoperative complications. These procedures are delayed until the aortic graft is well covered to prevent contamination.

SUPPORTIVE MEASURES

Good intraaortic catheter aortograms visualizing the entire aorta are obtained in each case and operation delayed 24-48 hours for rehydration and restoration of good renal function. Bronchitis is relieved and all patients given digitalis before operation to improve heart function and to prevent rhythm disturbances during operation. Anesthesia is obtained by nonmyocardial-depressant drugs and relaxation by muscle relaxants. The left lung is collapsed using double lumen balloon endotracheal tube. Intraarterial blood pressure, electrocardiography, and pulmonary arterial pressure are monitored continuously. Cardiac output, pulmonary wedge pressure, and systemic vascular resistance are measured intermittently by Swan-Ganz catheter. Blood gases, serum electrolytes, and plasma colloidal osmotic pressure are measured every 30 min. Detected abnormalities are appropriately corrected. Urine output is measured continuously by indwelling catheter.

Electrolyte solutions begun before operation are monitored during the procedure maintaining the CVP between 7 and 10 mm H_2O. The first liter is given as 5% dextrose and Ringer's lactate solution and the remainder as Ringer's lactate. Mannitol solution, 25 g, is given after induction of anesthesia. Blood replacement is by component technique using packed red blood cells, fresh-frozen plasma, and platelets. A unit of albumen and two units of fresh-frozen plasma are given at the start of operation and packed cells given as blood is lost, alternating 2 units of cells with 1 unit of fresh-frozen plasma and 10-16 units of fresh platelets are given as flow is restored in the grafts.

Temporary bypass is not employed during the period of aortic occlusion [1-3]. The proximal aortic clamp is slowly applied as nitroprusside and other agents are given to maintain normal blood pressure and pulmonary wedge pressure to avoid cardiac strain and rhythm disturbances. Similarly, at the end of reconstruction, the proximal clamp is slowly removed and these values maintained by administration of electrolyte solution, blood, and colloid solutions. Bicarbonate solution is given to correct the mild acidosis occurring after release of clamps, and calcium solution may be given to strengthen cardiac action. Heparin solution is never given, and autotransfusion techniques have not been used.

RESULTS

Of the 108 consecutive patients in this series, 97 (89%) survived. Death was due to hemorrhage from coagulopathies in 3 patients treated before availability of modern blood element transfusion techniques. Pulmonary insufficiency was the cause of death in 3 and infection in 2. The infection was due to peritonitis from ruptured stress ulcer in 1 and pneumonia in 1 patient on chronic hemodialysis. Death was due to stroke, renal failure, and wound infection in 1, myocardial infarction in 1, and unknown cause in 1 patient. Embolization and thrombosis did not occur despite not using heparin. No amputations were required, and peripheral occlusive lesions were not made worse. There were no ischemic disturbances of the gastrointestinal tract. The two principal areas of complication were renal and spinal cord function as discussed below.

Renal Function

Information regarding renal function and aortic and renal artery occlusion times is available in 102 patients (Table 2). Any elevation of serum creatinine after operation was considered evidence of disturbances in renal function.

Table 2
Correlation of Renal Function With Aortic Occlusion Time Required for Operation*

Occlusion Time (minutes)	Patients	Renal Dysfunction	Dialysis **
15 - 35	38	4	1
35 - 55	54	2	1
55 - 150	10	4	3
Total	102	10	5 +

** Two patients on chronic hemodialysis
\+ Death occurred in two patients
* Information available in 102 cases

Elevations were recorded in 10 patients. Hemodialysis was required in 5 patients, including 2 patients with chronic renal failure being maintained by this method. Death occurred in one of the latter and in one patient who had had normal renal function before operation. These disturbances occurred regardless of duration of renal artery occlusion; however, it was more common in patients with the longest occlusion time. Most of the latter patients had difficult and extensive procedures requiring a second operation to restore normal renal circulation. Considering the fact that many had rupture and extensive disease was frequent, this incidence of renal complications which caused death in only 2 patients is acceptable. A much higher incidence has been reported after replacement of aneurysms localized to the infrarenal aortic segment.

Cord Ischemia

Cord ischemia manifested by neurologic deficits of the lower body occurred in ten patients. This complication was predominantly in patients with lesions involving most of the descending thoracic and abdominal aorta and varied from mild transient deficits to permanent moderately severe problems. The deficit was mild and transient in four and moderately severe in six, four of whom survived. Two of the latter were rehabilitated and one lived effectively for 15 years. Two patients were treated recently, and motion in all muscle groups is present and increasing. Paraplegia was dependent upon a number of factors including postoperative hypotension, spinal cord infection, collateral circulation, and reattachment of intercostal and lumbar arteries. Transient deficits after operation were noted during hypotension from cardiac rhythm disturbances and permanent deficits from postural hypotension or myocardial infarction. Paraplegia developed in one patient 8 days after operation with the onset of bilateral herpes zoster. The complication was reduced to one-third with reattachment of intercostal and lumbar arteries. Of practical and predictable importance, paraplegia did not occur in patients with good collateral circulation manifested by large internal mammary epigastric arterial systems profusing intercostal arteries that were obstructed by the aneurysm, absence of visualized intercostal and lumbar arteries by aortography, prominent collateral circulation from the midsacral and iliolumbar arteries to the lumbar arterial system, and large arteries encountered while making the incision as in patients with coarctation of the aorta. This complication is perhaps the most dreaded by the patient, but fortunately permanent disability is relatively rare and modern rehabilitation techniques provide the opportunity to resume useful and happy lives of long duration. All patients are thoroughly informed of this possible complication, but to date none has rejected operation in favor of ultimate rupture.

Long-term followup was carried out 18 months ago in 77 survivors of operations done before this time. Current information was obtained in 73 (95%). Of those surviving operation, 51 (62%) were alive. An actuarial curve was constructed from this information and survival projected for a 6-year period and

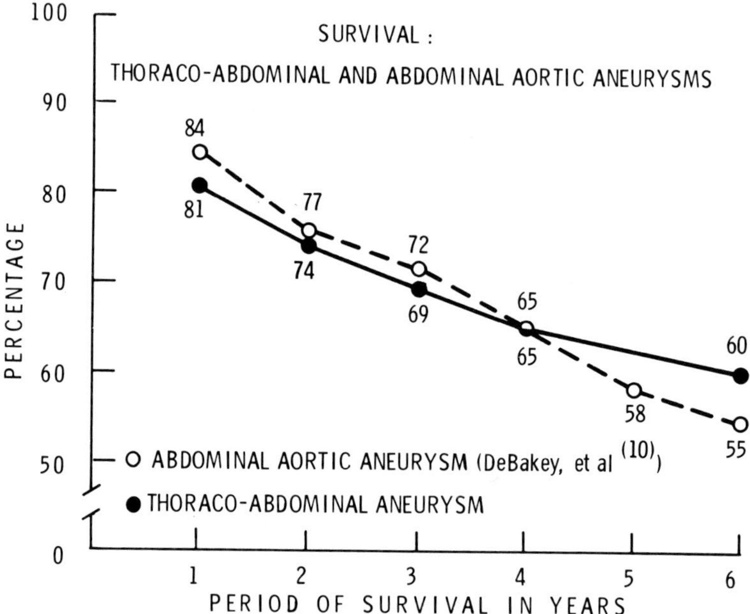

Fig. 10. Survival of patients with thoracoabdominal aortic aneurysms treated by inclusion technique compared to survival of patients with graft replacement infrarenal abdominal aortic aneurysm. [From Crawford ES, Snyder DM, Cho GC, et al: Progress in treatment of thoracoabdominal and abdominal aortic aneurysms involving celiac, superior mesenteric, and renal arteries. Ann. Surg. 188:404-422, 1978. Reproduced by permission of the J. B. Lippincott Company.]

compared to that of patients surviving simple infrarenal abdominal aortic resection [4]. Survival was the same (Fig. 10).

REFERENCES

1. Crawford ES: Thoraco-abdominal and abdominal aortic aneurysms involving renal, superior mesenteric, and celiac arteries. Ann. Surg. 179:763, 1974
2. Crawford ES, Rubio PA: Reappraisal of adjuncts to avoid ischemia in the treatment of aneurysms of descending thoracic aorta. J. Thorac. Cardiovasc. Surg. 66:693, 1973
3. Crawford ES, Snyder DM, Cho GC, et al: Progress in treatment of thoracoabdominal and abdominal aortic aneurysms involving celiac, superior mesenteric, and renal arteries. Ann. Surg. 188:404, 1978
4. DeBakey ME, Crawford ES, Cooley DA, et al: Aneurysm of abdominal aorta: Analysis of results of graft replacement therapy one to eleven years after operation. Ann. Surg. 160:622, 1964

5. DeBakey ME, Crawford ES, Garrett HE, et al: Surgical considerations in the treatment of aneurysms of the thoraco-abdominal aorta. Ann. Surg. 162:650, 1965
6. DeBakey ME, Ceech O Jr, Morris GC Jr: Aneurysm of thoraco-abdominal aorta involving the celiac, superior mesenteric, and renal arteries: Report of four cases treated by resection and homograft replacement. Ann. Surg. 144:549, 1956
7. Ellis FH Jr, Helden RA, Hines EA Jr: Aneurysm of the abdominal aorta involving the right renal artery: Report of case with preservation of renal function after resection and grafting. Ann. Surg. 142:992, 1955
8. Etheredge SN, Yee J, Smith JV, et al: Successful resection of a large aneurysm of the upper abdominal aorta and replacement with homograft. Surgery 38:1071, 1955
9. Javid H, Julian OC, Dye WS, et al: Complications of abdominal aortic grafts. Arch. Surg. 85:650, 1962

John H. Sanders, Jr., M.D.

Aortic Dissection

Acute aortic dissection has been recognized as a catastrophic event for centuries. The abrupt onset of searing back pain, with radiation to neck, chest, lumbar area, or abdomen, frequently allows the condition to be suspected by even telephone description. Its frequency probably approaches or surpasses that of ruptured abdominal aortic aneurysm, and until the last two decades its mortality approached 75% within the first week of diagnosis. The remaining patients would often succumb to extension of the hematoma or rupture of the false channel into the pericardium or left chest at a later date [11, 13, 16].

PATHOPHYSIOLOGY

The peak incidence of aortic dissection is in the 40-60-year age group, with males predominating. The majority will have a history of hypertension, often having ceased therapy, or will be markedly hypertensive at the time of admission. It is our impression that ascending aortic dissections tend to occur more often in younger individuals than do descending dissections. Virtually all patients with this condition will have some form of medial degeneration of the aorta, such as Erdheim's cystic medial necrosis. In younger individuals Marfan's syndrome, or a variant of it, is very likely to be present.

The initiating event in aortic dissection is rupture of the intima and inner media which allows access of blood flow to the degenerated portion of the media. The tear generally occurs where circumferential stress is greatest – in the midascending aorta on the outer portion of its greatest curvature – or where the descending aorta is tethered by the ligamentum arteriosum. Tears may occur in the transverse arch as well, but are less common. Progression of the dissecting hematoma is largely distal, but proximal extension is seen and may allow a descending dissection to rupture into the pericardium.

While systolic hypertension frequently accompanies acute dissection and may be instrumental in originating the intimal tear, it is the rapid rate of buildup of systolic pressure by the left ventricle, or dp/dt, which generates the impulse that allows the hematoma to dissect and progress distally. Anticoagulation, profound anemia, and hyperdynamic cardiac conditions facilitate this progression and increase the hazard of rupture through outer media and adventitia. Death most commonly results from pericardial tamponade – often caused by relatively slow weeping of blood through the membrane-thin outer layers of the diseased ascending aorta.

Aortic insufficiency occurs in approximately 25% of ascending aortic dissections from the inward displacement of the commissures of the valve – usually that between right and noncoronary cusps and that between noncoronary and left coronary cusps. This may be evidenced by a new diastolic murmur or by profound congestive heart failure. Healed dissections may present later with severe aortic insufficiency or with saccular aneurysms of the false lumen in the ascending, descending, or abdominal aorta.

DIAGNOSTIC CONSIDERATIONS

The majority of patients with aortic dissection experience excruciating pain of sudden, intense onset. The usual onset is upper back, but is varied enough that the condition may easily be mistaken for myocardial infarction, pancreatitis, biliary colic, renal colic, ruptured abdominal aneurysm, perforated peptic ulcer, or spontaneous pneumothorax. Because 20%-25% of patients may die within 12-24 hours of onset, overdiagnosis of aortic dissection is much safer than ruling out the myriad conditions it may mimic. A few patients with aortic dissection may have little or no pain and present with unexplained signs or symptoms related to the progressing hematoma. We have seen one patient with syncope and bloody pericardial effusion as her only findings referable to an undiagnosed ascending aortic tear.

Physical findings include the murmur of aortic insufficiency, unequal or absent pulses in the periphery, stroke, paraplegia, a cold extremity, hyperactive bowel sounds with mesenteric artery compromise, and occasionally a pulsatile abdominal mass suggestive of ruptured abdominal aneurysm.

On admission, patients often appear in great hemodynamic compromise with pallor, cold sweat, cyanosis, tachycardia, and tachypnea. Blood pressure, however, is usually above normal or becomes so with minimal volume replacement.

Initial Diagnostic Procedures

The plain chest film is helpful when findings of mediastinal widening, aortic root enlargement, tracheal deviation, depression of left mainstem bronchus, an aortic shadow outside a calcified knob, or pleural effusion are present. However, a normal chest film does not serve to rule out dissection and may miss as many as half of all patients with the condition.

An electrocardiogram and enzyme batteries should be obtained to rule out acute myocardial ischemia or infarction, although a dissection which occludes or narrows one of the coronary ostia may also produce such findings. A urinalysis may show hematuria with impending renal artery involvement.

At this point, the pursuit of other diagnoses is best left until after medical therapy for dissection has begun and aortography has been undertaken. A general goal should be to control hypertension and obtain a thoracic aortogram within 4 hours of admission of any patient suspected of harboring an aortic dissection. It is imperative that immediate access for arterial and venous pressure monitoring be made and blood pressure be controlled to limit hematoma progression. There are few, if any, conditions that mimic dissection that will be worsened by decreasing blood pressure and dp/dt, since left ventricular oxygen requirements are also reduced by this early therapy. Treatment can usually be effected by the time the angiography suite is prepared and renders the study far safer.

Angiography

Our policy has been to alert operating room personnel, the perfusionist, and the blood bank to prepare for a cardiopulmonary bypass procedure while the patient is being transferred to the radiology department. It is desirable to have an experienced cardiac intensive care nurse accompany the patient to help monitor and control blood pressure during the procedure. Until the conclusion of the procedure, the patient remains in the care of the cardiology and cardiac surgical services as a team effort.

The goal of angiography is to determine not only the presence and extent of an aortic dissection, but also the precise location of the intimal tear. For this reason, it is best to have the responsible surgeon review the films as they are developed so that additional views may be obtained if necessary and unnecessary runs avoided.

MEDICAL VERSUS SURGICAL THERAPY

Medical therapy should begin upon admission and should usually precede radiologic confirmation of the diagnosis. Dr. Myron Wheat's application in the early 1960s of available experimental data led to a drastic reduction in the early mortality of the condition [20, 21]. By using trimethaphan (Arfonad) to acutely lower systolic pressure to 90-120 mm Hg while decreasing dp/dt, he obtained a 100% early survival in six patients [12, 21]. The original Wheat-Palmer regimen is currently modified in most institutions by the use of nitroprusside instead of trimethaphan to lower systolic pressure effectively, while using propranolol intravenously or orally to eliminate reflex tachycardia and decrease dp/dt. Nitroprusside is supplanted later by alpha methyl-DOPA, and propranolol is continued orally as a lifetime medication.

While initial medical therapy is mandatory in all dissections, chronic medical therapy has a rather sharp attrition rate in certain instances [18]. DeBakey's description of his first 179 patients treated surgically classified the condition as it is most widely reported today (Fig. 1). In his and other papers, the relative urgency of repair of ascending dissections (types I and II) is contrasted with the relatively safe initial course of descending dissections (type III) [8, 17]. His surgical group had a high success rate initially (80% overall survival) with a relatively low attrition rate over time compared with Hirst's series of untreated patients [13]. Hume and Porter in 1963 and Daily in 1970 pointed out that with medical therapy alone, nearly 80% of patients with descending dissection would survive, contrasted with 20% of similarly treated patients with ascending aortic involvement [6].

Dalen et al. reported the Peter Bent Brigham Hospital experience in 1974 using a combined therapy based upon the different behavior of ascending and descending dissections. In this series, immediate surgical repair of ascending dissections led to a 77% survival [7]. Eighty percent of patients with descending dissection survived with medical therapy alone. Early surgical treatment of

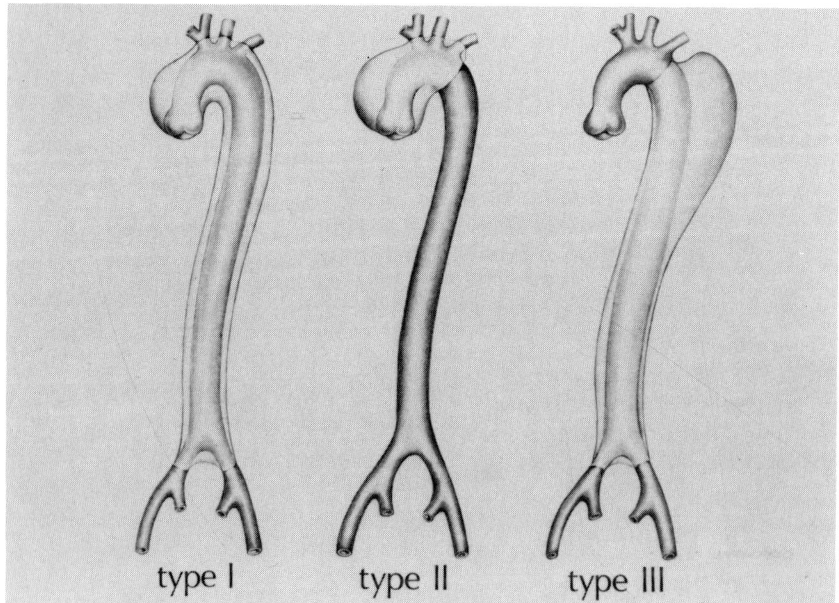

Fig. 1. DeBakey's classification of aortic dissections is still the most widely accepted [8]. Many groups prefer to classify dissections as ascending (types I and II) or descending (type III).

descending dissections in this and other studies has not significantly improved upon the early medical survival rate of approximately 80% [2]. However, surgically treated patients in both groups have a substantially better long-term prognosis than their medically treated counterparts. The controversy, then, really is limited to the question of surgery for the patient with descending aortic dissection.

Most patients with descending aortic dissection who succumb initially will do so from compromise of a major visceral artery or rupture into the thorax. Patients who at angiography have already thrombosed the false lumen are probably not at great risk for rupture or extension of the dissection if kept under good medical therapy. Those with an open or closed false lumen who develop a complication of the acute dissection – neurologic, visceral, arterial, or peripheral vascular changes – or who threaten to rupture as heralded by increased or recurrent pain, enlargement of the aortic shadow, or onset of pleural effusion should undergo urgent surgery.

A patient who has had successful medical therapy of an acute descending dissection and has reached the chronic stage must be watched for subsequent development of a saccular aneurysm of the false lumen. This generally occurs in the left chest, but may present as an abdominal aneurysm. While plain chest films are traditionally used for followup, we have found computerized axial tomography with intravenous infusion of contrast material to be a precise means of documenting the size and extent of aortic dissections. Accurate measurement of the size of true and false lumens at various thoracic and abdominal levels can be checked as an outpatient at convenient intervals. Enlargement of the aneurysm would be an indication for elective surgery in the patient with a chronic descending aortic dissection.

While few patients present with chronic ascending dissections because of the high initial mortality and rapid subsequent attrition, perhaps 5%-10% of acute patients may reach this state. Those who through good fortune do so are not necessarily candidates for repair unless a complication arises. Usually, aortic insufficiency in such a patient would be dealt with surgically when symptoms or progressive left ventricular enlargement occurred. As in descending dissections, progressive enlargement of the ascending aorta or formation of a saccular aneurysm would call for elective repair.

From a technical standpoint, one must be certain that major body branches of the aorta are visualized angiographically before attempting repair of a chronic aortic dissection. It is not uncommon to find a major branch arising from the false channel. We have seen one patient with chronic ascending dissection requiring aortic valve replacement in whom the major supply to renal, mesenteric, and cerebral vessels was by way of the false channel. In this case, both channels were deliberately left open at the aortic root to avoid disturbance of his double-barreled vascular system.

Patients in whom angiography demonstrates a site of entry in the transverse aortic arch or in whom the tear cannot be visualized accurately are best treated as having descending aortic dissections. However, this group should be followed more closely for complications, and the threshold for repeat angiography should be very low indeed.

CHOICE OF SURGICAL THERAPY

The surgical therapy of aortic dissection was initially limited to resection of the segment of aorta involved and replacement with a Teflon or Dacron graft prosthesis. When the aortic valve was insufficient, this was generally replaced with a prosthetic valve and the coronary arteries, if involved, were reimplanted into the graft. This led to a rather extensive surgical dissection and was a principal source of the major intraoperative cause of death – hemorrhage. Collins and co-workers demonstrated in 1973 that the aortic valve could be reconstructed in many instances of aortic dissection by resuspension of the valve commissures, reinforced with a Teflon felt ring inserted into the false lumen around the valve [5, 15] (Fig. 2). This reinforcement frequently eliminates the need to replace the valve and usually allows leaving the native coronary ostia intact. If this same sandwich technique is carried out for the distal segment of ascending aorta, the aorta can frequently be directly reconstructed without the need for graft material, or at most the interposition of a diamond-shaped patch of graft material. This technique effectively eliminates the need for extensive mobilization of the ascending aorta and allows the placement of all suture lines in a readily visible portion of the aorta. In the event of a large, unreconstructable ascending aorta, a ring of Teflon material can be placed within the false lumen at the proximal and distal ends of the dissection and graft interposed between (Fig. 2). This allows the construction of a much firmer aorta to which to sew a graft. The site of origin of the dissection is either resected or included in the repair. Other techniques which rely on a similar form of reconstruction utilize the placement of Teflon felt pledgets inside the true lumen of the aorta and outside the wall of the aorta to sandwich aortic tissue between them [4] (Fig. 3). Both of these techniques recreate much more normal tissue which can be sutured with less fear of significant hemorrhage at the discontinuance of cardiopulmonary bypass. In situations where the coronary vessels are involved and cannot be directly reconstructed, a button of aorta containing the coronary ostia may be sutured directly into the graft or a segment of saphenous vein may be used to bypass one or both coronary vessels, taking origin from the prosthetic graft material.

In the descending aorta, extensive replacement with prosthetic graft may involve excluding the segment of aorta from which the blood supply to the thoracic spinal cord arises. Here, too, the use of local reconstruction with intramural Teflon felt material and direct anastomosis or interposition of a small segment of graft helps lessen the risk of paraplegia.

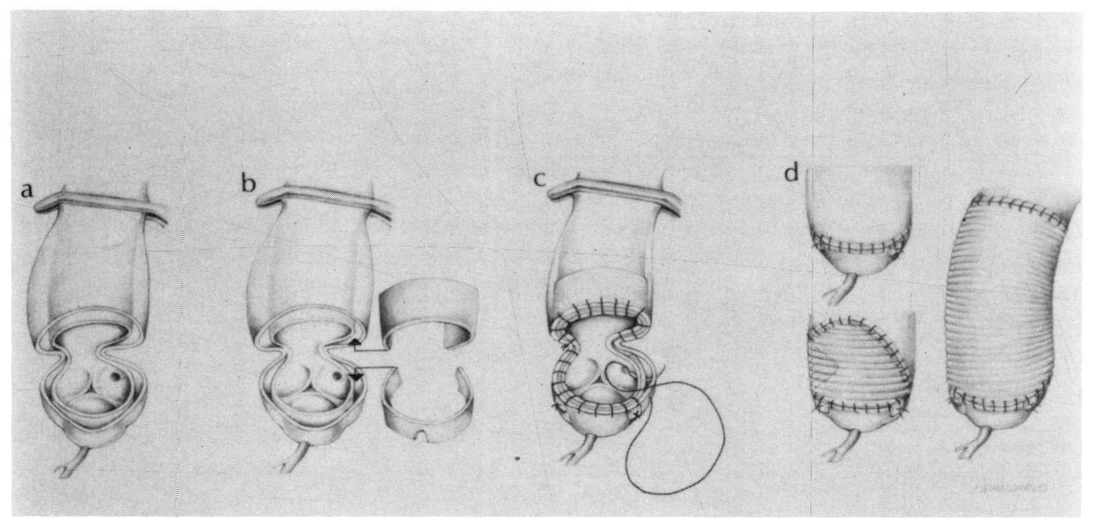

Fig. 2. Teflon felt sandwich technique of Collins [5]. (A) Ascending aorta is opened, showing intimal tear and loss of support of valve commissures. (B) Rings of Teflon felt are inserted into false lumen proximally and distally. (C) Pledgeted sutures resuspend valve commissures. Aortic walls are oversewn proximally and distally, with felt buttressing the false lumen. (D) Aorta is closed primarily, with diamond-shaped gusset of graft material, or with graft interposition depending on extent of dissection.

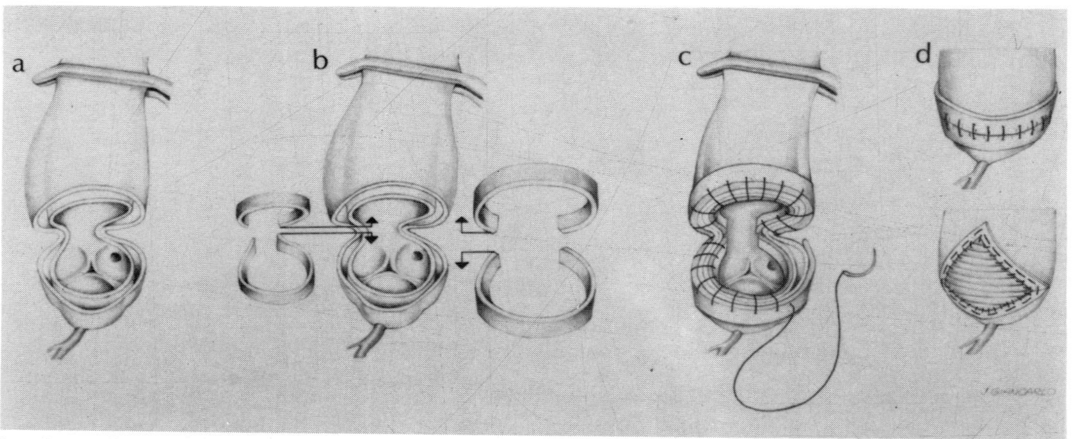

Fig. 3. Teflon felt sandwich technique of Berger [4]. (A) Ascending aorta is opened, showing intimal tear. (B) Rings of Teflon felt are placed inside the true lumen and outside the aortic wall. (C) Preliminary oversewing of proximal and distal cuffs creates a sturdy aortic wall and resuspends valve commissures. (D) Aorta is closed primarily or by use of an appropriate amount of graft material.

A significant advance in the repair of descending thoracic aortic dissections is the use of the heparin-bonded Gott shunt, eliminating the need for systemic heparinization [9, 14]. This bypass from the ascending aorta to the left femoral artery encounters far less intra- and postoperative hemorrhage than various systems of partial cardiopulmonary bypass. If such a shunt is combined with the use of a Swan-Ganz catheter for monitoring of left-sided filling pressures and the judicious administration of intravenous nitroprusside or nitroglycerin during the period of aortic cross-clamping, the danger of overloading the left ventricle is minimized.

One recent technique which offers promise in the treatment of aortic dissection is the ringed intraluminal graft described independently by Dureau and Ablaza [1, 10]. Both of these techniques call for the placement of a rigid-ring reinforced Dacron graft within the aorta which is held in place by heavy ligatures over both true and false lumens (Fig. 4). In this technique, the patient is placed on cardiopulmonary bypass in the instance of an ascending dissection or a heparin-bonded shunt is used for descending dissection. The aorta is cross-clamped, incised vertically, and the aortic tear enlarged. The prosthesis,

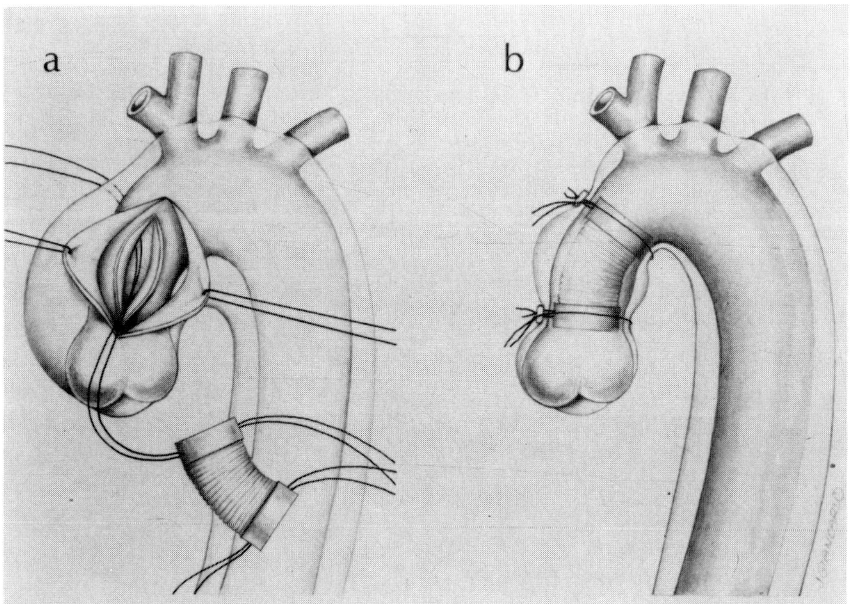

Fig. 4. Use of a ring-reinforced graft for repair of aortic dissection described independently by Dureau [10] and Ablaza [1]. (A) Aorta is opened longitudinally and the tear enlarged if necessary. Stay sutures are passed from the reinforcing rings of the prosthesis through all layers of the aortic wall. The prosthesis is seated, aided by the stay sutures. (B) Large ligatures bind all layers of the aorta to the prosthesis at both ends. The walls of the aorta are closed over the prosthesis, leaving the intimal tear isolated between the ligatures.

with its proximal and distal reinforcing rings, is placed within the lumen of the aorta and held in place with several tacking sutures. The external ligatures are tightened and the aorta is closed in the usual way. This technique offers a significant advantage in terms of time required and in the lack of dissection or mobilization of the aorta. Followup of this type of repair is short, however, and a major concern is that tight ligatures may cut through the aortic walls with time. If this form of repair does prove to be successful in the long run, it may prove to be a significant advance in the treatment of this difficult condition.

There are times when aortic dissection may present as an abdominal aortic aneurysm and more specifically as a rupturing abdominal aortic aneurysm. Under these circumstances, direct resection of the abdominal segment of the dissection is contraindicated. The thin, almost translucent outer layer of the aorta which forms the outer boundary of the false lumen is distinctly different in appearance from the thick-walled, chronic atherosclerotic aneurysm of the aorta. Resection of an abdominal aorta which is in fact an aortic dissection will leave the intimal tear patent proximally and the vessel will often prove to be unreconstructable when transected. Because of this, we currently recommend closure of the abdomen and immediate angiographic examination of the proximal aorta.

A final consideration is the means of dealing with occluded branches of the distal aorta secondary to an acute dissection. Initial attempts at fenestration of these branches to allow inflow from the true lumen were by and large fraught with failure [3]. At the present time, occluded branches of the distal aorta which occur with an acute dissection have been treated surgically. Often, closure of the site of origin of the dissection will allow the false lumen to thrombose and the hematoma to absorb. Over a period of several weeks or months, flow will gradually improve to many, if not all, of these branches. Where a major vessel such as a carotid is involved and neurologic symptoms are present, failure of the condition to resolve rapidly may necessitate an extraanatomical reconstruction such as a subclavian-to-carotid or carotid-to-carotid bypass. In the abdomen, where this is sometimes less practical, it may be necessary to attempt local reconstruction if no site exists as a donor for a bypass circuit. In these circumstances, it may be possible to suture a patch of Dacron material to the two layers of aorta in order to obtain a spot where a piece of tubular graft may take origin for supply to mesenteric or renal vessels.

CONCLUSION

There has been considerable progress in the treatment of aortic dissection. Much of this has stemmed from recognition that ascending and descending dissections behave differently and require different approaches. The immediate institution of good medical therapy aimed at decreasing the force of left ventricular contraction as well as systolic blood pressure has averted much of the immediate mortality which occurred in untreated patients. This has allowed orderly study with good angiography and the immediate repair of the more lethal ascending aortic dissection. A minority of patients with descending dissection will develop early complications, and they must be operated upon urgently. Those who develop late aneurysms can be operated upon electively. Operative techniques have gradually decreased in scope from complete resection of the involved aorta to local plastic procedures aimed at obliterating the false channel at the site of the tear. The heparin-bonded Gott shunt for the repair of descending aortic dissections has allowed this to be done with less morbidity from hemorrhage. Finally, recent studies of late postoperative patients have shown that patients who have undergone repair of aortic dissection may well have residual abnormalities, especially patent reentry points in the distal aorta [19]. Because of this, it is strongly recommended that patients who are treated by either medical or surgical means with initial success maintain careful surveillance under good medical therapy for life. By adhering to such a regimen we may be able to further decrease the mortality of this disease below its present 20% level.

REFERENCES

1. Ablaza SGG, Ghosh SC, Grana VP: Use of a ringed intraluminal graft in the surgical treatment of dissecting aneurysms of the thoracic aorta: A new technique. J. Thorac. Cardiovasc. Surg. 76:390, 1978
2. Applebaum A, Karp RB, Kirklin JW: Ascending vs. descending aortic dissections. Ann. Surg. 183:296, 1976
3. Austen WG, DeSanctis RW: Surgical treatment of dissecting aneurysm of the thoracic aorta. N. Engl. J. Med. 272:1314, 1965
4. Berger RL: A simplified plastic repair for aortic dissections. Ann. Thorac. Surg. 25:250, 1978
5. Collins JJ, Cohn LH: Reconstruction of the aortic valve: Correcting valve incompetence due to acute dissecting aneurysm. Arch. Surg. 106:35, 1973
6. Daily PO, Trueblood HW, Stinson EB, et al: Management of acute aortic dissections. Ann. Thorac. Surg. 10:237, 1970
7. Dalen JE, Alpert JS, Cohn LH, et al: Dissection of the thoracic aorta: Medical or surgical therapy? Am. J. Cardiol. 34:803, 1974
8. DeBakey ME, Henly WS, Cooley DA, et al: Surgical management of dissecting aneurysms of the aorta. J. Thorac. Cardiovasc. Surg. 49:130, 1965
9. DeMeester TR, Cameron JL, Gott VL: Repair of a through-and-through gunshot wound of the aortic arch using a heparinized shunt. Ann. Thorac. Surg. 16:193, 1973
10. Dureau G, Villard J, George M, et al: New surgical technique for the operative management of acute dissections of the ascending aorta: Report of two cases. J. Thorac. Cardiovasc. Surg. 76:385, 1978

11. Gore I, Seiwert VJ: Dissecting aneurysm of the aorta: Pathologic aspects: An analysis of eighty-five fatal cases. AMA Arch. Pathol. 53:121, 1952
12. Harris PD, Malm JR, Bigger JT Jr, et al: Follow-up studies of acute dissecting aortic aneurysms managed with antihypertensive agents. Circulation [Suppl I to vols 35 and 36] 183, 1967
13. Hirst AE Jr, Johns VJ Jr, Kime SW Jr: Dissecting aneurysm of the aorta: A review of 505 cases. Medicine (Baltimore) 37:217, 1958
14. Kärkölä P, Kairaluoma MI, Larmi TKI: A simple cannulation technique for perfusion problems in advanced aortic dissection. J. Thorac. Cardiovasc. Surg. 73:110, 1977
15. Koster K Jr, Cohn LH, Mee RBB, et al: Late results of operation for acute aortic dissection producing aortic insufficiency. Ann. Thorac. Surg. 26:461, 1978
16. McCloy RM, Spittell JA Jr, McGoon DC: The prognosis in aortic dissection: Dissecting aortic hematoma or aneurysm. Circulation 31:665, 1965
17. Parker FB Jr, Neville JF Jr, Hanson EL, et al: Management of acute aortic dissection. Ann. Thorac. Surg. 19:436, 1975
18. Pate JW, Richardson RL, Eastridge CE: Acute aortic dissections. Am. Surgeon 42:395, 1976
19. Thomas CS Jr, Alford WC Jr, Burrus GR, et al: The effectiveness of surgical treatment of acute aortic dissection. Ann. Thorac. Surg. 26:42, 1978
20. Wheat MW Jr, Harris PD, Malm JR, et al: Acute dissecting aneurysms of the aorta: Treatment and results in 64 patients. J. Thorac. Cardiovasc. Surg. 58:344, 1969
21. Wheat MW Jr, Palmer RF, Bartley TD, et al: Treatment of dissecting aneurysms of the aorta without surgery. J. Thorac. Cardiovasc. Surg. 50:364, 1965

R. M. Greenhalgh, M.A., M.Chir., F.R.C.S.

Small Aorta Syndrome

It is becoming evident that the term "atherosclerotic arterial disease" embraces a number of entities with differing etiological pathways. This disease, progressing to occlusion of peripheral or coronary arteries, is far less common in women than men, although this difference is diminished in women subjected to an early artificial menopause [3].

There are five separate groups of arterial disease that have been described, according to the situation and type of disease seen on the arteriogram [1]. By stenosing arterial disease we mean the most typical sort of arterial disease which affects the arteries supplying the lower limbs, in which the arteries are narrowed or even occluded by atheroma. By dilating disease we mean aneurysmal, baggy, and dilated arterial disease. To these one can add carotid stenoses and patients with intracranial aneurysms. The fifth group will be referred to as little women with blocked aortas [2] and may also be referred to as the small aorta syndrome.

"LITTLE WOMEN"

Presenting Data

We investigated a group of 27 "little women" who are apparently normal endocrinologically. Presenting data compare strikingly with other types of arterial disease (Table 1). These women presented at a mean age of 49 ± 7 years and all of them had smoked at least 20 cigarettes per day for 20 years or more. Thirty percent of them had already had a myocardial infarction. Each of them presented with a very clear history of bilateral buttock, thigh, and calf claudication which worsened to a point where they were prepared to undergo major arterial reconstructive surgery. Their age range was 34-59 years (Table 2) and they had a mean height of 61 ± 2 inches (Fig. 1.). They were not obese for their

Table 1
Patient Data

		MALE/FEMALE RATIO	AGE RANGE	MEAN AGE YEARS	HEAVY SMOKERS	MYOCARDIAL INFARCTION	DIABETES MELLITUS	HYPERTENSION	OBESE
145	STENOSING	13 : 1	40 - 70	61	98%	30%	12(8%)	29%	18%
69	DILATING	13 : 1	40 - 70	61	91%	36%	1	32%	24%
27	LITTLE WOMEN	-	34 - 59	49	100%	30%	1	0	0
43	CAROTID STENOSIS	10 : 1	45 - 75	61	93%	16%	1	48%	15%
22	INTRACRANIAL ANEURYSMS	0.7 : 1	25 - 70	53	50%	5%	0	55%	21%

Table 2
27 Young Little Women

Means and Standard Deviations	
AGE RANGE	34 to 59 years
MEAN AGE	49 ± 7 years
MEAN HEIGHT	61 ± 2 inches
MEAN WEIGHT	125 ± 15 pounds
IDEAL WEIGHT FOR THIS AGE AND HEIGHT	124 pounds
	(Scottish Widows' Model Weight Chart, 1971)

height and compared well with the ideal weight for this age and height as described by a life insurance company.

However, a comparison between height and weight was made with 50 control women who lived and were brought up in the same part of England. These 50 control women had no suggestion of arterial disease. They formed a consecutive series and in Table 3 one can see that the control women were both taller and heavier than the 27 "little women." It would seem that the "little women" constituting our "small aorta syndrome" were indeed small in stature in every respect.

Table 3
Heights and Weights Compared

Means and Standard Deviations	Height (inches)	Weight (pounds)
27 LITTLE WOMEN (Mean age 49 years)	61 ± 2.1	125 ± 15
50 CONTROL WOMEN (Mean age 52 years)	64 ± 2.4	144 ± 23
SIGNIFICANCE	t = 4.5 $p < 0.001$	t = 3.9 $p < 0.001$

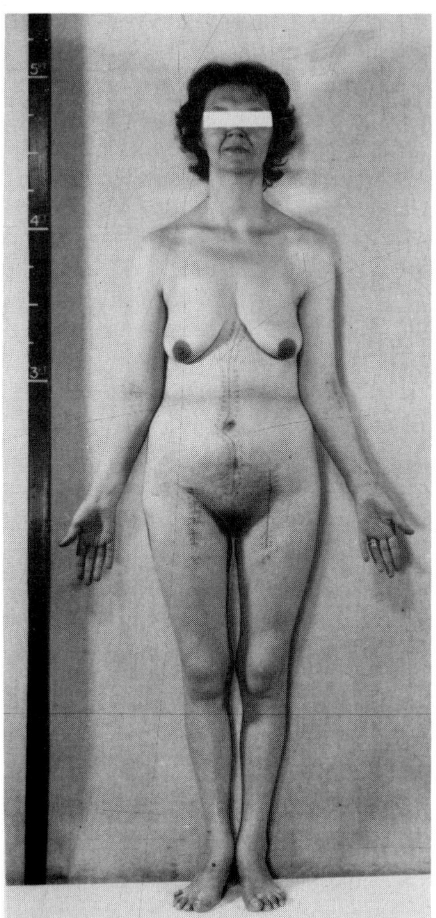

Fig. 1. Typical "little woman."

Arteriogram Findings

It was frequently necessary to perform a translumbar aortogram because often it was impossible to pass a catheter up from the femoral arteries beyond the aortic bifurcation. In Fig. 2 one can see a very typical aortogram of the "small aorta syndrome." The aorta is small below the renal arteries when compared with the vertebral column, but tapers down almost to a point at the bifurcation at its lower end. There was inevitably disease at and near the aortic bifurcation; below this the iliac arteries were of very narrow diameter but relatively normal. The femoropopliteal segment was always patent and free from disease.

In Fig. 3 one sees a later example of the same syndrome in which the disease at the lower end of the abdominal aorta has progressed to occlusion.

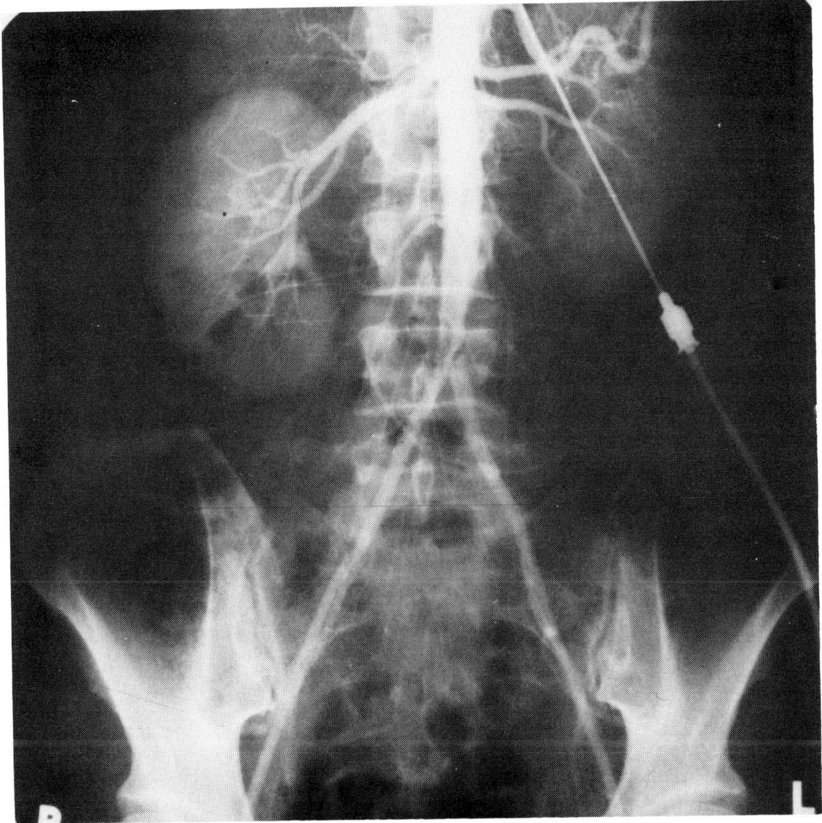

Fig. 2. Translumbar aortogram showing tapering of the lower abdominal aorta, with disease only near its bifurcation.

Serum Biochemistry

The fasting serum triglyceride and cholesterol levels are plotted in Fig. 4. The dotted lines refer to mean and two standard deviation positions of the control series. Clearly both triglyceride and cholesterol levels in the 27 female patients with "small aorta syndrome" are raised, but the cholesterol levels are especially high. In fact, 70% of our "little women" had a fasting serum cholesterol level above 270 mg/100 ml.

When the lipoprotein patterns in the "little women with blocked aortas" is compared with 50 control patients and 145 patients with stenosing arterial disease (Table 4), striking differences are noted between the groups. Seventy-eight percent of the 27 "little women" have an abnormal lipoprotein pattern, compared with 8% in the control series. The most commonly abnormal type is

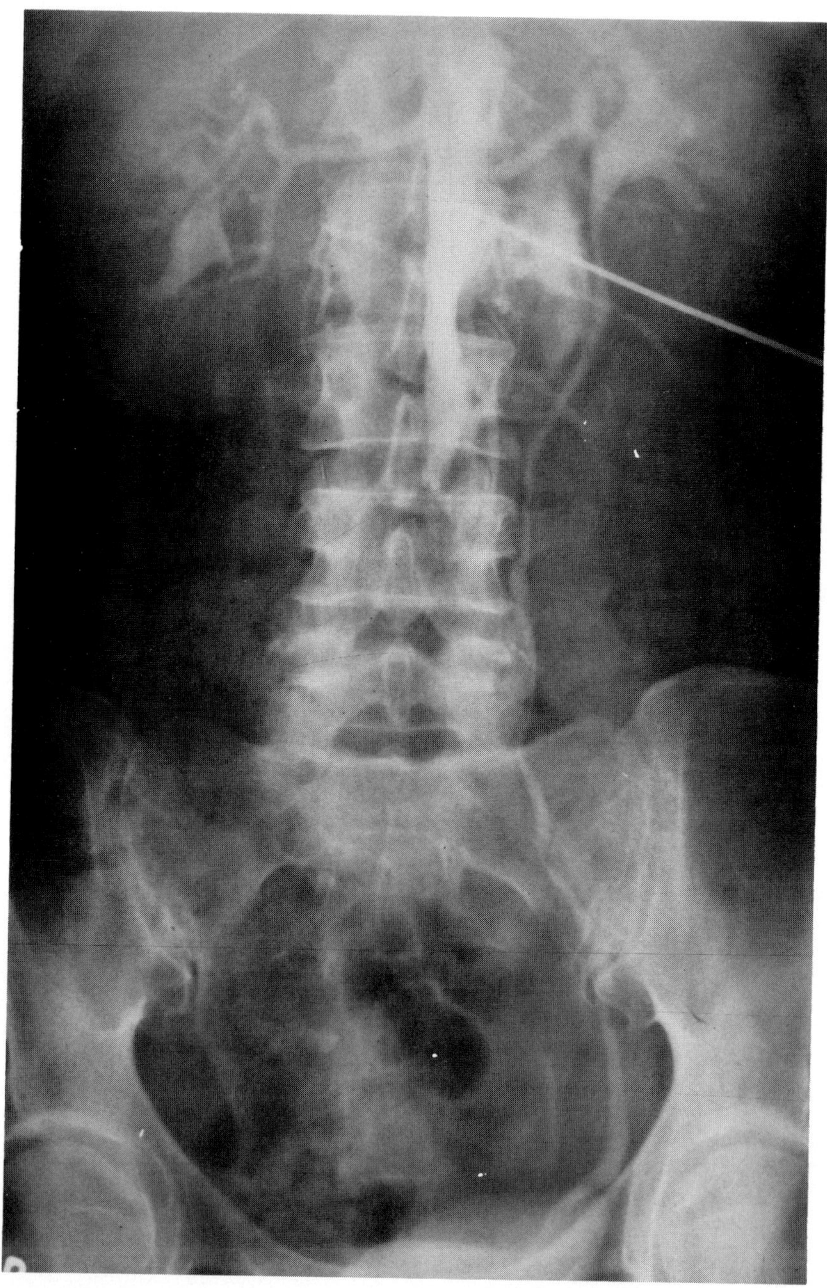

Fig. 3. More severe example. Here the disease at the bifurcation has progressed to occlusion.

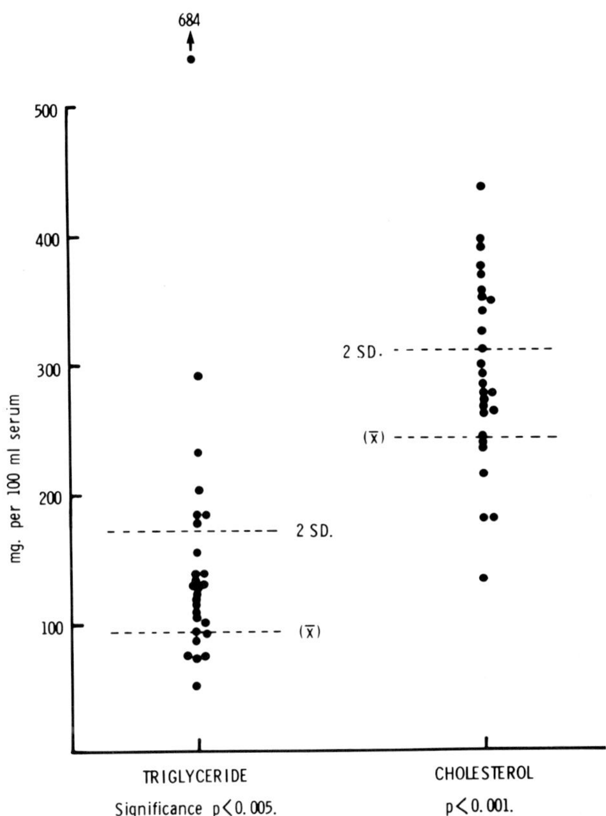

Fig. 4. Serum lipid concentrations in 27 female patients with small aorta syndrome.

type IIA (WHO classification 1970). Only 42% of the men had an abnormal lipoprotein type; of those, type IV was much the commonest abnormality. It should be remembered that type IV lipoprotein disorder indicates a raised level of very low density lipoprotein, with high levels of fasting serum endogenous triglyceride. On the other hand, type IIA represents a raised fasting low density lipoprotein, which implies a high level of fasting serum cholesterol on its own, without a raised triglyceride level.

MANAGEMENT OF THE SMALL AORTA SYNDROME

All 27 of these women came to major aortic reconstructive surgery. Occasionally the disease appeared to be so localized that a local aortic endarterectomy was performed, sometimes with a Dacron patch fashioned in the shape

Table 4
Lipoprotein Patterns in Little Women With Blocked Aortas

	TOTAL ABNORMAL	TYPE 11 a	TYPE 11 b	TYPE 111	TYPE 1V
50 CONTROL PATIENTS	4 (8%)	1	0	0	3
27 LITTLE WOMEN	21 (78%)	14	4	1	2
145 PATIENTS WITH STENOSING ARTERIAL DISEASE. (135 MEN)	61 (42%)	4	9	1	47
SIGNIFICANCE	F test $p < 0.001$.				

of an inverted Y so as to widen the aortic bifurcation and origin of the common iliac arteries. Unfortunately, occasionally the disease passed down the iliac vessels and it became difficult to get below it and achieve a suitable endpoint. On these patients a Dacron bifurcation graft to the external iliac arteries was performed. This was by far the commonest procedure we have performed for this condition. Very occasionally, the Dacron bifurcation graft was taken to the common femoral vessels through separate groin incisions.

It seems that in this group of "little women" forming the small aorta syndrome there is a clue somewhere to the etiology of the atherosclerotic disease process. Here we have a well defined syndrome of patients of one sex and similar height and with disease in exactly the same part of the arterial tree, with the rest of the arterial system apparently spared. The question, of course, is why atheroma should lay down in these patients at exactly that site alone, in the wrong sex and in the wrong age group. Perhaps if we are able to work out the cause of this, we may come closer to unraveling the whole atheroma problem.

REFERENCES

1. Greenhalgh RM: Biochemical abnormalities in gangrene and severe ischaemia of the lower extremities, in Bergan JJ, Yao JST (eds): Gangrene and Severe Ischemia of the Lower Extremities. New York, Grune & Stratton, 1978, pp 39-60
2. Greenhalgh RM, Taylor GW: Little women with blocked aortas. Br. J. Surg. 61:923-924, 1974
3. Sznajderman M, Oliver MF: Spontaneous premature menopause, ischaemic heart disease, and serum-lipids. Lancet 1:962-965, 1963
4. World Health Organization Memorandum: Classification of hyperlipidemia and hyperlipoproteinemia. Bull. WHO 43:891-908, 1970

Hassan Najafi, M.D., Hushang Javid, M.D.,
James A. Hunter, M.D., William S. Dye, M.D.,
Ormand C. Julian, M.D.

Occlusive Diseases of the Branches of the Aortic Arch

Arteriosclerosis, although a generalized disease, makes its most prominent appearance at the origin or bifurcation of the major arteries. In the brachiocephalic system, it causes stenoses and occlusions in the first centimeter or two of the branches arising from the aortic arch, at the origin of the vertebral arteries and the common carotid bifurcations. These lesions are seen far more commonly in males and predominantly in patients over the age of 50. In young women, however, the lesion, usually occlusive rather than stenotic, is secondary to nonspecific arteritis. In most instances, the process involves the proximal segments, sparing the cervical portion of these vessels. The significant implication of this pathologic pattern is its remarkable adaptability to surgical repair.

Fibromuscular hyperplasia has seldom been seen in the proximal segments of the brachiocephalic arteries. Aneurysms of these vessels, causing embolization, can produce cerebral vascular insufficiency or neurologic deficit. However, they are rare. Aortic dissection can also cause brachiocephalic occlusion with resultant cerebral ischemia or infarction. The management of such lesions consists of control of the dissection, rather than direct brachiocephalic reconstruction. An embolism lodging to the innominate bifurcation must be kept in mind as a rare lesion, as it should be removed promptly before irreversible brain damage has occurred.

Pathologic changes in the proximal 1-2 cm of the innominate, left common carotid, and left subclavian arteries interfere in varying degrees with the blood supply of the brain and the upper extremities. Consequently, a great variety of symptoms may result. These include some that are constant and progressive and others that are transient and recurrent. Among the intermittent symptoms are those that accompany isolated lesions at the origins of the internal carotid and the vertebral arteries. These include brief attacks of blurring of vision or blindness, dizziness, vertigo, headaches, diplopia, and transient paresthesia and paresis or incoordination of the extremities, usually unilaterally. More typical of lesions at the aortic arch branch origins are syncope and convulsions, which occur when the patient assumes an erect posture.

It has been estimated that 50%-70% of patients who suffer a major stroke are known to have had one or many of the above symptoms before the development of brain infarction, but it should be emphasized that these lesions do produce stroke as a first manifestation of the disease in an otherwise asymptomatic patient. This suggests that in an asymptomatic patient the objective evidence of significant brachiocephalic arterial occlusive disease may be sufficient to suggest surgical management.

Other clinical manifestations limited to brachiocephalic occlusive disease are facial atrophy, inequalities of the pulses of the cervical carotid arteries and arms, optic atrophy, presenile cataracts, and intermittent claudication of the arms.

The predominance of the ocular symptoms historically was responsible for the fact that ophthalmologists provided the earliest description of this syndrome. In 1908, Takayasu [11] described the course of a 21-year-old woman who lost her vision because of cataracts. In his description of the case, he noted a discrepancy in the pulses in the arms and neck. In 1959, Martorell [6] published an extensive review of the world literature which included 25 additional cases described in the Japanese literature, all occurring in young people and mostly females. In 1951, Shimizu and Sano [10] reported six examples of obstructions of the aortic arch vessels and called it "pulseless disease." Later the term "reverse coarctation" was suggested because the pulses are diminished or absent in the arms while present in the legs, the opposite of aortic coarctation.

Irrespective of terminology, two pathophysiologic mechanisms are responsible for the development of the wide range of clinical features described. The first is the diminished forward flow through the involved vessels and the second, described by Reivich et al. [9] in 1961, is the actual reversal of cerebral blood flow away from the brain.

The location of the lesion or lesions and their relative severity determine the symptoms and signs that will be presented by each patient. These are classifiable into those involving the upper extremities and those involving the brain. The most prominent symptom in the upper extremities is arm pain on exercise. The cerebral symptoms have a tendency to be intermittent. Light-headedness is frequent, but syncope occurring when the patient stands up is likely only in those instances of multiple vessel involvement. When there is subclavian or vertebral artery steal, the cerebral symptoms sometimes can be brought on by exercise of the involved arm.

The anatomical distribution of the lesions in our experience, extending from December 1955 to September 1977, is outlined in Table 1. Proximal subclavian occlusion by far has been the most common lesion and 224 patients were operated upon with a small percentage having had surgery on both subclavian arteries. The second most common lesion was that of obstruction or occlusion of

Table 1
Proximal Brachiocephalic Occlusive Disease,
December 1955 to September 1977

Location	No. of Patients	No. of Procedures	Stroke	Mortality
Subclavian artery	224	248	3 (1.2%)	5 (2%)
Common carotid	106	110	4 (3.6%)	3 (2.7%)
Vertebral artery	96	96	1 (1%)	1 (1%)
Innominate artery	38	38	2 (5%)	3 (7.8%)
Totals (averages)		492	10 (2%)	12 (2.4%)

the common carotid artery, which was rarely seen to be bilateral. This lesion was seen and operated upon in 106 patients. The third was the obstructive lesion involving the origin of the vertebral arteries seen in 106 patients, and in every instance the operation was performed only on one side. Finally, 38 patients presented with innominate artery stenosis or occlusion undergoing surgical reconstruction. Table 1 does not take into account the data relative to the small percentage of patients who had reconstruction of more than one artery such as concomitant innominate and left common carotid or ipsilateral subclavian and carotid reconstruction.

The consistently good results that follow the repair of operable lesions of the branches of the aortic arch encourage their surgical treatment often even in the absence of severe symptoms. As noted in Table 1 the incidence of stroke following brachiocephalic reconstruction in a series of patients undergoing 492 procedures was 2%. The hospital mortality in the same series was 2.4%. The less than 5% accumulative incidence of serious morbidity and mortality is quite acceptable when one takes into consideration the poor prognosis of the disease and the magnitude of the operations employed to improve cerebral circulation. Selection of the patient who should be advised to have an operation depends largely on the absence of any other systemic or atherosclerotic disease severe enough to comprise a contraindication and demonstration by angiography that the lesions are indeed reparable. Angiographic delineation of the aortic arch and its branches is best obtained by the use of a catheter passed retrograde from one of the femoral arteries. If this is not feasible retrograde brachial blowback or catheterization offers an excellent alternative. In several patients because of significant occlusive disease involving the arteries in all four extremities it has not been possible to carry out retrograde aortic root angiography by either the femoral or the brachial channels. In four such instances retrograde catheterization of the aortic arch has been successfully and safely achieved via a translumbar route. The indwelling catheter was left in place for arterial pressure monitoring during the reconstructive surgery in these patients.

Figure 1 demonstrates severe obstruction of the initial portions of all three major branches arising from the aortic arch in a 55-year-old female who also presented with severe aortoiliac occlusive disease precluding retrograde femoral artery catheterization. The arteriographic visualization was achieved by retrograde cannulation of the aortic arch through a percutaneous translumbar aortic needle. She underwent innominate and left carotid reconstruction using a Gore-Tex bifurcation graft designed and prepared at the operation (Fig. 2). The indwelling catheter used for angiography in this patient was left in place to allow blood pressure monitoring during the operation. The success of the innominate reconstruction was immediately apparent when the anesthesiologist could elicit a right arm cuff pressure equal to intraaortic pressure upon the release of the clamp on the innominate graft and restoration of flow into the right subclavian artery.

The armamentarium of surgical therapy of these lesions includes a variety of techniques such as endarterectomy, graft replacement, or bypass grafting [2, 3, 11, 12]. The most commonly employed method of restoration of flow is the implantation of a synthetic bypass graft. Thromboendarterectomy is reserved in this area for those lesions that are short and discrete. The earliest reconstruction of an atherosclerotic occlusion in our series was that of an innominate artery thromboendarterectomy carried out in March 1954 and reported in 1956. In 1961 this patient presented with recurrence of all of his cerebral symptoms. On this occasion the brachiocephalic lesions were more completely treated by the insertion of a Dacron bifurcation graft from the ascending aorta to the right common carotid and left subclavian arteries [5].

Table 2 summarizes our preferred procedures for the various lesions of the brachiocephalic arteries. Occlusion or severe obstruction of the innominate artery is managed by synthetic graft extending from the distal ascending aorta to the distal innominate artery or the proximal common carotid artery depending on the extent of the lesion. We prefer end-to-end innominate anastomosis and this has been possible in the majority of the patients. Temporary intraluminal shunt has not been utilized in recent years, and there have been no instances of cerebral complication in the past ten years. Innominate reconstruction is carried out through a full length median sternotomy with a slight extension of the incision into the base of the neck to allow for better exposure of the proximal subclavian and right common carotid arteries.

Occlusion of the right common carotid artery is managed by endarterectomy or graft replacement of this vessel. The entire right common carotid and the distal portion of the innominate artery can be isolated through a typical carotid endarterectomy incision extending down to the base of the neck. We have not found it necessary to manipulate the right clavicle in any of these patients. If

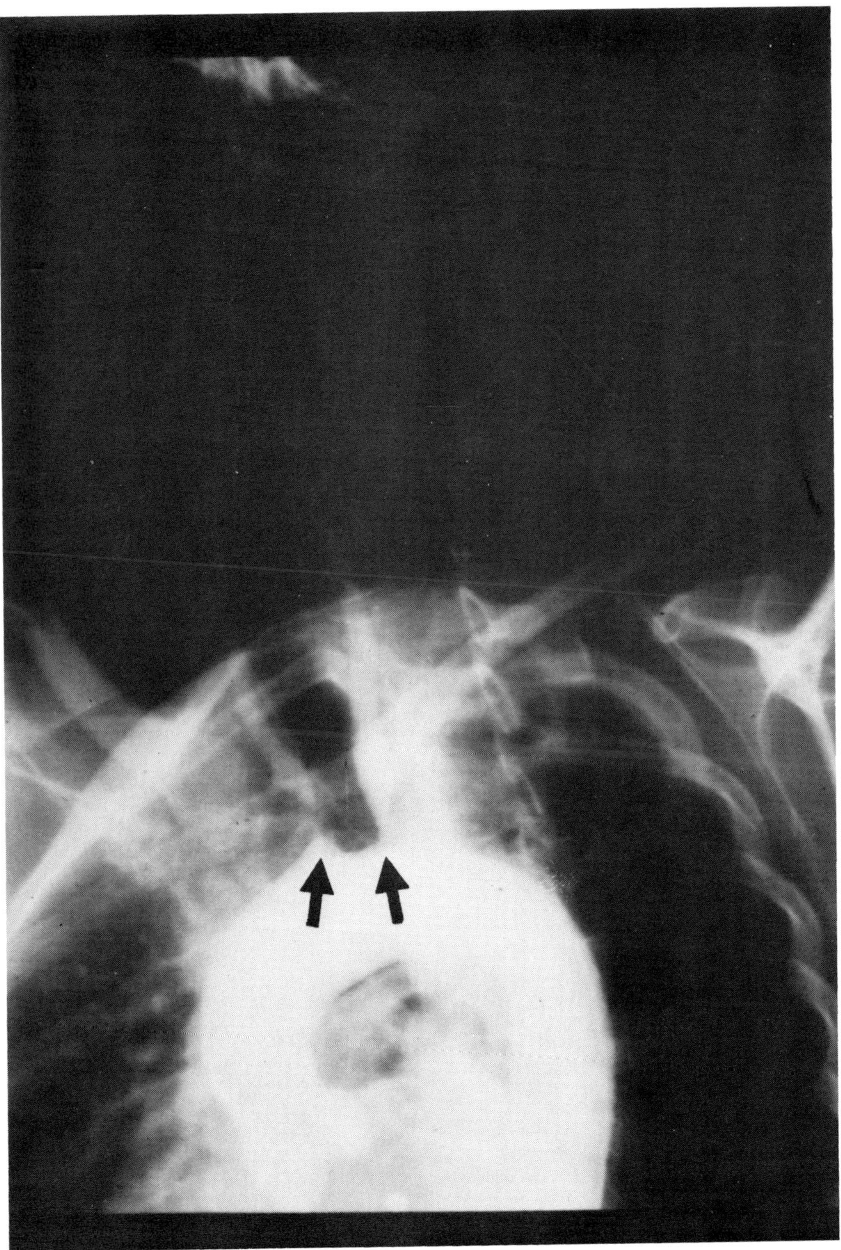

Fig. 1A. Aortic arch angiogram showing severe stenosis of the proximal innominate and left common carotid arteries (arrows). Distally, the arteries appear normal.

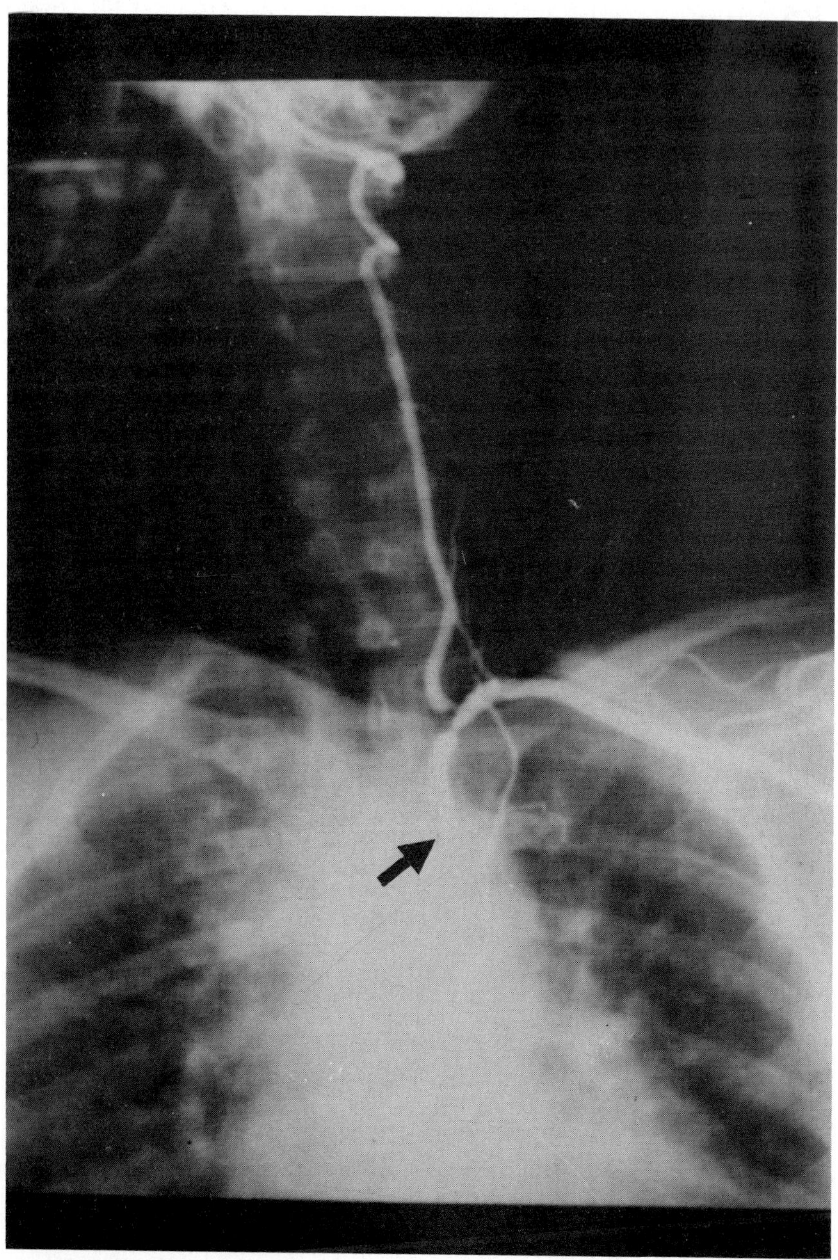

Fig. 1B. Selective left subclavian injection demonstrating severe stenosis of the origins of the subclavian and vertebral arteries. These injections were made via a long catheter inserted into the aortic arch through a translumbar aortic needle.

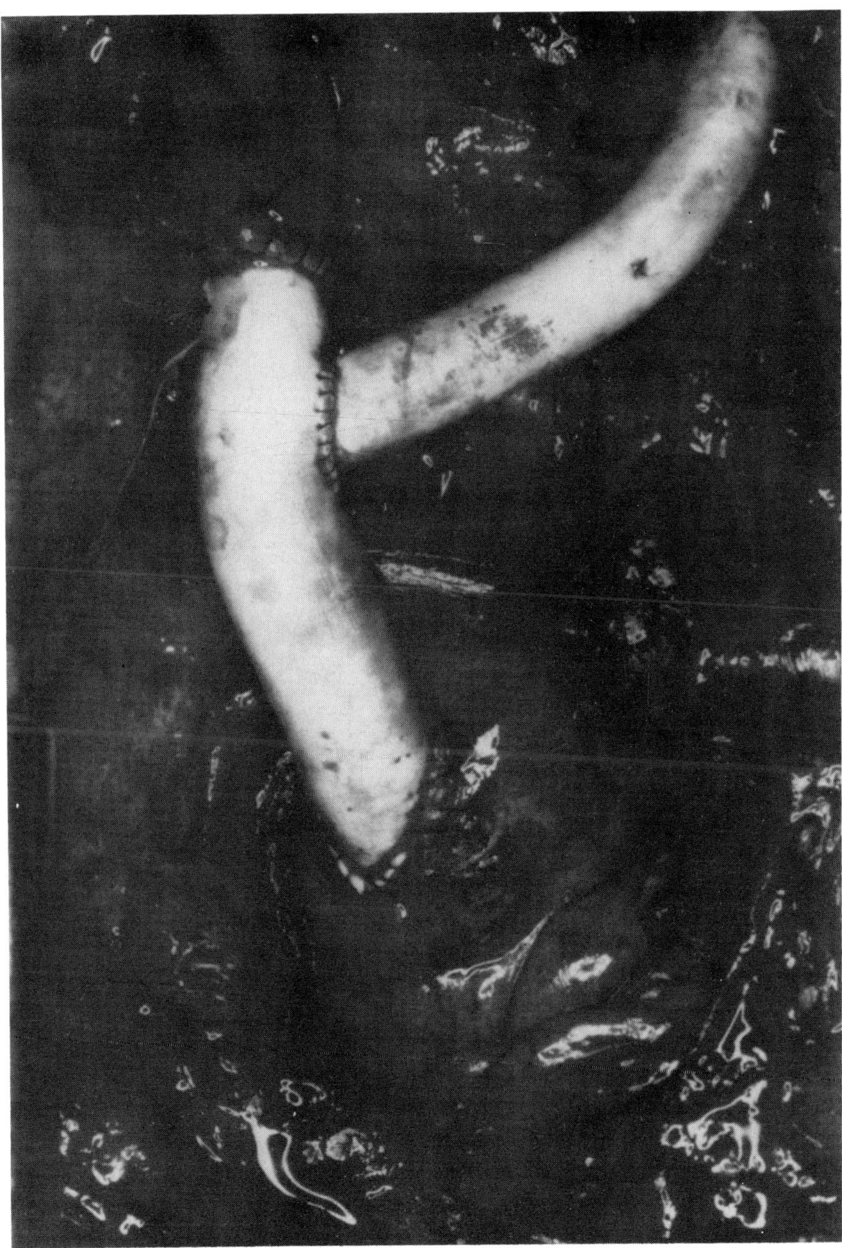

Fig. 2. Operative photograph demonstrating a Gore-Tex bifurcation graft extending from the distal ascending aorta to the innominate and left common carotid arteries in the same patient.

Table 2
Brachiocephalic Occlusive Disease: Surgical Management

Arterial Lesions	Procedures
Innominate	Ascending aorta to innominate or carotid bypass
Right carotid	Endarterectomy or graft replacement
Left carotid	Left subclavian—left internal carotid bypass
	Left carotid endarterectomy
Subclavian	Carotid subclavian bypass

endarterectomy is performed, liberal use of an elliptical patch angioplasty is encouraged for small carotid arteries. The alternative procedure consisting of subclavian-internal carotid bypass is best suited for the left common carotid occlusion. If the left subclavian artery is compromised by virtue of obstruction, occlusion, or calcification, then a total left common carotid endarterectomy can be carried out. Some of the technical details of this operation are demonstrated in Fig. 3.

Occasionally proximal brachiocephalic lesions are accompanied by obstructive atheroma at the common carotid bifurcations. The most fascinating example of this association occurred in an extremely overweight 53-year-old woman who presented with frequent transient ischemic attacks and repetitious syncopal episodes. On examination all of her peripheral pulses were absent except for the

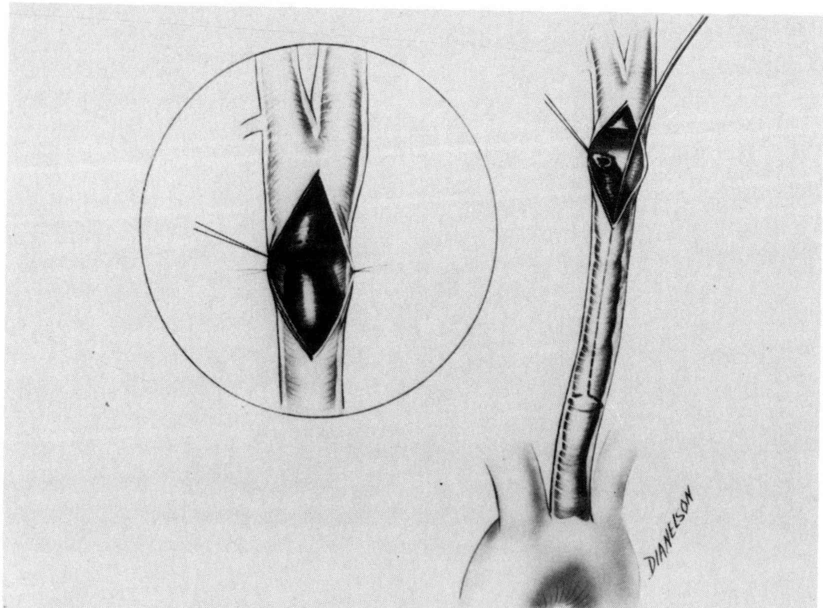

Fig. 3. Schematic drawing demonstrating some of the technical aspects of retrograde left common carotid endarterectomy.

left common carotid pulse. A loud bruit over the bifurcation of this artery led to a left percutaneous carotid arteriogram which revealed patent internal carotid but partially obstructed external carotid artery, accounting for the bruit. We had not as yet utilized translumbar cannulation of the aortic arch under these circumstances. Therefore the state of the distal arteries remained obscure and open to speculation. Because of her severe disability and extremely poor prognosis we elected to proceed with surgical exploration. Preparation and draping were carried out in such a manner to allow for extensive reconstruction including if necessary insertion of a graft extending from the ascending aorta to the distal brachiocephalic arteries. Accordingly the operation initially consisted of a right carotid exploration which revealed pulseless but normal internal and common carotid arteries with severe stenotic plaque at the carotid bifurcation. This of course encouraged the second phase of the procedure, which consisted of a sternotomy and exploration of the innominate artery. This vessel was occluded proximally but was otherwise perfectly normal. Consequently a 10 mm Dacron tube graft was anastomosed end-to-side to the distal ascending aorta using a partially occluding clamp. The distal end of the graft was then anastomosed to the distal divided end of the innominate artery, thereby restoring normal flow into the right subclavian and the right common carotid arteries. At this time a routine right carotid bifurcation endarterectomy utilizing a temporary intraluminal shunt completed the procedure. She is now 3 years postoperative, has remained asymptomatic, and has maintained normal right carotid and right arm pulses.

Proximal occlusion has occurred most frequently in the subclavian arteries in our series. Approximately two-thirds of the patients with subclavian occlusion presented with symptoms of cerebral vascular insufficiency. The symptom complex was that usually caused by vertebral basilar insufficiency. Arm symptoms and in particular intermittent claudication were seen in a small percentage of these patients. In almost every instance, except for patients with bilateral subclavian involvement, discrepancy in the quality and intensity of the upper extremity pulses and blood pressure was noted. Those with complete occlusion of the subclavian artery did not present with a systolic bruit, while severe proximal obstruction was associated with a loud bruit and in most instances a palpable thrill over the course of the involved subclavian artery.

Vertebral subclavian steal due to proximal obstruction or occlusion of the subclavian artery often is distinguishable clinically by a simple maneuver involving the use of two oscillometers (Fig. 4). An oscillometer is placed on each arm above the elbow. Digital compression of the common carotid artery in the neck will cause severe diminution or abolition of the oscillometric index of the same arm in the presence of subclavian occlusion compensated by reversal of vertebral flow. This observation must be controlled by an oscillometric tracing of the contralateral arm to be sure that a decrease in oscillation on the test side is not due simply to carotid sinus repressive reflexes [4].

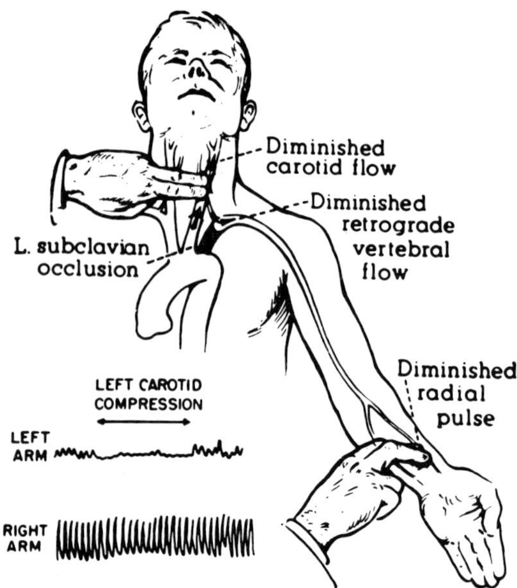

Fig. 4. Schematic drawing demonstrating the simple technique of carotid compression test for detection of subclavian steal phenomenon.

A totally isolated proximal subclavian occlusion is commonly asymptomatic and is unlikely to produce a stroke. When a lesion is asymptomatic it should not be considered as a surgical target. Factors influencing symptomatology include the size and patency of the opposite vertebral artery, the anatomy of the circle of Willis, other sources of collateral circulation to the arm, and other coexisting cerebral arterial lesions. Many patients with clinical syndrome of vertebral basilar insufficiency, whether it is secondary to subclavian steal syndrome or primary lesions of the vertebral arteries, have concomitant occlusive lesions in the carotid system. Experience has shown that carotid endarterectomy may so favorably influence the vertebral symptoms that further surgery on the subclavian or vertebral artery is not required [3, 7, 12]. The restoration of carotid circulation increases total cerebral blood flow, improves the collateral circulation to the posterior system, and so relieves the manifestation of ischemia. The importance of detailed serial arteriographic studies of both the carotid and subclavian vertebral systems under these circumstances is thus apparent.

In terms of surgical management a variety of operations have been applied. The operative procedure of choice, however, is that of a bypass graft extending from the common carotid to the distal subclavian artery. Although autogenous saphenous vein has been utilized as bypass conduit, a Dacron tube graft and more recently Gore-Tex graft has been employed with much greater frequency. If the common carotid artery is completely normal the flow through it into the brain will not be diminished by giving the proximal carotid artery the added load of subclavian artery supply. An extension of this technique has been applied to a number of patients presenting with proximal subclavian disease and significant lesion of the carotid bifurcation on the same side. Carotid endarterectomy is accomplished in the usual manner and subclavian flow is restored using a carotid-subclavian bypass [8]. Earlier in our experience we operated upon some 65 patients with left subclavian occlusion utilizing a tube graft from the proximal descending aorta to the left subclavian artery, all performed within the left hemithorax. This operation was successful in restoring circulation into the subclavian artery in every instance, but because of the major nature of the operation it was subsequently abandoned in preference to left carotid-subclavian bypass. We have, however, continued to use descending aorta-left subclavian bypass when no other alternatives have been available. Although we are very much aware of the preference many outstanding vascular surgeons have for endarterectomy under these circumstances, particularly in relation to the innominate artery [1], we have in general preferred the use of synthetic arterial implant as bypass conduits.

Regardless of individual preference, the surgeon engaged in operative management of lesions of the brachiocephalic arteries must be versatile and sufficiently imaginative to take full advantage of all available or inventive vascular techniques. This region of the arterial tree is particularly prone to a wide

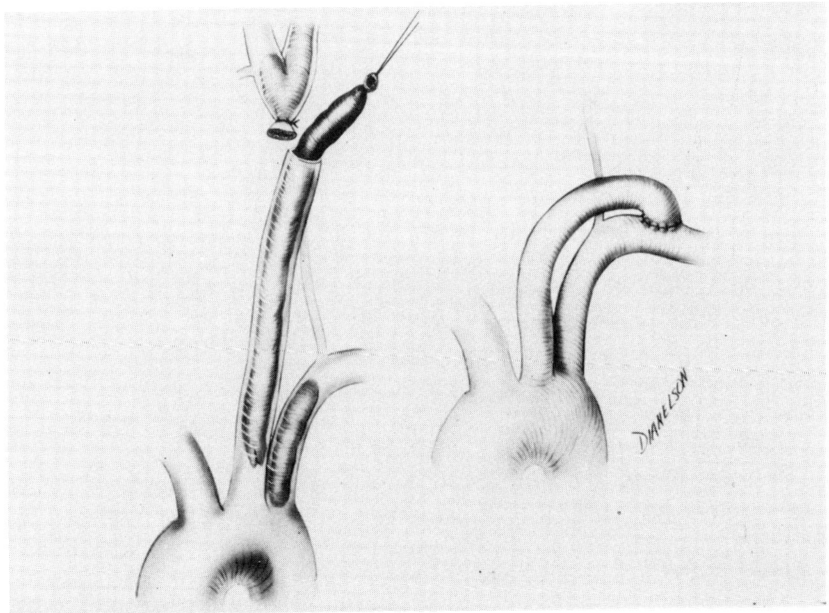

Fig. 5. Left carotid-subclavian bypass using the endarterectomized common carotid artery.

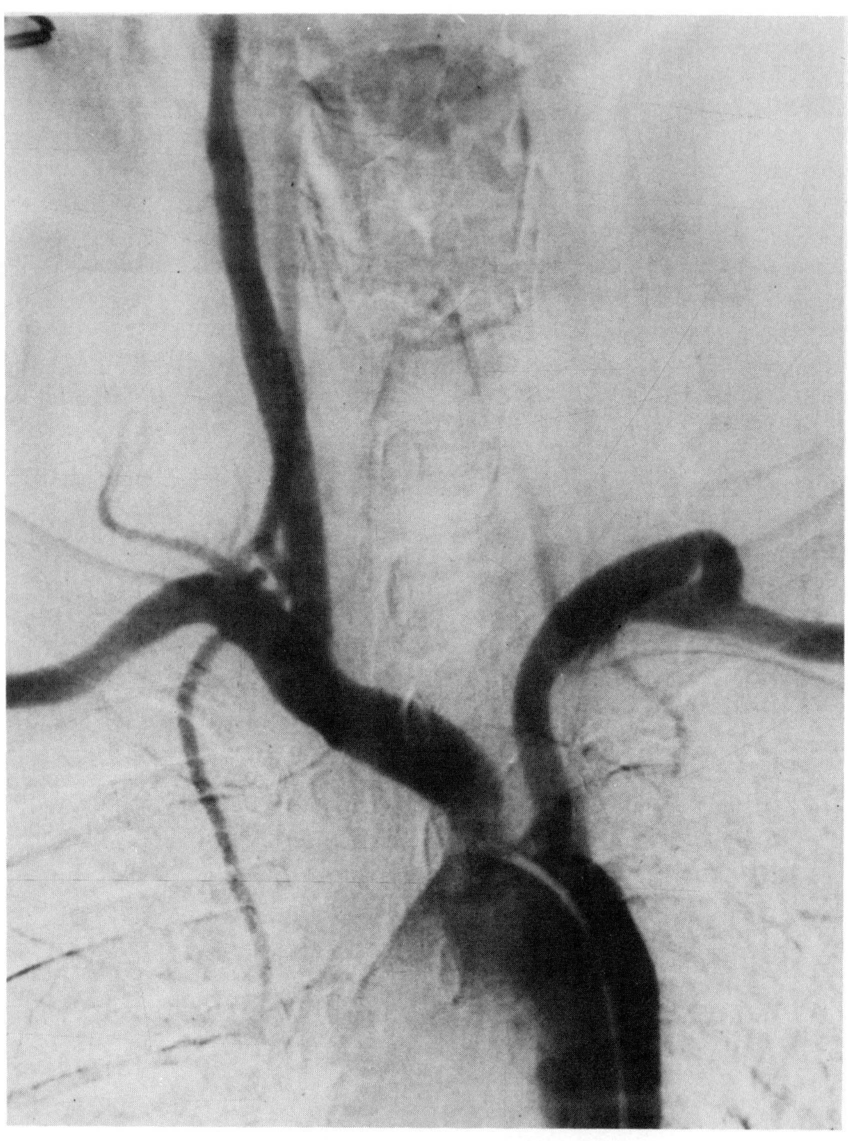

Fig. 6. Postoperative arch angiography demonstrating the patent left carotid-subclavian bypass.

spectrum of combinations of lesions, at times requiring a special and innovative surgical approach. This is best illustrated by a very symptomatic patient presenting with complete occlusion of the left internal carotid, left common carotid, and left subclavian arteries. Disabling symptoms of basilar arterial insufficiency in this patient were relieved by an extraordinary operation shown in Figs. 5 and 6. The totally occluded and useless left common carotid artery was endarterectomized and used as an autogenous conduit to restore normal circulation into the left subclavian and vertebral arteries. This operation is superior to crossover bypass from the other side of the neck and safer than aorta-left subclavian or axillary bypass reported by others.

REFERENCES

1. Carlson RE, Ehrenfeld WK, Stoney RJ, et al: Innominate endarterectomy: A 16 year experience. Arch. Surg. 112:1389, 1977
2. Crawford ES, DeBakey ME, Morris GC Jr, et al: Surgical treatment of occlusion of the innominate, common carotid, and subclavian arteries: A 10 year experience. Surgery 65:17, 1969
3. DeBakey ME: Successful carotid endarterectomy for cerebrovascular insufficiency. Nineteen-year follow-up. JAMA 233:1083, 1975
4. Javid H, Julian OC, Dye WS, et al: Management of cerebral arterial insufficiency caused by reversal of flow. Arch. Surg. 90:634, 1965
5. Julian OC, Javid H: Surgical management of cerebral arterial insufficiency. Curr. Prob. Surg. March 1971
6. Martorell F: El sindrome de obliteracion de los troncos supreaorticos. Angiologia 11:301, 1959
7. Najafi H, Cagle JE, Javid H, et al: Bilateral carotid arteriography: Its adequacy in cerebrovascular insufficiency evaluation. Arch. Surg. 98:53, 1969
8. Najafi H, Dye WS, Javid H, et al: Carotid bifurcation stenosis and ipsilateral subclavian steal. Arch. Surg. 99:289, 1969
9. Reivich M, Howling HE, Roberts B, et al: Reversal of blood flow through the vertebral artery and its effect on cerebral circulation. N. Engl. J. Med. 265:878, 1961
10. Shimizu K, Sano K: Pulseless disease. J. Neuropathol. Exp. Neurol. 1:37, 1951
11. Takayasu M: Case of queer changes in central vessels of retina. Acta Soc. Ophthalmol. Jpn. 12:554, 1908
12. Thompson JE, Patman RD, Talkington CM: Carotid surgery for cerebrovascular insufficiency. Curr. Prob. Surg. 15, December 1978

Jesse E. Thompson, M.D.

Elective Surgery for Abdominal Aortic Aneurysms

Since the report of Dubost, Allary, and Oeconomos [12] in 1951 of the first resection and homograft replacement of an atherosclerotic abdominal aortic aneurysm, great strides have been made in the treatment of this disease. The natural history of aortic aneurysms has been more clearly delineated, indications for operation have been more precisely defined, surgical management has become standardized, unusual manifestations and complications have been described, and operation is being performed with progressively lower mortality and morbidity rates. Because of the lethal nature of untreated aneurysmal disease from rupture, ideal therapy is elective surgical repair in all cases before rupture ensues. While this goal has not been achieved, continuing efforts toward earlier diagnosis have undoubtedly reduced the incidence of ruptured aneurysms.

The average age of patients operated upon for aortic aneurysms is about 65 years. The occurrence of numerous other diseases, especially complications of atherosclerosis, is a well-documented fact [11, 27, 32]. In our series 74% of the patients had one or more serious conditions. These included hypertension, diabetes mellitus, cardiac disease, renal disease, cerebrovascular disease, aortoiliac and femoral occlusive disease, and chronic obstructive pulmonary disease [32]. It is thus obvious that one is dealing with a group of elderly patients with multiple high-risk factors which must be evaluated critically when indications for elective operation are under consideration.

GENERAL PRINCIPLES OF MANAGEMENT

Diagnosis of abdominal aneurysm is usually easily made by the presence of a palpable pulsating mass or a line of calcium on an x-ray film, especially in the lateral projection. Recent employment of noninvasive techniques for confirmation of the diagnosis of aneurysm in questionable cases and for screening of patients with known atherosclerosis in other areas is a major advance and has lead to earlier and more accurate diagnosis in many instances. B-mode ultrasonic scanning (sonography) is the method most commonly used [6, 18, 22, 23]. Measurements of aneurysmal size on the scan have correlated closely with those made in the operating room. With this technique it is also possible to follow any increase in size of aneurysms which for one reason or another were not operated upon when first seen.

The question of performing aortography in cases of aortic aneurysm has been a controversial one. Since the advent of sonography, aortography is not necessary to establish the diagnosis of aneurysm. However, numerous reports attest to its usefulness in demonstrating lesions in the celiac, mesenteric, renal, cerebral, iliac, and femoral arteries [9, 26, 34]. It is particularly helpful in the presence of multiple renal arteries and in the rare instances of horseshoe kidney. When unsuspected aneurysmal or occlusive lesions are demonstrated, operative procedures may be better planned in advance. With increasing use of retrograde techniques through the femoral or axillary arteries under local anesthesia, risks and complications of aortography are at a very low level. At the present time we are utilizing preoperative aortograms in most cases of abdominal aneurysm.

In addition to the usual complete preoperative evaluation, patients with any degree of chronic obstructive pulmonary disease should undergo pulmonary function studies and then be given appropriate therapy preparatory to aneurysmectomy. This has been one of the most important improvements in the pre- and postoperative management of aneurysm patients. An intravenous urogram should be obtained in every case, as should a thorough cardiac evaluation.

INDICATIONS FOR OPERATION

Since the untreated abdominal aortic aneurysm carries a high incidence of fatal or serious complications (including rupture, whether retroperitoneal, intraperitoneal, duodenal, or caval), embolism into the lower extremities, and infection, the guiding premise is that most patients with unruptured aneurysms are candidates for elective surgical repair. A number of considerations enter in to lend credence to this statement as well as modify it. These include the natural history of aortic aneurysm with respect to the risk of rupture, the relationship of aneurysmal size to rupture, survival rates in untreated patients, the presence or absence of symptoms, the age of the patient, and the presence of multiple risk factors from associated medical conditions. Balanced against these items are the risk of operation and the survival rates following elective aneurysmectomy.

Studies by Bernstein and his associates have elucidated many aspects of the natural history of aortic aneurysms [5, 6]. Using B-mode scans, the mean growth rate of aneurysms ranging from 3 to 6 cm in diameter was found to be 0.4 cm per year [6].

Based on autopsy statistics, the rate of aneurysm rupture is approximately 28%, ranging from 15% to 50%. In five clinical series the rate of rupture was 31% [16]. Mortality in the patient with an untreated ruptured aneurysm is almost 100%. Size of the aneurysm has a dominant effect on rupture rate [5]. The mean rupture rate of aneurysms smaller than 5 cm in diameter appears to be about 5%. Aneurysms less than 6 cm in size have a mean rupture rate of 16%, but if they are 7 cm or larger, the rupture rate is 76%. There is thus a sharp and dramatic increase in the risk of rupture when an aneurysm attains a size of 6 cm [28]. Bernstein states that he has not observed rupture in an aneurysm that was less than 4 cm in size [5].

If associated medical conditions (e.g., malignancy, renal failure, etc.) make the risk of elective aneurysm repair overwhelming or impose an obligatory limitation on life expectancy of two years or less, operation should not be done. All other patients, regardless of age, should be considered for elective repair. This is especially true if the aneurysm is symptomatic (unruptured) or is greater than 6 cm in diameter. Many borderline situations exist, based on risk factors which make individual decisions difficult. In general, small asymptomatic aneurysms in younger patients should be operated upon. For older patients with small asymptomatic aneurysms and multiple risk factors it may be appropriate to follow the size of the aneurysm with sonograms. If the aneurysm enlarges and risk of rupture increases, operation may be performed, with acceptance of a higher operative risk. With time, as operative mortality has decreased, indications for operation in the older patient with multiple risk factors have been liberalized and contraindications have narrowed [28].

A special problem is the patient over the age of 80 with an aortic aneurysm. Until recently, operation was not recommended unless the aneurysm became symptomatic or ruptured and the patient was free of other serious diseases [4]. O'Donnell et al. [24], in a recent study, have recommended liberalization of indications in the octagenarian based on their operative mortality rate of 4.7%. They emphasized *physiological* rather than chronological age of the patient, acceptable long-term survival, and satisfactory quality of life following operation. For patients in this age group very careful selection must be made and all the necessary technical and support facilities must be available.

In view of all the above considerations it would appear that an aggressive surgical approach to the treatment of unruptured aortic aneurysms is justified. Further data relating to operative mortality and morbidity and long-term survival rates will be given below.

OPERATIVE TECHNIQUE

Skillful anesthetic management is of the utmost importance when operation is carried out on these elderly atherosclerotic patients. A Foley catheter is routinely placed in the bladder and a nasogastric tube inserted into the stomach.

An ECG monitor is used in every case. Central venous pressure and intraarterial lines may be used but are not routine. A Swan-Ganz catheter is occasionally employed in poor risk patients. Blood gases are checked routinely.

The technique of abdominal aneurysmectomy has become fairly well standardized. Minimal dissection is the essential feature. No effort is made to remove the aneurysm in toto as was done in the early days. The sac is simply opened, all clots are evacuated, and the lumbar arteries are sutured from within. This single step reduces tremendously operative complications. A preclotted knitted Dacron graft is then sutured into place with Dacron sutures, and the aneurysm wall, if sufficiently voluminous, covers the graft. Either a bifurcation or tubular graft may be used depending upon the aneurysm. Heparin is injected locally and systemically during clamping but is not employed postoperatively. Figures 1-3 illustrate the essential steps of a standard aneurysm repair. At times an end-to-side iliac anastomosis is performed rather than end-to-end because of a calcified posterior iliac artery wall. Occasionally the distal anastomoses are into the common femoral arteries.

One useful technical maneuver is shown in Fig. 4. A cuff of Dacron is slipped over the upper aortic anastomosis prior to clamp removal. This cuff supports the suture line, reduces bleeding, and isolates the anastomosis from small bowel.

Occasionally proximal control may be difficult, especially with inflammatory or ruptured aneurysms. One may obtain control at the level of the diaphragm manually, with a clamp, or with a special depressor. Another useful method is the insertion of a large Foley catheter through the aneurysm into the aorta above. Inflating the balloon controls bleeding temporarily and provides time for definitive control below.

Proper fluid therapy during and after aortic surgery is of critical importance in preventing hypotensive and renal complications. We previously reported [32, 33] in detail a regimen of fluid therapy for aortic surgery, which we have continued to use with certain refinements. Its basis is 5% dextrose in lactated Ringer's solution, and it is outlined in Table 1.

A liter of Ringer's is infused quickly at the beginning of anesthesia in order to promote urine flow. As a rule this solution is infused thereafter at the rate of about 500 ml per hour of operation. Blood is replaced volume for volume as lost. If packed red cells are used, each unit is accompanied by the infusion of two units of fresh-frozen plasma. This allows for adequate blood pressure levels without vasopressors and for good urinary output of at least 50 ml per hour. Postoperatively one reduces the Ringer's sharply, giving only enough to replace extrarenal losses and extracellular fluid which is sequestered in the operative site and legs. During the first 24 postoperative hours about 1 liter of Ringer's is used and the principal solution is dextrose in water, as in the second 24 hours.

One must use this regimen judiciously, as determined by the individual patient, in order to keep blood pressure and urinary output at appropriate levels but at the same time to avoid overload of the cardiovascular system. Hourly

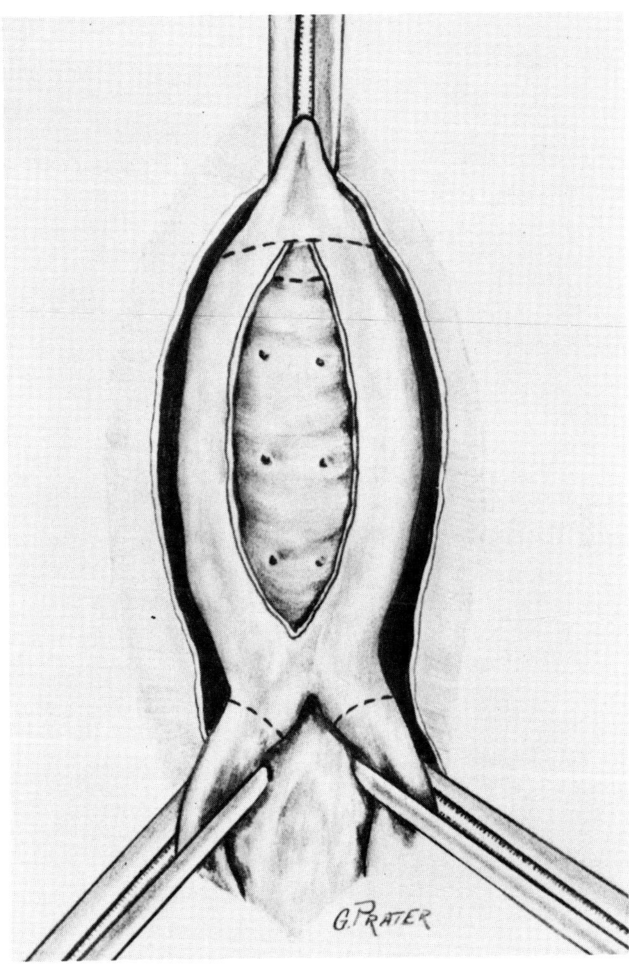

Fig. 1. First step in aortic aneurysm repair showing minimal dissection of aorta and iliac arteries and intrasaccular incision and exposure. No attempt is made to resect the aneurysm wall. [From Thompson JE, Hollier LH, Patman RD, et al: Surgical management of abdominal aortic aneurysms. Ann. Surg. 181:654, 1975. Used by permission of the J. B. Lippincott Company.]

urine output is routinely recorded and intraarterial and central venous pressures are monitored as indicated. It should be emphasized that the principal solution is 5% *dextrose* in lactated Ringer's. The osmotic effect of the dextrose in the Ringer's solution is very important, since if Ringer's solution only is used to keep the urinary output at satisfactory levels serious problems with fluid overload may result. The physiological basis of this regimen is the replacement of sequestered nonfunctional extracellular fluid with balanced salt solution in

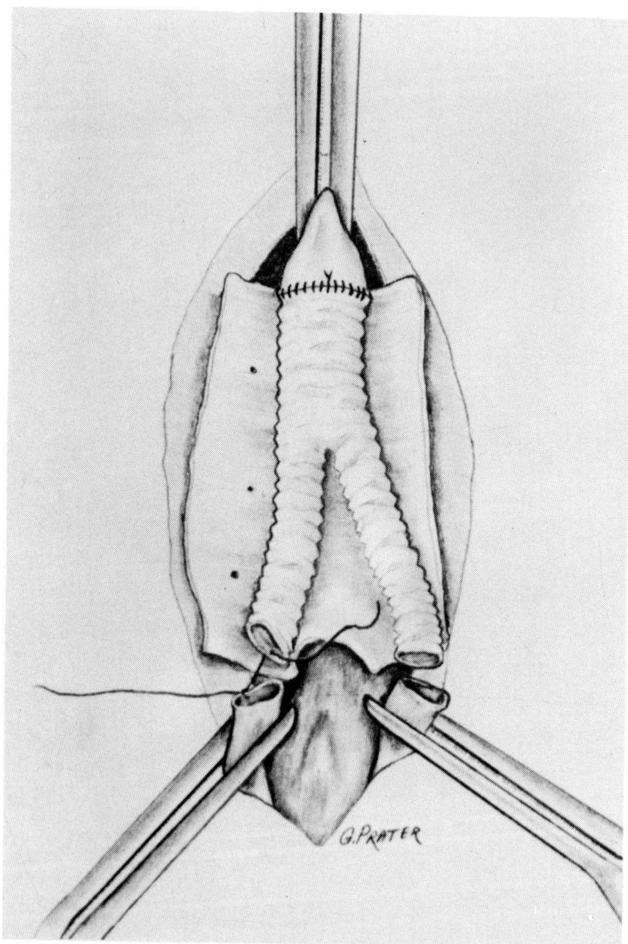

Fig. 2. Knitted Dacron graft is sutured to the proximal aortic stump with polyester sutures. Bleeding lumbar arteries are sutured from within the aneurysm sac. Right iliac anastomosis begun. [From Thompson JE, Hollier LH, Patman RD, et al: Surgical management of abdominal aortic aneurysms. Ann. Surg. 181:654, 1975. Used by permission of the J. B. Lippincott Company.]

order to maintain an effective circulating blood volume [25]. Other adjuncts such as plasma, plasma expanders, mannitol, etc. are not necessary.

All patients are placed in the intensive care unit for 3 days and are monitored continuously. Recent introduction of IPPB treatments, ultrasonic nebulization, and other innovations in respiratory tract therapy has been a significant feature of postoperative care. Occasionally a simple tube gastrostomy is constructed at the time of aortic operation to facilitate respiratory care in the elderly, obese, poor-risk, or pulmonary-cripple patient.

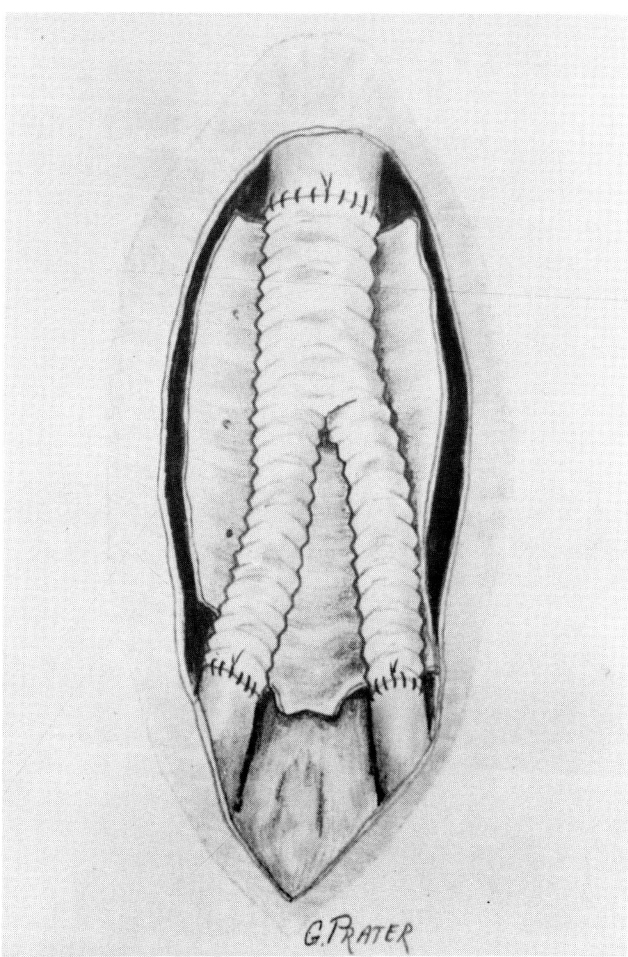

Fig. 3. Completed graft replacement for abdominal aneurysm. If the aneurysm wall is sufficiently voluminous, it is sutured over the graft, thus excluding the Dacron from direct contact with bowel and other viscera. [From Thompson JE, Hollier LH, Patman RD, et al: Surgical management of abdominal aortic aneurysms. Ann. Surg. 181:654, 1975. Used by permission of the J. B. Lippincott Company.]

All patients receive antibiotics prophylactically beginning the day prior to operation, continuing during operation and for 3 or 4 days postoperatively. At present the preferred antibiotic is sodium cephalothin or cefazolin. Topical antibiotic solution containing neomycin and bacitracin is used routinely during operation to flush the area of graft repair, the abdominal wound, and any groin incisions.

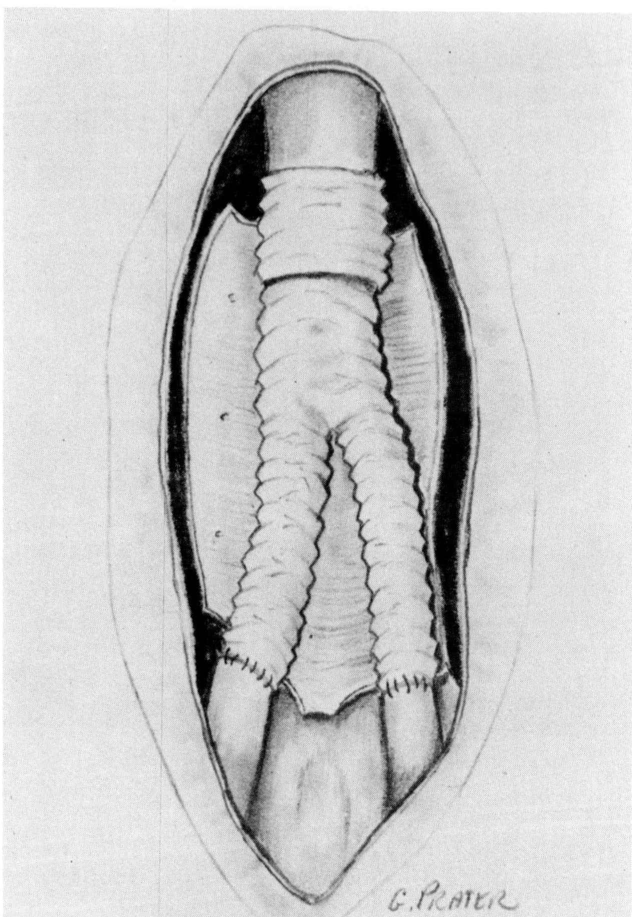

Fig. 4. Variant in the technique of upper aortic anastomosis, showing a cuff of Dacron placed over the suture line. This cuff reduces bleeding upon clamp removal, obviates postoperative hemorrhage, supports the suture line and proximal cuff of aorta when the latter is thin or aneurysmal, and isolates the suture line from small intestine, decreasing the possibility of aortoenteric fistulas. [From Thompson JE, Hollier LH, Patman RD, et al: Surgical management of abdominal aortic aneurysms. Ann. Surg. 181:654, 1975. Used by permission of the J. B. Lippincott Company.]

COMPLICATIONS

Serious complications peculiar to aortic surgery may result unless one is meticulous in surgical management. Ischemia of the legs may occur from embolization of debris or distal thrombosis [31]. Inadequate heparinization may

Table 1
Regimen of Fluid Therapy for Aortic Surgery (Liters)

	Operative	First 24 Hrs Postoperative	Second 24 Hrs Postoperative
Blood	As lost	0	0
5% dextrose in Ringer's lactate	3-4*	1	½
5% dextrose in water	½	2½	2

*Usual infusion rate *during operation* — 500 ml/hour.

be a factor, or the patient may have extensive distal disease requiring anastomosis into the femoral arteries or beyond. Gentleness in handling the aneurysm usually prevents distal embolization.

Renal failure is a serious complication which can usually be prevented by proper administration of fluids and avoidance of hypotension, especially at the time of declamping. In one series of 108 consecutive aneurysmectomies, there were no deaths from renal failure and no patient required dialysis [32].

Ischemia of the large bowel is a catastrophic event when it occurs [20]. The presence of a large "meandering mesenteric" should alert one to the possibility of major mesenteric vascular occlusion, and a bypass into the celiac or superior mesenteric systems may have to be constructed. As a rule the inferior mesenteric artery may be ligated with impunity unless it is large or unless its stump pressure is less than 40 mm Hg, when it may have to be reimplanted into the aortic graft [13]. Great care should be taken to avoid injury to the left colic artery arising from the inferior mesenteric during dissection of the aneurysm.

Spinal cord ischemia is a particularly devastating complication of aortic surgery [29]. Fortunately it is very rare following elective aneurysmectomy, being ten times more common in ruptured cases than in unruptured ones. Unfortunately its occurrence is largely unpredictable.

UNUSUAL MANIFESTATIONS

A number of unusual manifestations of abdominal aneurysm have been observed and recorded. Table 2 lists the more common ones. Awareness of these problems, recognition at the time of operation, and proper handling are imperative if such catastrophic complications as massive hemorrhage or loss of a kidney are to be averted. Appropriate methods of managing all these special problems have been reported and have undoubtedly resulted in reduced morbidity [8, 17].

Table 2
Unusual Manifestations of Aortic Aneurysms

Renal artery problems
Multiple, arising from aneurysm
Stenosis at origin
Renal vein variations
Retroaortic
Low-lying left vein
Circumaortic collar
Vena cava problems
Double vena cava
Left-sided cava
Aortocaval fistula
Horseshoe kidney
Inflammatory aneurysm

Renal artery problems are best recognized from preoperative aortograms and appropriate surgical plans can be made. Aberrant vessels may be implanted into the graft, or bypass grafts to the renal artery may be constructed to relieve occlusive lesions. Shunts may be used to perfuse the kidney in complicated resections [10].

Retroaortic left renal vein is the most common venous variant seen. Careful dissection is necessary for definition of the problem and avoidance of massive hemorrhage. Aortocaval fistulas are best repaired by a transaortic aneurysm approach; a major problem here is pulmonary embolism of debris from the aneurysm lumen.

Management of horseshoe kidney depends on the origin of the blood supply to renal tissue [7]. The renal arteries may arise in the usual location, from a single vessel below the kidney, from the iliac arteries, or as multiple arteries from the aneurysm itself.

Inflammatory aneurysm repair may be a very difficult technical problem because of the fibrosis and inflammation, making proximal control extremely difficult [15]. Intraaortic balloon tamponade may be required. The distal limbs may be sewn into the external iliacs or even the common femoral arteries if necessary.

RESULTS OF SURGICAL THERAPY

Operative mortality for elective aneurysm repair has progressively decreased in the past 25 years. Thus in our own experience [32] with 432 patients the operative mortality from 1954 to 1961 was 17%; from 1962 to 1967 it was 7.4%; and from 1968 to 1978 was 6.4% despite increasing liberalization of indications for operation, especially in the elderly atherosclerotic with multiple risk factors. Recent deaths have been largely cardiac and pulmonary in origin, whereas in the early days we lost patients from intestinal gangrene, anastomotic leaks, and renal failure, causes which were technical in nature or related to improper fluid management.

A survey of several representative series of elective aneurysm operations in the recent literature shows the operative mortality to range from zero to 9.8%, with a mean of about 5%. All authors report improvement with increasing experience [1, 3, 11, 19, 21, 27, 30, 32, 34]. No doubt these figures could be improved in many instances by more stringent selection criteria. However, the fate of those judged unfit for operation is such that the latter approach does not seem proper [28]. In fact, indications for operation have been broadened rather than contracted. An operative mortality rate in the range of 3%-7% appears to be reasonable and acceptable for these patients.

Several studies [2, 4, 5, 11, 14, 28, 30] have compared the long-term survival rates of patients with untreated aortic aneurysms with those of patients undergoing surgical resection and graft replacement. All are in substantial agreement that elective surgery prolongs life expectancy. Patients with untreated aortic aneurysms have a very poor outlook. Almost half die during the first year following diagnosis, about 75% are dead at 5 years, and all are dead at 10 years. The principal cause of death is rupture of the aneurysm. By contrast, of those operated upon, about 20% die during the first postoperative year, 50% are dead at 5 years, while about 25% are still alive at 10 years. The chief cause of long-term death in the operated group is cardiac disease. The 5-year survival rate for the normal population of similar age and sex is approximately 81%.

Since surgical therapy can be shown to increase life expectancy in patients with aortic aneurysms and fatal rupture can be prevented by elective resection, it is important, therefore, that diagnosis be made and definitive therapy carried out before this catastrophic event occurs. It is likewise imperative that operative mortality and morbidity be at the lowest possible levels if maximum benefit is to accrue from surgical management, since the limiting factors of coronary disease and other complications of atherosclerosis are still operative after aneursym removal. It has already been noted that mortality and morbidity rates related to operation have become progressively lower during the 28 years since Dubost's original operation. The important factors influencing this trend are earlier diagnosis using noninvasive techniques, refinements in operative technique, improvement in fluid management, innovations in anesthesia and intraoperative monitoring techniques, improvements in cardiac and pulmonary therapy, and the recognition and handling of unusual manifestations of aortic aneurysms.

Thus advances in all areas of clinical management have lowered the operative mortality to acceptable levels. While technical refinements may continue to occur to some degree, further improvement in mortality will most likely be dependent on earlier diagnosis with operation on smaller lesions, since the latter carry lower complication rates. At the same time, liberalization of indications for operation in the elderly patient with multiple risk factors tends to offset this trend and will keep the operative mortality at a certain irreducible minimum. Careful surgical judgment is necessary to render judicious decisions regarding operation in these marginal cases.

REFERENCES

1. Ameli FM, Gunstensen J, Jain K, et al: Surgical treatment of abdominal aortic aneurysm in Toronto: A study of 1,013 patients. Can. Med. Assoc. J. 107:1091, 1972
2. Baker AG Jr, Roberts B: Long-term survival following abdominal aortic aneurysmectomy. JAMA 212:445, 1970
3. Baker AG Jr, Roberts B, Berkowitz HD, et al: Risk of excision of abdominal aortic aneurysms. Surgery 68:1129, 1970
4. Bergan JJ, Yao JST: Modern management of abdominal aortic aneurysms. Surg. Clin. North Am. 54:175, 1974
5. Bernstein EF: The natural history of abdominal aortic aneurysms, in Najarian JS, Delaney JP (eds): Vascular Surgery. Miami, Symposia Specialists, 1978, p 441
6. Bernstein EF, Dilley RB, Goldberger LE, et al: Growth rates of small abdominal aortic aneurysms. Surgery 80:765, 1976
7. Bietz DS, Merendino KA: Abdominal aneurysm and horseshoe kidney. Ann. Surg. 181:333, 1975
8. Brener BJ, Darling RC, Frederick PL, et al: Major venous anomalies complicating abdominal aortic surgery. Arch. Surg. 108:159, 1974
9. Brewster DC, Retana A, Waltman AC, et al: Angiography in the management of aneurysms of the abdominal aorta. N. Engl. J. Med. 292:822, 1975
10. Cox JL, Sabiston DC Jr: The use of heparin bonded shunts for perfusion of the renal artery during resection of complex abdominal aortic aneurysms. Surg. Gynecol. Obstet. 147:859, 1978
11. DeBakey ME, Crawford ES, Cooley DA, et al: Aneurysm of abdominal aorta. Analysis of results of graft replacement therapy one to eleven years after operation..Ann. Surg. 160:622, 1964
12. Dubost C, Allary M, Oeconomos N: A propos du traitement des aneurysmes de l'aorte. Mem. Acad. Chir. Paris 77:381, 1951
13. Ernst CB, Hagihara PF, Daugherty ME, et al: Inferior mesenteric artery stump pressure: A reliable index for safe IMA ligation during abdominal aortic aneurysmectomy. Ann. Surg. 187:641, 1978
14. Foster JH, Bolasny BL, Gobbel WG Jr, et al: Comparative study of elective resection and expectant treatment of abdominal aortic aneurysm. Surg. Gynecol. Obstet. 129:1, 1969
15. Goldstone J, Malone JM, Moore WS: Inflammatory aneurysms of the abdominal aorta. Surgery 83:425, 1978

16. Gore I, Hirst AE Jr: Arteriosclerotic aneurysms of the abdominal aorta. Prog. Cardiovasc. Dis. 16:113, 1973
17. Hardy JD, Timmis HH: Abdominal aortic aneurysms: Special problems. Ann. Surg. 173:945, 1971
18. Hertzer NR, Beven EG: Ultrasound aortic measurement and elective aneurysmectomy. JAMA 240:1966, 1978
19. Hicks GL, Eastland MW, DeWeese JA, et al: Survival improvement following aortic aneurysm resection. Ann. Surg. 181:863, 1975
20. Johnson WC, Nasbeth DC: Visceral infarction following aortic surgery. Ann. Surg. 180:312, 1974
21. Key JA, Sokol DM: The symptomless abdominal aneurysm – A 15 year review. Can. J. Surg. 16:297, 1973
22. Leopold GR, Goldberger LE, Bernstein EF: Ultrasonic detection and evaluation of abdominal aortic aneurysms. Surgery 72:939, 1972
23. Mulder DS, Winsberg F, Cole CM, et al: Ultrasonic "B" scanning of abdominal aneurysms. Ann. Thorac. Surg. 16:361, 1973
24. O'Donnell TF Jr, Darling RC, Linton RR: Is 80 years too old for aneurysmectomy? Arch. Surg. 111:1250, 1976
25. Perry MO: The hemodynamics of temporary abdominal aortic occlusion. Ann. Surg. 168:193, 1968
26. Satiani B, Veazy CR, Smith RB III, et al: Preoperative aortography before abdominal aortic aneurysmectomy? Am. J. Surg. 44:650, 1978
27. Stokes J, Butcher HR: Abdominal aortic aneurysms. Factors influencing operative mortality and criteria of operability. Arch. Surg. 107:297, 1973
28. Szilagyi DE, Elliott JP, Smith RF: Clinical fate of the patient with asymptomatic abdominal aortic aneurysm and unfit for surgical treatment. Arch. Surg. 104:600, 1972
29. Szilagyi DE, Hageman JH, Smith RF, et al: Spinal cord damage in surgery of the abdominal aorta. Surgery 83:38, 1978
30. Szilagyi DE, Smith RF, DeRusso FJ, et al: Contribution of abdominal aortic aneurysmectomy to prolongation of life. Ann. Surg. 164:678, 1966
31. Tchirkow G, Beven EG: Leg ischemia following surgery for abdominal aneurysm. Ann. Surg. 188:166, 1978
32. Thompson JE, Hollier LH, Patman RD, et al: Surgical management of abdominal aortic aneurysms. Factors influencing mortality and morbidity – A 20 year experience. Ann. Surg. 181:654, 1975
33. Thompson JE, Vollman RW, Austin DJ, et al: Prevention of hypotensive and renal complications of aortic surgery using balanced salt solution: Thirteen year experience with 670 cases. Ann. Surg. 167:767, 1968
34. Volpetti G, Barker CF, Berkowitz H, et al: A twenty-two year review of elective resection of abdominal aortic aneurysms. Surg. Gynecol. Obstet. 142:321, 1976

H. Edward Garrett, M.D.
John Anderson, M.D.

Management of the Ruptured Abdominal Aortic Aneurysm

The management of the ruptured abdominal aortic aneurysm continues to present a challenge to the vascular surgeon, emergency room physician, and operating room personnel. In addition, the blood bank, intensive care, anesthesiology, and other supportive services within the hospital such as pulmonary medicine, nephrology, and hematology must be experienced in the management of these patients to achieve maximum survival. A prearranged plan of action by all concerned will yield the best results in the care of these critically ill patients.

The era of modern vascular surgery began almost 30 years ago with resection and graft replacement of the abdominal aorta by Oudot [21] and Dubost [13]. The accumulated experience has provided the vascular surgeon with improvements in instrumentation, grafts, and pre- and postoperative care and a better understanding of the natural history of aortic aneurysmal disease.

There has been consistent improvement in the mortality and morbidity associated with operative treatment of nonruptured abdominal aortic aneurysm but only modest improvement in the published series of ruptured abdominal aortic aneurysms. This experience confirms the highly lethal characteristics of the disease and the difficultics associated with treatment.

Certain important information concerning the natural history of abdominal aortic aneurysm and the accumulated experience in treatment of this lesion are worthy of review.

1. Approximately 95%-98% of abdominal aortic aneurysms originate below the renal arteries [9, 10].
2. Elective resection and graft replacement of the lesion is recommended in all cases unless associated disease contraindicates operation [9, 11, 28, 29].
3. Elective resection carries a low operative mortality [1, 29]; emergency resection of the ruptured aneurysm carries a high mortality (30%-80%) and morbidity [11, 17, 23, 28].

4. Aneurysms > 6 cm in diameter rupture more frequently than aneurysms < 6 cm, but small aneurysms rupture [10, 15].
5. The age of the patient, as an isolated consideration, is not a contraindication for operation [2].

A rational plan for management of the ruptured abdominal aortic aneurysm has evolved in most institutions and consists of the following general principles.

PREVENTION

If the number of patients dying from ruptured abdominal aneurysms is to be reduced, primary physicians must be alert and identify the asymptomatic lesions. These patients should be referred for possible operative treatment. The diagnosis may be evident by palpation of the abdomen in the nonobese patient. Anterior-posterior and lateral x-rays of the abdomen frequently disclose the lesion particularly if a thin rim of calcium is present in the aorta. Sonography of the abdominal aorta is highly accurate in making the diagnosis particularly in the obese patient in whom palpation of the aorta is difficult [22, 29]. Aortography is not particularly accurate in identification of an abdominal aortic aneurysm. The presence of laminated thrombus within the aorta at the site of dilatation produces a relatively smooth lumen and aneurysmal dilatation is not usually evident unless a calcified wall is present. Aortography may be valuable in evaluating associated occlusive disease, anatomical variations of renal arteries, and the status of iliac and femoral arteries [7].

Elective resection of asymptomatic abdominal aortic aneurysm is recommended in all patients in whom there is no severe contraindication to operation from associated disease. Occasional patients are reluctant to submit to operation, and it is important that they understand the relative risks involved, the importance of frequent followup, and that the associated risk factors, particularly hypertension, be controlled. Symptoms of rapid expansion or rupture such as abdominal pain, back pain, or hypotension requires immediate referral for operative treatment.

EMERGENCY ROOM MANAGEMENT

If transportation to another hospital is required, arrangements should be made by telephone for the surgical team to expect the patient and be prepared for immediate operation. Helicopter or ambulance may be preferable, depending on the distance and facilities. Antigravity suits have been utilized with apparent benefit under these circumstances [10, 14, 25]. The experience of a nurse, medic, or physician in attendance may be extremely beneficial to monitor blood pressure, intravenous infusions, and oxygen therapy.

A prearranged plan of action by the emergency room team should be activated upon arrival of the patient. At least two large intravenous cannulae should be inserted for infusion of blood, fluids, or medications. A central venous cannula placed into the internal jugular or subclavian vein can usually be inserted even if the patient is vasoconstricted from hypotension. A blood sample should be obtained immediately for hematocrit, type, and crossmatch of whole blood. Simultaneously the patient should be questioned and examined and the blood pressure obtained. As soon as possible, an intraarterial cannula for continuous blood pressure monitoring should be inserted into a radial artery and blood pressure and electrocardiogram displayed on a monitor. An indwelling Foley catheter should be inserted into the bladder and attached to a drainage bag. If the diagnosis is obvious by the presence of a pulsatile abdominal mass, immediate operation is indicated.

Whole blood should be available before the operation is started unless the patient is in extremis. Approximately 1 hour is required in most institutions for routine type and crossmatch of whole blood. However, a type and screening for major antibodies may be accomplished within 5 min and provides a safety factor of approximately 99% against transfusion reaction in patients who have not received blood previously. This method is useful in providing large amounts of whole blood rapidly for patients in hypovolemic shock from ruptured abdominal aneurysms.

OPERATIVE THERAPY

Patients with ruptured abdominal aortic aneurysms are prepared and draped before anesthesia is induced and intubation accomplished. The overall stability of hypovolemic and hypotensive patients tends to deteriorate with induction of general anesthesia. Whole blood is started and a vertical incision is made from xyphoid to pubis. No attempt is made to control bleeding from the wound. A large self-retaining retractor is inserted and the patient's transverse colon and small bowel are delivered onto the abdominal wall. Proximal control of the aorta is obtained immediately by one of several methods (Fig. 1). The aorta may be compressed by a manual occluder until such time as a vascular clamp can be placed proximal to the site of rupture. The clamp may be placed on the aorta immediately below the diaphragm through the gastrohepatic omentum if the aorta is palpable. If the hematoma is confined to the retroperitoneal space without communication with the peritoneal cavity, it is usually not entered until proximal control is obtained. If the aneurysm has ruptured into the peritoneal cavity, the hematoma is entered and either a Foley catheter or a finger of the surgeon is inserted into the aorta proximally until a vascular clamp can be placed below the renal arteries. Distal control is usually easily obtained at the common iliac arteries but again a Foley catheter may be inserted distally and inflated to

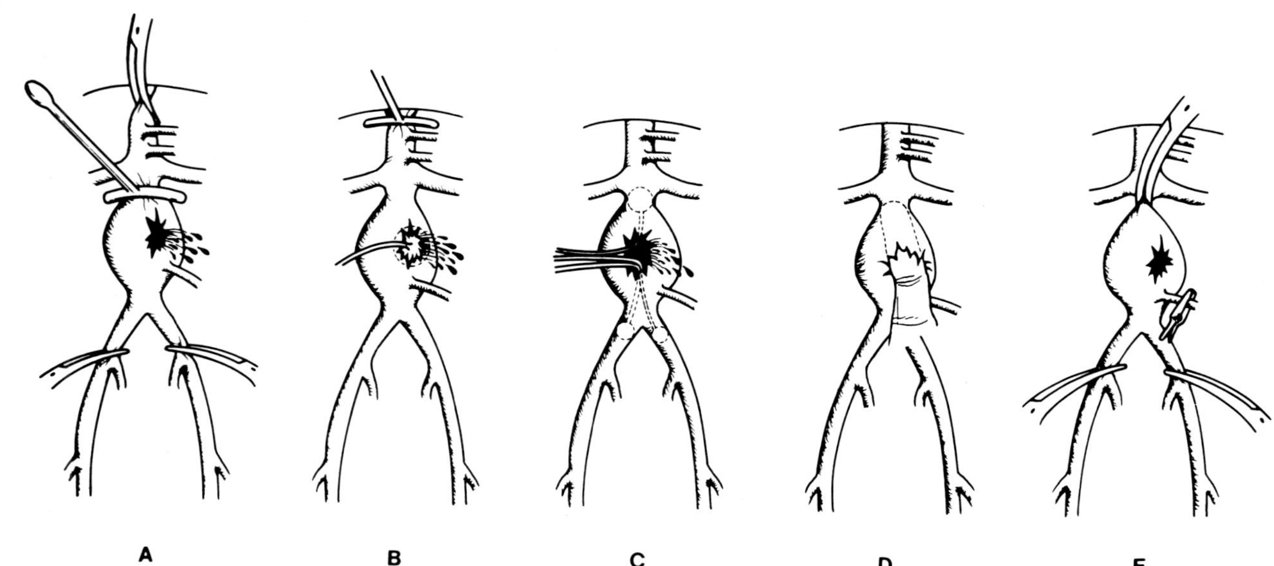

Fig. 1. (A) Drawing illustrating proximal and distal control of aorta by manual compressor and vascular clamps. (B) Drawing illustrating control of bleeding with compressor and balloon catheter. (C) Drawing illustrating control with proximal and distal balloon catheters. (D) Drawing illustrating initial control with finger of surgeon. (E) Drawing illustrating application of vascular clamps prior to resection of ruptured aneurysm.

achieve temporary control. Systemic heparinization is desirable once adequate control of bleeding is achieved.

An attempt is made to salvage as much blood as possible by use of some form of autotransfusion device. The Cell Saver (Haemonetics Corporation, Braintree, Mass. 02184) is one method of salvaging red cells which are aspirated in a heparinized solution, centrifuged, and retransfused within a short period of time. Once control of hemorrhage is achieved, no further dissection is performed until the patient's blood volume has been restored. All blood is infused through filters and is warmed to body temperature, if possible. The arterial blood pressure and central venous pressure are monitored throughout the procedure.

When the patient is relatively stable and vascular clamps are secure below the renal arteries and on the common iliac arteries, the aorta is incised circumferentially above the site of rupture and distally at the bifurcation or at the common iliac level. Lumbar arteries are controlled with suture ligatures and graft replacement is accomplished.

A tightly woven Dacron tube or bifurcation graft is selected. If the appropriate size of woven graft is unavailable, a knitted graft may be preclotted and flashed in an autoclave for 3 min. This preparation appears to seal the interstices of the graft and reduce or eliminate bleeding from the graft when the clamps are removed. The graft replacement is accomplished rapidly with continuous suture technique employing either monofilament polypropylene or braided Dacron suture material. Prior to completion of the distal suture line, appropriate flushing is accomplished, and on completion of the suture line the proximal clamp is slowly removed to avoid declamping hypotension. If satisfactory back flow is not obtained during the flushing procedure, Fogarty catheters may be introduced distally to retrieve any embolic material present [4]. Blood gas determinations are obtained after declamping and appropriate pH adjustments made. If the inferior mesenteric artery is large, back flow poor, or the sigmoid colon appears ischemic, reimplantation of the inferior mesenteric artery into the graft is performed.

The retroperitoneal space is then irrigated thoroughly with an antibiotic solution and inspected for bleeding. The wall of the aneurysm is sutured over the proximal suture line and the graft. Removal of the intima is unnecessary but does allow careful inspection of the orifices of the lumbar arterics for bleeding and removes atherosclerotic debris that theoretically might provide a culture media for infection. Retroperitoneal blood behind the sigmoid mesocolon is removed and the posterior peritoneum is closed with a continuous suture. It is important to separate the small bowel from the aortic suture line with a layer of viable periaortic tissue. If this is difficult, a cuff of Dacron graft may be placed around the proximal suture line prior to closure of the retroperitoneal space.

The peritoneal cavity is aspirated free of blood and clot; the small bowel and colon are inspected for viability and replaced in their anatomical positions. Wound hemostasis is obtained and closure accomplished according to the preference of thc surgeon. A Swan-Ganz catheter may be inserted for monitoring left atrial pressure if the patient is not entirely stable upon transfer to the Intensive Care Unit.

UNUSUAL TYPES OF RUPTURE

Practically all ruptured abdominal aortic aneurysms occur between the renal arteries and the bifurcation of the iliac arteries. However, occasionally a ruptured aneurysm of the internal iliac artery will be encountered [20], and on rare occasions a ruptured aneurysm of the upper abdominal aorta will occur requiring replacement of the major visceral branches [8].

The infrarenal aneurysm may rupture into the distal duodenum or proximal jejunum [18], left renal vein [26, 31], or inferior vena cava [3, 12]. In addition, certain anatomical variations may be present that complicate the operative management [16], such as persistent left vena cava, retroaortic left renal vein, horseshoe kidney, and visceral arterial branches arising from the aneurysm.

Primary aortoduodenal fistula occurs when an abdominal aortic aneurysm ruptures into the terminal portion of the duodenum. This complication should be suspected if upper gastrointestinal bleeding is associated with a demonstrable abdominal aortic aneurysm. If the bowel is densely adherent to the aneurysm at operation, aortoduodenal fistula is likely. Although primary repair of the bowel and excision and graft replacement of the aneurysm have been successful, the possibility of delayed graft infection is increased. Recently, closure of the duodenum and aorta with axillofemoral bypass as advocated for secondary aortoduodenal fistula has been recommended for this problem [5].

Fistula between the abdominal aortic aneurysm and the left renal vein may be encountered on rare occasions. Management consists of sacrifice of the left renal vein and graft replacement of the aneurysm.

Aortocaval fistula may be suspected before operation if a harsh continuous murmur is present over the abdomen, there is evidence of increased venous pressure in the lower extremities, or hematuria [6, 24]. Operative management consists of control of the aneurysm with vascular clamps, manual control of the vena cava above and below the fistula, and primary closure of the cava from within the wall of the aneurysm. Care must be taken to prevent atheromatous pulmonary emboli. Prophylactic placement of a vena caval clip between the fistula and the left renal vein is recommended.

COMPLICATIONS

Complications following operation for ruptured abdominal aortic aneurysm are not uncommon and may lead to death of the patient (Table 1). Certain complications occur more frequently following operation for ruptured aneurysm

Table 1
Complications Following Repair of Ruptured Abdominal Aortic Aneurysms in 120 Patients [17, 24, 30]

	No. of Cases	Incidence	Deaths	Mortality
Renal failure	37	31%	25	68%
Adult respiratory distress syndrome	32	26%	18	56%
Reoperation for bleeding	20	17%	16	80%
Myocardial infarction	16	13%	13	100%
Distal thrombosis	10	8%	6	60%

than operation for elective or expanding aneurysm. Management of these complications requires a high index of suspicion and the expertise of ancillary hospital services.

Hemorrhage. Retroperitoneal collection of blood following operation for ruptured aneurysm is not uncommon. Extensive raw surface, coagulation abnormalities following massive transfusion, and the presence of hematoma from the rupture site are contributing factors. Serial hematocrits, blood volume determinations, and palpation of the lateral abdomen may indicate blood loss in the retroperitoneal area. Any suggestion of instability of the patient from blood loss requires reexploration to control hemorrhage.

Bowel ischemia. Small bowel or colon ischemia following operation may be catastrophic. Careful inspection of the bowel prior to closure and palpation of the superior mesenteric artery may be helpful in detecting impending small bowel ischemia. Colon ischemia may follow ligation of a large inferior mesenteric artery, particularly if hypogastric perfusion is not adequate. Reimplantation of the inferior mesenteric artery should be considered if satisfactory blood supply is questionable. Accumulation of a large hematoma beneath the sigmoid mesocolon also may contribute to colon ischemia. Careful evacuation is essential prior to wound closure. Management of impending or overt colon ischemia requires early diagnosis by inspection and biopsy through a sigmoidoscope. Antibiotics, steroids, and reexploration to prevent rupture and retroperitoneal infection have been advocated in the treatment of this complication. Late stricture has been observed and should be considered if symptoms develop weeks or months after operation.

Renal failure. This complication occurs more frequently if prolonged hypotension occurs prior to operation. Successful management requires early recognition and treatment. Left atrial pressure monitoring with a Swan-Ganz catheter may be helpful in establishing optimum blood volume after operation and signal early renal failure. Nephrology consultation and early dialysis offer the patient the best chance of survival.

Adult respiratory distress syndrome. This pulmonary complication may be related to shock, massive transfusion, sepsis, pulmonary emboli, overhydration, renal failure, and other unknown factors. Early recognition through serial blood gas determinations and chest x-rays and treatment with various inhalation therapy techniques (PEEP, CPAP, IMV) supervised by pulmonary medicine offer the best chance for survival of the patient.

Arterial insufficiency of lower extremities. Thrombosis in the vascular prosthesis or in the lower extremities can be detected by frequent manual palpation of pulses or by employing a doppler ultrasound flow detector. Disappearance of previously present pulses usually requires exploration particularly if an extremity is threatened. This complication might be averted in some cases if routine distal embolectomy with a Fogarty catheter is performed as advocated by Bergan and Yao [4].

Other complications as listed in Table 2 may occur and require prompt therapy. The routine use of intensive care facilities with constant monitoring, preventive nursing care, and early recognition of possible complications is strongly advocated in the postoperative care of patients with ruptured abdominal aneurysm.

Spinal cord ischemia. Paraplegia may occur after elective resection of abdominal aortic aneurysm but is more common after emergency operation for ruptured aneurysm if prolonged hypotension is present. Unfortunately this complication cannot be predicted or prevented [27].

Table 2
Complications Following Operations for Ruptured Abdominal Aortic Aneurysms

Distal thrombosis	Coagulopathy
Renal failure	Pneumonia
Adult respiratory distress syndrome	Retroperitoneal hemorrhage
Myocardial infarction, Congestive Heart Failure	Gastrointestinal hemorrhage
Bowel ischemia	Paraplegia
Stroke	Sepsis, graft infection
Pulmonary embolus	Wound infection
Intestinal ileus/obstruction	Dehiscence

RESULTS

The results of operation for ruptured abdominal aortic aneurysms vary considerably in the published experience. Factors that influence mortality include age of the patient, associated diseases, condition of the patient at time of operation, length of cross-clamp or ischemic time, number of blood transfusions required, and complications of operation. Although there has been some improvement in operative mortality in recent years [19], elective resection of the unruptured aneurysm appears to offer the best chance of preventing deaths from ruptured lesions.

A review of a 2-year experience (1977-78) at Baptist Memorial Hospital, Memphis, is recorded in Table 3. The operations were performed by experienced vascular surgeons, and all operations for unruptured or expanding aneurysms were excluded. In 70% of the patients, symptoms were present over 6 hours. Those patients arriving in the operating room relatively stable (blood pressure > 80 mm Hg) had a 25% mortality, as compared with a 75% mortality observed in patients who were in prolonged shock. This experience is similar to other reports.

Sink [24] reviewed the literature and recorded 1239 ruptured abdominal aortic aneurysms (1964-1975) with 641 early deaths (52%). In many of the series, the condition of the patient at the time of operation was unclear. Table 4 clearly indicates the relationship between the stability of the patient and operative mortality.

Table 3
Ruptured Abdominal Aortic Aneurysms
(Baptist Memorial Hospital, Memphis, 1977-78)

Patients		Deaths	Mortality
Total group	28	13	46.4%
Stable (B.P. > 80 mm Hg)	16	4	25%
Unstable (B.P. > 80 mm Hg)	12	9	75%

Table 4
Mortality Statistics on Patients with Profound Shock Prior to Surgery

Year	Author	No. Patients	No. Deaths	Mortality
1968	Graham	55	37	67%
1969	Van Heeckeren	57	34	60%
1970	Darling	39	22	56%
1975	Sink	12	10	83%
1979	Garrett	12	9	75%
	Totals	175	112	69%

REFERENCES

1. Ameli FM, Gunstensen J, Jain K, et al: A study of 1013 patients. Can. Med. Assoc. J. 107:1091, 1972
2. Baker WH, Munns JR: Aneurysmectomy in the aged. Arch. Surg. 110:513, 1975
3. Beall AC, Cooley DA, Morris GC, et al: Perforation of arteriosclerotic aneurysms into inferior vena cava. Arch. Surg. 86:136, 1963
4. Bergan JJ, Yao JST: Modern management of abdominal aortic aneurysms. Surg. Clin. North Am. 54:175, 1974
5. Blaisdell FW, Hall AD, Lim RC Jr, et al: Aorto-iliac arterial substitution utilizing subcutaneous grafts. Ann. Surg. 172:775, 1970
6. Brewster DC, Ottinger LW, Darling RC: Hematuria as a sign of aorto-caval fistula. Ann. Surg. 186:766, 1977
7. Brewster DC, Retana A, Waltman AC, et al: Angiography in the management of aneurysms of the abdominal aorta – Its value and safety. N. Engl. J. Med. 292:822, 1975
8. Crawford ES, Snyder DM, Cho GC, et al: Progress in treatment of thoraco-abdominal and abdominal aortic aneurysms involving celiac, superior, mesenteric, and renal arteries. Ann. Surg. 188:404, 1978
9. Crisler C, Bahnson HT: Aneurysms of the aorta. Curr. Prob. Surg., Dec. 1972
10. Darling RC: Ruptured arteriosclerotic abdominal aortic aneurysms – A pathologic and clinical study. Am. J. Surg. 119:397, 1970
11. DeBakey ME, Crawford ES, Cooley DA, et al: Aneurysm of abdominal aorta – Analysis of results of graft replacement therapy one to eleven years after operation. Ann. Surg. 160:622, 1964
12. Doty DB, Wright CB, Lamberth WC, et al: Aortocaval fistula associated with aneurysm of the abdominal aorta: Current management using auto-transfusion techniques. Surgery 84:250, 1978
13. Dubost C, Allary M, Oeconomos N: Resection of an aneurysm of the abdominal aorta – Re-establishment of the continuity by a preserved human arterial graft, with result after five months. AMA Arch. Surg. 64:405, 1952
14. Gardner WJ, Storer J: The use of the G-suit in control of intra-abdominal bleeding. Surg. Gynecol. Obstet. 123:792, 1960
15. Gore I, Hirst AE Jr: Arteriosclerotic aneurysms of the abdominal aorta: A review. Prog. Cardiovasc. Dis. 26:113, 1973
16. Hardy JD, Timmis HH: Abdominal aortic aneurysms: Special problems. Ann. Surg. 173:946, 1971
17. Hicks GL, Eastland MW, DeWeese JA, et al: Survival improvement following aortic aneurysms resection. Ann. Surg. 181:863, 1975
18. Kleinman LH, Towne JB, Bernhard WM: A diagnostic and therapeutic approach to aorto-enteric fistulas: Clinical experience with 19 patients. Presented at the 33rd Annual Meeting of the Society for Vascular Surgery, Nashville, June 1979
19. Lawrie GM, Morris GL Jr, Crawford ES, et al: Improved results of operation for ruptured abdominal aortic aneurysms. Surgery 85:483, 1979

20. Lowry SF, Kraft RO: Isolated aneurysms of the iliac artery. Arch. Surg. 113:1289, 1978
21. Oudot J: La greffe vasculaire dans les thromboses du carrefour aortique. Pr. Med. 59:234, 1951
22. Shawker TH, Steinfeld AD: Ultrasonic evaluation of pulsatile abdominal masses. JAMA 239:419, 1978
23. Shumacker HF Jr, Barnes DL, King H: Ruptured abdominal aortic aneurysms. Ann. Surg. 177:772, 1973
24. Sink JD, Myers RT, James PM Jr: Ruptured abdominal aortic aneurysms: Review of 33 cases treated surgically and discussion of prognostic indicators. Am. Surg. 42:303, 1976
25. Stephenson HE Jr, Lockhart CG: Treatment of the ruptured abdominal aorta. Surg. Gynecol. Obstet. 144:855, 1977
26. Suzuki M, Collins GM, Bassinger GT, et al: Aorto-left renal vein fistula: An unusual complication of abdominal aortic aneurysm. Ann. Surg. 184:31, 1976
27. Szilagyi DE, Hageman JH, Smith RF, et al: Spinal cord damage in surgery of the abdominal aorta. Surgery 83:38, 1978
28. Szilagyi DE, Smith RF, DeRusso FJ, et al: Contribution of abdominal aortic aneurysmectomy to prolongation of life. Ann. Surg. 164:678, 1966
29. Thompson JE, Hollier LH, Patman RD, et al: Surgical management of abdominal aortic aneurysms: Factors influencing mortality and morbidity – A 20-year experience. Ann. Surg. 181:654, 1975
30. van Heeckeren DW: Ruptured abdominal aortic aneurysms. Am. J. Surg. 119:402, 1970
31. Yashar JJ, Hallman GL, Cooley DA: Fistula between aneurysm of aorta and left renal vein. Arch. Surg. 99:546, 1969

Julius Conn, Jr., M.D.

Colon Ischemia Following Abdominal Aortic Surgery

Ischemia of the colon is an unpredictable, often fatal, but fortunately rare complication of abdominal aortic surgery. When it develops, appreciation of its diverse clinical presentations is crucial to making a diagnosis. Only then can treatment be prompt, precise, and successful.

In the postaortic surgical patient, colon ischemia may be manifest as a transient ischemic event or as catastrophic gangrene. The former may begin with diarrhea and bleeding. This may proceed to uncomplicated healing, or the ischemic colon may heal with circumferential stricture. When transmural gangrene occurs, perforation, peritonitis, and abscess formation is to be expected [12, 27, 30]. Such infection is intolerable in patients with a fresh vascular suture line holding in place a prosthetic graft [17].

The overall mortality of colon ischemia following abdominal aortic surgery is reported to be 50%. However, if transmural gangrene occurs, the mortality is 90% [16, 17, 30]. Early recognition of the manifestations of ischemic colitis allows prompt, aggressive treatment which might help to lower the mortality of this dreadful aortic surgical complication.

INCIDENCE

Various authors place the incidence of ischemic colitis following abdominal aortic aneurysm or aortodistal reconstructions at 1.5%-10% [2, 13, 25-27, 30]. Ernst conducted a prospective study of such patients in order to clarify the true incidence of colon ischemia [10]. Colonoscopy was performed prior to operation and repeated in the early postoperative period.

Ischemic changes in the colon were seen in 4.3% of patients who had aortic reconstructions for occlusive disease and in 7.4% of those having graft replacement for aortic aneurysm. Colon ischemia never developed in patients whose preoperative arteriogram showed opacification of the inferior mesenteric artery from a meandering mesenteric artery.

HISTORICAL BACKGROUND

Early reports of resection and graft replacement of abdominal aortic aneurysms by Dubost in 1952 and DeBakey in 1953 mentioned ligation of the inferior mesenteric artery but did not describe colon ischemia [8, 9]. In fact, Moore, in 1954, presented the first report of ischemic colitis following resection of an abdominal aortic aneurysm [21]. This report retains relevance 25 years later. The patient developed moderate diarrhea in the immediate postoperative period. Six weeks later, he was discovered to have a stricture of the rectosigmoid colon 10 cm from the anal orifice. Grossly, the mucosa appeared to be chronic granulation tissue and biopsy revealed chronic proctitis. Moore noted that the inferior mesenteric artery was chronically occluded at the time of aneurysm resection. In spite of ligation of both internal iliac arteries the colon appeared normal prior to closure of the abdomen. The rectal stricture responded to conservative management, and the patient had an uneventful recovery. Movius reported a high incidence of diarrhea following aneurysm resection and two patients with rectal strictures 9 cm from the anus [24].

Ischemic colitis may present in the postoperative patient in any one of three distinctive patterns. The most benign form usually begins 3-10 days following surgery with tenesmus and diarrhea. The watery stools may be bloody, and occasionally patients may have tenesmus and pass blood mucous or stool within 24 hours of surgery. Frequently, no other signs of colon ischemia appear. However, in any one patient there is no assurance that this will be true. Patients with any sign of colon ischemia must be watched carefully for signs of colon gangrene and/or leakage. Proctoscopy or colonoscopy should be performed promptly. Dusky friable, edematous mucosa is characteristically seen. Within a few days the mucosa loses its normal texture and looks like a granulating wound with mucosal ulceration and inflammatory exudate [3, 4, 25, 30].

A barium enema, if done during the colonic ischemic event, will show spasm of the involved segment and "thumbprint" indentations which are characteristic of edematous ischemic bowel [7, 5, 12]. If the ischemia is severe, superficial ulcerations will be seen.

Patients with the mild form of ischemic colitis respond to fluid replacement and bowel rest. The ischemia only involves the mucosa, is transient, and heals without sequelae. However, development of delayed stricture formation must be kept in mind. When stricture occurs, simple diarrhea progresses to signs and symptoms of partial obstruction of the left colon or rectosigmoid. Such strictures usually occur 4-6 weeks after aortic surgery. Most respond to simple dilations but occasionally resection of the involved area is required. Stricture formation occurs as a result of the mucosa and submucosa destruction from the ischemic episode and subsequent healing by cicatricial contracture [2, 4, 27, 30].

The most feared complication of colon ischemia after aortic surgery is acute transmural gangrene of the colon. Patients with this may have nonspecific findings initially. They do fail to exhibit normal postoperative bettering, they remain distended, have a prolonged ileus, have marked but nonspecific abdominal pain and tenderness, and have a low grade fever and leukocytosis. Tenesmus and bloody diarrhea may or may not occur [2, 13, 20].

If diagnosis is not made at this time, high spiking fever, leukocytosis of 20,000-40,000, and progressive signs of peritoneal irritation will develop. Some patients with gangrene of the colon will have sudden or progressive cardiorespiratory failure, unexplained acidosis, or renal failure due to sepsis or peritonitis. In such situations, abdominal examination and early laboratory and x-ray findings are confused with routine postsurgical changes [13, 25, 29, 30].

Patients with colon necrosis will inevitably develop localized or generalized peritonitis, intraabdominal abscess, and death if untreated. In the presence of intraabdominal sepsis, infection of the vascular anastomosis may occur with catastrophic results.

The slightest suspicion of ischemic colitis following aortic reconstruction should prompt proctoscopy or colonoscopy without delay. If endoscopy is negative and the signs of colitis persist, a barium enema should be done [5, 10]. If mild colitis is seen, then conservative management with fluids, antibiotic, and serial observations are sufficient therapy.

If mucosal changes are identified the patient should be followed closely and then long term to insure that a stricture does not develop as the mucosa heals. A barium examination of the colon 8-12 weeks after symptoms have subsided should be done. Also, if a change in bowel habits or signs of obstruction develop, a colon contrast study is indicated.

Mild strictures can be dilated via the proctoscope if normal passage of stool does not provide sufficient dilation. Some strictures will fail to respond to conservative treatment, will remain symptomatic, and will require segmental resection of the colon. At that time, careful attention to the blood supply of the anastomosis and especial care to prevent peritoneal contamination must be a part of the operation [19].

If colitis is proven and the patient begins to develop evidence of peritoneal irritation or if perforation or peritonitis develops at any time, prompt laparotomy is mandatory. High dose, broad spectrum antibiotics should be given immediately, aerobic and anaerobic cultures should be obtained at the time of laparotomy, and contamination of the retroperitoneum minimized. Removal of the necrotic colon is essential. The proximal viable bowel may be brought out as an end colostomy. If possible the distal bowel is brought out as a mucous fistula, but when gangrene extends far into the pelvis the rectal stump must be oversewn [17, 20]. The peritoneum should be irrigated thoroughly with copious antibiotic solution or povidone iodine.

Restoration of continuity of the colon is dependent upon patient survival and should not be planned until all wounds are healed and there is no risk of further sepsis. Surviving patients must be watched long term, as risk of hemorrhage from a mycotic aneurysm is always present.

COLONIC VASCULAR ANATOMY

Complete knowledge of the vascular anatomy of the colon is critical to understanding and preventing postoperative ischemic colitis.

The inferior mesenteric artery normally arises from the ventral surface of the aorta at the level of the third lumbar vertebra. It passes laterally and downward at approximately 30° and gives origin to an ascending branch, the left colic, and then descends downward, giving off one to three sigmoidal branches before terminating as the superior hemorrhoidal artery. The left colic branches approximately 2 cm from the origin of the inferior mesenteric artery [1, 12, 14, 22, 23, 28].

In the course of aortic aneurysm resection, the inferior mesenteric artery and frequently one or both hypogastric arteries are sacrificed. Usually the inferior mesenteric artery is occluded and adequate collateral flow has already developed. Such major collateral blood supply of the left colon arises from the middle colic artery via the marginal artery of Drummond, which communicates with the left colic artery. However, in approximately 6% of individuals the left colic artery is completely absent. In this situation, the sigmoid artery is always large [4, 14].

Rather than being concerned about Sudek's critical point, the junction of the lowest sigmoid artery with the middle hemorrhoidal, the surgeon's area of greatest concern following aortic surgery should be the truly critical point at the splenic flexure where the marginal artery is often atretic or absent. It is true that the two most susceptible regions of the colon to ischemia are the rectosigmoid and the splenic flexure. Both areas depend upon collateral arterial flow when the inferior mesenteric artery or the hypogastric arteries are occluded. Interestingly, the middle colic artery is absent in 22% of the patients. In this situation, the right colic must supply the transverse and descending colon after ligation of the inferior mesenteric artery [22]. Another little known arterial collateral which should be protected is an anastomotic branch between the left and middle colic arteries in the root of the mesocolon [14].

The meandering mesenteric artery of the colon, the arc of Riolan, is a large collateral vessel that develops in response to stenosis of either the superior or inferior mesenteric artery. When present, it is large and tortuous. It connects the middle and left colic arteries and passes along the base of the mesocolon near the inferior mesenteric vein [22, 23]. Care must be taken to preserve this important collateral vessel.

The rectosigmoid blood supply is derived from the middle hemorrhoidal arteries. These are major branches of the hypogastric arteries. A fairly constant anastomosis between the superior hemorrhoidal and middle hemorrhoidal arteries is present. If both hypogastric arteries are occluded by atherosclerosis or ligated, the rectosigmoid may become ischemic. This is especially true if the middle colic-left colic anastomoses are deficient. Therefore, when feasible, the aortic reconstruction should include restoration of flow to at least one hypogastric artery [14, 18, 28, 30].

FACTORS INFLUENCING RISK OF COLON ISCHEMIA

Several factors increase the risk of ischemic colitis after aortic surgery. For example, preexisting stenosis of the superior mesenteric artery will decrease collateral flow. Prolonged hypotension may cause ischemic colitis because of low flow or indirectly by allowing vital collateral vessels to occlude. Prolonged cross-clamping of the infrarenal aorta may markedly reduce flow in the hypogastric arteries. Hemorrhage into or rough retraction of the mesocolon may cause thrombosis of the colon blood supply. Careless dissection or clamping of vessels in the retroperitoneal space or the mesocolon might reduce flow to the colon [25, 30].

Patients who have had previous bowel resections should be watched carefully for colon ischemia after aortic surgery, as important collateral channels may have been sacrificed at the original operation.

Of critical importance is proper attention to the inferior mesenteric artery at the time of aortic surgery. If it is found to be occluded by angiography or at the time of the operation, adequate collateral should be present as long as the left colic and sigmoid branches are preserved [3, 17, 19].

TECHNIQUES OF AVOIDANCE OF COLON ISCHEMIA

Preoperative angiography is helpful in identifying patients who might develop colon ischemia following aortic surgery. The angiogram may reveal stenosis of the superior mesenteric artery or a central anastomotic artery. The presence of significant disease in the superior mesenteric artery should alert the surgeon to the possible need for reanastomosis of the inferior mesenteric artery. The arteriograms might show inadequate communication between the middle colic and the left colic vessels. Angiographic demonstration of these findings is far more accurate in identifying high risk patients than palpatating pulses or trying to quantitate backbleeding from a divided artery [10, 11].

When the inferior mesenteric artery is patent, thought may be given to reimplantation of the artery. If colon ischemia is apparent during the procedure, reimplantation must be done. Unfortunately, following ligation of the inferior mesenteric artery, the gross appearance of the colon has not been reliable in predicting the eventual development of colon ischemia [2, 11, 15]. A dusky or pale, spastic left colon may be present after the aortic clamps are removed, but normal color and peristalsis may return within a short time. Conversely, what looks like a perfectly normal colon may develop ischemic colitis, stricture, or necrosis during the postoperative period [2, 19].

In trying to improve the diagnosis of impending colon ischemia, Ernst measured stump pressure in the inferior mesenteric artery. An inferior mesenteric stump pressure of at least 40 mm Hg or a IMA/systemic pressure ratio of 0.40 postresection of an abdominal aortic aneurysm was thought to preclude intestinal ischemia. Perfusion pressures in this range are higher than the critical closing pressure of 40 mm Hg and should provide adequate blood flow to the colon [11]. At this time, there is not enough quantitative data to allow correlation of various levels of stump pressure with the onset of colon ischemia after ligation of the inferior mesenteric artery.

Care must be taken to ligate the inferior mesenteric artery close to its takeoff from the aorta in order to preserve all of the branches (Fig. 1A). Others have used radioactive microspheres or intraoperative use of Doppler ultrasound to predict colon ischemia or infarction. These techniques have not proven to be of great value [15, 31].

To facilitate reimplantation of the inferior mesenteric artery, steps should be taken to preserve its proximal orifice. The proximal artery may be temporally controlled in continuity with a small, soft silastic sling or suture. Care must be taken to avoid injury to the left colic artery (Fig. 1A). If the artery must be reimplanted into the side of the aortic graft, an oval patch can be fashioned of aortic wall containing the origin of the inferior mesenteric artery (Fig. 1B). The patch is then easily anastomosed to the side of the graft by the terminolateral technique of Carrel [6] (Figs. 1B and 2A). This is a fast, easy technique of restoring flow to the colon. When the proximal inferior mesenteric artery is occluded or stenotic or if endarterectomy of the aortic patch is unsuccessful, reimplantation into the graft is facilitated by spatulating or "fish mouthing" the proximal artery (Fig. 2B).

CONCLUSIONS

Virtually every patient, following reconstructive surgery on the abdominal aorta, is at risk of developing colon ischemia. The inferior mesenteric artery is either already occluded or must be ligated during all operations done for

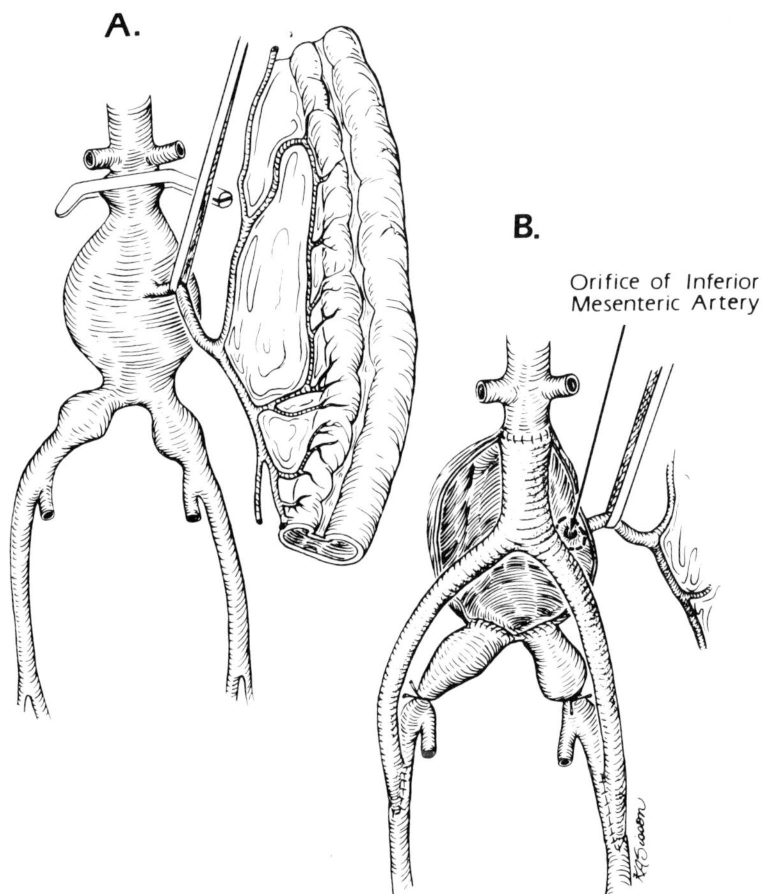

Fig. 1. (A) Soft sling on proximal inferior mesenteric artery. Left colic and sigmoidal branches preserved. (B) Aneurysm sac opened and orifice of inferior mesenteric still intact. Proximal and distal common iliac arteries ligated so as to preserve flow to hypogastric arteries when graft is placed. Dotted line shows area resected to fashion Carrel patch.

abdominal aortic aneurysm and at times following reconstructions done for occlusive disease. One or both of the hypogastric arteries are also often sacrificed or occluded when treating aortic disease. In spite of this, colonic ischemia is relatively uncommon, occurring in 1.5%-10% of patients undergoing aortic operations. Preservation of collateral arterial flow to the colon or reimplantation of the inferior mesenteric artery or restoration of flow to the hypogastric artery helps reduce the incidence of colon ischemia.

Unfortunately, there are few distinctive warning signs or symptoms of postoperative colon ischemia. Endoscopy, careful physical examinations, and a

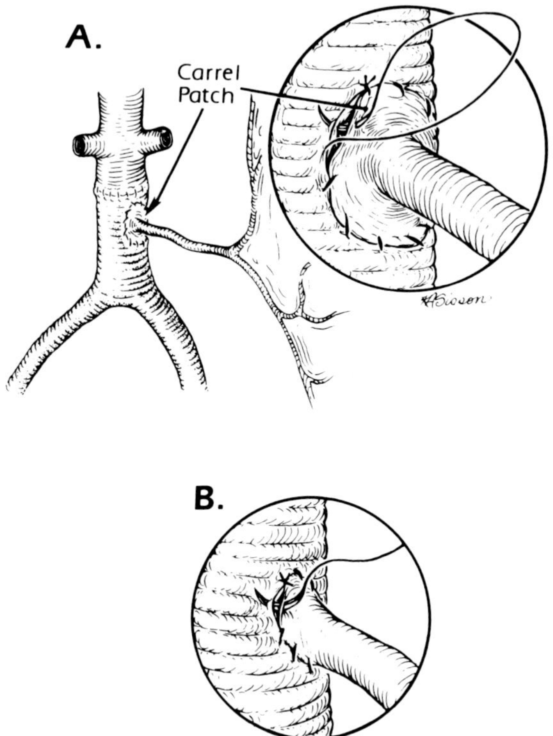

Fig. 2. (A) Patch of aneurysm wall with inferior mesenteric artery sutured to side of bifurcation graft. (B) Inferior mesenteric artery divided, spatulated, and sutured to graft wall.

high index of suspicion will lead to early diagnosis and prompt treatment. It is only with early corrective surgery that sepsis and ultimate death of the patient can be prevented.

REFERENCES

1. Ault GW, Castro AF, Smith RS: Clinical study of ligation of the inferior mesenteric artery in left colon resections. Surg. Gynecol. Obstet. 94:223, 1952
2. Bernatz PE: Necrosis of the colon following resection for abdominal aortic aneurysms. Arch. Surg. 81:373, 1960
3. Bertelsen S, Egeblad K: Necrosis of the colon and the rectum complicating abdominal aortic resection. Acta Chir. Scand. 134:151, 1968
4. Bicks RO, Bale GF, Howard H, et al: Acute and delayed colon ischemia after aortic aneurysm surgery. Arch. Intern. Med. 122:249, 1968

5. Boley S, Schwartz S, Lash J, et al: Reversible vascular occlusion of the colon. Surg. Gynecol. Obstet. 116:53, 1963
6. Carrel A: Technique and remote results of vascular anastomoses. Surg. Gynecol. Obstet. 14(3):246, 1912
7. Dalinka MK, Gohel VK, Schaffer B, et al: Gastrointestinal complications of aortic bypass surgery. Clin. Radiol. 27:255, 1975
8. DeBakey ME, Cooley DA: Surgical treatment of aneurysm of abdominal aorta by resection and restoration of continuity with homograft. Surg. Gynecol. Obstet. 97:257, 1953
9. Dubost C, Allary M, Oeconomos N: Resection of an aneurysm of the abdominal aorta. Arch. Surg. 64:405, 1952
10. Ernst CB, Hagihara PF, Daugherty ME, et al: Ischemic colitis incidence following abdominal aortic reconstruction: A prospective study. Surgery 80:417, 1976
11. Ernst CB, Hagihara PF, Daugherty ME, et al: Inferior mesenteric artery stump pressure: A reliable index for safe IMA ligation during abdominal aortic aneurysmectomy. Ann. Surg. 187:641, 1978
12. Fagin RR, Kirsner JB: Ischemic diseases of the colon. Adv. Intern. Med. 17:343, 1971
13. Goldschmidt Z, Durst AL, Romanoff H: Necrosis of the colon following elective resection of abdominal aortic aneurysms. Vasc. Surg. 9-10:141, 1975-76
14. Griffiths JD: Surgical anatomy of the blood supply of the distal colon. Ann. R. Coll. Surg. 19:241, 1956
15. Hobson RW II, Wright CB, Rich NM, et al: Assessment of colonic ischemia during aortic surgery by Doppler ultrasound. J. Surg. Res. 20:231, 1976
16. Johnson WC, Nasbeth DC: Visceral infarction following aortic surgery. Ann. Surg. 180:312, 1974
17. McBurney RP, Howard H, Bicks RO, et al: Ischemia and gangrene of the colon following abdominal aortic resection. Am. Surgeon 36:205, 1970
18. McKain J, Shumacker HB Jr: Ischemia of the left colon associated with abdominal aortic aneurysms and their treatment. Arch. Surg. 76:355, 1958
19. Miller JH, Bennett RC: Ischaemic strictures of the recto-sigmoid complicating resection of abdominal aortic aneurysms. Aust. N. Z. J. Surg. 37:345, 1968
20. Miller RE, Knox WG: Colon ischemia following infrarenal aortic surgery: Report of four cases. Ann. Surg. 163:639, 1966
21. Moore SW: Resection of the abdominal aorta with defect replaced by homologous graft. Surg. Gynecol. Obstet. 99:745, 1954
22. Morgan N, Griffiths D: High ligation of the inferior mesenteric artery during operations for carcinoma of the distal colon and rectum. Surg. Gynecol. Obstet. 108:641, 1959
23. Moskowitz M, Zimmerman H, Felson B: The meandering mesenteric artery of the colon. Am. J. Roentgenol. 92:1088, 1964
24. Movius HJ: Resection of abdominal arteriosclerotic aneurysm. Am. J. Surg. 90:298, 1955
25. Ottinger LW, Darling RC, Nathan MJ, et al: Left colon ischemia complicating aorto-iliac reconstruction. Arch. Surg. 105:841, 1972

26. Papadopoulos CD, Mancini HW, Marino AW Jr: Ischemic necrosis of the colon following aortic aneurysmectomy. Surgery 15:494, 1974
27. Smith RF, Szilagyi DE: Ischemia of the colon as a complication in the surgery of the abdominal aorta. AMA Arch. Surg. 80:806, 1960
28. Steward JA, Rankin FW: Blood supply of the large intestine: Its surgical considerations. Arch. Surg. 26:843, 1933
29. Young JR, Britton RC, DeWolfe VG, et al: Intestinal ischemic necrosis following abdominal aortic surgery. Surg. Gynecol. Obstet. 115:615, 1962
30. Young JR, Humphries AW, DeWolfe VG, et al: Complications of abdominal aortic surgery: II: Intestinal ischemia. Arch. Surg. 86:65, 1963
31. Zarins CK, Skinner DB, Rhodes BA, et al: Predictions of the viability of revascularized intestine with radioactive microspheres. Surg. Gynecol. Obstet. 138:576, 1974

Aortoiliac Occlusive Disease

J. F. Vollmar, M.D.
B. Heyden, M.D.

Experiences With Reconstructive Surgery of the Aortoiliac Segment

For reconstructive surgery of the aortoiliac segment some pathophysiologic aspects should be kept in mind:

1. Only one-fifth of patients suffering from arterial insufficiency of their lower extremities show occlusive lesions limited to the aortoiliac area [8]. In approximately 80% of patients there are concomitant lesions in the femoropopliteal segment or below the knee. This is especially true for patients with rest pain (stage III) and/or distal necrosis (stage IV).
2. In patients with such combined lesions the repair of the aortoiliac segments takes preference over all distal vascular interventions. The goal of such a central vascular repair is both restoring a full arterial "run-in or inflow" and elimination of a potential embolic source. Probably a remarkable number of concomitant distal occlusions are from embolic origin.
3. All aortoiliac reconstructions represent repair of large vessels under high flow conditions, with a sufficient runoff. This is even true in the presence of femoral artery occlusion: if the deep femoral artery is patent this vessel guarantees in most patients an excellent runoff (via profundaplasty).

On this basis aortoiliac surgery has become one of the most effective tools in the treatment of arterial occlusive diseases. Its long term results are significantly superior to those of the femoropopliteal segment. As a consequence no distal arterial repair should be performed before full patency of the aortoiliac segment has been proved or restored.

TECHNICAL ASPECTS – CHOICE OF PROCEDURE

In the last 20 years there has been much controversy concerning the choice of reconstructive procedure. In the meantime the extreme position of "strippers" and "grafters" has been overcome by a more knowledgeable evaluation of thromboendarterectomy (TEA) and bypass procedures. Now, both techniques are considered not as surgical alternatives but rather as complementary procedures for giving patients optimal vascular repair. From such a point of view the choice of procedure should be made in relation to the clinical findings (stages I-IV), the arteriographic patterns, and the general condition of the patient. Especially for aortoiliac repairs, the indications for surgery should be based on critical evaluation of several factors (Table 1) including the operative technique. As a guideline the "three S" principle should be kept in mind – the procedure should be *s*afe, *s*imple, and *s*hort.

Thromboendarterectomy (TEA)

In our hands this is the preferred procedure of repair of localized segmental occlusive lesions (types I and II; see Fig. 1) including unilateral iliac artery occlusions. In addition, TEA is the preferred technique in younger patients with free distal runoff. From a biological point of view TEA is superior to any synthetic graft.

As a technical principle, every TEA should be performed from one bifurcation to the next (Fig. 2). Usually a semiclosed technique is used. Spiral

Table 1
Three-Point Indication

I. CLINICAL INDICATION - should the patient be operated upon?

Degree of severity –			
	I	asymptomatic	None
	II	intermittent claudication: exercise limitation < 500 meters	Relative
	III	rest pain	Absolute
	IV	distal necrosis	Absolute

II. ANGIOGRAPHIC INDICATION - can the patient be operated upon? **(**local operability**)**

Points of importance are:
Location and extent of the occlusions; free inflow and run-off.
Vascular caliber.
Vascular wall calcifications.

III. GENERAL OPERABILITY - may the patient stand an operation?

Absence of relevant coronary, cerebral or renal vascular disturbance or other serious systemic illness (carcinoma, severe diabetes, etc.)

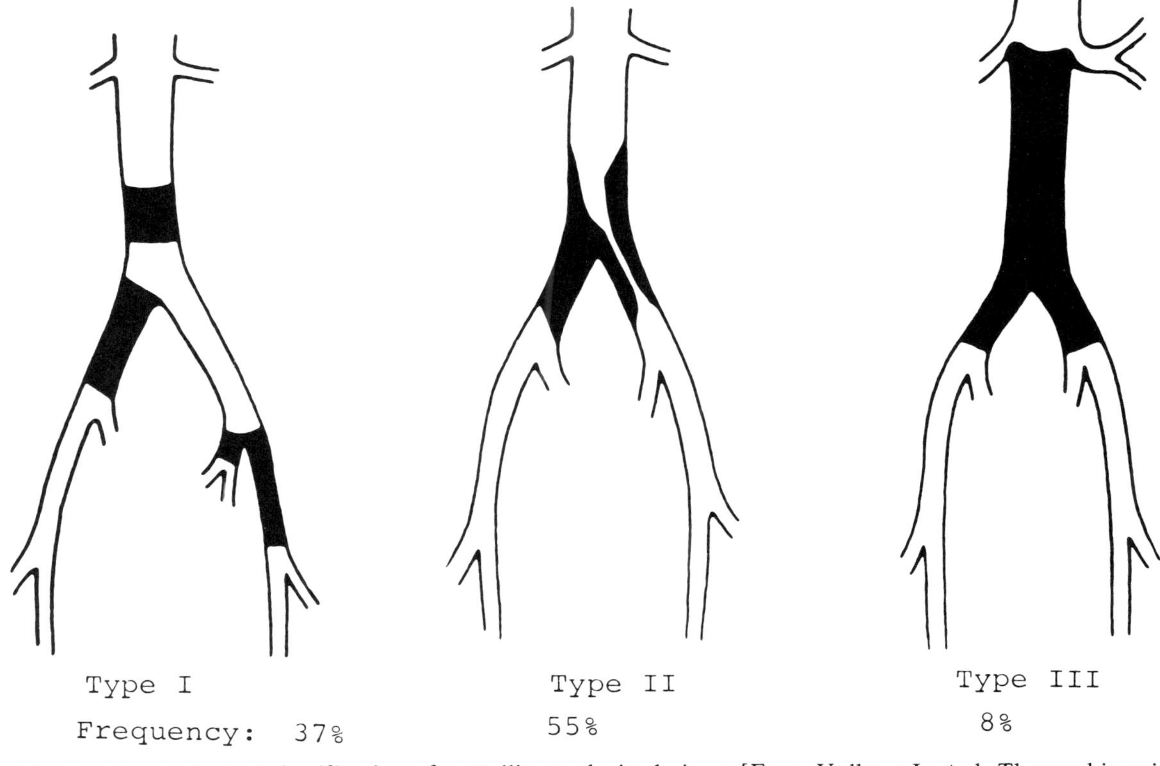

Fig. 1. Morphological classification of aortoiliac occlusive lesions. [From Vollmar J, et al: Thoraxchirurgie 13:453, 1965.]

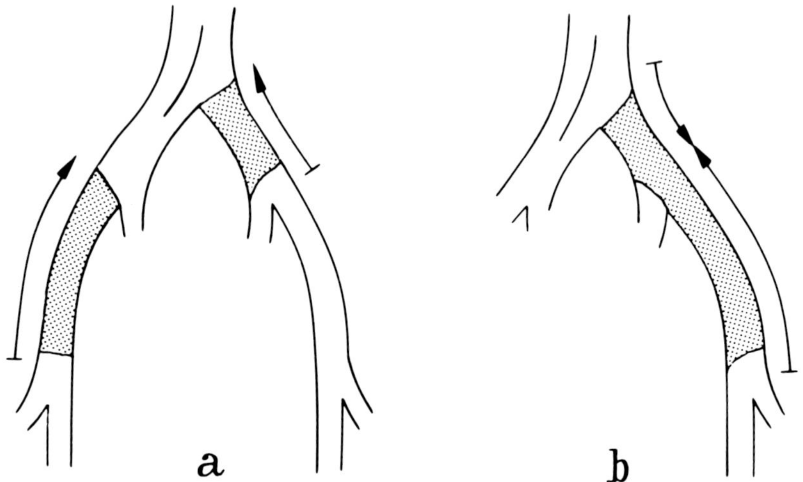

Fig. 2. Extension of semiclosed thromboendarterectomy (A) for segmental iliac artery occlusions and (B) for unilateral extensive occlusion. Principle: disobliteration from bifurcation to bifurcation.

dissection using rotation oblique rings has proved superior to all other recommended disobliterative techniques [7, 8] (Fig. 3).

As an example, in a patient with a localized stenosis of the aortic bifurcation and concomitant stenotic lesion in the right common iliac artery, the disobliteration is done between distal and proximal longitudinal arteriotomies (Fig. 4). The postoperative arteriogram demonstrates free patency and the characteristic widening of the disobliterated arterial segment (Fig. 5). In the case of unilateral common and/or external iliac artery occlusion the ring disobliteration is usually performed between femoral and aortic arteriotomies using two dissecting rings, from above and below (see Fig. 2B). The intimal core at the origin of the internal iliac artery gets broken by the retrograde introduction of the distal ring.

In male patients with complaints of disturbances in the sexual sphere the internal iliac inflow has to be restored by an additional open TEA of the iliac bifurcation. The vascular origin of impotence may be assessed by sonographic penile blood pressure measurement [2].

Other techniques of TEA may be applied under the following conditions:

1. For a segmental block of the external iliac artery with an intact proximal common and internal iliac artery, a transfemoral approach is preferred using a retrograde semiclosed TEA. A spiral dissection technique usually allows removal of the whole intimal core up to the level of the iliac bifurcation without difficulties. An additional exposure of the iliac bifurcation is usually unnecessary (Fig. 2A).

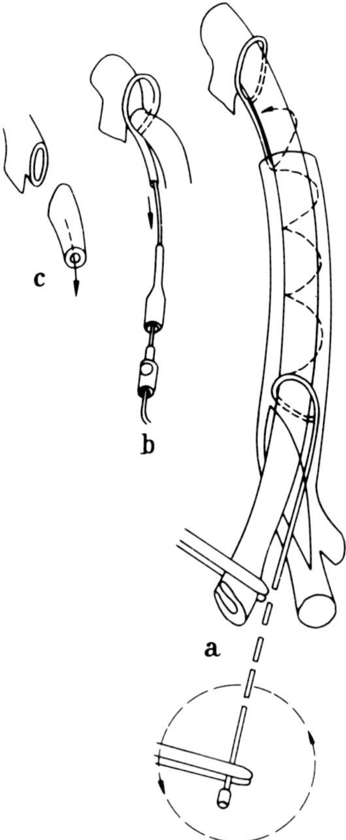

Fig. 3. Technique of transfemoral retrograde ring disobliteration. (A) Spiral dissection of the occlusive cylinder by intramural introduction of an oblique ring. (B) Using a cutting wire at the level of the iliac bifurcation if the intimal core is fixed (compare Fig. 6).

2. In high-risk patients extensive iliac artery occlusions may be repaired in a similar way via a transfemoral approach using a cutting ring at the iliac or aortic bifurcation. This special instrument (Fig. 6) allows a cutdown of the intimal core without exposure of the central vessels.
3. If there is an additional superficial femoral artery block with a free patent segment in the popliteal artery a combined balloon and ring disobliteration, the Rififi technique, may be used [7] (Figs. 7 and 8). The primary introduction of the balloon catheter through the occluded femoral segment, with inflation of its tip in the popliteal artery, prevents dislodgment of embolic material to the distal arteries. After spiral dissection of the occluded segment by a ring the simultaneous retraction of both instruments usually

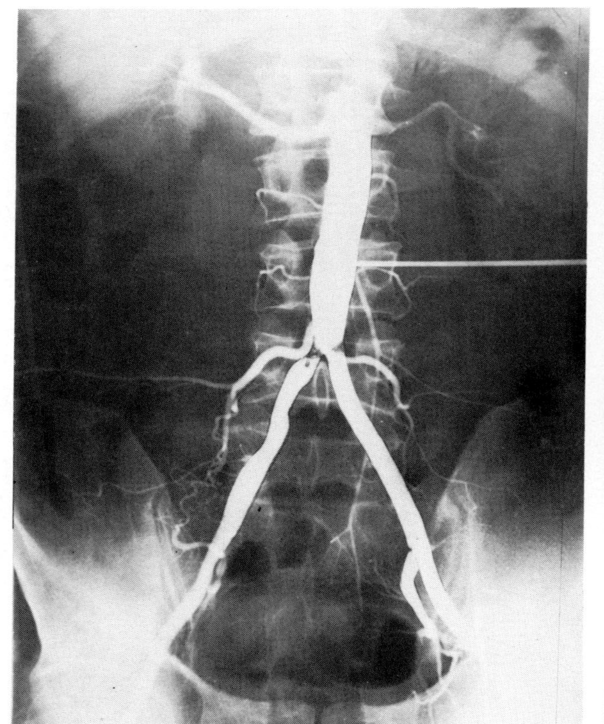

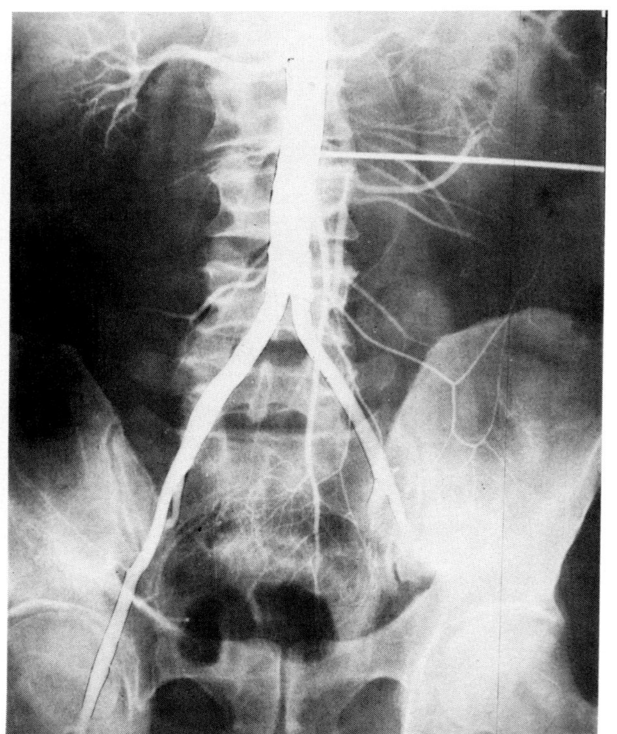

Figs. 4 and 5. Severe stenoses on the aortic bifurcation with intimal plaques in the right common iliac artery. Repair by aortoiliac ring disobliteration. Full restored lumen with characteristic widening of the artery 3 years later. [From Vollmar J: Rekonstruktive Chirurgie der Arterien (vol 2). Stuttgart, Thieme, 1975.]

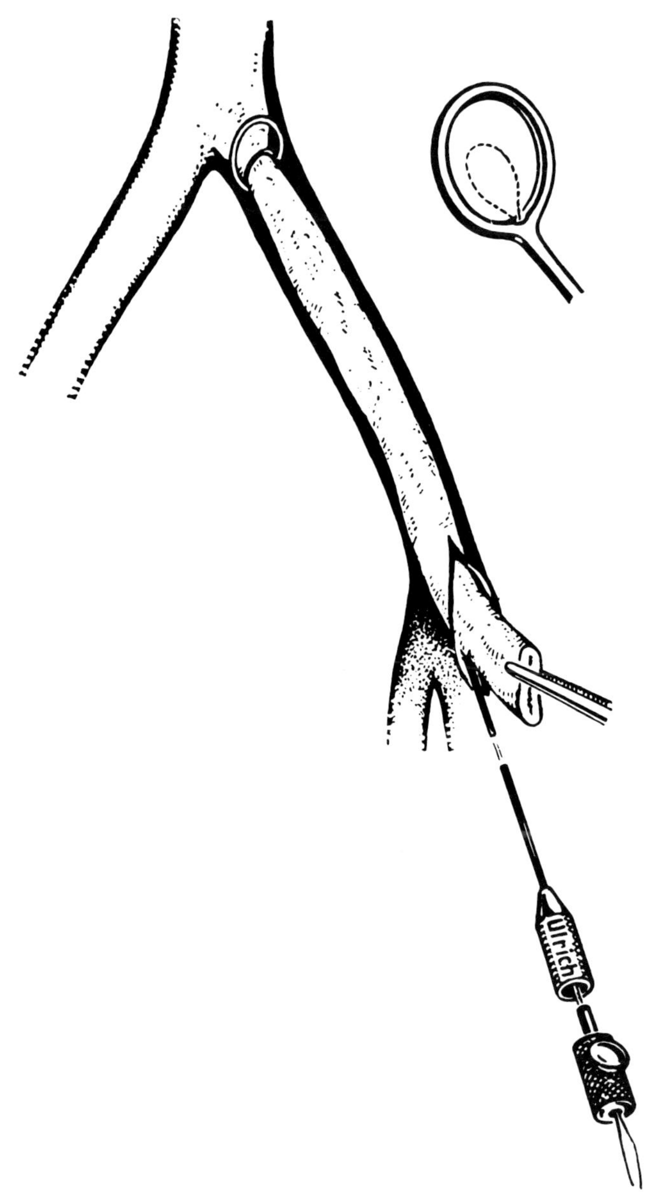

Fig. 6. Ring disobliterotome (manufacturer, Fa. H. C. Ulrich, Ulm, West Germany). Following spiral dissection of the occlusive cylinder up to the aortic bifurcation the intimal core is cut off by snare and removed through the distal arteriotomy. Main indications: semiclosed disobliterations of the pelvic artery or the aortic bifurcation in high risk patient. [From Vollmar J: Rekonstruktive Chirurgie der Arterien (vol 2). Stuttgart, Thieme, 1975.]

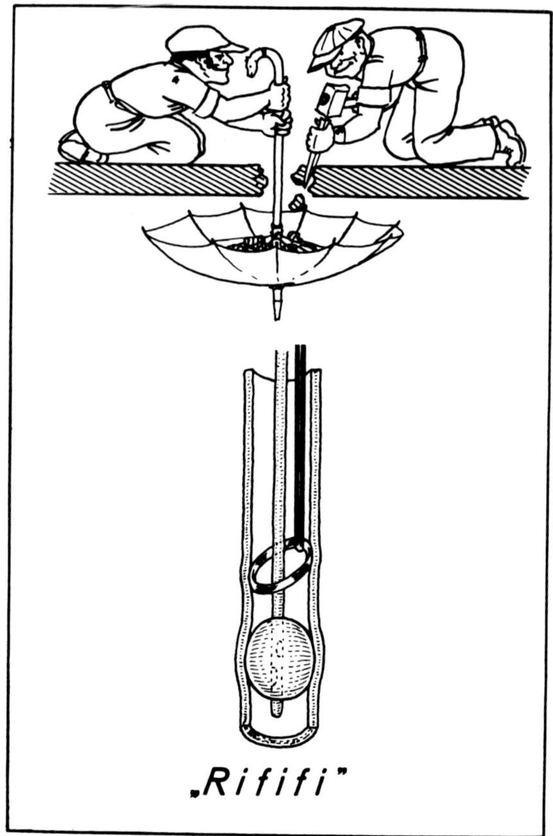

Fig. 7. Principle of the "Rififi" technique. Orthograde or retrograde ring disobliteration under the protection of an occluding balloon catheter.

allows a smooth distal breakoff of the occlusive cylinder and its complete removal through the central arteriotomy.

CASE REPORT

In this 72-year-old high risk patient with distal necrosis of the left foot the arteriogram demonstrated a two-level occlusion of the external iliac, common femoral, and superficial femoral arteries. A transfemoral Rififi disobliteration technique was used in both proximal and distal directions with full restoration of the arterial lumen (Fig. 9).

For this type of vascular repair the surgeon should always be prepared to clean up the lumen, if necessary, through an additional distal or proximal

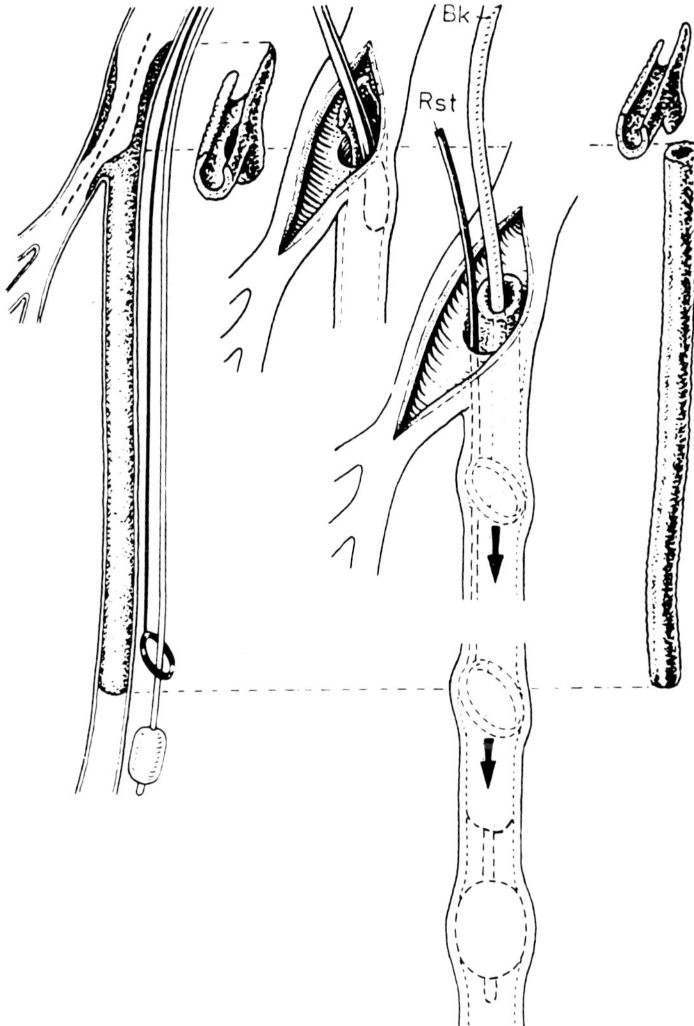

Fig. 8. Technique of the combined ring-balloon disobliteration. Rififi technique for the femoropopliteal vascular segment. Bk = balloon catheter; Rst = ring-stripper.

arteriotomy. Most failures of semiclosed TEA are caused by technical faults due mainly to incomplete removal of the occluding cylinder. Therefore every orthograde or retrograde semiclosed disobliteration should have intraoperative control by arteriography or by vascular endoscopy [9, 10].

Vascular endoscopy is useful in all disobliterative interventions on large arteries and veins. It offers a three-dimensional inspection of the whole vascular lumen, requires only a few minutes, and is performed prior to closure of the

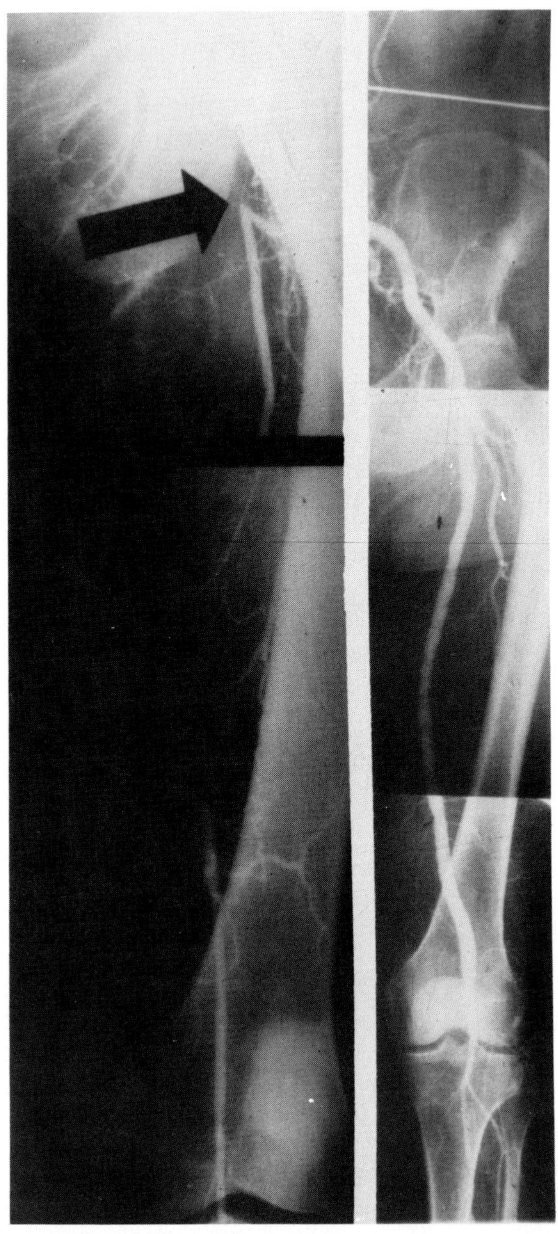

Fig. 9. Extensive occlusion of the left external iliac, common femoral, and superficial femoral artery in a 72-year-old high risk patient (rest pain with distal necrosis on his left foot). (A) Preoperative arteriogram. (B) X-ray after transfemoral Rififi disobliteration with full restoration of the arterial lumen.

arteriotomy (Fig. 10). The main indication for intraoperative arteriography is control of bypass procedures and all types of small vessel repairs (diameter below 6 mm; Table 2).

If after TEA a full lumen restoration has been proven, the same good final results as in bypass procedures may be expected both in the iliac and in the femoral level.

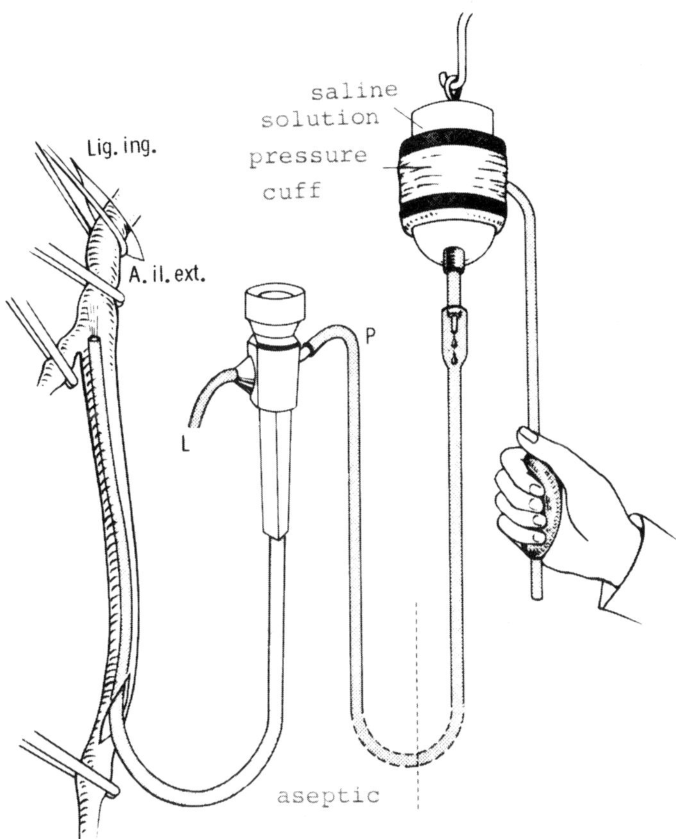

Fig. 10. Principle of vascular endoscopy (femoral popliteal segment). Central and distal occlusion of flow by vascular clamps. Retrograde introduction of a flexible fiberendoscop (manufacturer, Olympus). L, cold light source; P, perfusion attachment. The lumen of the reopened vascular segment is tested and inspected under continuous fluid perfusion and with a pressure of 80-100 mm Hg.

Table 2
Synopsis of Intraoperative Lumen Control

	endoscopy	angiography
lumen control	three dimensional	one dimensional
afforded time	minimal (5 - 10min.)	greater (10 - 15min.)
costs	minimal (4 - 10 $)	increased (40 - 60 $)
application	limited a) vascular lumen >5mm b) not for bypass grafts	unlimited
secondary vascular repair	easy (on open vessel)	more difficult
complications	< 0,1 %	< 0,1%

BYPASS PROCEDURES

In recent years bypass procedures using straight or bifurcated Dacron or Teflon prostheses have become the most frequently utilized reconstructions (80%) for repair of aortoiliac occlusive lesions [1]. Their main advantage is technical; i.e., easy performance with reduced operating time and therefore reduced risk for the patient. Therefore the bypass procedure is chosen especially in elderly high risk patients and in the presence of the following angiographic patterns:

1. Bilateral extensive diseased aortoiliac segment.
2. High occlusion of the infrarenal aorta.
3. Recurrent occlusion after TEA.

The availability of new improved synthetic vascular prostheses such as velour knitted Dacron grafts with high porosity and a more physiological diameter ratio between mainstem and limbs (14/8/8 mm) has remarkably reduced the frequency of healing complications including anastomotic aneurysms and deep wound infections [5].

Some technical aspects of graft insertion may be mentioned which make the procedure short, safe, and simple. For bifurcation grafts an anterior approach through a long median laparotomy is preferred. The patient is turned on the operating table to the right. In this position, facing the operator, the eventrated small bowel is easily kept in position. After covering the bowel by a simple plastic sheet, two big retractors are inserted according to the V principle (Fig. 11). The use of a plastic bag causes additional troubles and should be avoided.

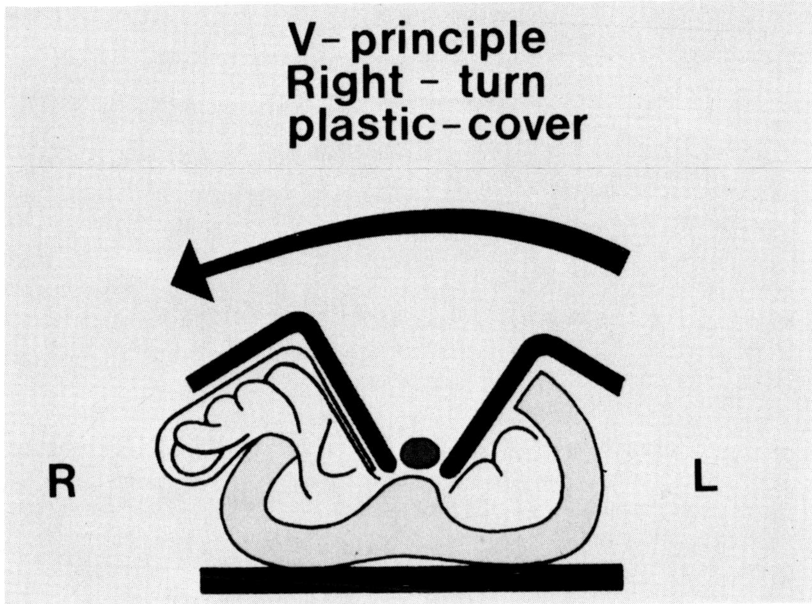

Fig. 11. V principle for the exposure of the infrarenal aorta.

As a rule, the upper anastomosis should be performed as high as possible, i.e., immediately below the left renal vein. A second important point is to trim the mainstem of the bifurcated graft very short both for end-to-side and end-to-end-anastomoses (Fig. 12). This type of insertion guarantees a high position of the graft bifurcation, usually 2-3 cm higher than the patient's own aortic bifurcation, preventing any kinking of the limbs. A low anastomosis and a long mainstem of the prosthesis result frequently in kinked prosthetic limbs which favor early thrombosis.

After completion of the proximal anastomosis, the waiting time for graft preclotting is used for the exposure of the common femoral artery in both groins. For preventing any damage to the inguinal lymph nodes and lymph vessels a longitudinal lateral groin incision is preferred, shifting the entire subcutaneous fat tissue – including the lymph nodes – in a medial direction (Fig. 13). If the femoropopliteal segment is patent, a long end-to-side anastomosis of the prosthetic limb with the common and superficial femoral artery is performed, usual length 4-5 cm.

In the presence of concomitant occlusive lesions of the femoral segment the prosthetic limb is routinely inserted into the deep femoral artery using a long end-to-side anastomosis according to the principle of a profundaplasty [3, 11]. This means tapering of an 8 mm prosthesis down to the diameter of the receptor artery, usually 4-6 mm (Fig. 14). Mechanical dilatation of the deep femoral artery has proved an excellent approach to overcoming any pronounced

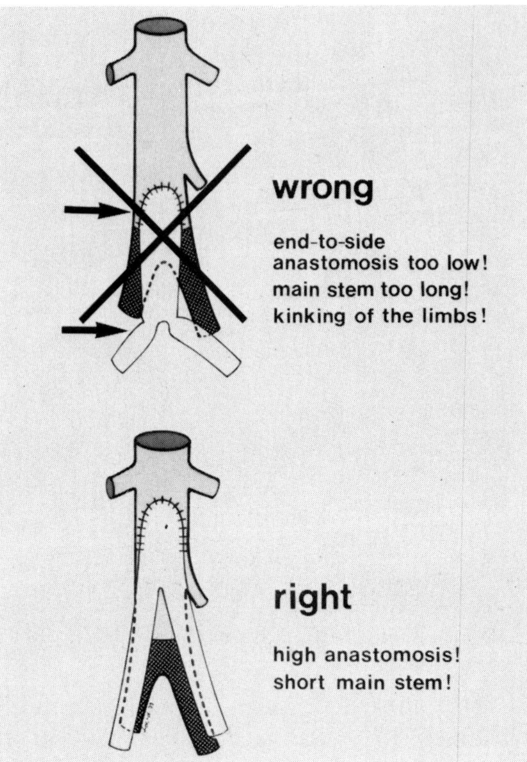

Fig. 12. Trimming of the mainstem for bifurcated graft, upper anastomosis.

diameter discrepancy. In addition, every profundaplasty should be combined by a lumbar sympathectomy (L3-L5).

The modified type of profundaplasty, i.e., long arterial incision beyond the first bifurcation widening of this vascular segment by patch or long end-to-side graft insertion, results in a "conic adaption" of the large run-in or inflow vessel (common femoral artery or graft) to the small runoff vessel (deep femoral artery) [3, 4, 11].

From a hemodynamic point of view conicity of the vessel means increase of flow velocity, i.e., an additional protective factor against suture line thrombosis.

The effect of simultaneous lumbar sympathectomy on the deep femoral artery flow is not yet clearly understood. In combination with conventional femoropopliteal reconstruction lumbar sympathectomy has little or no effect on flow rate. However, as an additional measure with profundaplasty its effect on blood flow is impressive, probably due to remarkable reduction of flow resistance [3, 4, 11] (Fig. 15).

In a retrospective study, including 403 limbs of stages II-IV, the triad procedure (aortoiliac reconstruction plus profundaplasty plus lumbar

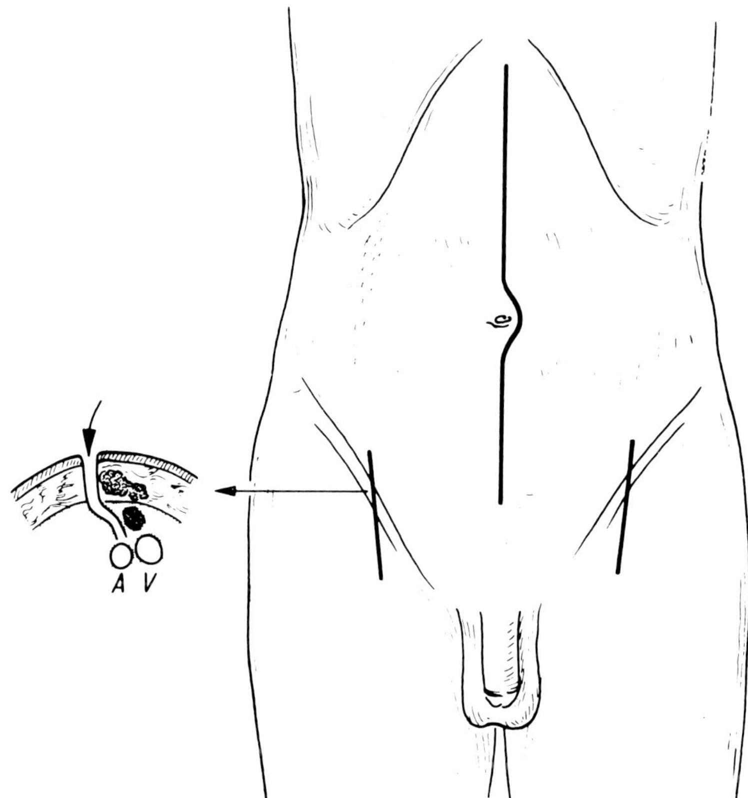

Fig. 13. Incisions for aortofemoral bifurcation bypass. Exposure of the femoral bifurcation by a surgical slightly slanted cut 1 cm lateral to the artery. In this manner the subcutaneous and subfascial lymphatics are left medial to the incision (avoidance of postoperative lymphatic complications). [From Vollmar J: Rekonstruktive Chirurgie der Arterien (vol 2). Stuttgart, Thieme, 1975.]

sympathectomy; group II) showed a cumulative patency rate of 77% versus 39% in the total repair (group I; Fig. 16). In limb salvage operations (stages III-IV) the corresponding figures for amputation rate were 8% and 39% and for the need of reoperation 7% and 23% [3].

Following limb salvage operation 19% of the extremities in total-repair group I returned to stage I (asymptomatic) and 43% to stage II (mild rest claudication). The corresponding figures for group II (triad procedure) were 44% and 46%. In addition, the rate of major amputations following interventions for limb salvage was 36% for group I and only 8% for group II.

On the basis of these results in Europe there is an increased trend toward giving up the time-consuming two-level repair and restricting the surgical activities mainly to restoration of aortoiliac inflow by a triad procedure.

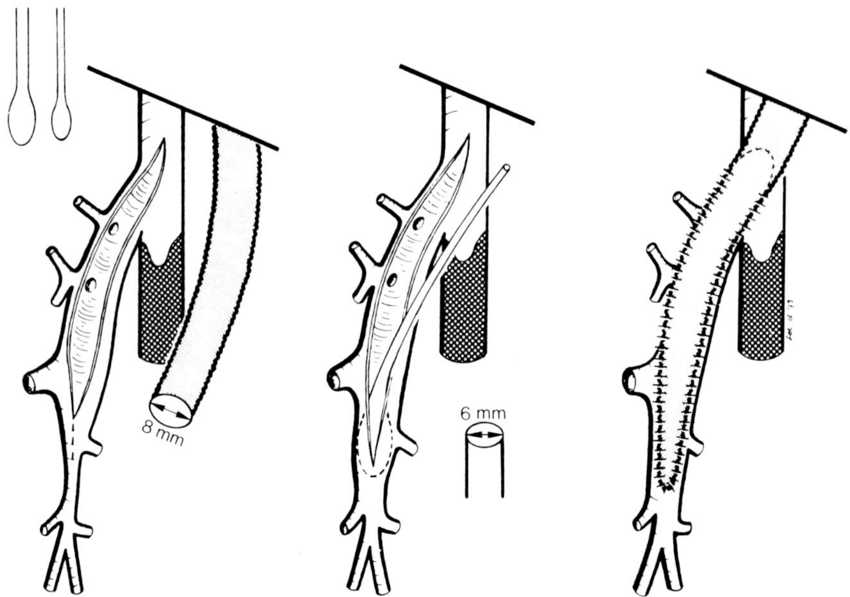

Fig. 14. Technique of profundaplasty. Long end-to-side insertion of the prosthetic limb in the deep femoral artery resulting in a "conic adaption" of the big run-in or inflow vessel to the small runoff vessel. In addition, for the avoidance of pronounced discrepancy in vessel diameters the distal deep femoral artery may be dilated using special olive-shaped dilatators.

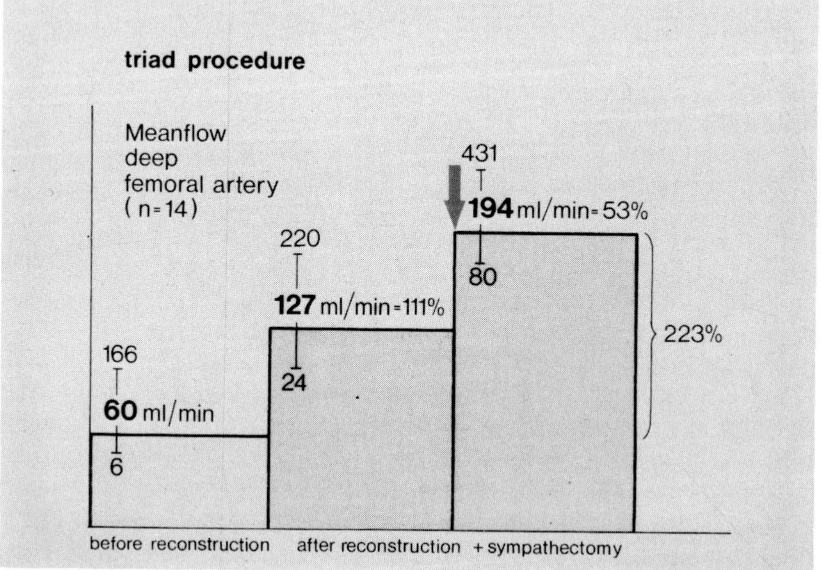

Fig. 15. Changes in flow rate of the deep femoral artery by triad procedure.

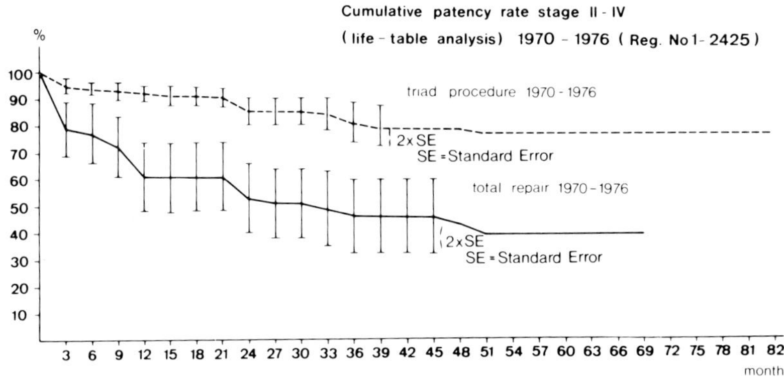

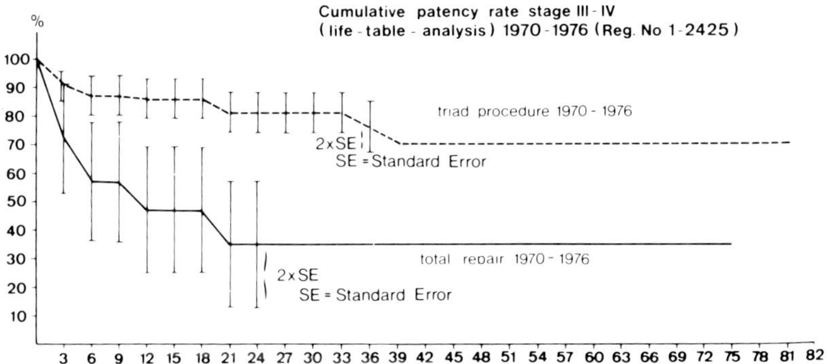

Fig. 16. Triad procedure versus total repair.

For a successful partial repair in patients with a two-level occlusion some prerequisites must be fulfilled. These include, first of all, an intact deep femoral artery system with sufficient collateral runoff, i.e., patency of the "recipient segment" of popliteal artery.

Nevertheless, there is still a good place for total repair. This more extensive and time-consuming intervention is justified and necessary under the following conditions:

1. Hopelessly diseased deep femoral artery.
2. Patent deep femoral artery but insufficient collateral runoff, i.e., occlusion of the "recipient segment" of the popliteal artery and/or concomitant occlusions of two or more crural vessels.

But these circumstances were present only in 12% of 337 evaluated combined occlusions. Therefore total repair may be restricted to few exceptional cases. If a previous triad procedure remains insufficient a staged distal revascularization may be added.

RESULTS AND OUTLOOK

For a followup period of 10 years the patency rates for TEA and Dacron bypass grafts are nearly identical, i.e., 90% for 5 years and 84% for 10 years (Fig. 17). These figures are based on an evaluation of 1071 patients with predominantly isolated aortoiliac lesions operated upon between 1959 and 1974 at the University Clinic at Heidelberg [6]. Operative mortality for good risk patients averaged 2%-4%. This is mainly influenced by the experiences of the vascular surgeon, i.e., selection of patients and quality of vascular repair. The death rate approaches 50% for the 10 years following surgery. In comparison with the spontaneous course of arterial occlusive diseases, the amputation rate can be reduced in the operative group by approximately half (14% versus 7%).

Postoperative complications

Early reocclusions following TEA bypass procedures [7, 8] (frequency 4.2%) are mainly caused by technical faults. Immediate reinterventions allow, in over 90% of cases, full restoration of the arterial pathway. Deep wound infections [1, 6-8] (frequency 0.5%-1.0%) predominantly concern the groin incision; 90% of the infected grafts have to be removed under the protection of a new aseptic bypass procedure (such as iliopopliteal obturator bypass or axillofemoral graft). The infection rate of 1% in 2000 operations was not changed by the routine use of antibiotics. Therefore we give antibiotics only in patients with manifest infections according to the antibiogram.

Anastomotic aneurysms were observed after use of synthetic grafts with a frequency of 1.7%-6%. The most frequent location was the groin. An increasing number of aneurysms was observed beyond a 10-year followup.

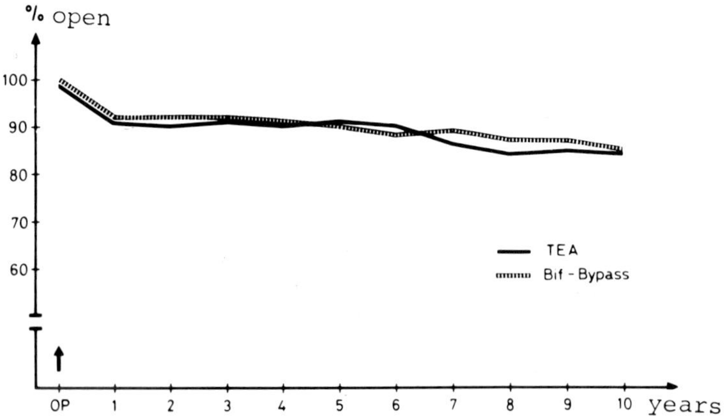

Fig. 17. Final results of aortoiliac reconstructive procedures [according to Schulz et al., 1977].

REFERENCES

1. Brewster DC, Darling RC: Optimal methods of aortoiliac reconstruction. Surgery 84:739-748, 1978
2. Gaylis H: The assessment of impotence in aorto-iliac disease using penile blood pressure measurement. S. Afr. J. Surg. 16:39-46, 1978
3. Heyden B, Voss EU, Vollmar J: Repair of combined occlusive lesions of the aorto-iliac and femoro-popliteal segment. J. Cardiovasc. Surg. (in press)
4. Rocher A, Basyn ML, Joos FE: Blood flow measurements in arterial surgery of lower limb. J. Cardiovasc. Surg. 16:384, 1975
5. Sauvage LR, Robel SB, Wood SJ, et al: Geometric comparison of aortic bifurcation prostheses to the normal and atherosclerotic human aorta, and clinical triad of a vertical seamed bifurcation prosthesis. Surgery 81:22-32, 1977
6. Schulz Z, Laubach K, Preissler P: Zur Wahl des Operationsverfahrens im aorto-iliacalen Gefässabschnitt. Langenbecks Arch. Chir. 344:41-52, 1977
7. Vollmar J: Rekonstruktive Chirurgie der Arterien (vol 2). Stuttgart, Thieme, 1975
8. Vollmar J, Laubach K, Campana JM: Die chirurgische Behandlung der chronischen Arterienverschlüsse im aorto-iliakalen Gefässabschnitt. Thoraxchirurgie 13:453-478, 1965
9. Vollmar J, Junghanns K: Die Endoskopie der Arterien, in Ottenjann R (ed): Fortschritte der Endoskopie. Stuttgart-New York, Schattauer, 1970
10. Vollmar J, Storz LW: Vascular Endoscopy. Possibilities and limits of its clinical application. Surg. Clin. North Am. 54:111, 1974
11. Voss EU, Heyden B, Vollmar J: Le traitement chirurgical des obstructions étagées aorto-iliaques et fémoro-poplitées. Angéiologie 31:3-8, 1979

Luis A. Queral, M.D., William R. Flinn, M.D.
John J. Bergan, M.D., James S. T. Yao, M.D., Ph.D.

Sexual Function and Aortic Surgery

Aortoiliac arterial occlusive disease was noted to affect adversely pelvic blood flow in 1940, when Leriche [16, 17] described the syndrome related to thrombotic obliteration of the abdominal aortic bifurcation. Symptomatology of male patients included inability to keep a stable erection and lower extremity fatigue. In 1960, Scheer [24] called attention to impotence as a symptom of pelvic arterial disorders and stated that impotence often heralded the symptoms of claudication. Recently, several authors have described sexual dysfunction subsequent to aortoiliac reconstruction [11, 19, 25]. May, DeWeese, and Rob [19] emphasized the importance of maintaining hypogastric artery blood flow in order to avoid postoperative erectile impairment. Others have advocated a technique of sparing of sympathetic nerves during aortic exposure and have claimed this to be important in preserving erectile function [6, 25]. It is clear that sexual dysfunction may be related to neurogenic factors as well as a decrease in blood supply.

SEXUAL DYSFUNCTIONS

In the male, sexual dysfunctions include impotence and retrograde ejaculation. The former is closely related to adequacy of blood supply, and the latter is mostly neurogenic in origin. In patients with aortoiliac disease, the incidence of impotence is high (more than 30% of cases).

Unlike males, females appear to be largely immune to surgically induced adverse sexual effects for two main reasons: (1) Feminine sexual sensation

Supported in part by the Dr. Scholl Foundation and the Northwestern University Vascular Research Fund.

depends locally in great part upon the intact somatic pudendal nerve and its efferent sensory nerve fibers. The pudendal nerves are situated close to the periosteum of the pelvic bones, covered and protected by a thick layer of endopelvic fascia, and are unlikely to be disturbed during arterial operative procedures. (2) Collateral arterial blood supply to the gynecological organs is immense, and female sexual malfunction secondary to vascular insufficiency is unknown. In contrast, neural injury and alterations in arterial pelvic hemodynamics can occur as sequelae of arterial reconstruction in males, and these lead to ejaculatory malfunction and erectile impairment, respectively. Therefore since female sexual function does not appear to be influenced by vascular surgery, subsequent discussion will be limited to the preoperative assessment of males.

Causes of Sexual Dysfunction

A thorough knowledge of the causes of impotence is essential to understanding of male sexual dysfunction. Impotence is defined as the inability to attain or sustain penile erection to a degree necessary to achieve satisfactory coitus. Normal sexual function in an adult male requires normal anatomy, appropriate androgenic secretion at the time of puberty, normal endocrine function, and intact nerve and vascular supply to the genitalia. Thus developmental, endocrinologic, neurologic, or vascular disorders may be organic causes of impotence. When no apparent cause can be established for complaints of impotency, a psychogenic etiology is deduced.

Table 1 summarizes the causes of impotence. For vascular surgeons, several factors affecting sexual function are important in the evaluation of impotence. These are diabetes mellitus, the influence of various pharmacological agents, blood supply to the genital organs, and postsurgical effects.

Table 1
Causes of Impotence

Developmental	*Trauma*
Hypospadias	Pelvic trauma with membranous urethra damage
Endocrinological	*Pharmacological agents*
Eunuchoidism	*Postsurgical*
Hypopituitarism	Abdominal-perineal resection
Hypothyroidism	Aortofemoral reconstruction
Cushing's syndrome	
Diabetes mellitus	
Neurological	
Spinal cord injury	
Sacral spinal cord tumor	
Tabes dorsalis	
Multiple sclerosis	

Diabetes mellitus is a common, chronic disorder with metabolic, neural, and vascular components. The metabolic manifestations of this disease are closely related to the degree of insulin insufficiency present, since the pathways of carbohydrate, lipid, and protein metabolism require the presence of this hormone. Neuropathy is a frequent complication of diabetes and the vascular component of the disease manifests as both accelerated atherosclerosis and microangiopathy. Impotence occurs in about one-fourth of all diabetic males under 40 years of age. This extremely high incidence of sexual malfunction in diabetics makes an evaluation of etiologic criteria prior to aortofemoral reconstruction desirable. The first step in evaluation of the impotent diabetic is to differentiate organic from psychogenic causes. Table 2 lists a number of criteria which can aid in this differentiation. The separation of neuropathic from vasculogenic causes is also important, and Table 3 lists some of the differences between them. The separation of organic from psychogenic causes is sometimes difficult and psychiatric consultation may be necessary for clarification. On the other hand, the separation of neurogenic from vasculogenic causes of impotence may be impossible to achieve because a large number of patients have both.

Pharmacologic agents which interfere with the parasympathetic component of erection can produce impotence [10]. The major group of drugs involved are ganglionic blocking agents, belladonna derivatives, tricyclic compounds, phenothiazines, and monoamine oxidase inhibitors and cimetidine.

Vascular causes of impotence. Insufficient arterial blood supply to the penis results in either inability to obtain or incapacity to maintain an erection.

Table 2
Criteria Differentiating Organic from Psychogenic Impotence in the Diabetic Patient

Criteria	Organic	Psychogenic
Onset	Gradual (2-18 months)	Rapid (less than 30 days)
Pattern	Complete	Intermittent
Partner specificity	None	May be present
Nonintercourse behavior	No erection during masturbation	Erection during masturbation
Morning erection	Absent	Present
Relation of onset to emotional stress	Absent	Present
Testicular pain on palpation	Decreased	Normal
Sexual drive (libido)	Retained	Varied
Nocturnal tumescence	Absent	Present
Cystometrograms	Neurogenic bladder	Normal

Table 3
Criteria Differentiating Neurogenic from Vasculogenic Impotence in the Diabetic Patient

Criteria	Neurogenic	Vasculogenic
Erections	Absent	Present but short-lived
Penile pressure	Normal	Decreased
Testicular pain on palpation	Decreased	Normal
Cystometrogram	Neurogenic bladder	Normal
Masturbatory ejaculations	Absent	Present
Pupillary abnormalities	Present	Absent
Impaired gastric emptying	Present	Absent
Orthostatic hypotension	Present	Absent
Neurogenic ulcers	Present	Absent
Angiographic appearance of internal iliac arteries and main branches	Patent	Occlusive disease

This functional ischemia can result from obstruction of the aortic bifurcation, internal iliac artery occlusive disease, or an obliterative process of the distal branches of the internal pudendal artery. Patients with the Leriche syndrome are readily identified from their symptoms of impotence, buttock and lower extremity claudication, and the physical findings of diminished or absent femoral pulses [17]. The impotence has been described as a progressive inability to maintain a stable erection, rather than the inability to initiate erection. Sexual incapacitation often precedes symptoms of lower extremity ischemia. It is not unusual for patients to experience buttock claudication and erectile malfunction prior to thigh and leg claudication [24].

In addition to occlusive disease of the internal iliac artery as a cause of impotence, shunting of blood away from the pelvic region has also been related to impotence. In patients with unilateral external iliac artery occlusion and contralateral internal iliac artery stenosis, the ipsilateral internal iliac artery may act as the main supply to the lower limb. With greater demand for blood from the thigh and calf muscles, a condition of "steal phenomenon" has been described by Michal et al. [21] and by Barker [1]. This "pelvic steal" with collateral flow to the ischemic extremity deriving from a hypogastric artery shunting pathway may contribute to impotence [5].

Objective Evaluation

Arteriography is essential to establish the diagnosis of impotence of vascular origin. Retrograde catheter arteriography will visualize the internal iliac artery and its major branches, and an oblique view is often helpful to determine the degree of stenosis. Without special attention to visualization of the penile arteries, most arteriograms will not disclose the diseased state of the penile arteries. Recently, Ginestig and Romieu [9] have advocated selective arteriograms via the internal iliac artèry to demonstrate the pelvic arterial supply. In order to improve the visualization of penile arteries, these authors suggest an indwelling catheter to empty contrast media from the bladder.

Anatomically, blood supply to the penis is derived from the deep artery, the dorsal artery, and urethral artery (Fig. 1). Both deep and dorsal arteries of the penis are terminal branches of the internal pudendal artery, which is a large branch of the internal iliac artery. The vessel is longer in males than females. The deep artery of the penis, which is a smaller branch, is always more laterally placed than the dorsal artery of the penis (Fig. 1). The urethral artery is the terminal branch of the perineal artery, which is another branch of the pudendal artery (Fig. 1). Thus the entire penile supply derives from the internal iliac artery.

The blood supply to the pelvic region is abundant. The internal iliac artery has eight major branches (Fig. 1). Because of this, unless selective angiography is performed, it is unlikely that small arteries like the deep or dorsal penile arteries will be visualized on routine arteriography.

In a survey of 38 patients who had aortoiliac occlusive disease or aortic aneurysm, correlation of symptoms of impotence and 36 available arteriograms was as illustrated in Table 4. Most patients had routine arteriography; therefore status of patency of penile arteries could not be ascertained.

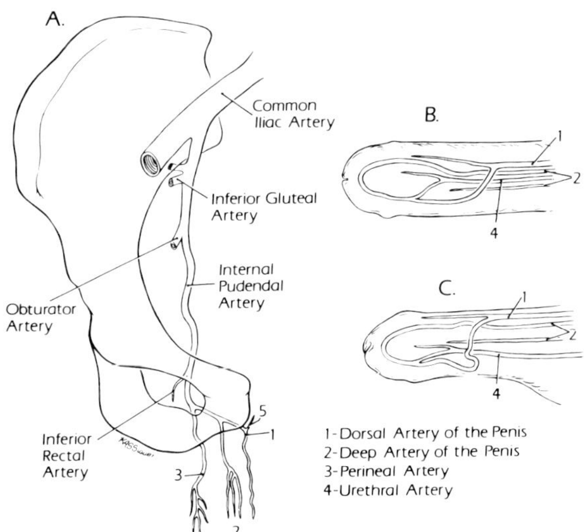

Fig. 1. Major blood supply to the penis is from the deep and dorsal penile arteries and the urethral artery. All these arteries are branches of the internal pudendal artery, which is a large branch of the internal iliac artery.

Table 4
Relationship Between Sexual Function and Arteriographic Findings of the Common and Internal Iliac Arteries in 36 Patients

	Stenosis of Common Iliac or Internal Iliac Arteries:		
	Unilateral	*Bilateral*	*Normal*
Potent	6	9	3
Impotent	4	12	2

Penile arterial pressure measurement. There are various methods of measuring penile blood flow, either by pulse waveform recording or by measurement of systolic pressure. Table 5 summarizes reported techniques to accomplish this aim. Of the various techniques reported, the Doppler ultrasound method is simplest and easiest to use. It is ideal for office or bedside use.

Penile systolic blood pressure is measured in a way similar to recording brachial pressure. It is done by applying a 2.5 cm pneumatic cuff around the base of the penis. The cuff is connected to an aneroid sphygmomanometer. Using the 10 kHz ultrasound Doppler probe as a sensor over the dorsal penile artery, systolic pressure is determined at the return of flow signal during deflation of the cuff (Fig. 2). Recording of penile pressure is done in a supine position.

The penile systolic pressure is then divided by the brachial systolic blood pressure to formulate a penile-brachial index (PBI). In normal males, the penile

Table 5
Techniques of Measuring Penile Flow and Pressure Reported by Various Investigators

Author	Year	Technique	Parameter
Canning et al. [3]	1963	Impedance plethysmograph	Pulse waveform
Britt et al. [2]	1970	Strain-gauge plethysmograph	Pulse waveform; reactive hyperemia test
Gaskell [8]	1971	Spectroscope (oxyhemoglobin)	Systolic pressure
Macvar et al. [18]	1973	Doppler ultrasound	Flow velocity waveform
Carter [4]	1978	Doppler ultrasound	Systolic pressure
Engel et al. [7]	1978	Doppler ultrasound	Systolic pressure
Kempczinski [15]	1979	Doppler ultrasound and pulse volume recorder	Systolic pressure; volume pulse waveform; reactive hyperemia test
Queral et al. [22]	1979	Doppler ultrasound	Systolic pressure

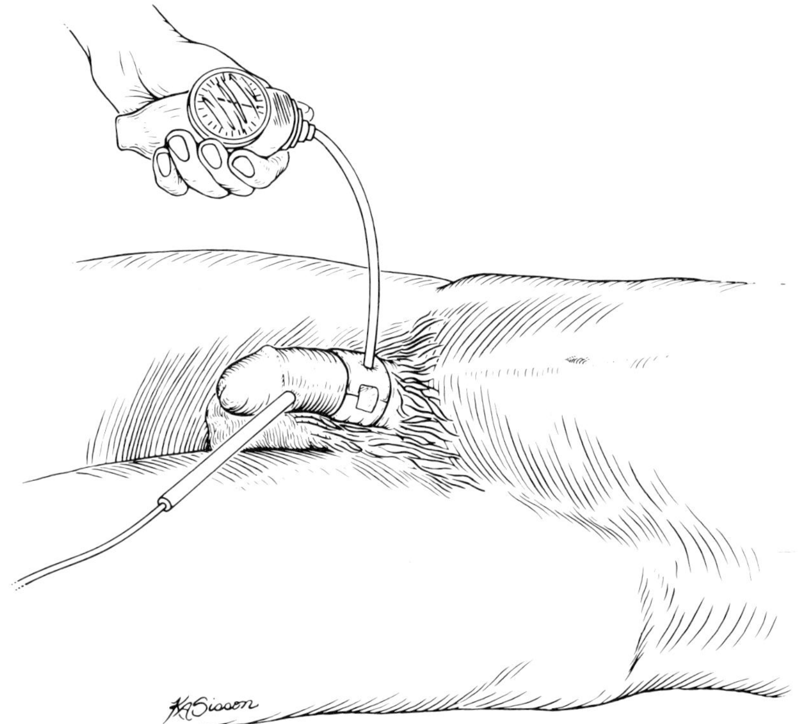

Fig. 2. Technique of recording penile systolic pressure using the Doppler ultrasound technique. [From Queral LA, et al: Pelvic hemodynamics after aorto-iliac reconstruction. Surgery (in press), 1979. Used by permission of the C. V. Mosby Co.]

pressure is close to the brachial pressure, and therefore the penile pressure index is about 1.0. Penile systolic pressure 20 mm Hg lower than brachial systolic pressure is considered abnormal [8].

Thirty-eight patients who underwent reconstructive surgery for aortoiliac occlusive disease of aortic aneurysm were studied by recording of their penile pressure [22]. In these 38 patients, the penile blood pressure was significantly lower for those patients who had impotence as compared to those who did not (Fig. 3). Patients with impotence all had a PBI less than 0.60. However, there was an overlap between the two groups, since the impotent group included patients with low libido secondary to old age as well as patients with diabetes and neurogenic impotence whose penile pressures were normal.

At present, a PBI less than 0.60 is considered compatible with impotence of vascular origin. The Northwestern University finding was similar to that reported by Kempczinski [15], who found a penile-brachial index of 0.58 ± 0.26 in patients who had vasculogenic impotence. Also, in an independent survey by Engel et al. [7] from the Northwestern University Department of Urology, a

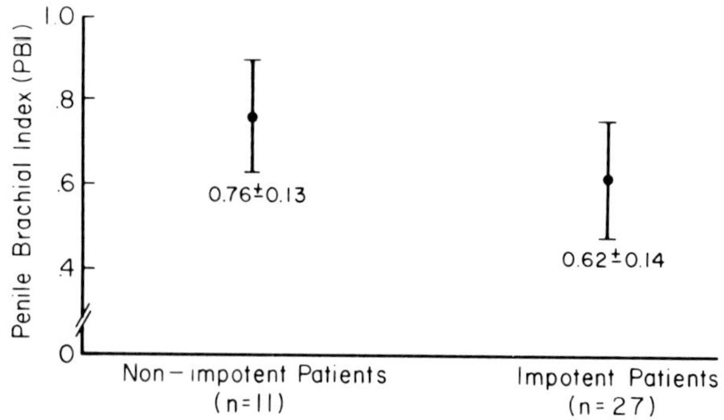

Fig. 3. Penile-brachial index (PBI) in patients with normal potency and impotent patients ($p<0.05$). [From Queral LA, et al: Pelvic hemodynamics after aorto-iliac reconstruction. Surgery (in press), 1979. Used by permission of the C. V. Mosby Co.]

penile-brachial index of 0.59 ± 0.11 was found in patients with impotence who had peripheral arterial disease.

When the PBI of 38 patients was compared to arteriographic findings, there were variable correlations. Of 12 patients with a preoperative PBI less than 0.6, 7 had hemodynamically significant stenosis of both common and internal iliac arteries and 5 had severe stenosis of only one hypogastric vessel. Of the remaining 26 patients who had a preoperative penile-brachial index greater than 0.6, 15 had unilateral stenosis of the common or internal iliac arteries and 11 exhibited bilateral significant stenosis of the hypogastric arteries. If a PBI of 0.75 or greater were chosen as the lower limit of normal, there were 11 patients who fell into this category; 5 of these 11 patients had normal iliac arteries, 6 had unilateral iliac occlusive disease, and none had bilateral iliac occlusive disease.

Nocturnal penile tumescence (NPT). The recording of nocturnal penile tumescence by means of strain-gauge plethysmography in combination with polysomnographic parameters is now standard. This establishes the presence of organic cause of impotence [13]. In a sleeping laboratory, the presence of nocturnal penile tumescence during the REM phase of sleep indicates psychogenic cause of impotence. On the other hand, absence of such erections on three consecutive nights of testing is convincing evidence of the organic nature of the patient's impotence. When NPT was compared with penile systolic pressure measurement, Karacan et al. found systolic pressure was lower in diabetic patients with abnormally diminished NPT than in nondiabetics with normal NPT. The NPT appears to be a useful test when used in conjunction with penile pressure measurement, especially in diabetic patients [14].

Diagnostic Scheme for Patients With Impotence

A detailed history and careful physical examination should help to establish the diagnosis of vasculogenic impotence. Both penile-brachial index and NPT help to guide the patient to further diagnostic workup. Figure 4 illustrates the diagnostic scheme for workup of patients with impotence.

EFFECT OF AORTIC SURGERY ON SEXUAL FUNCTION

The effect of aortic surgery on sexual function is well known but little discussed. Several groups have described their experience with patients undergoing aortic surgery [11, 19, 22, 23]. Contributing factors to postoperative impotence are either neural or failure to maintain adequate blood supply to the genitalia. The incidence of impotence following aortic surgery as reported by various investigators is listed in Table 6.

In an effort to assess the effect of aortic surgery on pelvic hemodynamics, a study of 38 patients who underwent various types of aortic reconstruction has been completed in our laboratory [22]. This study was done by measuring penile pressure before and after surgery and relating its changes to alterations in sexual function. The significant findings were as follows: (1) Surgical inter-

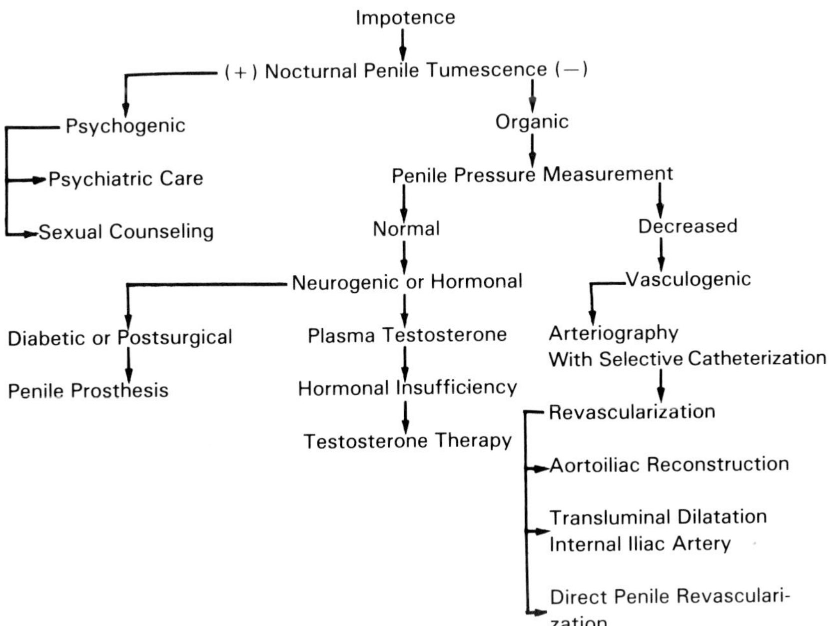

Fig. 4. Diagnostic scheme for patients suspected to have impotence.

Table 6
Incidence of Sexual Dysfunction After Aortic Surgery as Reported by Various Authors

Author	Year	No. of Patients	Incidence
May et al. [19]	1969	70	21% after aneurysmectomy 34% after aortofemoral surgery
Sabri & Cotton [23]	1971	9	77%
Harris & Jepson [12]	1965	6	33%
Hallbook & Holmqvist [11]	1970	31	45%
Weinstein & Machleder [25]	1974	25	10%

vention did not affect the PBI in 16 patients (42%), resulted in an increase in PBI in 14 patients (37%), and a decrease in 8 patients (21%). (2) When penile erectile capability was related to the penile pressure measurements, the erectile capability of patients whose PBI was unaffected by surgery remained unchanged in all cases except one (Fig. 5). This one patient unaccountably regained erectile function after surgery without apparent improvement in penile blood pressure.

Of the 14 patients who had a significant increase in PBI after surgery, 3 had no preoperative erectile problems, and these noted little change in sexual function after surgery. Of the 11 remaining patients, 8 were preoperatively impotent. These had return of erectile function after surgical correction of their aortoiliac disease.

None of the eight patients who had a decrease in PBI after aortoiliac reconstruction had ability to achieve penile erection afterwards (Fig. 5). This includes two patients who had normal erectile function preoperatively and who lost this capability after the surgical event.

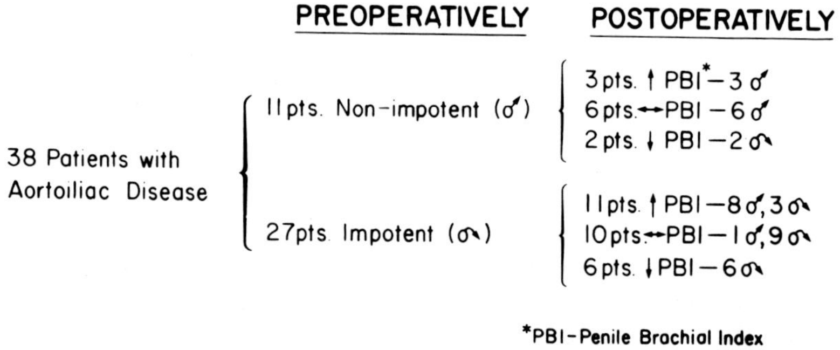

PREOPERATIVELY POSTOPERATIVELY

38 Patients with Aortoiliac Disease

11 pts. Non-impotent (♂)
3 pts. ↑ PBI* – 3 ♂
6 pts. ↔ PBI – 6 ♂
2 pts. ↓ PBI – 2 ♂↘

27 pts. Impotent (♂↘)
11 pts. ↑ PBI – 8 ♂, 3 ♂↘
10 pts. ↔ PBI – 1 ♂, 9 ♂↘
6 pts. ↓ PBI – 6 ♂↘

*PBI–Penile Brachial Index

Fig. 5. Effect of aortic surgery on potency and penile brachial pressure. None of the eight patients who had a decrease in PBI regained sexual potency after surgery. [From Queral LA, et al: Pelvic hemodynamics after aorto-iliac reconstruction. Surgery (in press), 1979. Used by permission of the C. V. Mosby Co.]

Of the 22 patients who underwent aortoiliac or aortofemoral reconstruction 12 had end-to-end anastomosis at the aorta. This group included 6 patients with severe occlusive disease of the external iliac artery. All 6 of these patients had a decreased PBI after surgery, and all are impotent. Clearly, the aortic transection and simultaneous reconstruction to the femoral level effectively bypassed the internal iliac arterial system.

This study confirmed the observation by May et al. [19], who emphasized the importance of maintaining blood flow to the hypogastric system during aortic surgery by making the anastomosis of distal graft limb above the level of the external iliac artery. They also advised that, if necessary, the hypogastric arteries should be thromboendarterectomized to provide as favorable a restoration of pelvic flow as possible.

The Northwestern University study indicates that patients with aortoiliac occlusion usually improve their pelvic blood flow, as indicated by penile blood pressure measurement. However, patients with extensive external iliac occlusive disease which prevents retrograde flow should have end-to-side anastomosis of their aortobifemoral graft in order to preserve blood flow to the iliac arteries.

DISCUSSION

From the current survey, it is evident that impotence is common in patients with aortoiliac arterial occlusive disease. Assessment of such impotence requires a thorough knowledge of its causes. The influence of pharmacologic agents and diabetes mellitus are important as contributing factors in impotence. Differentiation between organic and psychogenic impotence can be made readily by the nocturnal tumescence test and penile blood pressure measurement. In most centers, a sleep laboratory is available for the examination of impotence. It is advisable that patients who have impotence be carefully evaluated by a urologist, a vascular laboratory, and, if necessary, a psychiatrist.

The present study indicates that simple penile pressure recorded by Doppler ultrasound is sufficient to establish a diagnosis of vasculogenic impotence. The diagnostic criterion of a PBI of 0.60 or less is reliable and is comparable to that found by other investigators [7, 15]. It can be stated that the PBI below 0.60 provides a guideline for establishment of the diagnosis of vasculogenic impotence.

In addition to its diagnostic use, penile blood pressure is also useful to supplement arteriographic findings. The lack of correlation between PBI and arteriographic findings in the iliac system found in the present survey is not surprising. First, selective arteriography was seldom used; therefore the status of the penile arteries was unknown. Second, the presence of adequate collateral flow or the failure of routine arteriography to determine hemodynamically significant stenosis may contribute to the discrepancy seen. In patients who have a low penile-brachial index and in whom routine arteriography fails to show significant stenosis of the internal iliac artery, a selective internal iliac arteriogram should be performed to evaluate the status of penile arteries. It is obvious that diseased penile arteries may account for impotence and the low penile blood pressure reading.

The effects of aortic surgical procedures on pelvic hemodynamics are of interest. Analysis of arteriographic findings and corrective surgical procedures revealed three general patterns corresponding to three possible effects of surgery on pelvic hemodynamics. In 16 patients whose penile pressure was unchanged, surgical reconstruction consisted of end-to-side anastomosis of femorofemoral graft, and these reconstructions did not affect inflow to the internal iliac artery. The second group were those patients who had an increase of penile pressure caused by surgical augmentation of the inflow to the hypogastric system. These 14 patients underwent bypass reconstruction which resulted in an increased pelvic flow from retrograde perfusion through patent external iliac arteries. Finally, in patients whose penile pressure decreased, the surgical reconstruction interfered with inflow to the pelvic vessels. This was evident in patients who underwent aortofemoral graft replacement with end-to-end proximal anastomosis and who had severe external iliac artery disease. Because of the presence of severe external iliac artery disease, retrograde flow was not possible and preoperative antegrade flow was interrupted by complete transection of the aorta. Six patients in the present study fell into this category. All these patients became impotent after surgery. The untoward effect on erectile capability may have been avoided if the aortic anastomosis were fashioned in end-to-side manner, permitting antegrade perfusion of the internal iliac artery or, alternatively, anastomosing one internal iliac artery to a limb of the aortobifemoral graft if the aortic disease warranted an end-to-end anastomosis.

It is recognized that impotence is a result of multiple factors and improvement of penile pressure by aortic surgery does not necessarily lead to erectile capacity. However, the reverse is true: a decrease of penile pressure after surgery renders a patient impotent. Both the arteriogram and penile pressure measurement assist in planning of the vascular reconstruction. Perfusion of the hypogastric artery should be made optimal. A diseased external iliac artery which prevents retrograde flow should be noted. Especially when there is a normal preoperative penile-brachial index, every effort must be made to preserve inflow to the hypogastric system. When aortofemoral grafting is contemplated, a proximal aortic anastomosis fashioned in end-to-side manner is advisable to preserve antegrade flow to the internal iliac artery.

It is apparent that penile pressure measurement plays an important role in the evaluation of organic impotence. It aids surgeons in planning the type of reconstruction for aortoiliac arterial occlusive disease. With the current enthusiasm for the femoropudendal bypass to relieve impotence, penile pressure measurement should provide a simple method to document objectively the success of the operation.

REFERENCES

1. Barker WF: Major Problems in Clinical Surgery (vol 4). Philadelphia, W. B. Saunders, 1966, p 67
2. Britt DB, Kemmerer WT, Robison JR: Penile blood flow determination by mercury strain-gauge plethysmography. Invest. Urol. 8:673, 1970
3. Canning JR, Bowers LM, Lloyd FA, et al: Genital vascular insufficiency and potency. Surg. Forum 14:298, 1963
4. Carter SA: Role of pressure measurements in vascular disease, in Bernstein EF (ed): Noninvasive Diagnostic Techniques in Vascular Disease. St. Louis, C. V. Mosby, 1978, p 280
5. Darling RC: In discussion of May et al. [19]
6. DePalma RG, Levine SB, Feldman S: Preservation of erectile function after aorto-iliac reconstruction. Arch. Surg. 113:988, 1978
7. Engel G, Burnham S, Carter MF: Penile blood pressure in the evaluation of erectile impotence. Fertil. Steril. 30:687, 1978
8. Gaskell P: The importance of penile blood pressure in cases of impotence. Can. Med. Assoc. J. 105:1047, 1971
9. Ginestig JF, Romieu A: Radiologic Exploration of Impotence. The Hague, Martinus Nijhoff Medical Division, 1978
10. Goodman L, Gilman A: Pharmacological Basis of Therapeutics (ed 4). New York, MacMillan & Co., 1970
11. Hallbook T, Holmqvist B: Sexual disturbance following dissection of the aorta and the common iliac arteries. J. Cardiovasc. Surg. 11:255, 1970
12. Harris JD, Jepson RP: Aorto-iliac stenosis: A comparison of two procedures. Aust. N. Z. J. Surg. 34:211, 1965
13. Karacan IA: Clinical value of nocturnal erection in the prognosis and diagnosis of impotence. Med. Aspects Human Sexuality 4:27, 1970
14. Karacan I, Ware JC, Dervent B: Impotence and blood pressure in the flaccid penis. Relationship to nocturnal penile tumescence. Sleep 1:125, 1978
15. Kempczinski RF: Role of the vascular diagnostic laboratory in the evaluation of male impotence. Am. J. Surg. (in press)
16. Leriche R: De la resection du carrefour aorticoiliaque avec double sympathectomie lombaire pour thrombose arteritique de l'aorta; le syndrome de l'obliteration terminoaortique par arterite. Pr. Med. 48:601, 1940
17. Leriche R, Morel A: The syndrome of thrombotic obliteration of the aortic bifurcation. Ann. Surg. 127:193, 1948
18. Macvar T, Baron T, Clark SS: Assessment of potency with the Doppler flowmeter. Urology 2:396, 1973
19. May AG, DeWeese JA, Rob CE: Changes in sexual function following operation on the abdominal aorta. Surgery 65:41, 1969
20. Michal V, Kramar R, Pospichal J: Femoro-pudendal bypass, internal iliac thromboendarterectomy and direct arterial anastomosis to the cavernous body in the treatment of erectile impotence. Bull. Soc. Int. Chir. 4:343, 1974
21. Michal V, Kramar R, Pospichal J: External iliac steal syndrome. J. Cardiovasc. Surg. 19:355, 1978

22. Queral LA, Whitehouse WM Jr, Flinn WR, et al: Pelvic hemodynamics after aorto-iliac reconstruction. Surgery (in press), 1979
23. Sabri S, Cotton LT: Sexual function following aorto-iliac reconstruction. Lancet 2:218, 1971
24. Scheer A: Impotence as a symptom of arterial vascular disorder in the pelvic region. Munch. Med. Wochenschr. 102:1713, 1960
25. Weinstein MH, Machleder HI: Sexual function after aorto-iliac surgery. Ann. Surg. 181:787, 1975

Ralph G. DePalma, M.D.
Kalish Kedia, M.D.
Lester Persky, M.D.

Vascular Operations for Preservation of Sexual Function

Increased interest exists in the preservation of normal sexual function in patients undergoing vascular procedures. Vascular surgeons for decades have recognized patients presenting with impotence and lower extremity ischemia due to aortoiliac atherosclerosis [10]. They will also now examine patients referred with primary complaints of erectile dysfunction which may be due to a newly recognized entity called vasculogenic impotence [23]. The problem of diagnosing and treating these patients is unraveling the myriad causes of impotence. Despite the complexity of this area, the vascular surgeon seeking to prevent sexual disability should recognize the interplay among psychic factors, neural function, and blood flow. Sexual disabilities are frequently seen in men who are candidates for aortic surgery and in diabetics requiring distal vascular reconstructions. Sexual disabilities are not, however, limited to men alone; women with aortoiliac obstructive disease may report lack of vaginal lubrication and orgasmic failure when lubrication and orgasm were previously present in stable relationships. These complaints can be relieved by aortic bypass to relieve lower extremity ischemia, just as normal function can be restored in many instances in men.

This report describes the anatomy and current physiologic concepts of the penile erectile mechanism; it also outlines approaches for preservation of normal sexual function in patients with vascular disease. Vascular operations which seek to preserve or restore sexual function are of recent origin [3, 14, 15]. The choice of procedures for particular patients depends upon the anatomy and physiology of disturbed erectile function, as well as an absolute need to correct life threatening aneurysmal or occlusive disease. Techniques currently described will here be considered both in terms of prospects for success and limiting factors. A background of information about the mechanisms of normal erection is required to understand current thinking about the treatment of vasculogenic impotence.

BACKGROUND INFORMATION

Anatomy

If neural pathways are intact, normal penile erection is a function of adequate arterial inflow. The arterial blood supply of the penis originates in the internal pudendal artery, the smaller of the two terminal branches of the internal iliac artery. The paired internal pudendal arteries in the male exit from the pelvis between the pyriformis and coccygeus muscles, cross the ischial spine, and enter the perineum through the lesser sciatic foremina. As they course to the base of the penis, they pass along the lateral wall of the ischiorectal fossa. At this point the exit of the artery from the pelvis is situated about 4 cm above the lower margin of the ischeal tuberosity. Figure 1 shows the emergence of the vessel and

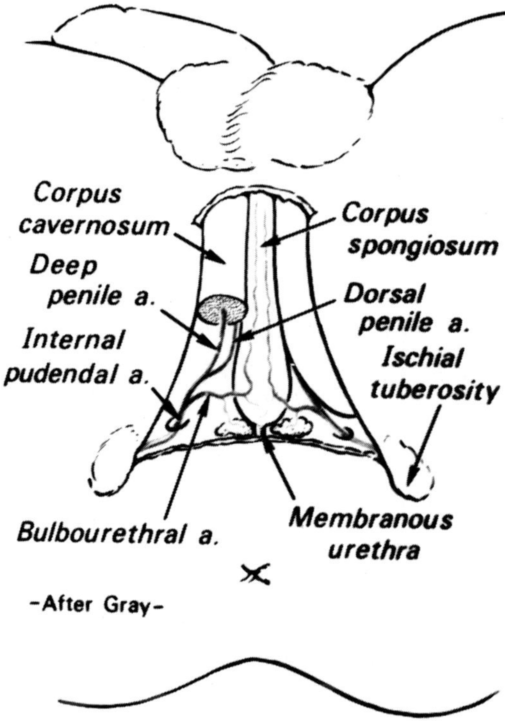

Fig. 1. View of course of internal pudendal artery and branches; lithotomy position. Note exit of main trunk anterior to ischeal tuberosity.

its course in the deep perineal layer. At the point where the artery emerges anterior to the ischeal tuberosity, audible Doppler signals can be detected and recorded with the subject in lithotomy position.

Variations in blood supply occur when the internal pudendal artery is smaller than usual or does not have its usual branches. An accessory pudendal may arise from the internal pudendal before its exit from the greater sciatic foramen. When this occurs, the vessel passes along the lower part of the bladder and the side of the prostate to the root of the penis. Thus a small internal pudendal may end as the artery of the urethral bulb; the dorsal and deep arteries of the penis are then derived from the accessory pudendal. The incidence of such variations is not yet known; however, as more subselective angiographic visualizations of this area are obtained, these variations in blood supply will become better characterized.

Figure 2 shows the usual disposition of the terminal branches of an internal pudendal artery as it supplies the cavernous bodies of the penis and urethral bulb. An angiographic projection [6] of these distal vessels can be obtained in the oblique position used for lateral cystourethography (Fig. 3). Note that in examining the penis by palpation, or with a Doppler ultrasonic flow detector probe, pulsatile impulses are normally obtained from both dorsal arteries, the paired cavernosal arteries, and along the corpus cavernosum urethrae inferiorally.

Terminal branches of the penile arteries and the penile vessels themselves communicate with the cavernous spaces via valvelike structures variously called polsters, Ebner pads, or coussinets [1]. These contain smooth muscle and are positioned so as to facilitate blood flow between the arteries and the cavernous spaces. Under normal circumstances, the smooth muscle fibers of the pads are contracted in the flaccid state; the arteriolar lumen is thus obstructed and blood

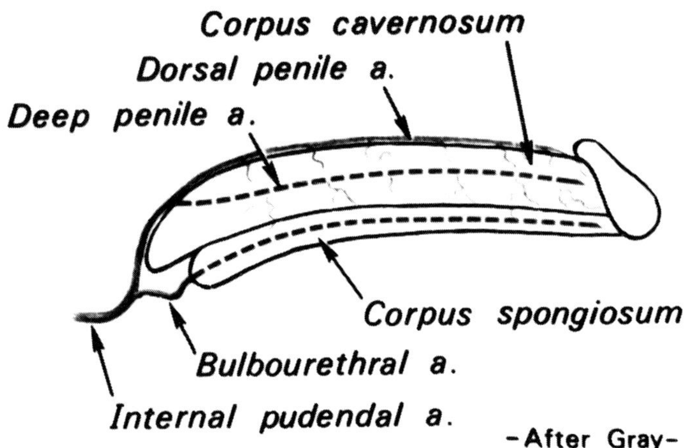

Fig. 2. Anatomy of terminal branches of one internal pudendal artery within penis. Note existence of three paired vessels.

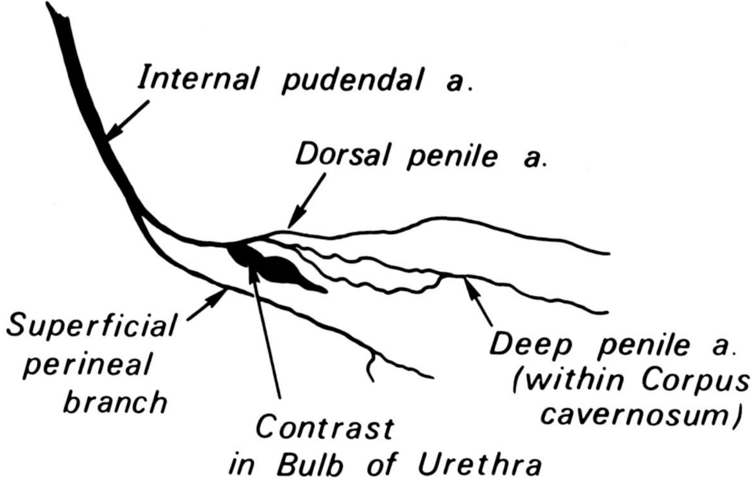

Fig. 3. Idealized normal subselective angiogram (after J-F Ginestie). Note filling of dorsal and deep penile arteries. The arteries of the corpus spongiosum not visualized.

is diverted into the penile veins. In normal erection, relaxation of the smooth muscle fibers of the pads and circular fibers of the arteriolar tunica media permit an increased blood flow into the cavernous bodies.

Physiology

The process of shunting blood into the cavernous penile structures is under neural control. Penile erection depends on the integration of afferent signals in both the thorocolumbar and sacral erection centers [25], intact autonomic nerves to the penis, and an adequate arterial blood supply. In the past it was believed that an element of venous occlusion was important in producing erection. Though polsterlike occlusive structures can be seen in veins [1], the venous element in erectile function is no longer considered the dominant factor producing erection. Newman and associates [17] observed that venous blockade induced a cyanotic and edematous penis, not normal penile erection. Reflex contraction in the muscles about the bulb was also considered responsible for pumping blood into the corpora and maintaining erection; however, patients with flaccid paralysis of these muscles also experience erections. These observations support dominance of the arterial supply ultimately producing a functional penile erection.

The importance of arterial inflow is also supported by direct observations in animals and man. The experimental mechanical constriction of the aorta during erection causes immediate detumescence even when stimulation of the nervi erigenti continues [22]. The rate of perfusion of the corpora correlates with the degree of penile erection in both patients [16] and human volunteers [17]. Once obtained, an artificially produced erection can be maintained by lower flow rates. In studies done by Michal and Pospichal [16], penile erection occurred at cavernous infusion rates of 46-160 ml/min, depending upon size. Only 60% of the initial infusion rate was required to maintain erection. These workers believe that the presence or absence of dorsal penile artery pulsation during artificial erection under general anesthesia is important in diagnosing intrinsic disease of the penile arteries. They observed that four normally potent controls had readily palpable pulsation of both dorsal penile arteries; in 30 impotent patients, 7 had no pulsation, 18 exhibited pulses in only one penile artery, and 5 exhibited bilateral pulses. These findings correlated with subselective angiograms performed in the same patients.

SCREENING FOR VASCULOGENIC IMPOTENCE

The data about normal penile erection, while emphasizing the complex nature of stimuli initiating this process, direct attention to the need for adequate arterial inflow. This basic physiology must be considered in evaluating recent findings of unique, poorly understood pathology which has been demonstrated in penile vessels and corporal bodies. Varying degrees of pathological changes have been described after the age of 38 years [20] in the organs of men who died from a variety of causes. These histological changes consist of replacement of the smooth muscle of Ebner pads by collagen, calcification of pads and arterial walls, as well as stenoses and occlusions of penile arteries. The severity of these changes is thought to correlate with age and the presence of diabetes. Clearly more morphologic information must be obtained in a large number of individuals and, if possible, correlated with functional state and angiographic appearances. The implication of these findings is that certain intrinsic penile vascular changes might limit normal erection, even with adequate inflow.

In spite of incomplete knowledge about the importance of changes in the intrinsic vascular structures of the penis, surgeons attempting to preserve or restore normal sexual function will recognize two primary areas underlying vasculogenic impotence. The first, and most obvious, is atherosclerosis of the aortoiliac system; the second, and more subtle, is isolated arteriopathy of the internal pudendal arteries or of its distal branches. Provided neural function is intact, the selection of an ideal vascular procedure to obtain normal erectile function entails a precise anatomic diagnosis and the penile capability to respond to increased flow. When small vessel disease exists, subselective angiography is required for adequate diagnosis; when the aorta and common iliacs are mainly involved, traditional lumbar aortography is often adequate to obtain information about the large pelvic vessels. Before a decision to perform angiography, however, the surgeon must first determine that vasculogenic impotence is a reasonably probable diagnosis.

Our experience indicates that certain aspects of the history, physical examination, and noninvasive examination deserve emphasis when approaching these patients. The information obtained can sharpen the indications for angiography. A careful history is the most important initial step. Levine [12] uses four basic questions which help to distinguish between psychological, organic, or ambiguous patterns of erectile dysfunction:

1. *What is the physiologic impairment?* Is it the inability to obtain an erection, the inability to maintain an erection during intercourse, or some combination?
2. *How firm does the penis become?* Not firm at all, slightly firm but erection not self-supporting, decreased firmness with coitus still possible, or fully turgid?
3. *Is the impairment constant or episodic?* Under what circumstances is the pattern not present: with other partners, with masturbation, with sleep, upon awakening, during the day, when engaging in other erotic activity?
4. *What life events were occurring when the dysfunction initially appeared?*

Classic organic dysfunction is recognized by the gradual onset of inability to achieve firm erection in the setting of an otherwise satisfactory relationship, uncomplicated by traumatic life events. Flaccidity of one of the corporal bodies may even suggest unilateral ischemia. When organic impotence is misdiagnosed or treated inappropriately, both partners can develop severe psychological problems which often require formal psychiatric evaluation. The surgeon himself should evaluate the attitudes of both partners about sexual disability. He can then help them understand if organic erectile dysfunction persists or even develops postoperatively. Even if organic disability is irreversible, its clear recognition is quite important in relieving anxiety.

The history should also include careful inquiry into the duration and severity of known risk factors for atherosclerosis: cigarette smoking, hyperlipidemia, hypertension, and glucose intolerance [8]. The importance of unrecognized or poorly controlled diabetes cannot be overemphasized. All patients with a historical pattern of organic impotence should be given a 3 hour glucose tolerance test. Effective treatment of unrecognized diabetes can occasionally reverse an organic pattern of erectile dysfunction. If diabetes is already under effective treatment, impotence is not likely to be altered by medical therapy. Historical and physical evidence of peripheral neuropathy should be sought in these patients. A history of penile or perineal sensory changes, retrograde ejaculation, ejaculation without sensation or without erection all suggest neuropathy. The neuropathic state in many diabetics [4] can be confirmed by cystometric studies.

Alcohol abuse and antihypertensive drugs are among the most common organic causes of erectile dysfunction. When isolated renal artery disease contributes to hypertension, drug therapy used to treat it may cause impotence.

Impotence will be relieved if surgical correction of renal artery hypertension removes the need for drugs. All of these etiologic factors must be sought and altered if possible.

The physical findings of hypertension, absent or decreased extremity arterial pulsations, and femoral bruits suggest the probability of vasculogenic impotency due to aortoiliac atherosclerosis. Vasculogenic impotence may, however, occur without these signs when only the pelvic or pudendal vessels are involved. In addition to examination of the extremities, the Doppler ultrasound flow detector is useful to examine the internal pudendal artery as it exits from the pelvis and branches into the penis. This can be done easily as part of the physical examination.

Pulse volume recordings have proved extremely valuable in the office setting for estimating penile perfusion. The following method for penile pulse volume recordings has been developed: The penis is first wrapped with a fine plastic material such as Handiwrap for sanitary purposes. A digital plethysmographic cuff is placed snugly about the base of the flaccid penis and inflated with an amount of air sufficient to attain *mean arterial pressure*. Inflation of the cuff to mean arterial pressure (diastolic brachial blood pressure plus one-third of pulse pressure) yields reproducible recordings. Since the penis is compressible in the nonerect state, this procedure is preferred; cuff inflation techniques (either fixed volume or pressure) effective in bony members may not be as easily reproducible for PVR recordings of the penis. Permanent PVR recordings are obtained at a chart speed of 25 mm/sec. The chart deflection, rate of systolic upstroke, and presence or absence of dichrotic notches are recorded. For a review of plethysmographic technique, see Raines [18] and Winsor [26]. Representative recordings from individuals reporting normal potency are shown in Fig. 4.

Penile plethysmography has replaced nocturnal penile tumescence monitoring in our practice as a most satisfactory means of initial vascular screening for vasculogenic impotence. It is rapid, simple, and inexpensive. Nocturnal penile tumescence studies are useful for pre- and postoperative evaluations in cases of ambiguous impotency or hospitalized patients. Kempczinski [9] recently described vascular laboratory screening procedures applied to screening for impotence. These are based on measurement of distal penile blood pressure in the preputial artery and determinations of penile-brachial systolic gradients. Penile volume wave forms with simultaneous recording of the wave form in the right index finger were obtained in the normal and postischemic reactive hyperemic states. He used these procedures to identify patients with normal penile blood flow who would not benefit from direct surgery. Unfortunately, the procedures described did not rule out significant ischemia as a cause of impotence, especially in patients over 40 years of age. We have found that distal blood pressure measurements in the preputial artery may vary widely because the Doppler signal of this small vessel varies. We no longer use this technique. Further, subselective angiography shows that this vessel may not be important in erection; it rarely visualizes in normal men.

PVR RECORDINGS

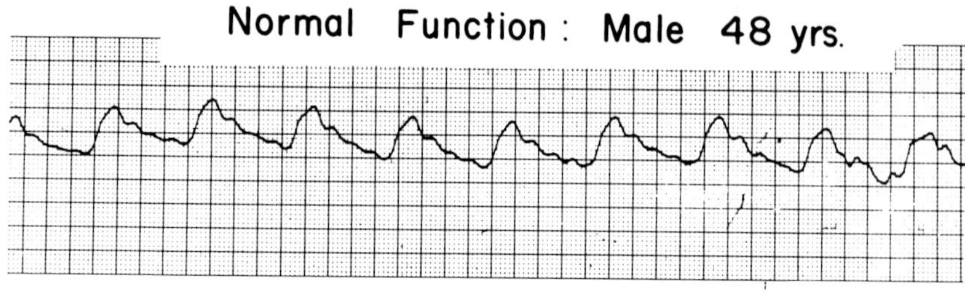

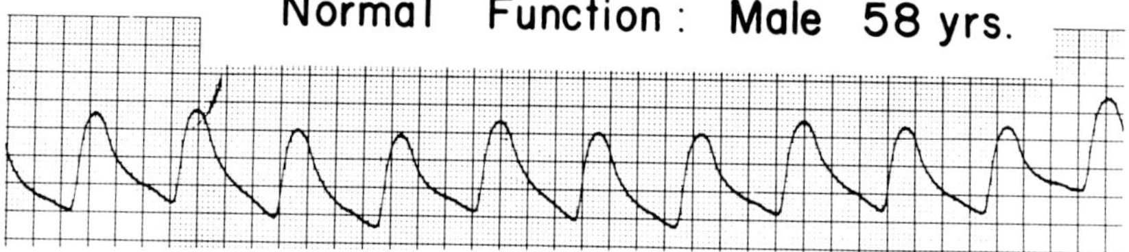

Fig. 4. PVR recordings obtained with digital Buffington plethysmographic cuff inflated to mean arterial pressure. Two middle-aged men with normal function. Note systolic crest time less than 5 mm at chart speed 25 mm/sec, amplitude greater than 5 mm in height, and dicrotic notch in upper recording.

We presently consider penile plethysmography the most unique adaptable screening method for penile inflow. It measures the contributions of all vessels at the root of the penis while the organ is flaccid. PVR recordings also appear to correlate with increased flow in the erect penis. Our observations indicated that improved PVR tracings, using criteria similarly applied to extremity measurements, correlated with restoration of normal potency. Pulse volume recordings also correlated with severity of pelvic angiographic patterns of occlusive disease; more data will be needed to estimate the importance of collaterals in determining overall arterial input. The contributions of each of the main internal iliac arteries are clearly recognizable. Further experience is needed in correlating PVR tracings with subselective angiographic patterns of small vessel disease in the penis itself.

OPERATIONS TO PRESERVE OR RESTORE ERECTILE FUNCTION

Operations which maintain or restore normal sexual function fall into three general categories: reconstruction of large vessels, direct penile revascularization, and prosthetic devices. While progress in prosthetics is beyond the scope of this discussion, prosthetic devices must not be ignored in the total care of these patients. Prosthetics are among the most valuable adjuncts available. We have used an inflatable prosthesis [21] in our own patients with diabetic neuropathy and in those whose distal pudendal atherosclerosis progressed after an initial aortic reconstruction temporarily restored potency. In spite of preliminary exciting reports, the potential of direct penile revascularization and exact techniques of performance have not yet been delineated. Its use is limited, especially in diabetics and older men with possible intrinsic pathology in the Ebner pads or cavernosal spaces which might not respond even to adequate penile inflow. Table 1 summarizes our current experience with large and small vessel revascularization in relation to erectile function surviving patients followed from 6 months to 6 years. Table 2 shows the data contrasting normal and abnormal function by age and number of late deaths. We have described details of dissection principles to minimize damage to the autonomic plexi [3] and to prevent embolization of atheromatous debris into the internal iliac arteries [2]. Previously [3] we have included only nondiabetic patients in analyses; because of the frequency of diabetes, both aortoiliac reconstruction and penile revascularizations now include diabetic patients in total results.

Aortoiliac Reconstruction

These operations have been performed for lower extremity ischemia or abdominal aneurysms; preservation or restoration of sexual function were secondary aims. In one instance, impotence was the presenting complaint in a

Table 1
Procedures, Ages, and Results of Various Reconstructions

Procedure	Number	Average Age ± SD [Years] (Range)	Potent Post-operatively	Later Erectile Dysfunction*
Aortoiliac reconstruction				
Limited nerve sparing dissection	37	58.2 ± 7.7 (42-72)	25	3
Conventional dissection	22	65.4 ± 7.3 (52-81)	2	1
Iliac endarterectomy	3	55 (45-62)	3	1
Femorofemoral bypass	9	63.1 (48-72)	5	—
Inf. epigastric to corpora cavernosa	7	58 (46-69)	5	1

*Impotence 6 months or more after report of normal erectile function.

Table 2
Comparison of Ages and Late Deaths

Procedure	Number	Average Age at Operation ± SD (Range) [Years]	Late Death*
Aortoiliac reconstruction			
Normal postop erectile function	33	57.7 ± 8.0 (43-72)	2†
Postop erectile dysfunction	38	64.9 ± 6.6 (52-81)	7
Corpora revascularization			
Normal postop erectile function	7	52 (46-58)	0
Postop erectile dysfunction	2	68.5 (68-69)	0

*Died 6 months or more after surgery.
†Both due to carcinoma of lung.

man with a previously undetected aneurysm which caused sudden occlusion of the internal iliac artery. Preoperative aortograms using conventional techniques were obtained in all cases. It was possible to classify the outflow patterns in the internal iliac arteries in 49 of them.

The prognostic significance of preoperative angiographic patterns of the pelvic vessels is demonstrated in Fig. 5. The angiographic patterns relate both to conventional and limited dissections in patients needing aortoiliac reconstruction. Group 1 patients were preoperatively potent, postoperatively impotent. These two patients had extensive unilateral internal iliac disease, and they either sustained atheroembolism or exhibited iliac aneurysm formation. One man, aged 52, was treated urgently for ruptured abdominal aortic aneurysm, underscoring the point previously made [5] that the best circumstances for preservation of sexual function exist in elective cases. The second patient, aged 55, was operated upon urgently for rest pain and peripheral manifestations of atheroembolism involving both lower extremities. Both patients were distressed by their postoperative sexual disability.

Group 2 patients demonstrated bilateral, diffuse, internal iliac disease with maintenance of lower extremity flow by partially occluded common and external arteries. This pattern has a particularly poor prognosis; in addition, it may be associated with the later onset of impotence after an initially favorable result. Group 3 patients, with preservation or no change in sexual function, exhibited either mild internal iliac artery disease or none at all. Group 4 patients were

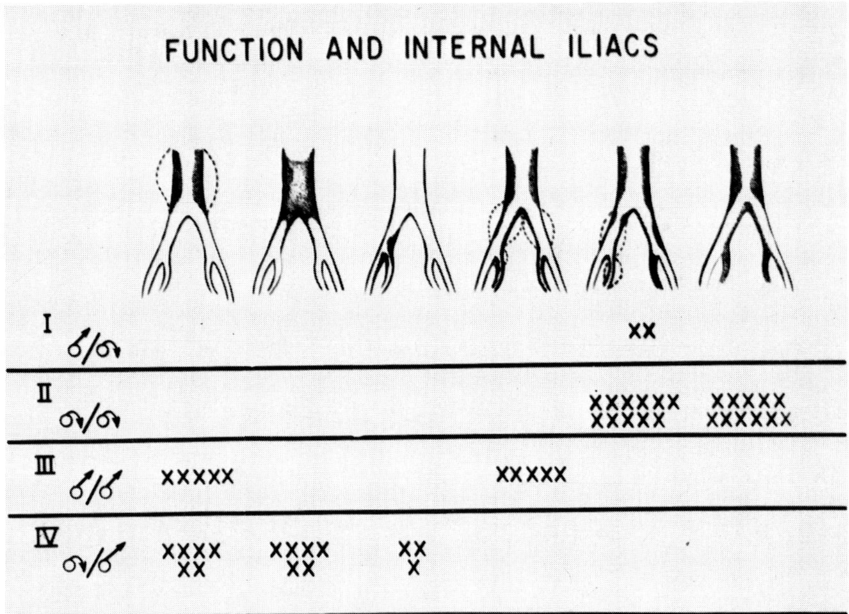

Fig. 5. Pre- and postoperative erectile function and representation of angiographic patterns of aorta and branches in 49 patients. *X* represents a single patient.

often younger, exhibiting the classic Leriche syndrome [10] due to aortic thrombosis. When neural function remains intact postoperatively, this situation is favorable for restoration of normal postoperative function. Characteristically, the distal circulation is spared, though the internal iliac vessels may not fill in a retrograde fashion during conventional angiography.

We have continued to question these patients and their wives about their sexual function on followup examinations. We have observed that impotence can occur later presumably due to progression of disease in the internal iliac system. This has been documented by flat waveforms on penile plethysmography. The inflatable prostheses have been used successfully in two of the three instances in which this occurred.

Femorofemoral Reconstruction and Localized Iliac Endarterectomy

The decision to perform either femorofemoral bypass or local internal iliac endarterectomy was based on preoperative angiographic findings showing either occlusion or high grade stenosis of one common iliac artery or of the origin of one internal iliac artery. The third angiographic pattern in Fig. 5 typifies this picture. The bypass operations were done only to relieve lower extremity ischemia. For this purpose, femorofemoral bypass offers simplicity, low mortality, and long-term patency [5]. It completely avoids an intraperitoneal approach and the potential neural damage of aortoiliac dissection. In all instances, preexisting sexual function was preserved; in one of nine cases, enhanced postoperative sexual function was reported. Endarterectomy of localized lesions of these internal iliac artery can be accomplished extraperitoneally. Anterior longitudinal dissection in the region of the common iliac bifurcation identifies nerve fibers and permits their retraction for endarterectomy. These operations were done primarily for complaints of impotence.

Figure 6 illustrates a favorable internal iliac lesion in a 62 year old man complaining of recent erectile dysfunction. The erectile dysfunction was associated with a flat preoperative PVR recording; postoperatively, waveforms approached normal configurations (Fig. 7). This patient subsequently reported satisfactory erections and coital frequency of three or four times weekly. An interesting ancillary note is that the arteriographic examination (Fig. 6) revealed stenosis of one of the inferior epigastric artery origins. The implications of involvement of this artery with plaque will be discussed subsequently in considering direct penile revascularization.

Direct Corporal Revascularization Procedures

Leveen [11], Genestie and associates [6], and Michal [13] have described direct anastomoses of one of the inferior epigastric arteries to the corpora. Although initial results were encouraging, Waterhouse and Laungani [24] and Leveen [11] reported uniform later closure of these grafts. Instead of this particular technique, we have implanted both inferior epigastric arteries into the corpora at the base of the penis just above the pubic bone (Fig. 8). Our experience with this operation to date is summarized in Table 2. Patients ranging in age from 46 to 69 have been operated on and followed up to 2 years. There have been two instances of onset of erectile dysfunction associated with closure of graft. In two of these cases, late graft failure was documented by angiography and flattened PVR recordings (Fig. 9).

This procedure is limited by the possible atheromatous involvement of inferior epigastric arteries to be used for the revascularization procedure (Fig. 10). These occlusive lesions were found in both inferior epigastric arteries of a 43 year old diabetic with hypertension and a 30 year history of cigarette smoking. He required femoropopliteal reconstruction for rest pain of the left foot; simultaneously inferior epigastric artery implants were attempted. Both vessels were diseased; one was marginally suitable for implant. The patient reported initial erectile function postoperatively, but lost erectile function within weeks. He is now awaiting a prosthetic implant.

The other limitations of direct corporal revascularization include the technical difficulties of direct anastomoses of the epigastric arteries to the relatively

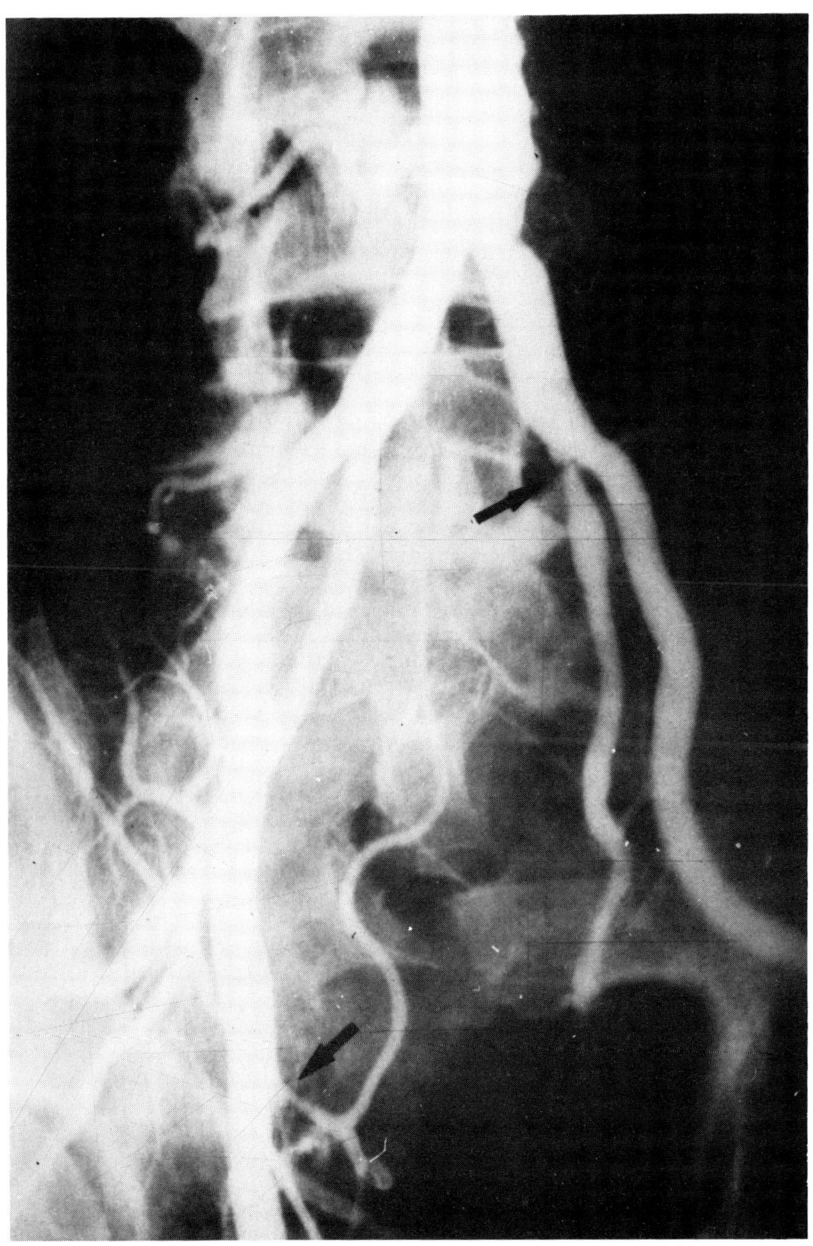

Fig. 6. Aortogram in 62 year old impotent male. Note isolated lesion of origin of left internal iliac artery at arrow and lesion at origin of right inferior epigastric artery.

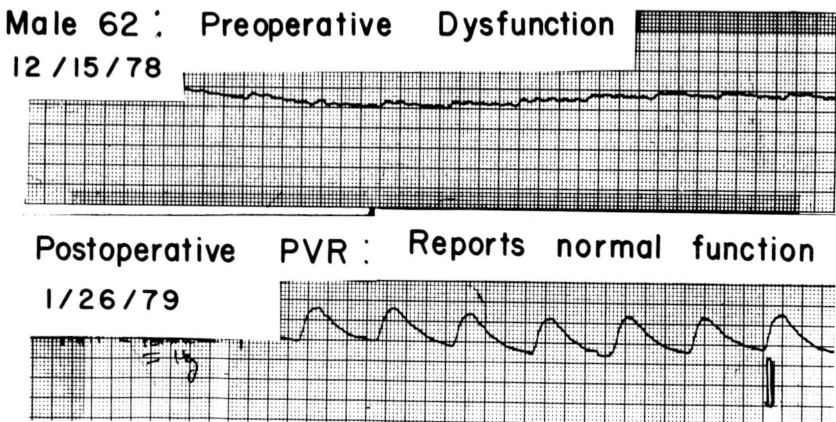

Fig. 7. Pre- and postoperative PVR recordings in 62 year old patient whose angiogram is shown in Fig. 6. Patient reported normal function after left common and internal iliac endarterectomy. See text.

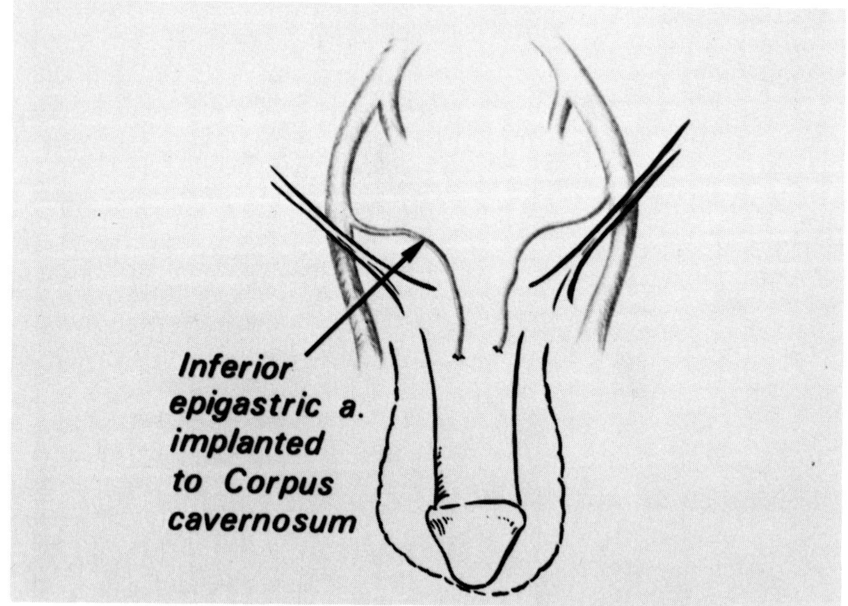

Fig. 8. Schema of technique of bilateral inferior epigastric artery-corpora bypass developed by Dr. Kalish Kedia. Note bilateral implants.

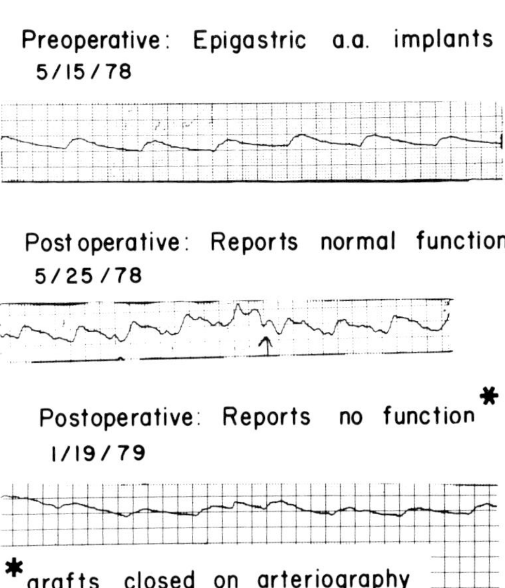

Fig. 9. PVR recordings obtained with digital Buffington plethysmographic cuff inflated to mean arterial pressure. Recordings obtained preoperatively improved by procedure shown in Fig. 8; patient reported normal erectile function. Loss of function coincided with abnormal recording shown for January 19, 1979.

thick walled corpora and positional changes in the course of the graft which might cause kinking and subsequent failure. The group from Montpellier [6, 7] performing this procedure recommended postoperative anticoagulation in these patients. This has not been our practice. Direct vein grafts from the femoral artery to the corpora have also been reported; priapism can be a problem due to high flow in the large caliber conduit. This has not been seen in the inferior epigastric artery anastomoses performed by us. Rossi and Zorgniotti [19] reported a saphenous vein bypass procedure in which the proximal anastomoses were made to the inferior epigastric artery; potentially this procedure would avert the complication of priapism. Finally, Michal [13] reported direct anastomoses of one of the inferior epigastric arteries to the dorsal penile artery with good results in 10 of 18 patients.

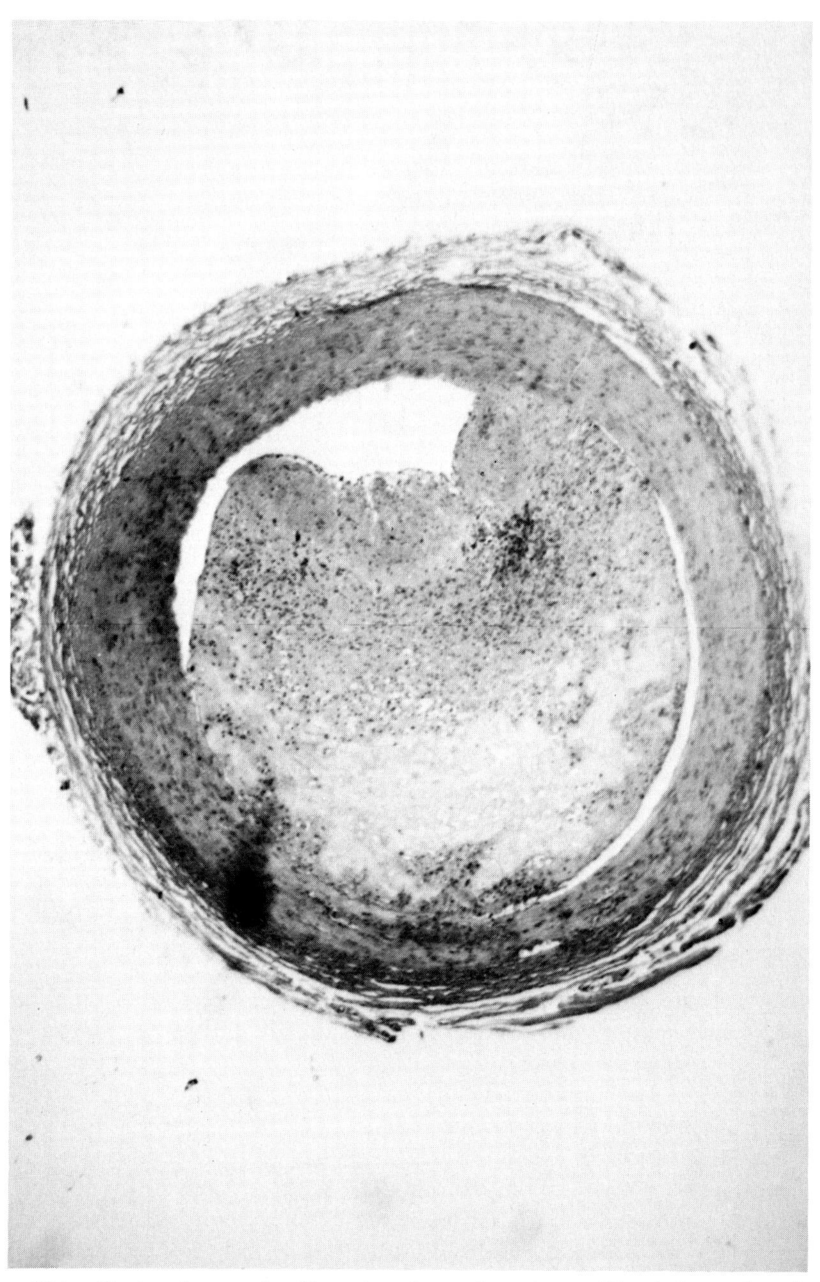

Fig. 10A. Photomicrograph. Hematoxyln and eosin × 70. Atherosclerotic plaque in midportion of left inferior epigastric artery of 43 year old diabetic male smoker; artery not suitable for bypass.

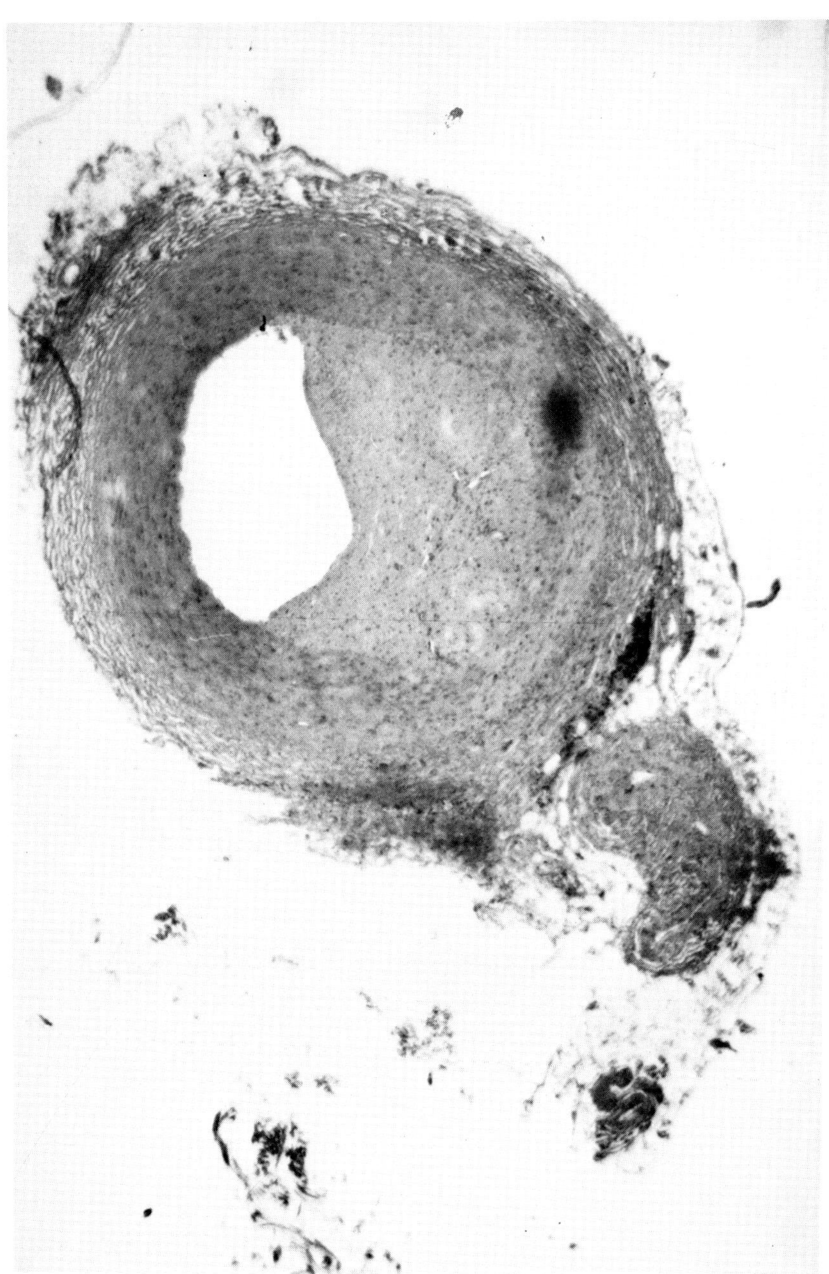

Fig. 10B. Photomicrograph. Hematoxyln and eosin × 70. Atherosclerotic plaque in distal portion of right inferior epigastric artery, same patient. Graft shortly failed.

FUTURE PROSPECTS

Vasculogenic impotence is now a recognized entity. This will evolve into a challenging area for vascular surgery. As yet the concept is novel. It can be seen that screening approaches, arteriographic techniques, and surgical procedures are still evolving. There is little doubt that vasculogenic impotence will receive intense attention in the future, due to our older population and changing societal attitudes toward sexual function. Much remains to be learned about the etiologies and the treatment of vasculogenic impotence.

Men with aortic disease may now be offered the prospect – not the promise – of preserved or restored sexual function. Prosthetic devices can be offered if the effort is not successful. At the least, the problem will be clearly understood by both partners and much anxiety relieved. Traumatic interruption of pelvic or penile blood supply also offers important opportunities. A variety of approaches for penile revascularization exists for patients with vasculogenic impotence as a primary complaint; their long-term potential is not yet documented. Progress in this area depends upon refinements of subselective angiography, study of the pathology of small penile vessels and corpora, application of microvascular techniques, and better management of disease processes signaled by onset of vasculogenic impotence. In surgical treatment, several clinics have reported early encouraging results of small vessel direction revascularization. Our experience suggests cautious optimism qualified by limiting factors discussed previously. At present, direct vascular anastomoses to dorsal penile arteries deserve careful scrutiny.

This area also offers broad preventive considerations. The possibility of the internal pudendal artery being a target for early atherosclerosis is a novel observation; the complaint of organic impotence might be the first signal of significant vascular disease elsewhere. All these men deserve careful screening to detect unrecognized atherosclerotic involvement of their coronary or peripheral arterial vessels. Interventions which preserve or restore normal sexual function improve the quality of life. Normal sexual function might also provide an important motivation for controlling other gratifications such as cigarette and dietary indiscretions which can intensify the atherosclerotic process.

REFERENCES

1. Conti G: L'erection due penis humain et ses bases morphologico-vasculaires. Acta Anat. 14:17, 1952
2. DePalma RG: Aorto-iliac dissection principles for prevention of post-operative sexual dysfunction, in Zorgniotti AW (ed): Vasculogenic Impotence: Proceedings of the First International Conference on Corpus Cavernosa Revascularization. Springfield, Ill., Charles C. Thomas, in press

3. DePalma RG, Levine SB, Feldman S: Preservation of erectile function after aortoiliac reconstruction. Arch. Surg. 113:958, 1978
4. Ellenberg M: Impotence in diabetes: The neurologic factor. Ann. Intern. Med. 75:213, 1971
5. Flanigan DP, Pratt DG, Goodreau JJ, et al: Hemodynamic and angiographic guidelines in selection of patients for femoro-femoral bypass. AMA Arch. Surg. 113:1257, 1978
6. Ginestie JF: Results of corpus cavernosum revascularization, in Zorgniotti AW (ed): Vasculogenic Impotence: Proceedings of the First International Conference on Corpus Cavernosa Revascularization. Springfield, Ill., Charles C. Thomas, in press
7. Ginestie JF, Ramieu A: Radiologic Exploration of Impotence. The Hague, Martinus Nijhoff, 1978
8. Gordon T, Kannel WB: Predisposition to atherosclerosis in the head, heart and legs: The Framingham study. JAMA 221:661, 1972
9. Kempczinski RF: Role of the vascular laboratory in the evaluation of male impotence. From the 7th Annual Symposium on Vascular Surgery, Palm Springs, Calif., March 1979
10. Leriche R, Morel A: The syndrome of thrombotic obliteration of the aortic bifurcation. Ann. Surg. 127:193, 1948
11. Leveen HH: Experiences and techniques utilized to revascularize the penis, in Zorgniotti AW (ed): Vasculogenic Impotence: Proceedings of the First International Conference on Corpus Cavernosa Revascularization. Springfield, Ill., Charles C. Thomas, in press
12. Levine SB: Marital sexual dysfunction: Erectile dysfunction. Ann. Intern. Med. 85:342, 1976
13. Michal V: Revascularization procedures of the cavernous bodies, in Zorgniotti AW (ed.): Vasculogenic Impotence: Proceedings of the First International Conference on Corpus Cavernosa Revascularization. Springfield, Ill., Charles C. Thomas, in press
14. Michal V, Kramar R, Pospichal J: Femoro-pudendal bypass, internal iliac thromboendarterectomy and direct arterial anastomosis to the cavernous body in the treatment of erectile impotence. Bull. Soc. Int. Chir. 33:343, 1974
15. Michal V, Kramar R, Pospichal J, et al: Gefabchirurgie erektirer impotenz. Sonderdruck Sexualmed. 5:15, 1976
16. Michal V, Pospichal J: Phalloarteriography in the diagnosis of erectile impotence. World J. Surg. 2:239, 1978
17. Newman HF, Northrup JD, Devlin J: Mechanism of human penile erection. Invest. Urol. 1:350, 1964
18. Raines JK: Mechanics of air plethysmography in arterial disease: The pulse volume recorder, in Bernstein EF (ed): Noninvasive Diagnostic Techniques in Va scular Disease. St. Louis, C. V. Mosby Co., 1978, pp 157-161
19. Rossi G, Zorgniotti AW: Experience with corpus cavernosum revascularization, in Zorgniotti AW (ed): Vasculogenic Impotence: Proceedings of the First International Conference on Corpus Cavernosa Revascularization. Springfield, Ill., Charles C. Thomas, in press

20. Ruzbarsky V, Michal V: Morphological changes in the arterial bed of the penis with aging: Relationship to the pathogenesis of impotence. Invest. Urol. 15:194, 1977
21. Scott FB, Bradley WE, Timm GW: Management of erectile impotence: Use of implantable inflatable prosthesis. Urology 2:80, 1973
22. Semans JH, Langworthy OR: Observations of the neurophysiology of sexual function in the male cat. U. Urol. 40:836, 1938
23. Zorgniotti AW (ed): Vasculogenic Impotence: Proceedings of the First International Conference on Corpus Cavernosa Revascularization. Springfield, Ill., Charles C. Thomas, in press.
24. Waterhouse RK, Laungani G: Results of corpus cavernosum revascularization, in Zorgniotti AW (ed): Vasculogenic Impotence: Proceedings of the First International Conference on Corpus Cavernosa Revascularization. Springfield, Ill., Charles C. Thomas, in press
25. Weiss HD: The physiology of human penile erection. Ann. Intern. Med. 76:793, 1972
26. Winsor T: Segmental plethysmography, in Winsor T (ed): Peripheral Vascular Diseases: An Objective Approach. Springfield, Ill., Charles C. Thomas, 1959, pp 157-179

F. William Blaisdell, M.D.
S. N. Carson, M.D.

Alternatives to Direct Surgery of Aortoiliac Disease

Over the past 25 years, developments in the field of reconstructive vascular surgery have followed certain predictable lines. Earlier attempts to treat aortoiliac occlusive disease consisted of a direct attack on the disease with endarterectomy introduced into this country by Wylie in 1951 [28]. At first, endarterectomy was limited to short segments, but as it became clear that atherosclerosis was generally progressive and more diffuse than seen on arteriography, it was realized that extensive aortoiliac endarterectomy was usually required for an optimal result. As better materials were developed for use as vessel substitutes, bypass grafting procedures as popularized by DeBakey [9] became the most popular method of treatment. These procedures permitted the more rapid bypass of diseased arterial segments and proved to be of greatest value when occlusive disease was extensive.

The concept of extraanatomical bypass (which was developed after these first two procedures) evolved from the need to reroute and restore circulation after a complication such as prosthetic graft infection had developed. Freeman and Leeds in 1952 described what we consider to be the first case of extra-anatomical bypass which used endarterectomized superficial femoral artery for a femorofemoral bypass [15]. Subsequently Vetto popularized this operation by describing successful experience with ten cases in 1962 [26].

We first applied the extraanatomical bypass in 1960 [2] when infection caused the destruction of an abdominal aorta Dacron graft anastomosis. The graft was removed, the aorta ligated below the renal arteries, and a thoracic aorta-to-femoral artery graft was placed, followed by a femorofemoral graft. However, this procedure proved less than optimal because it required a thoracotomy in a desperately ill patient. Abandoning the concept that a large donor artery was required, we found that a small artery such as the axillary artery could accommodate the entire cardiac output, a concept which was essential to the development of the more practical axillofemoral procedure for bypassing the abdominal aorta [3, 4].

Recently, there has been increasing evidence that in comparable groups of patients extraanatomical bypass grafts function nearly as well as conventional aortic bypass grafts and can be carried out with considerably less risk [1, 8, 14, 17, 20].

INDICATIONS FOR ALTERNATIVE PROCEDURES

Femorofemoral Bypass

In our opinion, femorofemoral bypass grafting is an underutilized procedure. Vetto, who originally popularized the operation [26], rarely used arteriography at that time and felt that a palpable pulse in one groin was sufficient to permit the corresponding femoral artery to be used as a donor vessel to bypass iliac occlusive disease of the opposite side. In his experience, femorofemoral bypass grafts rarely failed because of progression of disease on the donor side. In fact, Vetto believes that higher flows through the donor iliac artery generated by a femorofemoral bypass may actually prevent the progression of arteriosclerosis. Certainly the general experience has been that femorofemoral bypass grafts have compared favorably in terms of longevity with aortofemoral bypass grafts [5, 6, 17]. For this reason, we believe that femorofemoral bypass is appropriate whenever there is a normal femoral pulse in the contralateral groin and when arteriography demonstrates that occlusive disease does not compromise patency of the donor vessels by 50% or more [13]. It should be noted, however, that significant common femoral outflow occlusion may well result in a normal pulse even in the presence of extensive proximal iliac disease. Therefore we believe that arteriography is indicated prior to carrying out a femorofemoral procedure except in the most emergent circumstances.

It is of some interest to note that while noninvasive Doppler analog recordings may predict some successful femorofemoral bypasses, postoperative Doppler pressures and electromagnetic flow rates recorded at operation do not correlate well with patency rates or relief of symptoms [14]. Clearly, this serves to emphasize the need to have thorough preoperative selection criteria for evaluating inflow (as already mentioned) as well as for the evaluation of the degree of recipient limb outflow disease.

The optimal situation in which femorofemoral bypass can be utilized is when one limb of an aortobilateral-femoral bypass has occluded. Under these circumstances, the proximal anastomosis of the femorofemoral graft can be used to enhance flow through the remaining patent limb. The exposure for both anastomoses of the femorofemoral graft may also be used to patch stenotic outflow lesions of the profunda or superficial femoral artery. In most instances it is not necessary to reenter the abdomen, with all its potential complications, in order to deal with this type of graft occlusion.

Axillofemoral Bypass

In most series, the indications for axillofemoral bypass have been in patients with advanced systemic disease or perigraft infection, or in cases presenting adverse technical problems. For this reason most of the published reports do not permit comparison of long-term results for axillofemoral bypass with those of conventional aortofemoral bypass procedures. Recently, series by LoGerfo [18] and Ray and Sauvage [20] have suggested that when axillofemoral bypass and aortofemoral bypass are carried out in similar patient populations, the results are comparable. A less successful experience has been reported by Moore [12]. Differences in patient populations, indications for surgery, graft materials and willingness to reoperate immediately on acutely thrombosed grafts tend to make such series impossible to compare adequately [10, 12, 17, 19]. A recent review of these discrepant reports has been conducted by Rutherford [21], who points out that part of the reason for differing results lies in the way patency rates are reported.

While it is probable that the longer axillofemoral graft makes it more vulnerable to accidents leading to occlusion, an advantage of the axillofemoral graft is that the graft is readily accessible for thrombectomy. Usually this is a relatively minor procedure in the superficially placed graft and most often is performed using local anesthesia.

In the final analysis, we believe that no mortality is acceptable when dealing with aortoiliac occlusive disease, since occlusive disease confined to this level should not threaten life and rarely in itself threatens limb. Yet all large series to date document a 2%-5% mortality for aortofemoral bypass procedures. Hence the primary rationale for using conventional procedures is the greater long-term patency. The advent of new graft materials appears to be associated with better graft healing and a lower graft thrombosis rate. Recent series document greater longevity for a progressively higher percentage of these extraanatomical grafts, and all document their increased safety. No doubt further developments in graft materials will help potentiate these trends toward conservative operations [7, 28].

In our opinion, extraanatomic arterial bypass grafting should be used when the risk of standard operations is high due to associated disease or anticipated technical problems. The most common indication for these operations is the presence of severe pulmonary or cardiac disease, and an absolute indication is infection or possibility of infection along the proposed path of placement of conventional grafts [22, 24]. Another nearly absolute indication is acute myocardial infarction or acute pulmonary disease in a patient who has developed severe ischemia of the extremities which requires emergent operation. Under these circumstances, bypass procedures can be performed under local anesthesia or light general anesthesia with less risk than is associated with conventional procedures or with amputation.

An additional report has focused attention on the use of axillofemoral bypass [16] of aortic aneurysms in patients too ill to tolerate abdominal operations. In the study, thrombosis within the aneurysm was initiated by iliac interruption in eight out of ten patients while limb flow was maintained using the bypass.

CONTRAINDICATIONS TO EXTRAANATOMIC BYPASS PROCEDURES

There are very few contraindications to the use of extraanatomic bypass grafting procedures. Those which exist are essentially the same contraindications as for any vascular reconstructive procedure: inadequate inflow or outflow vessels, or infection along the proposed route of the graft.

Blood pressure should be carefully measured in both arms and the subclavian area should be auscultated, a decreased blood pressure in one arm contraindicating use of the corresponding axillary artery as the donor vessel. A bruit or decreased brachial artery pressure should be further evaluated with arteriography to rule out disease of the proximal subclavian artery. Noninvasive vascular studies using plethysmography or Doppler exam of the upper extremities may also be helpful. Any stenosis of the innominate or subclavian artery of 50% or more rules out the use of the proximal axillary artery as a source of inflow for the graft.

A patent profunda femoral artery is the minimum requirement to provide outflow to an axillofemoral or femorofemoral graft. If preoperative arteriography has not adequately visualized the outflow tract, operative arteriography must be performed to ensure that this requirement will be met and that runoff will be adequate.

OPERATIVE TECHNIQUE

Although these procedures have been carried out successfully under local anesthesia, light general anesthesia is usually optimal. Graft materials may consist of autogenous vein, woven or knitted Dacron, or the newer PTFE grafts. Generally, we have favored a knitted Dacron graft – most recently of the velour type – because of its size, ready availability, and proven durability. Knitted Dacron tubes 10 mm in diameter are considered optimal for use as axillofemoral grafts, although 8 mm Dacron tubes have been used successfully as well. Eight or ten millimeter Dacron tubes are also optimal for femorofemoral grafts. If there are two operating teams, bypass procedures can be performed in less than 1 hour.

Femorofemoral bypass is the procedure of choice when dealing with an aortoiliac or aortofemoral graft in which vessels of only one limb are patent. The common femoral artery is the most accessible donor vessel, but the external iliac or deep femoral artery can also be used. A Dacron tube can be carried preperitoneally by tunneling under the inguinal ligament, or by tunneling subcutaneously across the pubis to the opposite vessel.

Anastomoses are made with an obliquely cut end of the Dacron graft; this cut helps avoid narrowing at the anastomosis. Experience orienting the graft in a transverse direction or at a reverse oblique angle from the femoral artery has not seemed to limit flow, nor has it seemed to increase the graft thrombosis rate. Since the reconstruction parallels flexion creases, the graft rarely kinks or obstructs.

Axillofemoral bypass has been used by choice when there is occlusive disease of both iliac systems in an appropriate patient or when infection is present. The axillary artery is a satisfactory inflow vessel if no proximal occlusive disease of the corresponding subclavian artery is present. Verification of patency by arteriography is optimal but not essential. The axillary artery itself is rarely diseased, and its proximal one-third (i.e., between the clavicle and pectoralis minor muscle) is the segment of choice for proximal anastomosis. The first portion of the artery is fixed to the chest wall so that the anastomosis does not flex with motion of the arm. In addition, there is only one small collateral branch from this segment, the highest thoracic artery. The tunnel for the graft is created behind the subclavian vein deep to the pectoral musculature downward and laterally to the midaxillary line, where a small counterincision at about the level of the eighth to tenth rib facilitates development of a tunnel that can be carried subcutaneously or deep to the external oblique fascia. This tunnel is best carried posterior to the anterior axillary line at the waist so that angulation or kinking is less likely to occur when the patient sits or bends. End-to-side anastomosis to the common femoral or profunda femoral artery is then carried out in conventional fashion. If the ipsilateral axillary artery is diseased, the contralateral artery can be used, in which instance the graft is brought down to the level of the ipsilateral anterior iliac spine and curved transversely across the lower abdomen to the opposite femoral artery.

The procedure which maximizes longevity of the axillofemoral graft is a combination of axillofemoral and femorofemoral bypass grafting. This doubles the flow in the axillofemoral section of the graft and improves long-term patency of the graft over that obtained with unilateral axillofemoral procedures [8, 26]. In carrying out this procedure, one bypass graft is first placed between the axillary artery and the corresponding femoral artery. A second graft is then anastomosed to the first, as close to the lower anastomosis as possible and is carried to the opposite femoral vessel subcutaneously or preperitoneally.

This reconstruction provides total substitution for the infrarenal abdominal aorta and permits retrograde perfusion of the hypogastric artery if one or both external iliac arteries are patent. This method of bilateral reconstruction also permits the contralateral side to continue to receive flow should one distal limb of the graft thrombose.

POSTOPERATIVE MANAGEMENT

The only special postoperative precaution for bypass grafting is prevention of flexion of the thighs within the immediate postoperative period. Vital signs should be monitored carefully; the pulse in the graft and the status of the feet should also be monitored. Doppler pressures are recorded in foot vessels both pre- and postoperatively, since a significant improvement or stabilization of Doppler pressures is expected if the surgery has been successful. No special medications are administered. If antibiotics are indicated for management of graft infection, they should be initiated 24 hours prior to operation, continued intravenously during the procedure, and then the administration should be extended for 24-48 hours postoperatively.

All of our bypass graft patients are placed on antiplatelet-aggregating drugs, since this therapy has the theoretical advantages of preventing arterial clot and slowing the progression of arteriosclerosis. Enteric-coated aspirin is administered orally starting on the second to third postoperative day and is continued indefinitely at a dosage of 300 mg daily.

COMPLICATIONS

The complications of extraanatomic bypass procedures are similar to those associated with any other major vascular operation. These consist primarily of thrombosis and infection. If thrombosis should occur, reoperation is easily done under local anesthesia. However, restoration of patency must be verified by operative angiography involving both anastomoses and the entire graft. If infection occurs, this is generally an indication to remove the graft, ligate the inflow and outflow vessels, and accept amputation as the ultimate treatment if this becomes necessary. This is preferable to risking the patient's life due to hemorrhage from a suture line.

An important theoretical consideration relates to whether small arteries such as the axillary or femoral arteries can supply adequate amounts of blood to the lower half of the body without some type of "steal" phenomenon developing. Our experience with several hundred operations in which the axillary artery was used to supply blood flow to the lower half of the body has repeatedly verified the safety of this type of bypass procedure. No cases of steal have been documented, upper extremity ischemia has not occurred, and when the operation has been technically successful the circulation in the lower extremities has subsequently improved.

At first we feared the patient might constrict an axillofemoral graft by wearing tight clothing or by applying direct pressure on the graft while asleep. But these fears were apparently unwarranted, since despite warnings to the contrary patients have continued to wear belts and have obviously slept lying directly on the grafts without causing constriction. We have not seen any graft thromboses that could be directly related to this type of compression. In fact, intentional attempts to occlude the graft by digital pressure during arteriography are usually unsuccessful. This leads us to believe that in the presence of stable cardiac output and normal blood pressure it is very difficult to occlude one of these long grafts sufficiently to produce thrombosis.

RESULTS

Acute graft failures do not occur if arteriography demonstrates good flow in the graft and if anastomoses are free from technical defects. We believe that all graft failures which occur in the immediate postoperative period are due to technical errors and as such are preventable.

Late failure cannot be accurately predicted, since occasionally a patient with very poor outflow has ultimately done well. However, long-term patency seems to correlate with persistence of good flow. When flow is high through the superficially placed graft, the graft remains soft, thin, and compressible. In this circumstance, long-term patency has been the rule. But when flow rate through the graft is low, the graft becomes firm to palpation due to a thickening of the neointima. We postulate that graft failure is due to disruption of the neointima as described by Wesolowski [12] or to actual embolism or thrombosis in portions of the thickened intima as it becomes disrupted at the sites of flexion. A few of our grafts have remained patent for prolonged periods even though flow through them has been negligible. This supports the hypothesis that accidents to neointima tend to produce most of the closures. It is our impression that the thicker the neointima, the greater the likelihood of these accidents occurring.

As regards femorofemoral grafts, long-term patency has been excellent and comparable to that for aortoiliac bypass, a 5-year patency rate of 74%. Even when one or more outflow vessels are occluded, the femorofemoral grafts have done comparably as well as aortofemoral grafts.

The patency rate is lower for axillofemoral grafts and is similar to our experience with femoropopliteal Dacron bypass grafts, with a failure rate of 50% at 2 years. The advent of the newer velour prostheses offers promise of more rapid graft healing and improved patency. Our experience with these newer prostheses, while favorable to date, has not been sufficient to document conclusively whether or not they constitute a significant advance in long-term patency in the extraanatomic position. The risk of extraanatomic bypass operations is low, and any mortality seen has been related to the presence of systemic disease rather than to the operative procedure itself. We have not as yet used axillofemoral grafts in a series comparable to that of our aortofemoral grafts. All of our axillofemoral graft patients had either serious systemic disease or life-threatening graft infection.

In LoGerfo's experience with 88 aortobilateral iliac or femoral grafts and 56 axillobilateral femoral grafts performed electively for the management of occlusive disease of the abdominal aorta or iliac vessels, the long-term patency has been excellent [18]. Their results indicated that the axillobilateral femoral graft, when used in an older population, had a lower operative mortality than did conventional aortic bypass procedures, and had a similar long-term patency rate to conventional procedures, 76% at 5 years. They found, however, that axillofemoral grafting required more frequent reoperation to obtain this patency rate.

With better-defined criteria for patient selection and a greater understanding of the hemodynamic properties of subcutaneous grafts [11, 14, 25], future reports on the use of these procedures utilizing new graft materials are expected to show even better patency rates. Furthermore, as uses for such grafts are expanded, future reports will undoubtedly focus on the improved quality of life rendered these surgical patients.

REFERENCES

1. Baker R, Parker JC: Femoro-femoral crossover grafts. Br. J. Surg. 59:701, 1972
2. Blaisdell FW, DeMattei GA, Gauder PJ: Extraperitoneal thoracic aorta to femoral bypass graft as replacement for an infected aortic bifurcation prosthesis. Am. J. Surg. 102:583-585, 1961
3. Blaisdell FW, Hall AD: Axillary-femoral bypass for lower extremity ischemia. Surgery 54:563-568, 1963
4. Blaisdell FW, Hall AD, Lim RC Jr, et al: Aortoiliac arterial substitution utilizing subcutaneous grafts. Ann. Surg. 172:775-780, 1970
5. Brief DK, Alpert J, Parsonnet V: Crossover femorofemoral grafts: Compromise or preference: A reappraisal. Arch. Surg. 105:889, 1972
6. Brief DK, Brener BJ, Parsonnet V: Crossover femoro-femoral grafts followed up five years or more. Arch. Surg. 110:1294, 1975
7. Campbell CD, Brooks DH, Siewers RD, et al: Extraanatomic bypass with expanded polytetrafluoroethylene. Surg. Gynecol. Obstet. 148:525, 1979
8. Davis RC, O'Wara ET, Mannick JA, et al: Broadened indications for femoro-femoral grafts. Surgery 72:990, 1972
9. DeBakey ME, Crawford ES, Morris GC, et al: Late results of vascular surgery in the treatment of arteriosclerosis. J. Cardiovasc. Surg. 5:473, 1964

10. DeLaurentis DA, Sala LE, Russell E, et al: A twelve year experience with axillo-femoral and femoro-femoral bypass operations. Surg. Gynecol. Obstet. 147:881-887, 1978
11. Ehrenfeld WR, Harris JP, Wylie EJ: Vascular steal phenomena: An experimental study. Am. J. Surg. 116:192, 1968
12. Eugene J, Goldstone J, Moore WS: Fifteen year experience with subcutaneous bypass grafts for lower extremity ischemia. Ann. Surg. 186:177, 1976
13. Flanigan DP, Pratt DG, Goodreau JJ, et al: Hemodynamic and angiographic guidelines in the selection of patients for femoro-femoral bypass. Arch. Surg. 113:1257-1262, 1978
14. Flanigan DP, Yao JST: Crossover femoro-femoral grafting in patients with severe lower extremity ischemia, in Bergan JJ, Yao JST (eds): Gangrene and Severe Ischemia of the Lower Extremities. New York, Grune & Stratton, 1978
15. Freeman NE, Leeds FH: Operations on large arteries. Calif. Med. 77:229, 1952
16. Leather RP, Shah D, Goldman M, et al: Nonresective treatment of abdominal aortic aneurysms by acute thrombosis and axillofemoral bypass. Presented at the SVC/ICVS Meeting, June 1979, Nashville
17. LoGerfo FW, Mannick JA, et al: A comparison of the late patency rates of axillobilateral femoral and axillounilateral femoral grafts. Surgery 81:33-40, 1977
18. Mannick JA, Williams LE, Nalseth DC: The late results of axillofemoral grafts. Surgery 68:1038, 1970
19. Ray LI, O'Connor JB, Davis CC, et al: Axillofemoral bypass: A critical reappraisal of its role in the management of aortoiliac occlusive disease. Am. J. Surg. 138:117, 1979
20. Rutherfored RB: Extra-anatomic bypass in lieu of major aortic surgery. Presented at the Society for Clinical Vascular Surgery VII Symposium, March 1979, Palm Springs
21. Shaw RW, Baue AE: Management of sepsis complicating arterial reconstructive surgery. Surgery 53:75-86, 1963
22. Sheiner NW: Peripheral vascular surgery: Alternate anatomical pathways and the use of allograft veins as arterial substitute. Curr. Prob. Surg. 15:5-76, 1978
23. Spanos PK, Gilsdorf RB, Sako Y, et al: The management of infected abdominal aortic grafts and graft enteric fistulas. Ann. Surg. 183:397, 1976
24. Sumner DS, Strandness DE: The hemodynamics of the femoro-femoral shunt. Surg. Gynecol. Obstet. 134:629, 1972
25. Vetto RM: The treatment of unilateral artery obstruction utilizing femoro-femoral graft. Surgery 52:342, 1962
26. Welsh P, Repetto R: Intraoperative blood measurements following revascularization of the lower extremities with chronic arterial occlusive disease. J. Cardiovasc. Surg. 19:515, 1978
27. Wesolowski SA: The healing of vascular prostheses. Surgery 57:319, 1965
28. Wylie EJ: Thromboendarterectomy for arteriosclerotic thrombosis of major arteries. Surgery 32:275, 1952

Leonardo T. Lim, M.D.

Management of Aorto-Vena Caval Injury

Since the first successful repair of an abdominal aortic laceration from a stab wound by Wildegans in 1926, there have been an increasing number of reports of such cases with improved survival [1, 2, 5, 9, 12, 13, 17, 18]. At present, effective and logical steps in the management of this highly lethal form of vascular trauma have evolved.

Injuries to the abdominal aorta are rare, comprising 1%-5% of all vascular injuries. They are often due to penetrating injuries from gunshots and stab wounds, and carry mortality rates of 50%-65%. Most aortic wounds are fatal at the scene of the accident because of rapid and exsanguinating hemorrhage. About 15%-20% of patients manage to arrive alive in hospitals within an hour of the incident, thus allowing resuscitation and surgical intervention.

In contrast to aortic injury, not much attention has been focused on injuries to the inferior vena cava. These are seen more often, are equally life threatening, and require complex and challenging surgical care. Unlike aortic injury, the low pressure vena cava when injured has a much greater chance of spontaneous tamponade from a retroperitoneal hematoma. Resumption of torrential bleeding during surgical exploration is characteristic of this lesion. Ineffectiveness of proximal and distal control in achieving hemostasis is due to abundant venous lumbar collaterals.

The mortality rate for aorto-vena caval trauma is influenced by many factors: speed of patient transport, degree and duration of shock, availability of adequate blood, number of associated organ injuries, anatomic location of the injury, and effectiveness of the surgical team. An efficient, coordinated, well rehearsed resuscitative effort and deliberate surgical intervention to achieve quick and effective hemostasis is of utmost importance in order to achieve a successful outcome.

It is the purpose of this communication to present a standardized method of approach to the management of aorto-vena caval trauma as practiced at the Cook County Hospital in Chicago. We have found this helpful in our hands. Cases presented illustrate important points.

ACUTE AORTIC TRAUMA

Diagnosis and Resuscitation

A presumptive diagnosis of aortic injury or solid viscus rupture (liver and spleen) should be made in patients who arrive in shock from a penetrating or blunt abdominal trauma. The probability of aortic injury is enhanced when a penetrating wound is seen close to or at the midline or when a bullet is determined to have crossed the anatomic location of the abdominal aorta. A quick abdominal needle paracentesis should reveal nonclotting blood. If paracentesis is negative, one should always look for the two other common conditions that produce shock: cardiac tamponade and tension pneumothorax. These are usually caused by high abdominal or lower chest penetrating injuries. Absence of breath sounds in the hemithorax after establishment of an upper airway justifies the placement of a chest tube, while the presence of increasing central venous pressure in a hypotensive patient with a lower chest or upper abdominal wound should indicate pericardial tamponade, and immediate diagnostic needle pericardiocentesis should be done. It is important to be aware of these two injuries because the mode of therapy in each is different from that of aortic trauma.

Immediate endotracheal intubation, placement of upper extremity large bore venous lines, drawing of blood for typing and cross-matching, and central venous catheter and Foley catheter placement are done.

Ringer's lactate is used as initial resuscitation fluid rather than non-type-specific uncross-matched blood. Such blood will often cause a complex uncontrollable bleeding diathesis. Fresh whole blood replacement is desirable but often impossible to obtain. Frozen red cells with equivalent platelets and fresh-frozen plasma may be added to maintain normal coagulation. The distinct advantages of frozen red cell blood banking are the indefinite preservation of fresh highly competent red cells, normal potassium content, less cellular aggregates, and, most important, better availability of an adequate quantity of blood. The practice of discarding stored ACD preserved blood limits availability of this transfusate.

Often no other diagnostic study is possible to aid in diagnosis of aortic injury in these critically ill patients. Emergent exploration for vascular control is carried out as part of the intensive resuscitation. Occasionally, if a patient remains stable, arteriography is helpful in defining a vascular injury. Patients with severe back injuries from blunt trauma and rapid deceleration injuries are suspected to have aortic tears and may benefit from diagnostic arteriography [19].

Aortic Control and Exposure

As indicated above, immediate surgical intervention for vascular control is needed in patients with aortic injury as part of the resuscitation effort. Any patient sustaining blunt or penetrating injury who is in profound shock or has refractory hypovolemic shock will require immediate exploration. A seventh interspace left thoracotomy for initial descending thoracic aortic exposure and cross-clamping in patients who are moribund with no obtainable blood pressure is useful. This thoracotomy has the advantage of preserving the tamponade effect of an intact peritoneal cavity [15]. Blood volume is then increased by transfusion to perfuse the coronaries and brain. This is then followed by a xyphoid to symphysis pubis long midline incision for direct exposure of the abdominal visceral organs. Distal aortic control follows. This is easily done.

For patients in moderate shock with systolic pressure of 50-80 mm Hg, an initial laparotomy using a long midline incision is useful. The chest is prepped and exposed for possible incision extension, when necessary. Immediate proximal control of the aorta at the diaphragmatic crura is accomplished quickly and effectively by an occluding aortic compressor [6] (Fig. 1). There is no need to isolate the aorta for placement of a vascular clamp. Thus unnecessary blood loss

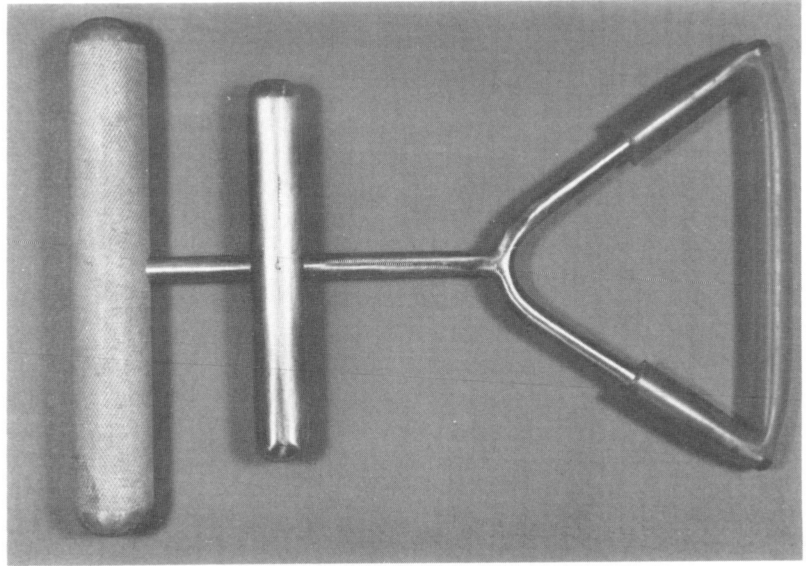

Fig. 1. Aortic compressor device.

is prevented and inadvertent injury to surrounding structures by a hasty dissection is obviated. A quick search for the aortic injury is done and direct pressure over the rent will effectively control bleeding. The use of an intraluminal occluding balloon catheter may be employed if the injury is easily identified. Otherwise, direct pressure over the aortic wound will suffice. It is at this time, when hemorrhage is controlled, that one should pause to allow replacement of intravascular volume. Once adequate blood volume and blood pressure are obtained, one can then proceed in obtaining a more permanent proximal and distal control and exposure of the aortic injury.

Exposure of the infrarenal aorta is similar in trauma to that of aortic aneurysm surgery. The posterior peritoneum is incised at the root of the mesentery from the ileocecal area to the ligament of Treitz. The entire infrarenal aorta distal to the left renal vein is seen.

Suprarenal aortic injury carries a mortality rate of 70%-90% because of relative inaccessibility of the aorta. Visceral organ ischemia contributes also. Irreversible shock from exsanguinating hemorrhage and renal failure are the most frequent causes of death. The surgical approach that has given best exposure is mobilization of the splenic flexure, spleen, pancreas, and left kidney. This is done by incising along the left lateral peritoneal gutter. The entire organ complex is then rotated across the midline to the right utilizing the retropancreatic fusion fascia, thus exposing the entire suprarenal aorta and all its visceral branches. Figure 2 depicts this method of suprarenal aortic exposure. It differs slightly from previously described exposure by Buscaglia et al. [5] and Lim et al. [11] in that the left kidney is included in the mobilization. Exposure of the suprarenal abdominal aorta requires an initial thoracic incision for proximal descending thoracic aortic control. Otherwise, direct pressure on the aorta during mobilization may allow rebleeding because of displacement of direct control on the aortic wound. Experience shows that this method of exposure is adequate except for a retropancreatic portal-superior mesenteric vein injury. In those instances, a resection of the neck of the pancreas is necessary.

Surgical Management

Most aortic injuries can be repaired by primary closure with cardiovascular monofilament sutures. The use of a saphenous vein patch is advisable if primary repair causes significant stenosis of 40% or more. The use of a synthetic Dacron graft [8] may be necessary if a large segment of aorta is lost. Prophylactic antibiotic and copious peritoneal saline irrigation should be instituted because of frequent associated organ injuries. Colon injuries, in particular, should be exteriorized and colostomy done. They should never be repaired primarily. Occasionally, if significant peritoneal soilage and sepsis is present, aortic ligation and extraanatomic bilateral axillofemoral bypass grafts may be necessary.

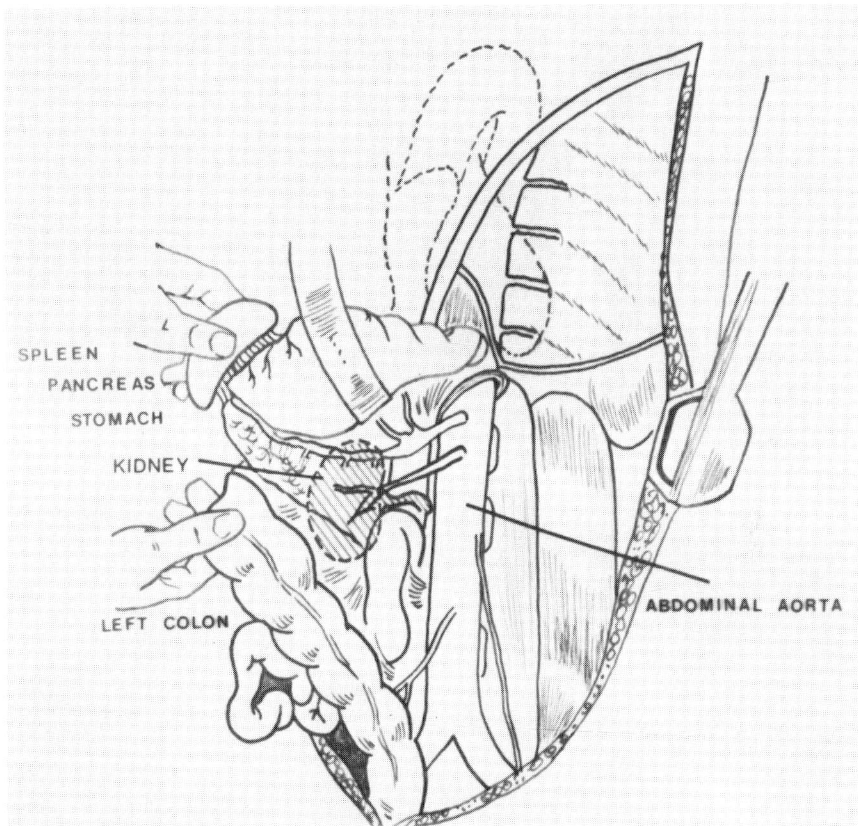

Fig. 2. Thoracoabdominal incision and reflection of entire left abdominal viscera for maximum exposure of suprarenal aorta.

CHRONIC ABDOMINAL AORTIC INJURY

Missed injuries to the abdominal aorta are more difficult to manage because of dense fibrosis, proximal aortic dilatation, and pseudoaneurysm formation. Missed aortic injuries happen because of initial incomplete abdominal exploration.

Aortocaval Fistula

Aortic injuries that involve the adjacent inferior vena cava with formation of an arteriovenous fistula may be missed because only a small overlying hematoma may be noted. The blood is shunted into a low pressure venous system and decreases hematoma size [10, 14, 20].

Illustrative case. An 18 year old male was admitted in high output cardiac failure. He had had an abdominal exploration two years previously for a gunshot wound and no vascular injury had been noted. A loud continuous abdominal bruit was readily observed at the present admission. An aortogram (Fig. 3A) revealed a large aorto-vena caval fistula at the renal artery and vein level. At exploration, dense fibrosis was present. Dilatation of the aorta and vena cava at the fistula site was seen. A false aneurysm of the left renal artery was as seen in Fig. 3B. Lateral closure of the vena cava laceration was done with resection of the fistula and closure of the aortic laceration. The left renal artery was resected and repaired with a bypass graft.

Similarly, the angiogram in Figure 4A is of a patient who had an abdominal exploration done for a stab wound from an ice pick injury 4 years previously. Dense fibrosis (Fig. 4B) was encountered over the site of aortic and caval injury. Figure 4C shows the traumatic arteriovenous fistula dissected after proximal and distal vascular control.

UNUSUAL AORTIC INJURY

Unusual injuries to the abdominal aorta may be found. Missile embolism from an aortic injury with distal embolization is sometimes seen and should be suspected when a missile is noted to migrate in subsequent x-rays or when the missile is not found in injuries where there is no exit wound. The unilateral absence of a distal extremity pulse should suggest embolization. Missile embolus can also be missed when roentgenograms are limited to the chest and abdomen.

Illustrative case. Figure 5A demonstrates such a case. A 28 year old male was admitted to the Vascular Service because of intermittent claudication of the left leg two weeks after he was discharged from another hospital after treatment of a gunshot wound to the lower anterior chest. No exit wound was noted at that time. A chest and abdominal x-ray revealed no missile. Indeed, the missile had embolized into the popliteal artery as shown in the arteriogram, and did not cause symptoms until the patient started to have intermittent claudication. The embolus was successfully removed through an arteriotomy in the popliteal artery (Figure 5B) which was closed with a vein patch.

Aortoenteric fistula from trauma rarely happens. It may occur in missed contused aortic wall injury secondary to blast effect of a missile. This cannot be appreciated readily without arteriography. The small bowel may adhere to the injury and later form an aortoenteric fistula.

A rare case of traumatic aortojejunal fistula was encountered in a 33 year old male who was seen in the emergency room with recurring episodes of massive hematemesis and no evidence of external trauma. Emergent endoscopy did not show any gastroduodenal or esophageal lesion. An immediate abdominal aortic

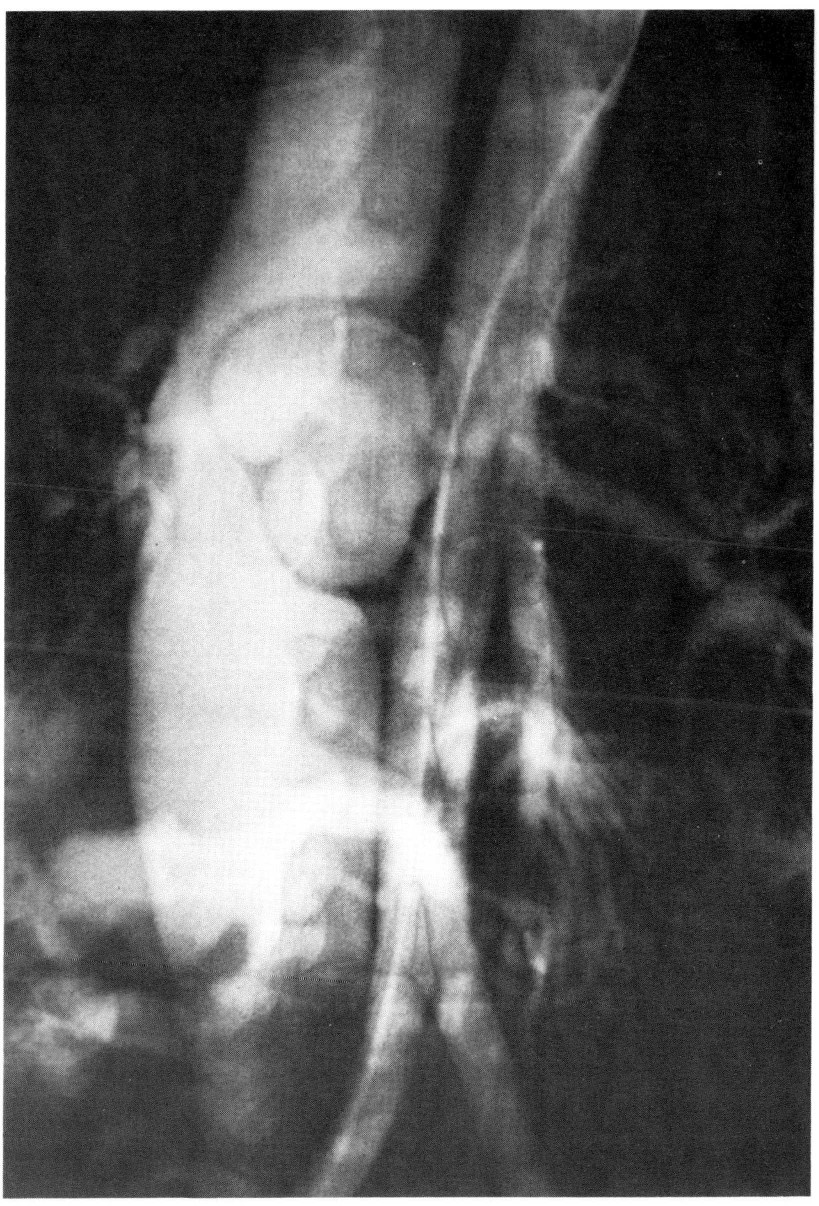

Fig. 3A. Large traumatic aorta-vena cava fistula from gunshot wound.

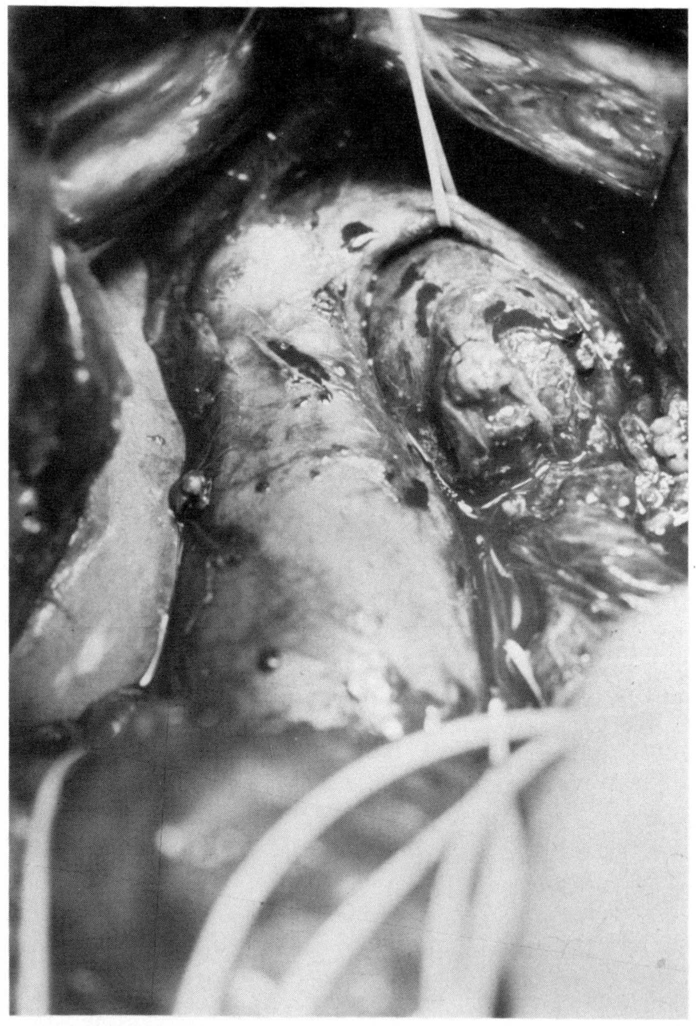

Fig. 3B. Note marked dilatation of inferior vena cava and aneurysmal formation of aorta at site of arteriovenous fistula.

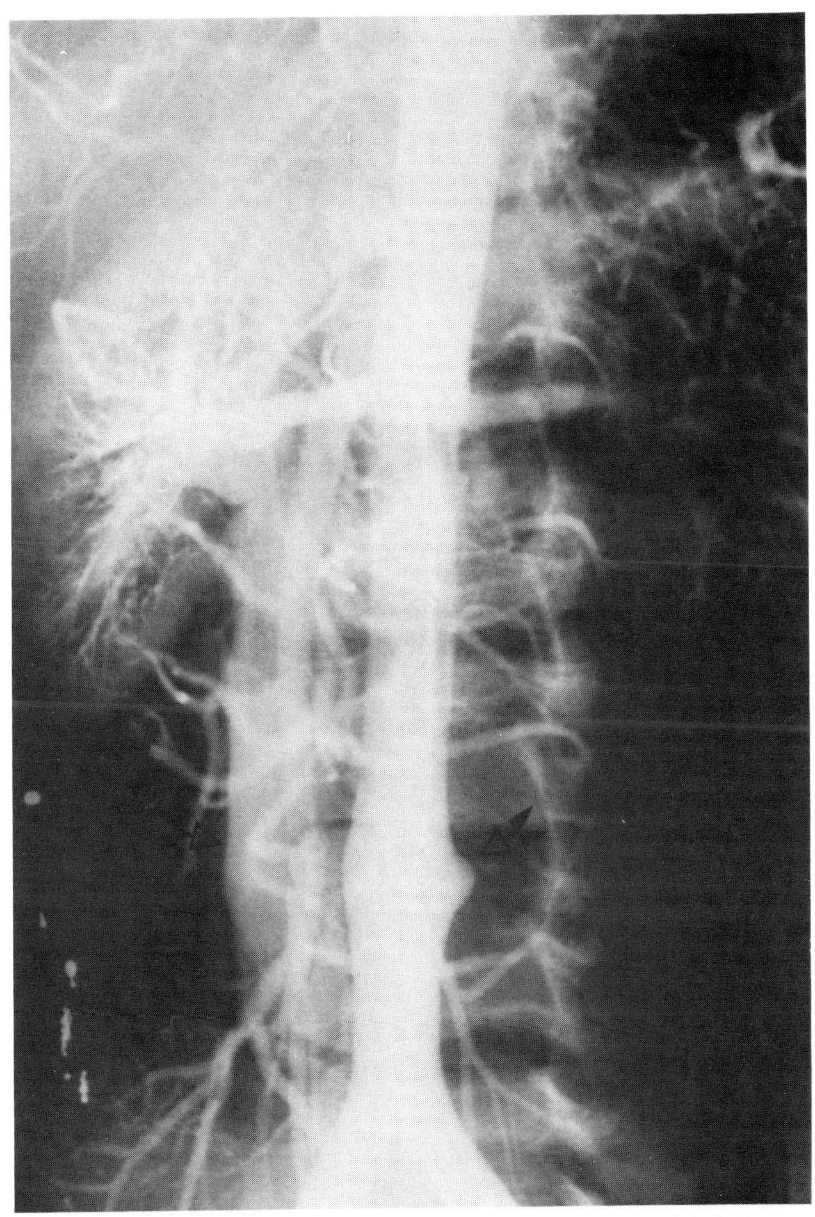

Fig. 4A. Flush aortogram. Note simultaneous visualization of inferior vena cava. Arrow points to fistula site.

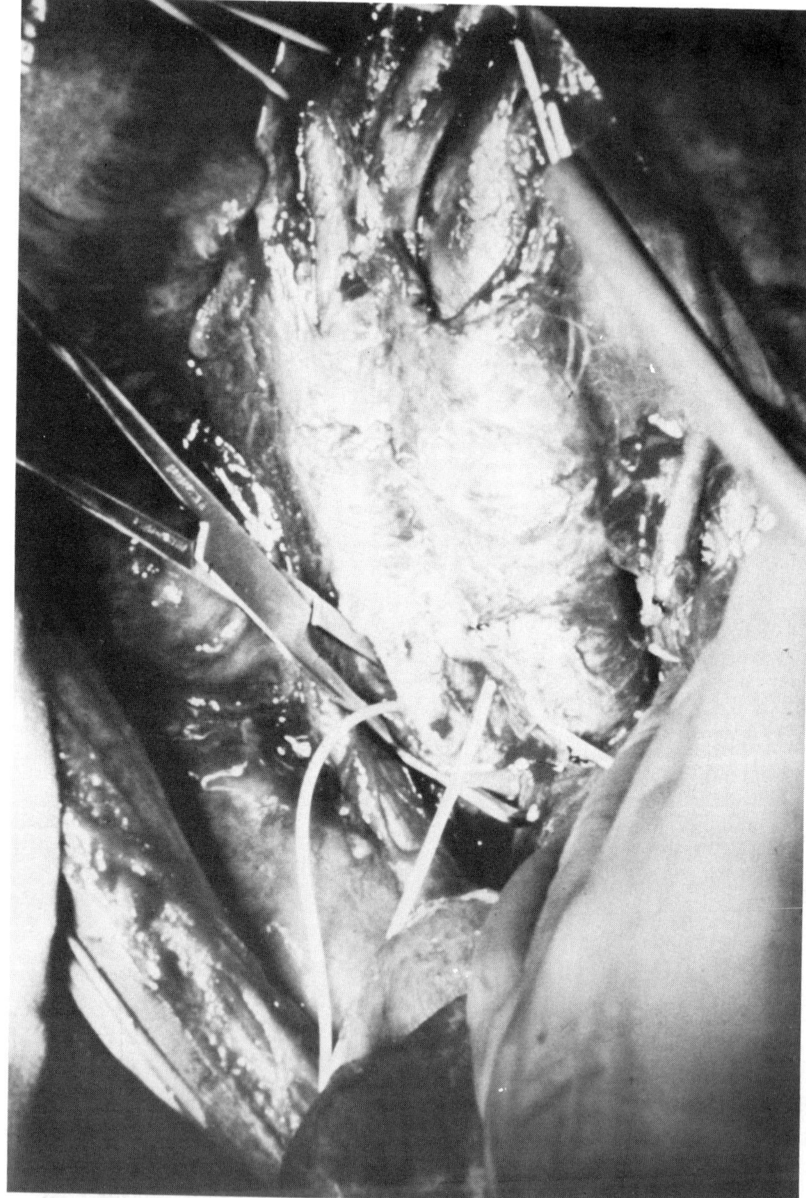

Fig. 4B. Note dense fibrosis around aorta and vena cava injury.

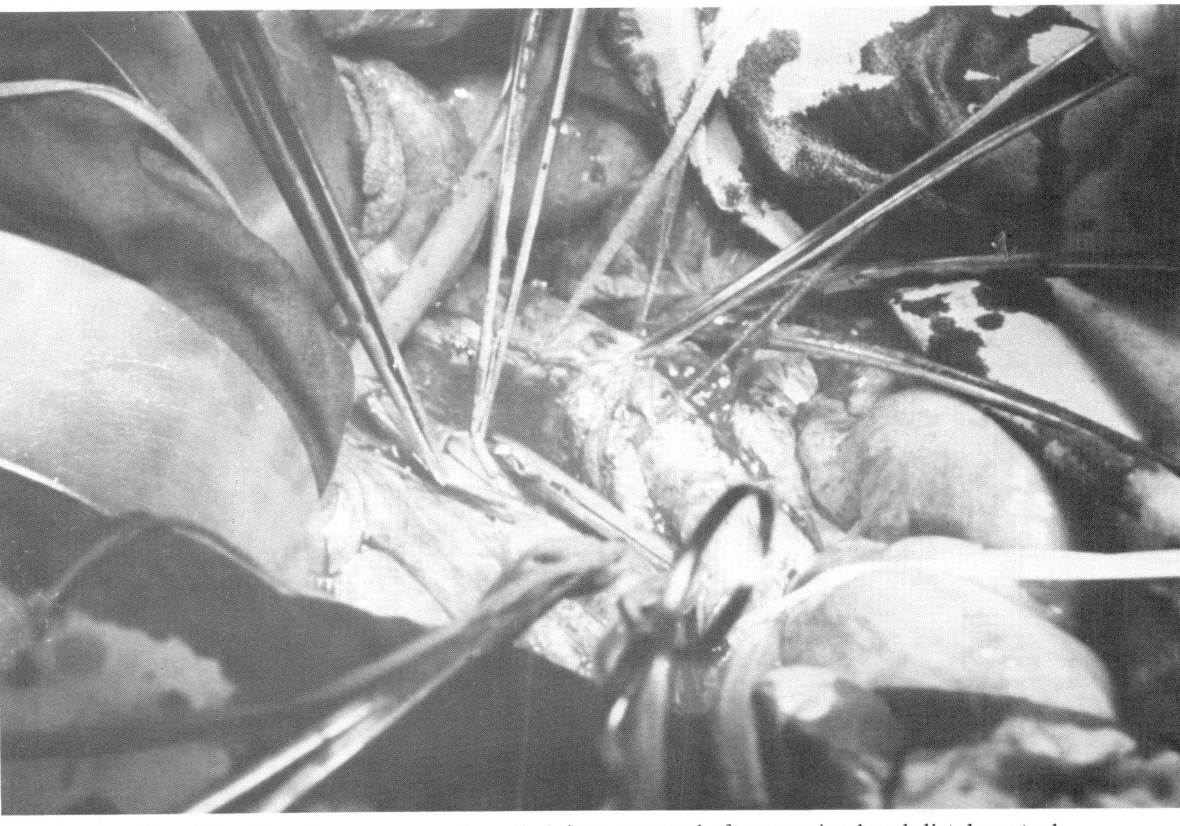

Fig. 4C. Site of vena cava and aortic injury exposed after proximal and distal control.

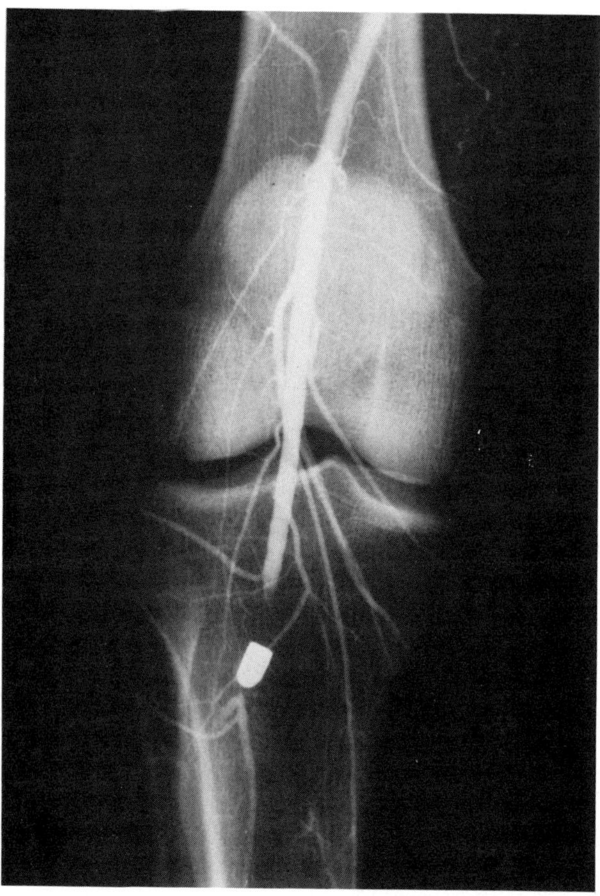

Fig. 5A. Missile embolus to popliteal artery from gunshot wound to aorta.

arteriogram was done for diagnosis. A straight radiopaque, 2.5 inch long foreign body that looked like a sewing needle was noted to move with passage of the arteriogram catheter. This indicated the location to be partially inside the aorta (Fig. 6A). Abdominal exploration indeed revealed a 2.5 inch long rusted milliner needle that traversed from the proximal jejunum at the ligament of Treitz to the anterior wall of the abdominal aorta (Fig. 6B). Closure of the jejunal fistula and primary repair of the aortic laceration was done (Fig. 6C). The patient denied ever swallowing a sewing needle, but because of the rusty condition of the needle the injury must have happened many years before. The needle was lodged at the proximal jejunum and gradually eroded into the aorta, forming an aortojejunal fistula.

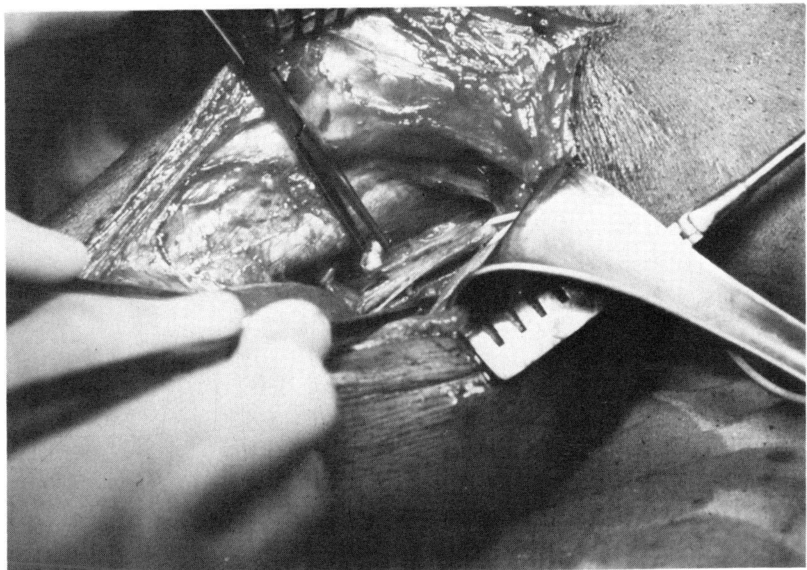

Fig. 5B. Operative photograph showing .22 caliber missile removed from popliteal artery.

INJURIES TO THE INFERIOR VENA CAVA

Less attention has been directed to management of inferior vena caval injury than aortic injury. Like aortic injury, massive bleeding is the main cause of death in caval trauma. Fifty percent of such patients are admitted in shock, and the reported mortality rate is 40%. Surgical management is as formidable as aortic injury.

There are two features which differentiate caval from aortic injury. First, spontaneous tamponade is common in most vena cava injuries. The retroperitoneal hematoma that forms is able to tamponade effectively the bleeding that arises from the low pressure venous system. Thus a large number of patients with vena cava injury are able to arrive alive in the hospital. The second difference is in difficulty of controlling the bleeding from vena cava locations because lumbar veins with enormous blood flow, when not controlled, may easily allow exsanguination.

Management

Resuscitation is done in patients with cava injury in a fashion similar to those with aortic injury. Few diagnostic tests are needed. Few are possible. Major efforts are directed toward resuscitation, establishing adequate airway, and restoring intravascular volume.

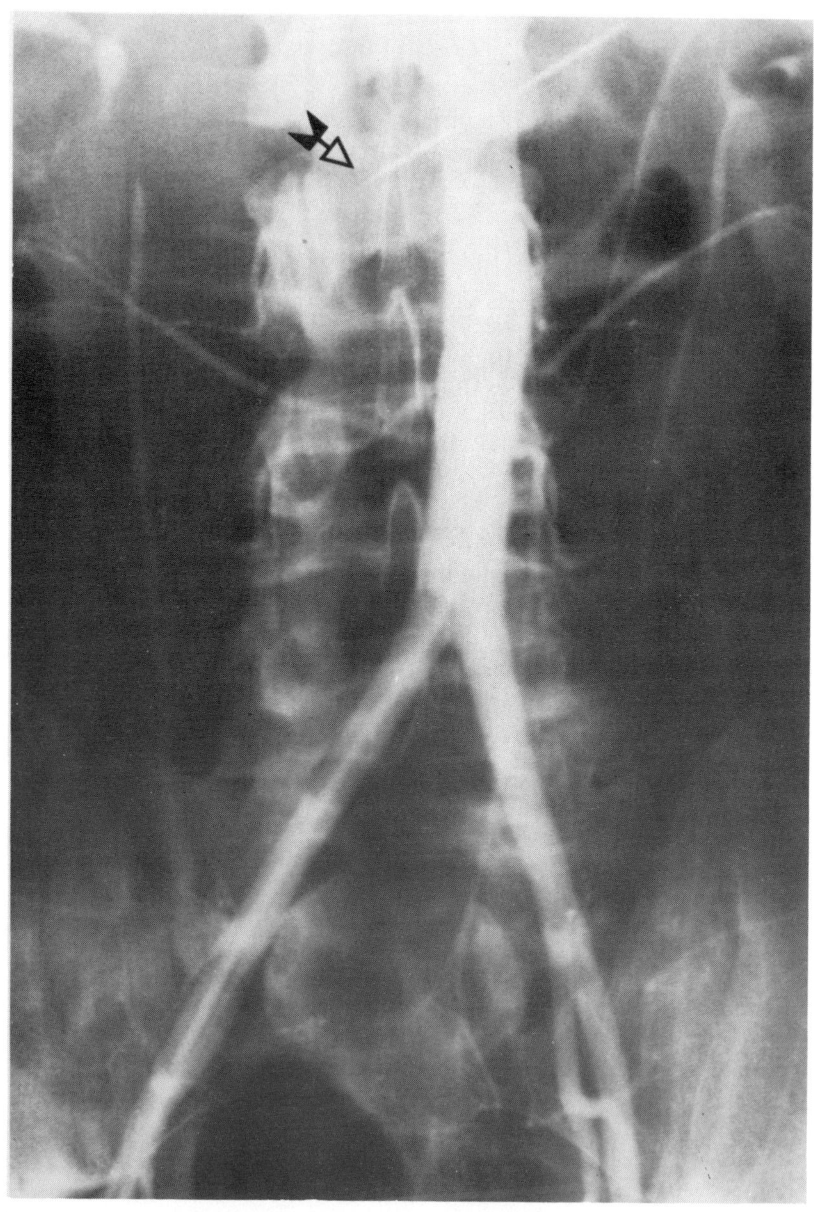

Fig. 6A. Emergency aortogram showing needle inside the aorta on a 33 year old patient with massive upper gastrointestinal bleeding.

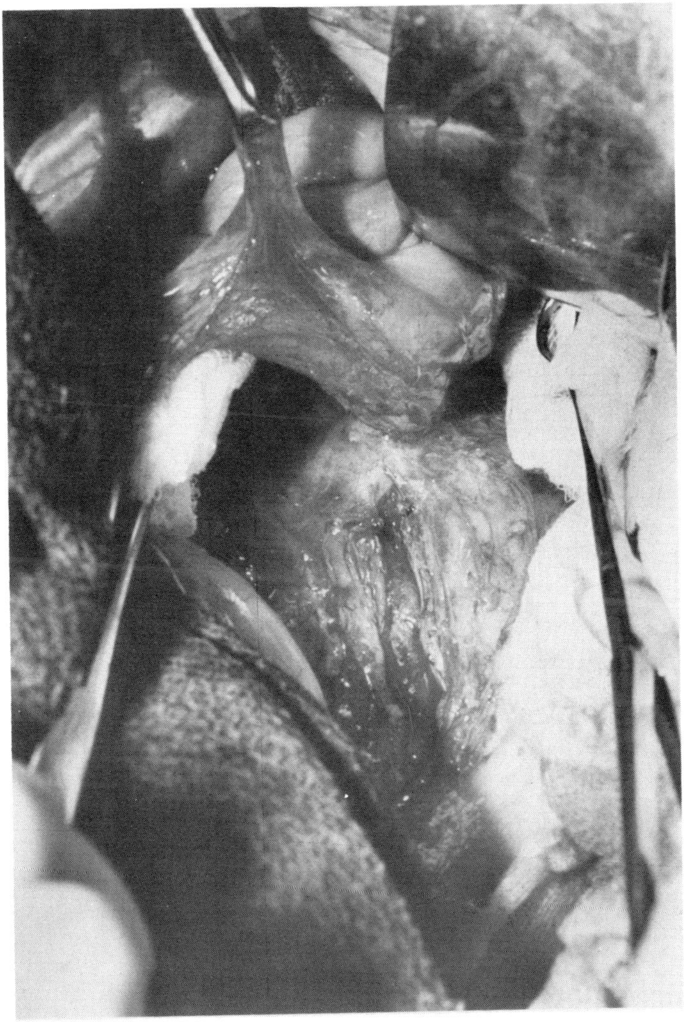

Fig. 6B. Operative photograph demonstrates site of aortojejunal fistula.

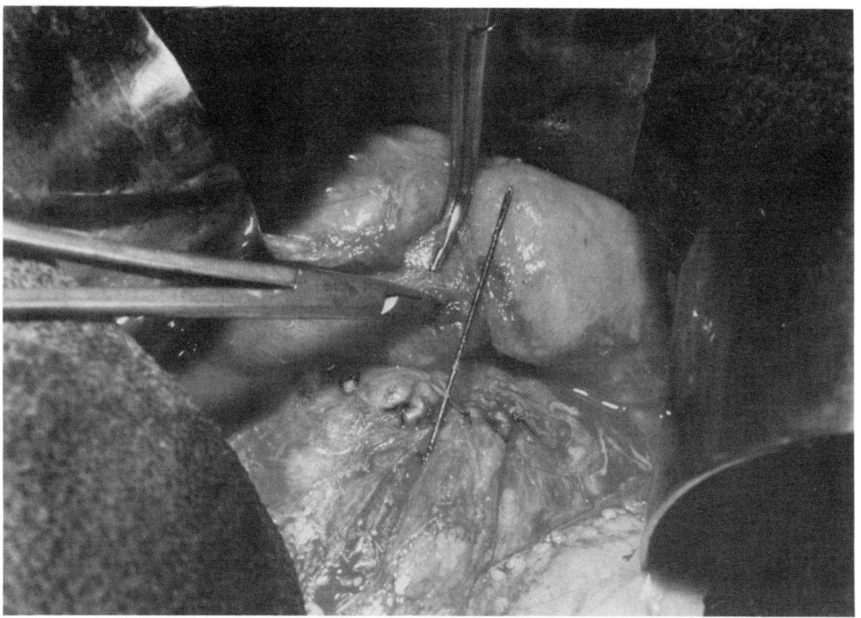

Fig. 6C. Rusty seamstress needle at aortojejunal fistula site.

A long midline incision is made. Often a contained retroperitoneal hematoma with no active bleeding is encountered. No attempt should be made to disrupt this hematoma until adequate fluid volume replacement has been made and provisions for vascular control are available. Associated injuries to the intraperitoneal organs may be cared for at this time to minimize soilage from hollow viscus injuries. Retroperitoneal hematomas should be explored to prevent the possibility of missing injuries to retroperitoneal structures. The inferior vena cava is exposed by reflection of the right colon and duodenum. Direct digital pressure is applied immediately to the site of the injury. Proximal and distal pressure is inadequate to control enormous venous collateral flow. The placement of a partially occluding Satinsky clamp over the caval laceration is often difficult because the vein wall is collapsed, thin-walled, and separated. Visibility is often poor because of enormous bleeding. A simple and effective technique of direct control of the caval laceration is the sequential application of Allis clamps as shown in Fig. 7. With one hand applying direct digital control over the laceration, the first Allis clamp is applied immediately above the site of the most superior caval laceration. A gentle lifting motion of this forcep will allow coaptation of the lacerated wall immediately inferior to it. A second Allis clamp is then applied to hold the vein walls together. A succession of Allis clamps are placed until all the lacerations are completely held together. Primary closure suture is then done easily.

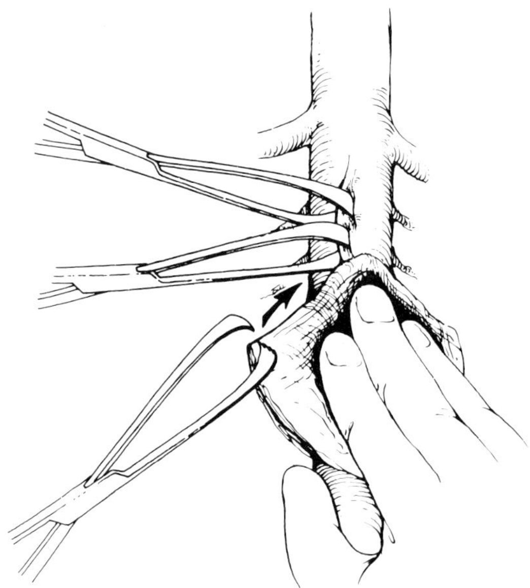

Fig. 7. Simple, rapid, and effective method of vascular control on vena caval laceration by sequential application of Allis clamps.

Injury to the suprarenal retrohepatic vena cava is not readily accessible. It is usually associated with penetrating or blunt liver injuries with involvement of the hepatic veins and retrohepatic vena cava. Isolation of the vena cava with placement of vascular clamps is not possible at this location. A temporary intracaval shunt as described by Buchberg, Timmis, Rosanova, and Larkin and first clinically used by Schrock, Blaisdell, and Matherson is useful. The intracaval shunt channels caval blood flow through the injured segment and thus provides a bloodless field for the identification and repair of the caval injury. The procedure is accomplished by placement of a large (28 French) catheter introduced from the right atrium to the inferior vena cava [3, 4, 7]. A vascular occluding tape is encircled around the intrapericardial portion of the inferior vena cava and the inferior vena cava just above the renal veins. A Pringle's maneuver is simultaneously applied by placement of vascular clamps to interrupt portal vein and hepatic artery flow. In initial experience, the catheter was introduced from above through the right atrium. In later experience, it was found that introduction from below at the infrarenal vena cava is easy. This minimizes the problems of air embolism and does not require placement of pursestring sutures over the right atrium. Figure 8A illustrates a current method of intracaval shunt placement. Figure 8B shows an operative photograph of a retrohepatic caval injury

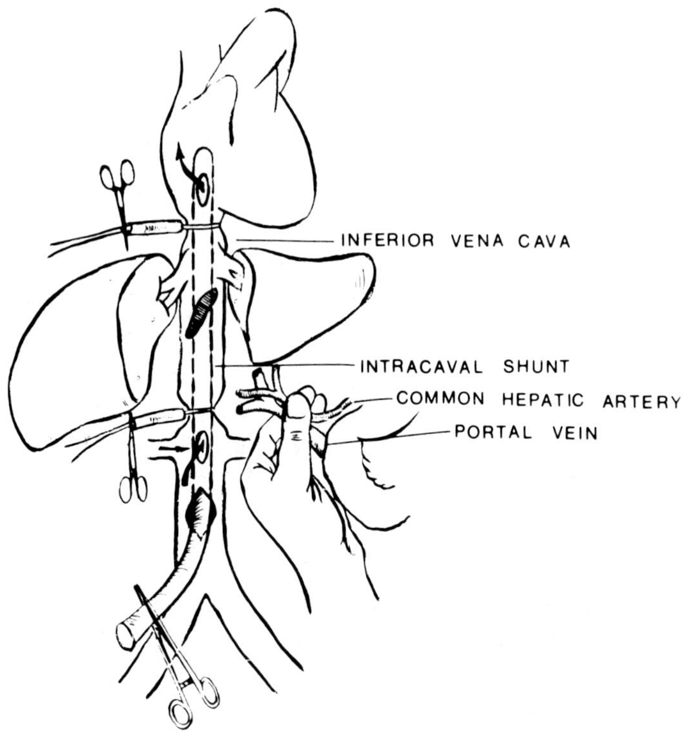

Fig. 8A. Use of intracaval shunt for retrohepatic vena cava injury.

exposed in a bloodless field with the use of the intracaval shunt. It is not always necessary to resect the liver to gain access to the cava. The liver may be gently rotated after incision of its peritoneal attachments. More often, however, there is an associated massive liver injury and a resection may be required.

Repair of injuries to the inferior vena cava is most often accomplished by lateral suture. Extensive injuries with large segment loss in the infrarenal vena cava may require ligation. The site of ligation ideally should be just below the renal veins to prevent the formation of a cul de sac where a stagnant column of blood may allow thrombosis and pulmonary embolization. Prosthetic grafts for venous repair are not recommended because of thrombosis. Use of autogenous veins, the saphenous and internal jugular vein, as patches or paneled grafts is effective. In extensive injuries of the suprarenal vena cava, ligation is not tolerated and is often fatal. Every attempt should be made to repair the cava in this location. Occasionally, it may be necessary to harvest the infrarenal vena cava and transpose this superiorly to bridge the suprarenal caval defect.

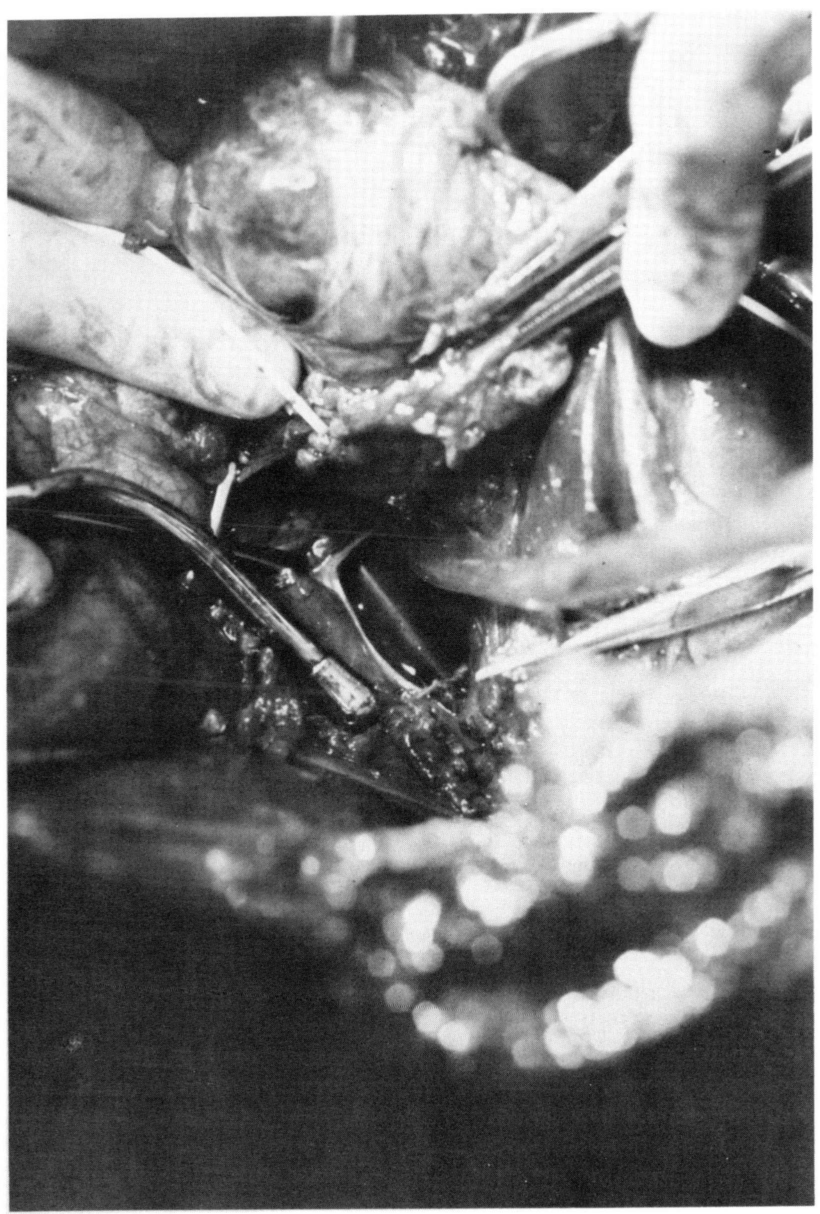

Fig. 8B. Operative photograph showing a retrohepatic vena cava laceration over a temporary intracaval shunt.

CONCLUSION

Injuries to the abdominal aorta and inferior vena cava carry high mortality because of shock from massive blood loss and associated multiple organ injuries. To achieve patient survival, the need for quick transport and a well organized plan for resuscitation by a cohesive trauma team are essential. The availability of blood is crucial, and the use of emergency surgery for vascular control should be a part of the resuscitative armamentarium. Vascular control is obtained by methods that depend upon the patient's state of shock and anatomic level of aortic injury. The need for an initial thoracic incision for proximal control of suprarenal aortic injury and the method of exposure by reflection of the right colon, pancreas, spleen, and kidney en mass to the right has been effective and useful.

The incidence of missile embolism, though uncommon, is real, and a high index of suspicion should be raised on an unaccountable disappearing missile. The routine practice of including the retroperitoneal organs in abdominal exploration for trauma as well as the exploration of retroperitoneal hematomas should prevent the possibility of missed injuries. Dense fibrosis and dilatation of the aorta and vena cava is common in chronic aortic and vena caval injury. This makes late surgery more difficult.

In inferior vena caval injury, spontaneous tamponade should be utilized in continuing volume resuscitation efforts prior to vascular exploration. Direct caval pressure over the injury and progressive application of Allis clamps over the lacerated caval wall to obtain vascular control of the laceration has been particularly useful in achieving quick hemostasis with minimal blood loss. Lastly, the intracaval shunt placement for exposure and repair of retrohepatic vena caval injury has saved lives in an otherwise often fatal injury.

REFERENCES

1. Allen TW, Reul GJ, Morton JR, et al: Surgical management of aortic trauma. J. Trauma 12:862, 1972
2. Beall AC Jr: Penetrating wounds of the aorta. Am. J. Surg. 99:770, 1960
3. Bricker DL, Morton JR, Okies JE, et al: Surgical management of injuries to the vena cava: Changing patterns of injury and newer techniques of repair. J. Trauma 2:725, 1971
4. Brown RS, Boyd DR, Matsuda T, et al: Temporary internal vascular shunt for retrohepatic vena cava injury. J. Trauma 11:736, 1971
5. Buscaglia LC, Blaisdell FW, Lim RC: Penetrating abdominal vascular injuries. Arch. Surg. 99:764, 1969
6. Conn J Jr, Trippel OH, Bergan JJ: A new atraumatic aortic occluder. Surgery 64:1158, 1968

7. Davis EA, Falk G, Yarnoz M, et al: An improved technique for the repair of the intrahepatic inferior vena cava and hepatic veins. J. Trauma 11:738, 1971
8. Fromm SH, Carrasquilla C, Lucas C: The management of gunshot wounds of the aorta. Arch. Surg. 101:388, 1970
9. Hardy JD, Raju S, Neely WA, et al: Aortic and other arterial injuries. Ann. Surg. 181:640, 1975
10. Hughes CW, Jahnke EJ Jr: The surgery of traumatic arteriovenous fistulas and aneurysms: A five year follow-up study of 215 lesions. Ann. Surg. 148:790, 1958
11. Lim RC Jr, Trunkey DD, Blaisdell FW: Acute abdominal aortic injury: An analysis of operative and post-operative management. Arch. Surg. 109:706, 1974
12. Mattox KL, McCollum WB, Jordan GL, et al: Management of upper abdominal vascular trauma. Am. J. Surg. 128:823, 1974
13. Perdue GD Jr, Smith RB: Intra-abdominal vascular injury. Surgery 64:562, 1968
14. Pemberton JD, Seefield PH, Barker NW: Traumatic arteriovenous fistula involving the abdominal aorta and the inferior vena cava. Ann. Surg. 123:508, 1946
15. Richards AJ, Lamis PA, Rogers JP Jr, et al: Laceration of abdominal aorta and study of intact abdominal wall as tamponade: Report of survival and literature review. Ann. Surg. 164:321, 1966
16. Starzl TE, Kaupp HA, Beheler HM, et al: Penetrating injuries of the inferior vena cava. Surgery 51:195, 1962
17. Stone HH, Oxford WM, Austin JT: Penetrating wounds of the abdominal aorta. South. Med. J. 66:1351, 1973
18. Thal ER, Perry MO: Peripheral and Abdominal Vascular Injuries. Philadelphia, W. B. Saunders, 1977
19. Tomatis LA, Doornbos FA, Beard JA: Circumferential intimal tear of aorta with complete occlusion due to blunt trauma. J. Trauma 8:1096, 1968
20. Williams CL, Robinson DW: Traumatic abdominal aorta-inferior vena cava fistula with immediate repair. Ann. Surg. 154:998, 1961
21. Yajko RD, Trimble C: Arterial bullet embolism following abdominal gunshot wounds. J. Trauma 14:200, 1974

Thomas W. Kornmesser, M.D.
Otto H. Trippel, M.D.
Sidney P. Haid, M.D.

Acute Occlusion of the Abdominal Aorta

"We do not know when arterial surgery began but it developed slowly during many centuries."

Charles Rob, 1972 [13]

One of the most dramatic and catastrophic medical events occurs upon acute occlusion of the abdominal aorta. Diagnosis and treatment should be prompt in order to salvage both the affected extremities and the patient as a whole.

Sabaneyev [15] in 1895 reported the first attempt at removal of an aortic saddle embolus, and Bauer [1] successfully accomplished this feat in 1913. In 1950 Oudot [12] described resection and replacement of the aorta, and in 1962 Blaisdell and Hall [2] introduced the concept of extraanatomic bypass. It was in 1963, however, that the true "breakthrough" in the treatment of acute arterial occlusion occurred with the monumental contribution of Fogarty and his colleagues [6], the balloon catheter for extraction of thrombus from the arterial system.

In the past 15 years, experience has accumulated but little that is new has been added. This paper will attempt to summarize our data and reaffirm the premise that aggressive surgical management is indicated.

DIAGNOSIS

Acute aortic occlusion presents with pallor, paresthesia, paralysis, pain, poikilothermy, and pulselessness just as any other acute arterial occlusion. The extent and severity of the symptoms may not be the same in both legs and depends primarily upon the presence or absence of collaterals and upon whether total or near total occlusion is present. This status of the collateral bed can be assessed with the use of the Doppler ultrasound. An unrecordable pressure at the ankle is ominous and suggests immediate surgical intervention is necessary, as does the presence of nerve ischemia – i.e., anesthesia or especially loss of motor function.

Differentiation of the etiology of the acute aortic occlusion is necessary preoperatively to plan the appropriate treatment. Embolus is the most common etiology and is heralded by no past history of chronic occlusive disease, the presence of atrial fibrillation, and/or myocardial infarction. A past history of rheumatic fever or myocardiopathy would also be helpful, as would previous embolic events. Approximately 45% of embolus patients reported by Darling had a recurrent embolus [4]. Most of these occurred during the discontinuation of recommended anticoagulant treatment.

Acute thrombosis of the aorta will generally present with a history of some arterial insufficiency. Only about 6% of the patients with aortoiliac occlusion present with acute occlusion as their first symptom [5]. Examination can reveal an abdominal mass and/or chronically ischemic extremities. Arteriography will often be helpful.

An acute aortic dissection can usually be differentiated by the history of severe chest pain. Also, chest x-ray will frequently show mediastinal widening. These findings, accompanied by severe hypertension, will commonly point out this diagnosis.

Acute venous occlusion can, on occasion, cause such a severe decrease in arterial flow that differentiation from arterial occlusion is difficult. However, edema should be the differentiating factor. The temperature of the skin should be warm, although in phlegmasia cerulea dolans the leg is cold secondary to the severe artificial insufficiency that is present [17].

The presence or absence of blunt abdominal trauma is important historical data to obtain. The cardinal findings of paraplegia and loss of distal pulses in this situation should alert one to this entity of traumatic occlusion [19].

CLINICAL MATERIAL

Between February 1969 and the present, we have seen 22 patients with acute aortic occlusion. This series includes 12 males and 10 females between the ages of 42 and 87.

The most common etiology was a sudden embolus, one of which was diagnosed on microscopy as myxoma. Five patients developed acute thrombus; two of these were acute occlusions of aortic aneurysms (Table 1).

There were seven deaths, all cardiac in origin and all from the group with saddle embolus. There was no instance of limb loss in any of the patients treated.

The most common operative procedure was bilateral embolectomy from the groin with Fogarty catheters. Four patients underwent aortofemoral bypasses, and one patient required a primary axillary femoral bypass.

Table 1
Etiology

Saddle embolus	17
Myocardial infarction	(7)
Atrial fibrillation	(5)
Unknown (no myocardial infarction or atrial fibrillation)	(4)
Myxoma	(1)
Acute thrombosis	5
Abdominal aortic aneurysm	(2)
Distal aortic occlusive disease	(3)

There were three patients in which removal of a saddle embolus from the groin was unsuccessful. These all required a secondary surgical procedure. Two patients had a saddle embolus in addition to chronic occlusive disease. These patients required axillary femoral bypass. One of the patients died postoperatively.

The third patient with a failed embolectomy required a transabdominal aortic embolectomy. This patient was found to have embolized an atrial myxoma to the aortic bifurcation, left renal artery, and parenchyma of the right kidney (Fig. 1). This patient required a long hospital stay which included dialysis and extensive physical therapy.

It is of interest that three patients had no surgical treatment. One of these patients died shortly after initial evaluation. The other two patients were recovering from their acute ischemic event when first seen and required no immediate surgical intervention. One patient was lost to followup and the other was seen recently 6 years postembolus and was doing well with no surgery.

DISCUSSION

The so-called saddle embolus is the most common cause of acute aortic occlusion with severe ischemia. The source of the embolus is uniformly the heart. These patients either had atrial fibrillation (chronic or acute), acute myocardial infarction, or, as in one case, a myxoma. The frequency of arterial embolism to the aortic bifurcation is about 9% of all embolic events [4, 18].

The mortality for acute aortic occlusion secondary to embolus is high primarily because of the presence of severe associated cardiac disease. Thompson [18] noted this in his group of patients, as did we. Our mortality was quite high, 7 of 17. It is pointed out by Levy [11] that the attendant disease process is the cause and not the surgical procedure itself.

The timing of embolectomy does appear important and suggests that the best results are obtained by early intervention [11]. However, late embolectomy should not be withheld, as exemplified by our series and as discussed by

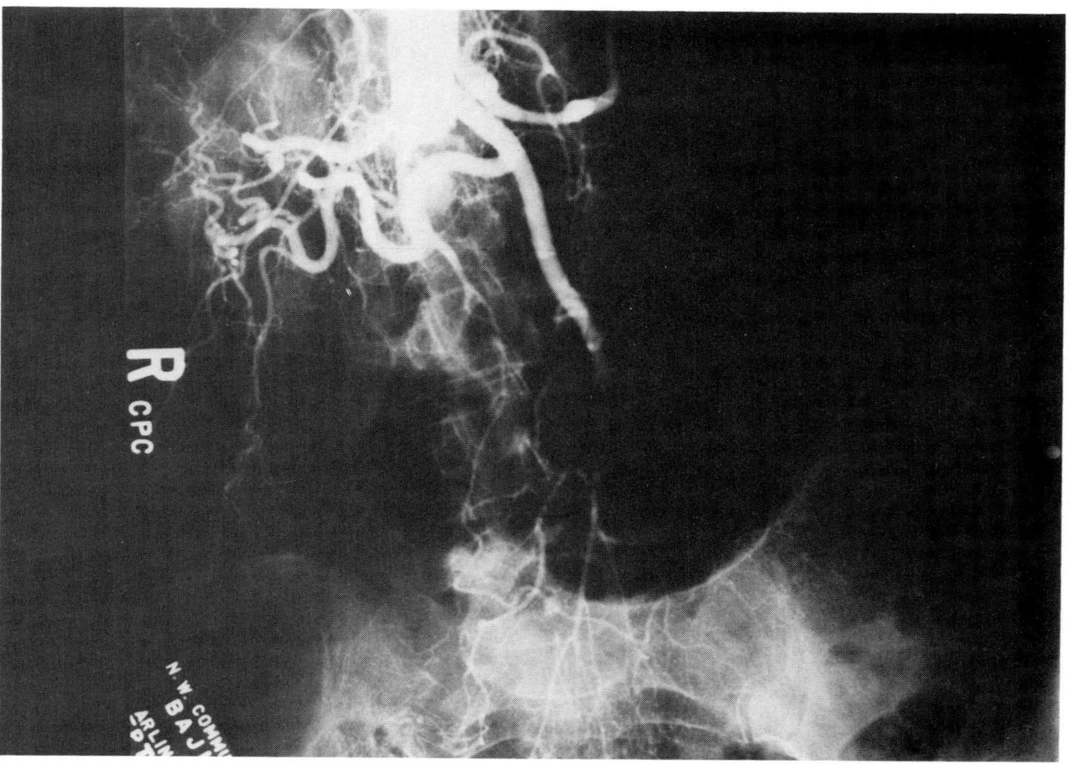

Fig. 1. Transaxillary aortogram demonstrating occlusion of the infrarenal aorta, the left renal artery, and parenchymal branches of the right renal artery. On microscopy this was found to be myxomatous embolus.

Thompson [18]. One patient in our series did not have surgical intervention until 7 days postevent; a successful result was obtained (Table 2). We could not document any "golden period" for surgery.

Intracardiac tumors are uncommon, but their frequency varies in different series. About 50% of the intracardiac tumors are myxomata. They are histologically benign but can provide serious consequences. The most common clinical presentation is peripheral embolization [9]. The tumor usually originates from the atria [9] but can also arise in the ventricle [20]. These often embolize only a small portion but can rarely embolize the whole tumor [10] to the aorta, as presumably occurred in our one case.

Sudden occlusion of an abdominal aortic aneurysm (Fig. 2) is a rare complication and an unusual cause of aortic occlusion [8, 16]. The majority of these patients have distal occlusive disease as well as an aneurysm present, and this appears to be the common denominator in this unusual group. The size of the aneurysm apparently varies significantly. The mortality rate of this particular entity is quite high, as noted in the literature, most deaths being cardiac in origin [8, 16].

Other causes of acute aortic occlusion include blunt abdominal trauma and dissecting aneurysm, both of which are unusual. Abdominal aortic occlusion secondary to blunt trauma does occur [3, 14, 19]. The cause is related to the force of the trauma and the fact that the aorta is relatively fixed to the vertebral column and to the lumbar vessels. This is more likely to be a precipitating event when severe atherosclerosis is present, but it can occur in a normal vessel [14].

Acute neonatal occlusion is mentioned only for completeness. The etiology of this is varied but includes dehydration, sepsis, hypersensitivity, umbilical sepsis, and thrombus of the umbilical artery [7].

Once the diagnosis of acute aortic occlusion is made, the patient is immediately given heparin to prevent proximal and distal propagation of thrombus. This also helps in the prevention of further embolization. An intravenous bolus of 10,000 units is our recommended dosage.

The operative management depends primarily upon the etiology. These patients are generally quite ill and unable to tolerate any large procedure. An

Table 2
Interval From Onset of Symptoms to Treatment

Time (Hours)	No. of Patients	Success	Failure (Deaths)
0 - 12	10	8	2
12 - 24	5	2	4
> 24	5	4	1

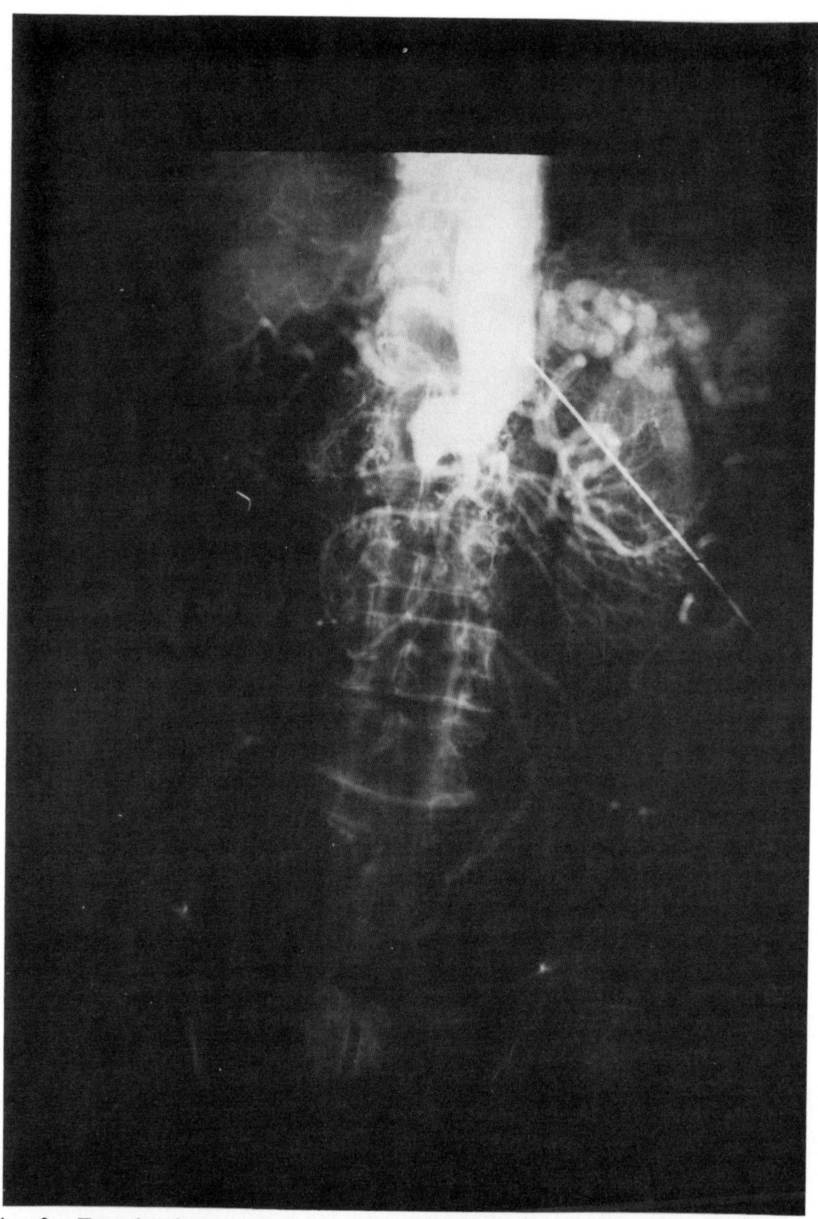

Fig. 2. Translumbar aortogram with visualization of only the neck of an abdominal aortic aneurysm, the remainder having spontaneously thrombosed.

embolectomy from the groin with Fogarty catheter can generally be performed under local anesthesia and is tolerated well. If this is not successful, transabdominal embolectomy, aortofemoral bypass, or axillary femoral bypass needs to be considered, depending upon the patient's condition. If the etiology is other than embolus, one must plan the surgical management accordingly. The use of either anatomic or extraanatomic bypass may be necessary.

Postoperatively, the patients who have embolized are anticoagulated to prevent future embolization. Heparin is generally started 6-8 hours after surgery, maintained for a minimum of 1 week, and then the patient is converted to coumadin. Care must be taken to prevent periods of inadequate anticoagulation.

CONCLUSIONS

Although the clinical picture is quite familiar to practicing clinicians, varying etiology requires careful planning of the best therapeutic approach. With aggressive surgical management, salvage of useful, functioning, pain-free limbs is to be expected despite a continued high mortality due primarily to associated severe cardiac disease. Nonetheless, restoration of adequate circulation remains a superior alternative to the spector of major amputation.

REFERENCES

1. von Bauer F: Embolies aortae abdominalis operation heilung. Cbl. Chir. 2:1945-1946, 1913
2. Blaisdell FW, Hall AD: Axillary femoral artery bypass for lower extremity ischemia. Surgery 54:563-565, 1962
3. Dajee H, Richardson IW, Iype MO: Seat belt aorta: Acute dissection and thrombosis of the abdominal aorta. Surgery 85:263-267, 1979
4. Darling RC, Austen WG, Linton RR: Arterial embolism. Surg. Gynecol. Obstet. 122:106-114, 1967
5. Faerbairn JF II, Bernatz PE: Acute arterial occlusion, in Faerbairn JF II, Juergens JL, Spittel JA Jr (eds): Peripheral Vascular Diseases. Philadelphia, W. B. Saunders, 1972, p 256
6. Fogarty TJ, Cranley JJ, Krause RJ, et al: A method for extraction of arterial emboli and thrombi. Surg. Gynecol. Obstet. 116:241-245, 1963
7. Gupta PK, Bargava SK: Thrombotic occlusion of the aorta in the newborn. Ind. J. Pediatr. 34:325-327, 1967
8. Johnson JM, Gaspar MR, Movius HJ, et al: Sudden complete thrombosis of aortic and iliac aneurysms. Arch. Surg. 108:792-794, 1974

9. Koikkalainen K, Kostiainen S, Luosto R: Left atrial myxoma revealed by femoral embolectomy. Scand. J. Thorac. Cardiovasc. Surg. 11:33-35, 1977
10. Kulkarni M, Jessiman I McD, French S: Entire left atrial myxoma presenting as a saddle embolus. Thorax 24:629-631, 1969
11. Levy JF, Butcher HR Jr: Arterial emboli: An analysis of 125 patients. Surgery 68:968-973, 1970
12. Oudot J.: La grebbe vasculaire dans les thromboses du carre four aortique. Pr. Med. 59:234-236, 1951
13. Rob CG: A history of arterial surgery. Arch. Surg. 105:821-823, 1972
14. Rybak JJ, Thomford NR: Acute occlusion of the infrarenal aorta from blunt trauma. Am. Surgeon 35:444-447, 1969
15. Sabaneyev IF: The problem of vascular suture. Russk. Chir. Arch. 2:132-140, 1895
16. Saha SP, Nunn DB: Sudden thrombotic occlusion of abdominal aortic aneurysm. Am. Surgeon 40:246-247, 1974
17. Strandness DE, Sumner DS: Hemodynamics for Surgeons. New York, Grune & Stratton, 1975, p 426
18. Thompson JE, Sigler L, Rout PS, et al: Arterial embolectomy: A 20 year experience with 163 cases. Surgery 67:212-220, 1970
19. Welborn MB, Sawyers JL: Acute abdominal aortic occlusion due to nonpenetrating trauma. Am. J. Surg. 118:112-116, 1969
20. Young RD, Hunter WC: Primary myxoma of the left ventricle with embolic occlusion of the abdominal aorta and renal arteries. Arch. Pathol. 43:86-91, 1947

Renovascular Hypertension

John H. Laragh, M.D.
David B. Case, M.D.

The Renin System for Understanding and Managing Renovascular Hypertensions

If human renal hypertension were always obliging enough to conform precisely to the Goldblatt experimental model, it would be cured invariably by nephrectomy or surgical repair of the stenotic vessel. While distinct success achieved by surgery in some patients demonstrates the validity of the model, the failure in others suggests that there may be more than one model. In addition, the radiographic demonstration of renal artery stenosis in some normotensive patients compounds the conceptual difficulty.

The critical nature of this problem stems from the seriousness of the disease and from the considerable risk attending its surgical correction; surgical mortality as high as 10% and a 12%-15% incidence of postoperative graft closures have been reported. There is a pressing need for a better means of selecting surgical and medical therapy among patients with renal and renovascular hypertension, who account for 10%-15% of clinical hypertension. This paper will summarize some recent studies and approaches at our center, suggesting that useful diagnostic and therapeutic guidelines, together with sharper insights into the more exact mechanisms of renal hypertension, may be found by reanalysis in terms of our present understanding of the renin-angiotensin-aldosterone (RAA) system.

It is well established that the RAA axis can provide central controls over arterial blood pressure [28, 29, 31]. Briefly, as diagrammed in Fig. 1, renin, released into the bloodstream from renal juxtaglomerular cells, acts upon a liver-derived plasma substrate to produce angiotensin I, which is enzymatically

Supported by SCOR Grant HL 18323.

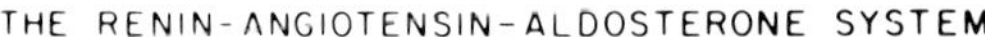

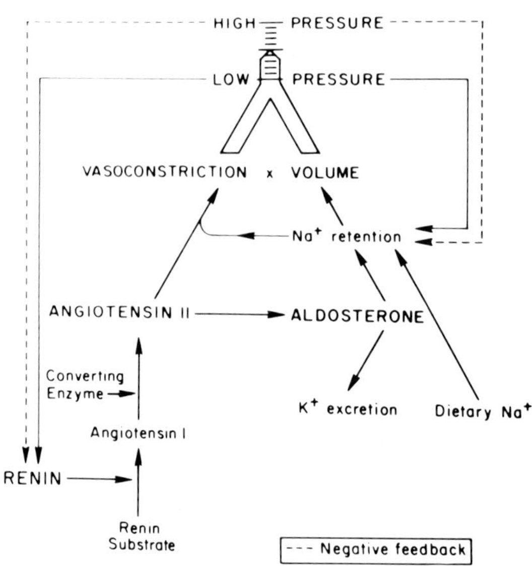

Fig. 1. Renin-angiotensin-aldosterone system and the cybernetics of sodium and volume homeostasis. The vasoconstriction-volume hypothesis for control of blood pressure. [Reprinted from Laragh JH, Letcher RL, Pickering TG: Renin profiling for diagnosis and treatment of hypertension. JAMA 241:151-156, 1979.]

converted to the active pressor agent angiotensin II. Angiotensin II raises blood pressure by virtue of its powerful vasoconstrictive effect. But beyond that, angiotensin II also stimulates adrenal cortical synthesis and secretion of aldosterone, which in turn increases renal sodium retention and accumulation of fluid, thereby raising effective blood volume and adding its influence to the increase of blood pressure. The increased sodium retention also amplifies vascular receptor response to angiotensin which serves to further enhance the pressor effect. Cyclical feedback and homeostasis is mediated directly or indirectly by the heightened blood pressure itself, which suppresses renin release, reduces sodium reabsorption, and promotes natriuresis.

It would appear logical to suspect that renal hypertension would be accompanied by derangements in the renin system and that the association might suggest parameters of diagnosis, prognosis, and therapy. A number of investigators have examined the possibility but were unable to show a consistent relationship between circulating renin levels and clinical [1-4, 15, 17, 24, 42, 43, 47] or experimental [9, 16, 21, 23, 25, 26, 35, 41] renovascular hypertension. Moreover, aldosterone secretion is invariably increased in patients with severe or malignant hypertension [30], but is often "normal" in patients with surgically curable renovascular disease.

Recently, we reinvestigated the problem, this time with results somewhat closer to the objective of finding useful surgical indicators. We reasoned that the level of arterial pressure is the outcome of the patient's vascular capacity and the volume contained within, and is the product of rather individualized forces. A vasoconstrictive force that might be normal for one patient would be inappropriate for another with different capacity and volume characteristics. It was proper, we felt, to determine the "normalcy" of the patient's renin activity levels not to standards derived from the community, but rather from the patient's individual physiologic situation. Perhaps "appropriate" is a better word than "normal" in this context.

A reasonable way of doing this, we concluded, was to relate the renin level to the daily rate of sodium excretion used as an indirect measure of vascular filling. When this was examined in 24 patients operated on for renovascular hypertension [44], we found 14 with inappropriately high peripheral plasma renin activity. Of these 14, one technical failure of surgery occurred due to closure of the graft, but all of the remainder were cured by the procedure. This suggested that renin activity, when it is high, related to a proper physiologic index, such as the rate of sodium excretion, can furnish a reliable prediction of curability. Doubtless if such an index were employed elsewhere, it would be found that many patients cured by nephrectomy and presumed by traditional standards to have had normal renin levels did indeed have a relative physiologic excess of the hormone.

However, that the physiologic renin level is not the only indicator of surgical curability and that the sodium index may incompletely reflect physiologic aspects can be seen in five of our patients who had normal renin levels, even when indexed against sodium excretion, but who were cured or improved by surgery nonetheless.

Animal Models

The search for the relationship between the renin system and renovascular hypertension took us back to animal models, in which the renovascular hypertensive process can be more precisely controlled. Two such models of experimental Goldblatt hypertension can be employed. In the two-kidney model, a renal artery is clamped but the other kidney is untouched; the animal will have increased renin in the peripheral plasma and in the clipped kidney but reduced renin in the intact kidney. In the one-kidney type, a renal artery is clamped and the other removed; this animal will have low or normal renin in the plasma and low renin content in the kidney.

When we gave an intravenous infusion of a specific peptide inhibitor of angiotensin II to both these models [8], blood pressure was promptly reduced to normal only in the two-kidney animals, demonstrating the vasoconstrictive origin of their hypertension. The one-kidney animals did not respond with any drop of blood pressure when the angiotensin-mediated vasoconstriction was blocked, suggesting that their hypertension was supported by other factors, later to be proven to be volume.

When the one-kidney animals were depleted of sodium, angiotensin blockade produced a marked drop in blood pressure. But when the same animals were sodium-repleted and studied 24 hours later, the angiotensin inhibitor again had no effect [20]. Therefore hypertension in the one-kidney animal is sustained by sodium and excess volume, and angiotensin dependency can be demonstrated only when the volume factor is eliminated. The renin-angiotensin vasoconstrictive factor in the one-kidney model, one might postulate, reflects the fact that the one-kidney animal needs hypertension to maintain glomerular filtration, which in the absence of volume support is supplied by vasoconstriction.

Figure 2 sketches the relationships. In the two-kidney model, unabated release of renin induces a systemic hypertension to which the normal kidney responds with marked secretion of sodium and water. But the one-kidney Goldblatt rat cannot react in this way because the normal kidney has been removed and the circulation in the clipped kidney is compromised. The degree to which volume increases before it can restore sufficient pressure to suppress renin secretion beyond the clamp is extreme enough to constitute a systemic hypertensive state characterized by normal renin levels and high volume.

Human Counterparts

Can the above mechanisms explain renal hypertension in man? One can propose a human counterpart of the one-kidney Goldblatt rat in the patient with one stenosed kidney and the other so compromised by occult disease that it cannot excrete sodium and water normally. As in the one-kidney rat, in order to shut off renin secretion to normal or even low levels, an expanded sodium/volume state is required. Thus when low or normal peripheral renin activity is observed in the hypertensive patient with an apparent reduction in flow to one kidney, bilateral disease should be suspected.

The same mechanism may be operative when normal or subnormal renin values occur in patients with chronic bilateral kidney disease. They may be unable to excrete sodium normally and the resulting volume-induced hypertension may suppress renin secretion. The sodium/volume basis for their hypertension is demonstrated by the evidence that vigorous hemodialysis corrects the hypertension in most such patients. In a minor fraction, a renin basis for their hypertension is indicated by an appropriately high plasma renin, and it is established by the fact that bilateral nephrectomy corrects the hypertension [5, 34, 45, 46].

The two-kidney animal model has its obvious counterpart in the patient with unilateral renovascular hypertension and one normal kidney. The normal kidney,

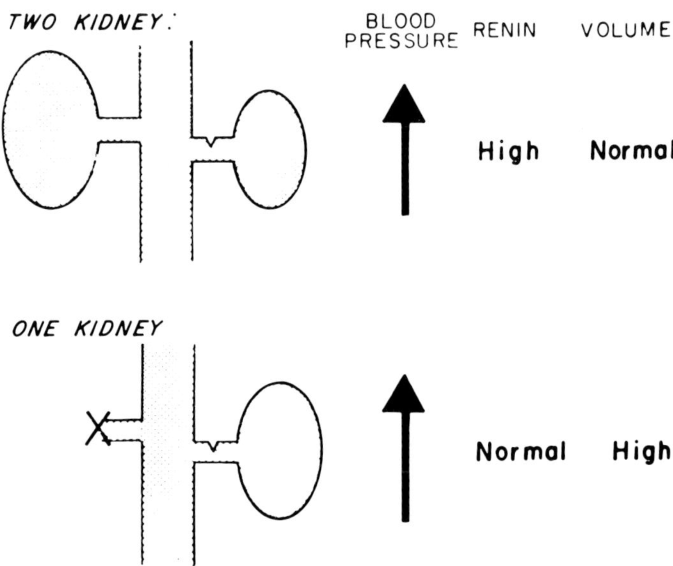

Fig. 2. Animal models of renovascular (i.e., Goldblatt) hypertension. Although comparable blood pressure elevation occurs in the Goldblatt hypertension of either the one-kidney or two-kidney type, different mechanisms are involved. Volume overexpansion is implicated in the one-kidney type, whereas renin-initiated vasoconstriction appears largely responsible for the two-kidney type. [Reprinted from Laragh JH, Sealey JE, Bühler FR, et al: The renin axis and vasoconstriction volume analysis for understanding and treating renovascular and renal hypertension. Am. J. Med. 58:4-13, 1975.]

hypersecreting sodium and water with the increased pressure, cancels volume retention as a factor in the hypertension and thereby impedes the feedback on renin secretion.

CLINICAL IMPLICATIONS

What are the clinical implications of this construction? First, when the patient with suspected renovascular hypertension has normal plasma renin levels, the possibility of bilateral disease must be entertained. In these patients, volume expansion sustains the hypertension and suppresses renin secretion. Nephrectomy is surely contraindicated, for removal of any functioning renal mass would only aggravate the problem. Renal artery reconstruction is indicated instead.

We now employ three criteria that utilize renin measurements for identifying the surgically curable patient with Goldblatt hypertension. The first of these is that the circulating plasma renin level should be high. As explained earlier, our evaluation of normalcy stems not from community values but from an individual physiologic index plotted against the patient's daily rate of sodium excretion, an imperfect index, to be sure, but one that will have to suffice until a better practical means of physiologic assessment is developed.

Peripheral renin concentration is the product of renal secretion and hepatic removal. The practical application of our first criterion bases itself on the conviction that the peripheral renin level is a true indicator of renal renin production. The conviction is armed by our study of these patients in which we demonstrated that the clearance rate of renin is a constant fraction of the peripheral level of renin in hypertensive patients, irrespective of the absolute level of renin secretion.

The second criterion narrows the picture somewhat by the requirement that the contralateral kidney be completely "normal." The critical "normal" feature is complete endocrine suppression of renin secretion. Thus this kidney responds appropriately to the perceived systemic hypertension and "turns off" renin secretion. A presumably normal but actually diseased kidney that in fact is incompletely suppressed because of occult bilateral disease adds some renin to the circulation and may well account for some of the surgical failures after nephrectomy.

Endocrine suppression of renin in the contralateral kidney can be shown by renal vein measurements. When the suppression is complete, the renal vein renin from the uninvolved kidney will be equal to that in arterial blood, while the renin in the vein of the involved kidney will be considerably higher. Renal vein concentration on the involved side minus arterial input ($V–A$) should be close to zero [27, 42, 44]. For practical purposes, the level of renin in the inferior vena cava is equal to that in the arterial system.

The relationships are illustrated in Fig. 3. In the attempt to discover how much renin two kidneys normally add to the circulation in the hypertensive state, we studied 43 patients with essential hypertension [39]. We found that their renal vein level is about 25% higher than in the periphery. From a technical standpoint, this rather small increment means that identification of complete suppression of renin secretion is never positive, but only suspected. This means that the measured values should be used only as weighted factors in the clinical analysis, without diminishing the theoretical importance of contralateral suppression.

Because of the technical difficulty in proving contralateral suppression, we sought and identified a third criterion for predicting surgical curability. This is the degree of ischemia in the suspected kidney. We have shown that this also can be quantified with relatively noninvasive renin measurements that provide an estimate of renal plasma flow [39, 44]. The rationale for this estimate is based

RENAL VEIN RENIN DIAGNOSTIC PATTERNS

ESSENTIAL HYPERTENSION

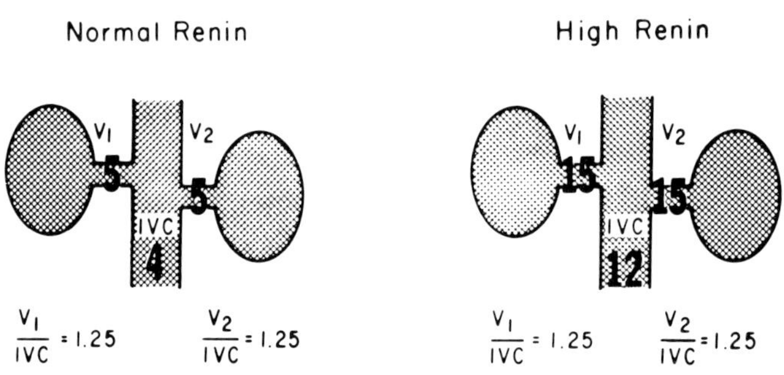

RENOVASCULAR HYPERTENSION

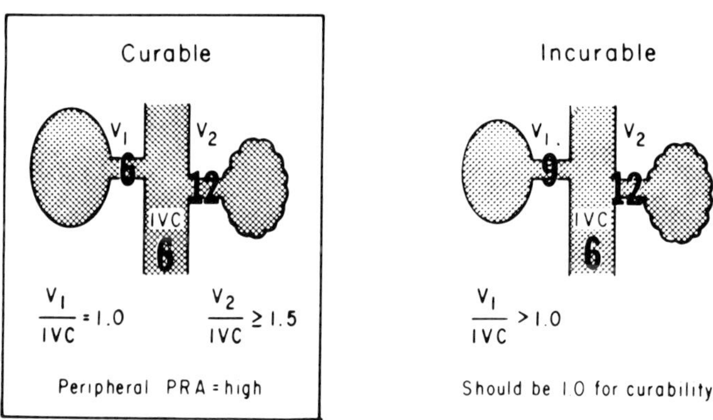

Fig. 3. Renal vein renin diagnostic patterns. Reliable diagnosis of surgically curable renovascular hypertension depends upon an understanding of the normal physiologic relationship in which the renin level in each renal vein is about 25% greater than either the peripheral arterial or the venous level (top, left). The upper right corner illustrates that this relationship persists at a higher setting in bilateral involvement. In surgically curable unilateral renovascular hypertension (bottom, left), the uninvolved kidney is under endocrine suppression and secretes no renin. Accordingly, the involved kidney is solely responsible for supporting the plasma renin level. Therefore the renal vein plasma renin from this kidney must be at least 50% higher than the peripheral renin value. In occult bilateral disease, renin is also secreted by the unsuspected kidney (bottom, right). Surgical curability is impossible in this situation and removal of the suspect kidney is contraindicated, while vascular repair promises only partial benefit. [Reprinted from Laragh JH, Sealey JE: Renin-sodium profiling: Why, how and when in clinical practice. Cardiovasc. Med. 2:1053-1075, 1977.]

on the above finding that among essential hypertensive patients with presumed normal symmetrical renal plasma flow the renal vein renin increment $(V\text{–}A)$ on each side is 25% above arterial input. Under steady-state conditions, this reflects a constant and appropriate hepatic removal rate. In the renovascular patient in whom renin secretion from the normal contralateral kidney is completely suppressed, the involved kidney must secrete renin $(V\text{–}A)$ that is 48% or greater than arterial input in order to maintain a constant arterial level. This 48% increase would be expected only if renal plasma flow were normal in the involved kidney. However, in the presence of reduced renal plasma flow in the involved kidney renin is secreted into a smaller renal venous volume, thereby raising the renal vein renin concentration. Therefore using the Fick principle the extent to which renal vein renin in the involved kidney exceeds 48% is a measure of the degree of its ischemia.

Scoring System

None of the three criteria alone can designate the surgically curable patient. The first, a high peripheral renin, is a nonspecific index of vasoconstriction and attends many conditions other than renovascular hypertension. The second criterion, a normally functioning contralateral kidney, and the third, ischemia in the involved kidney, are drawn from renal vein renin measurements, the sensitivity and precision of which are sometimes inadequate to calculate meaningful differences. In addition, blood samples may not have been collected from ideal locations under steady-state conditions [40].

However, taken together, the three criteria can provide a high order of predictability. We have evolved a scoring system which assigns certain values to each. Table 1 provides the details. A score of 5 or more suggests curable renovascular hypertension. To attain this value, two of the criteria must be positive if any one is negative. Also, if the total $(V\text{–}A)/A$ from both kidneys is less than 0.48, a value not possible under steady-state conditions, the score is canceled and the renal vein study is repeated.

CLINICAL APPLICATIONS

We have already shown that among our 23 study subjects operated on for Goldblatt hypertension, all who had high peripheral plasma renin levels (the first criterion) were cured, except for one in whom a technical failure was found. The application of the other two criteria is plotted in Fig. 4.

Among those patients cured or improved by surgery, the contralateral kidney showed little or no net secretion of renin. The fractional production of renin by the involved kidney, $(V\text{–}A)/A$, was always greater than 0.48, with one exception. The exception suggests that the measurement of $(V\text{–}A)/A$ may

Table 1
Combination Analysis of Renal Vein and Peripheral Renin by Weighted Scoring as a Discriminatory Tool to Identify Potentially Curable Patients With Renal Arterial Disease

Criterion	Score
Peripheral plasma renin activity	
Elevated	3
Normal	0
Subnormal	—3
Stenotic kidney (V-A/A)	
>0.70	4
0.48-0.69	23
<0.48	—
Contralateral kidney (V-A/A)	
<0.23	
0.24-0.38	1
>0.38	—3

Interpretation: maximum, 10 points. Indication for surgery, 5 points. Indication for repeat study, $(V_1\text{-}A)/A + (V_2\text{-}A)/A < 0.48$ when peripheral renin is elevated.

identify sampling errors, since a low value would indicate that the catheter was not in the renal vein or that a sudden change of renin secretion had occurred.

In patients who failed to improve after surgery, either contralateral renin suppression or increased $(V\text{–}A)/A$ in the suspect kidney could not be demonstrated. In three patients, $(V\text{–}A)/A$ in the suspect kidney was quite high, but renin secretion in the other kidney was not suppressed. In four patients, contralateral suppression could be shown, but not ischemia on the other side.

It should also be noted that demonstration of complete contralateral suppression of renin secretion is not by itself enough to establish normalcy of the contralateral kidney. It is important also to demonstrate a normal serum creatinine level (less than 1.2 mg%). In the presence of elevated creatinine levels, one should suspect bilateral kidney disease, and in this situation a nephrectomy removing the suspect renin secreting kidney might not be appropriate or indicated. On the other hand, such a patient might well be a candidate for an attempted repair of a compromised renal artery.

A note of caution should be added here to indicate that there are two rare clinical conditions which might yield renal vein increments up to but not exceeding 0.48 in the suspect kidney. One is the patient with a renin-secreting tumor without reduced total blood flow [32, 38]. Another might be found in patients with segmental ischemia produced by stenosis of branch renal arteries [37] insufficient to reduce total kidney flow. In both circumstances, renin secretion in the contralateral kidney would be suppressed and the suspect

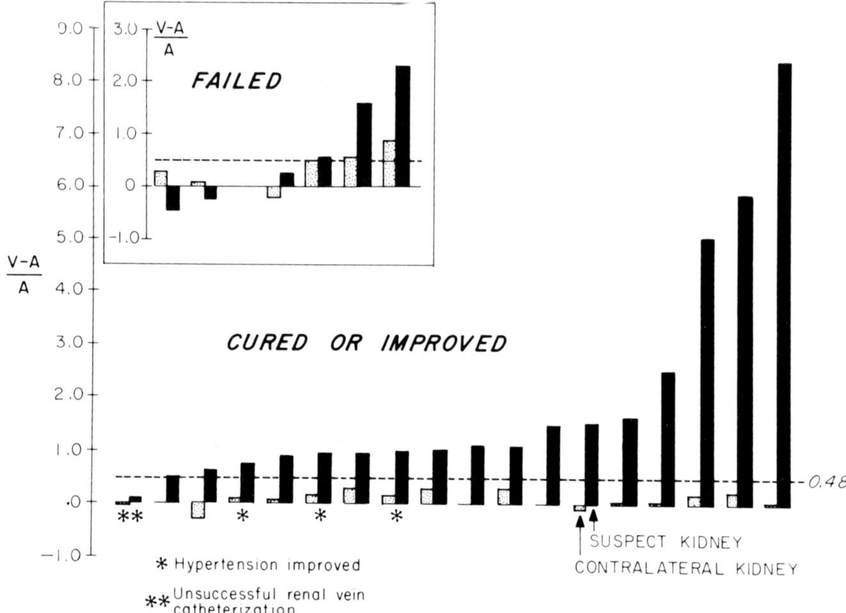

Fig. 4. Contralateral suppression and ipsilateral ischemia as indices of surgical curability. Fractional renal vein renin increment $(V–A)/A$ from the suspect (black bars) and contralateral (stippled bars) kidneys are shown for 23 patients suspected of having renovascular hypertension. All but one (a patient with a graft closure) of the patients who had $(V–A)/A$ in excess of 48% from the suspect kidney and a suppressed value from the contralateral kidney were cured. In contrast, the unsuccessful group exhibited either abnormally high $(V–A)/A$ from both kidneys or did not exhibit an elevated value from the suspect kidney. [Reprinted from Laragh JH: Indicators of renin dependency and of surgical curability in renal hypertensions, in: Proceedings of the Sixth International Congress of Nephrology, Florence, 1975. Basel, Karger, 1976, pp 334-347.]

kidney, maintaining the steady state alone, should be producing at least the sum of the levels found in both kidneys as in patients with essential hypertension.

While this new method of analysis holds great promise for improving our ability to understand and treat many forms of human renal hypertension, at this time it should be used in addition to, rather than in lieu of, accepted and basic approaches to these clinical problems.

SCREENING FOR RENOVASCULAR HYPERTENSION

We have recently reviewed our experience with 47 patients with proved renovascular hypertension who met the criteria for curability as described previously [12]. When tested on normal sodium intake, all 47 ambulatory patients with Goldblatt hypertension had plasma renin levels of 5 ng AI/ml/hour or greater measured in the upright position. This now provides a dividing line in the spectrum of renin measurements below which renovascular hypertension is unlikely. However, in the same study 20 of 64 patients with normal or high-renin essential hypertension also had plasma renin values greater than 5. Thus the renin measurement in addition to the usual and accepted clinical criteria can now be used practically to screen patients for the more definitive yet invasive tests previously described.

The Use of Drug Responses for Diagnosis

Besides renin measurements, a body of knowledge has now developed which indicates that the responses to specific pharmacological probes can provide important information about the degree of renin dependency of the hypertension in individual patients. This concept was initiated with the realization that beta-adrenergic blocking drugs such as propranolol lower blood pressure largely by blocking renin secretion and lowering plasma renin levels. Accordingly, a good therapeutic response to propranolol, when given alone, provides encouragement to the physician to proceed with a workup for renovascular disease.

This concept has gained considerable strength in the past several years with the introduction of other types of antirenin system drugs which produce responses parallel to those observed with beta-adrenergic blocking agents. The first of these new drugs, Sar-1-Ala-8-angiotensin II (saralasin), is a competitive antagonist of the hormone angiotensin II and lowers blood pressure by competing for receptor sites in the blood vessel wall. This compound identifies renin-dependent hypertension by producing depressor responses when given as a short intravenous infusion [6, 7]. However, it is now clear that saralasin grossly underestimates renin participation in blood pressure since it is a weak agonist and has pressor properties of its own which may substitute for the pressor action of angiotensin [13]. This problem with saralasin has been solved with the introduction of two newer agents which block not the action of angiotensin II but its formation by blocking the enzyme which converts angiotensin I to the active pressor hormone. The first of these was a nonapeptide (teprotide). Using this compound intravenously led to correction of part or all of the hypertension in high renin and in most normal renin patients and was without significant activity in the low renin group [14, 18]. More recently, a newer converting enzyme inhibitor called captopril has been developed; this compound is highly active orally. The experience to date with this compound completely retraces that obtained with the single intravenous injections of teprotide but has added the additional dimension of time, since with captopril it has been possible to control hypertension over the long term in direct proportion to the renin participation.

Recent studies from our center [10, 12] have demonstrated that there is another response to angiotensin blocking drugs which has as great or even greater potential in discriminating correctable renovascular hypertension. While patients are on normal sodium intake and in the seated position, renin levels rise to much higher levels in renovascular patients than in those with essential hypertension even with similar pretreatment renin values and induced reductions in pressure. Thus virtually all Goldblatt patients had depressor responses (a 9% or greater drop in diastolic pressure) and reactive hyperreninemia (to about 15 ng AI/ml/hour or greater) to saralasin and both converting enzyme inhibitors. In contrast, only a very few patients with essential hypertension had both of these responses. This "uncorking" of renin secretion by angiotensin blockers in renovascular hypertension is a simple and rather specific test which may gain a place in the routine workup of hypertensive patients when these drugs are introduced for general use.

This "uncorking" of renin may also prove to be valuable in increasing the sensitivity and specificity of a renal vein renin study. Thus we and others [36] have recently found that the antihypertensive response to captopril is accompanied by a great enhancement in the renin secretion from the involved side, whereas the renin from the contralateral kidney remains suppressed. This provocative test may prove quite useful in sorting out complicated cases and in characterizing the abnormal renin secretion which is the culprit in renovascular hypertension. Thus antirenin pharmacological probes can be used not only to demonstrate the renin dependency of the hypertension, but also to increase the precision in discriminating its unilaterality and therefore its surgical approachability.

ANGIOTENSIN BLOCKADE AS AN ALTERNATIVE TO SURGERY

With the development of an orally active converting enzyme inhibitor which specifically blocks the renin system [33], it is now possible to treat cases of Goldblatt hypertension with a degree of effectiveness never achieved by other oral agents. In addition, the drug captopril appears to have only minimal toxicity and distinct palatability [11, 19]. This pharmacologic innovation has led to the most attractive major medical alternative to surgery, since the drug is uniquely effective in renovascular hypertension, but is also effective in other underlying forms of essential hypertension. Long-term studies will be required to determine whether medical therapy with agents such as captopril will match up to the record of surgical correction.

RENAL ARTERY DILATATION AS AN ALTERNATIVE TO SURGERY

Very recently, Gruntzig and his associates have described a new technique for intravascular dilatation of arteries and arterioles using balloon catheter dilatation [22]. Their group has already described successful dilatation of stenotic renal arteries using the transvascular approach. This has led to complete correction of hypertension in a small series of patients. This new technique may prove to be especially useful when applied presurgically in selected patients, especially in high-risk patients, and it may also be valuable in patients with obvious bilateral disease with reduced renal function. In this latter group of patients where surgery is contraindicated or risky, repeated balloon dilatations theoretically offer a very attractive alternative. More work is needed on this interesting new approach, but the physician should be immediately aware of its potentialities. The long-term success and the risk of this new procedure requires more information.

REFERENCES

1. Amsterdam EA, Couch NP, Christlieb AR, et al: Renal vein renin activity in the prognosis of surgery for renovascular hypertension. Am. J. Med. 47:860, 1969
2. Bath NM, Gunnells JE, Robinson RR: Plasma renin activity in renovascular hypertension. Am. J. Med. 45:381, 1968
3. Bourgoignie J, Kurz S, Catanzaro FJ, et al: Renal venous renin in hypertension. Am. J. Med. 48:332, 1970
4. Brown JJ, Davies DL, Lever AF, et al: Variations in plasma renin concentration in several physiological and pathological states. Can. Med. Assoc. J. 90:201, 1964
5. Brown JJ, Düsterdieck G, Fraser R, et al: Hypertension and chronic renal failure. Br. Med. Bull. 27:128, 1971
6. Brunner HR, Gavras H, Laragh JH: Angiotensin II blockade in man by Sar[1]-ala[8]-angiotensin II for understanding and treatment in high blood pressure. Lancet 2:1045, 1973
7. Brunner HR, Gavras H, Laragh JH, et al: Hypertension in man, exposure of the renin and sodium components using angiotensin II blockade. Circ. Res. [Suppl] 1:35, 1974
8. Brunner HR, Kirshman JD, Sealey JE, et al: Hypertension of renal origin. Evidence for two different mechanisms. Science 174:1344, 1971
9. Carpenter CCJ, Davis JO, Ayers CR: Relation of renin, angiotensin II, and experimental renal hypertension to aldosterone secretion. J. Clin. Invest. 40:2026, 1961

10. Case DB, Atlas SA, Laragh JH: Reactive hyperreninemia to angiotensin blockade identifies renovascular hypertension. Clin. Sci. Mol. Med. (in press)
11. Case DB, Atlas SA, Laragh JH, et al: Clinical experience with blockade of the renin-angiotensin-aldosterone system by an oral converting enzyme inhibitor (SQ 14,225, Captopril) in hypertensive patients. Prog. Cardiovasc. Dis. 21:195, 1978
12. Case DB, Laragh JH: Reactive hyperreninemia in renovascular hypertension after angiotensin blockade with saralasin or converting enzyme inhibitor. Ann. Intern. Med. 91:153, 1979
13. Case DB, Wallace JM, Keim HJ, et al: Usefulness and limitations of Saralasin, a partial competitive agonist of angiotensin II, for evaluating the renin and sodium factors in hypertensive patients. Am. J. Med. 60:825, 1976
14. Case DB, Wallace JM, Keim HJ, et al: Possible role of renin in hypertension as suggested by renin-sodium profiling and inhibition of converting enzyme. N. Engl. J. Med. 296:641, 1977
15. Dustan HP, Tarazi RC, Frolich ED: Functional correlates of plasma renin activity in hypertensive patients. Circulation 41:555, 1970
16. Eyler WR, Clark MD, Garman JE, et al: Angiography of the renal areas including a comparative study of renal arterial stenoses in patients with and without hypertension. Radiology 78:879, 1962
17. Fitz A: Renal venous renin determinations in the diagnosis of surgically correctable hypertension. Circulation 36:942, 1967
18. Gavras H, Brunner HR, Laragh JH, et al: An angiotensin converting enzyme inhibitor to identify and treat vasoconstrictor and volume factors in hypertensive patients. N. Engl. J. Med. 291:817, 1974
19. Gavras H, Brunner HR, Turini GA, et al: Antihypertensive effect of the oral angiotensin converting-enzyme inhibitor SQ 14,225 in man. N. Engl. J. Med. 298:991, 1978
20. Gavras H, Brunner HR, Vaughan ED Jr, et al: Angiotensin-sodium interaction in blood pressure maintenance of renal hypertensive and normotensive rats. Science 180:1369, 1973
21. Gross F: The renin-angiotensin system in hypertension. Ann. Intern. Med. 75:777, 1971
22. Gruntzig A, Vetter W, Meier B, et al: Treatment of renovascular hypertension with percutaneous transluminal dilatation of a renal-artery stenosis. Lancet 1:801, 1978
23. Holley KE, Hung JC, Brown AL, et al: Renal artery stenosis. A clinical-pathologic study in normotensive and hypertensive patients. Am. J. Med. 37:14, 1964
24. Judson WE, Helmer OM: Diagnostic and prognostic values of renin activity in renal venous plasma in renovascular hypertension. Hypertension 13:79, 1965
25. Kaufman JJ: Results of surgical treatment of renovascular hypertension: An analysis of 70 cases followed from 1 to 6 years. J. Urol. 94:211, 1965
26. Kaufman JJ: Surgery of renal and adrenal hypertension, in Kendall, Karafin

(eds): Practice of Surgery. London, Harper & Row, 1971

27. Laragh JH: Curable renal hypertension – Renin, marker or cause? JAMA 218:733, 1971
28. Laragh JH: Vasoconstriction-volume analysis for understanding and treating hypertension. The use of renin and aldosterone profiles. Am. J. Med. 55:261, 1973
29. Laragh JH, Baer L, Brunner HR, et al: Renin, angiotensin and aldosterone system in pathogenesis management of hypertensive vascular disease. Am. J. Med. 52:643, 1972
30. Laragh JH, Sealey JE, Sommers SC: Patterns of adrenal secretion and urinary excretion of aldosterone and plasma renin activity in normal and hypertension subjects. Circ. Res. 18/19 [Suppl 1]:158, 1966
31. Laragh JH, Sealey JE: The renin-angiotensin-aldosterone hormonal system and regulation of sodium, potassium and blood pressure homeostasis, in Orloff J, Berliner RW (eds): Handbook of Physiology, Baltimore, Waverly Press, 1973, p 831
32. Lee MR: Renin-secreting kidney tumours. A rare but remedial cause of serious hypertension. Lancet 2:254, 1971
33. Ondetti MA, Rubin B, Cushman DW: Design of specific inhibitors of angiotensin converting enzyme. New class of orally active and antihypertensive agents. Science 196:441, 1977
34. Onesti G, Swartz C, Ramirex O, et al: Bilateral nephrectomy for control of hypertension in uremia. Trans. Am. Soc. Artif. Intern. Organs 14:361, 1968
35. Page IH, McCubbin JW: Renal Hypertension. Chicago, Year Book Medical, 1968
36. Re R, Novelline R, Escourrou M-T, et al: Inhibition of angiotensin-converting enzyme for diagnosis of renal artery stenosis. N. Engl. J. Med. 298:582, 1978
37. Schambelan M, Glickman M, Stockigt JR, et al: Selective renal-vein renin sampling for segmental renal lesions. N. Engl. J. Med. 290:1153, 1974
38. Schambelan M, Howes EL, Stockigt JR, et al: Role of renin and aldosterone in hypertension due to a renin-secreting tumor Am. J. Med. 55:86, 1973
39. Sealey JE, Bühler FR, Laragh JH, et al: The physiology of renin secretion in essential hypertension: Estimation of renin secretion rate and renal plasma flow from peripheral and renal vein renin levels. Am. J. Med. 55:391, 1973
40. Sealey JE, Gerten-Banes J, Laragh JH: The renin system: Variations in man measured by radioimmunoassay or bioassay. Kidney Int. 1:240, 1972
41. Simon N, Franklin SS, Bliefer KH, et al: Clinical characteristics of renovascular hypertension. JAMA 220:1209, 1972
42. Stockigt JE, Noakes CA, Collins RD, et al: Renal-vein renin in various forms of renal hypertension. Lancet 1:1194, 1972
43. Strong CS, Hunt JC, Sheps SG, et al: Renal venous renin activity; Enhancement of sensitivity of lateralization by sodium depletion. Am. J. Cardiol. 27:602, 1971

44. Vaughan ED Jr, Bühler FR, Laragh JH, et al: Renovascular hypertension. Renin measurements to indicate hypersecretion and contralateral suppression, estimate renal plasma flow, and score for surgical curability. Am. J. Med. 55:402, 1973
45. Vertes V, Cangiano JL, Berman LB, et al: Hypertension in end-stage renal disease. N. Engl. J. Med. 280:978, 1973
46. Weidman P, Maxwell MH, Lupu AN, et al: Plasma renin activity and blood pressure in terminal renal failure. N. Engl. J. Med. 285:757, 1971
47. Winer R, Lubbe WF, Simon M, et al: Renin in the diagnosis of renovascular hypertension. JAMA 202:139, 1967

James C. Stanley, M.D.

Morphologic, Histopathologic, and Clinical Characteristics of Renovascular Fibrodysplasia and Arteriosclerosis

Clinically important renal artery occlusive lesions are relatively uncommon. Although the exact incidence of renovascular stenotic disease remains unknown, it is the most common cause of surgically correctable hypertension. Mural pathology of the renal artery encompasses a number of distinct entities, including fibrodysplastic and arteriosclerotic stenoses, dissections, arteriovenous fistulae and malformations, as well as aneurysms. Arterial fibrodysplasia and arteriosclerosis are the most prevalent of these diseases. Specific comments concerning these lesions must be individualized because of marked differences in their biologic character and clinical importance.

ARTERIAL FIBRODYSPLASIA

Dysplastic renovascular disease probably affects less than 1% of the general populace. However, it may be the most common cause of remedial renovascular hypertension. Dysplastic renal artery lesions represent a heterogeneous group of stenoses categorized according to the principal level of vessel involvement [13]. Included are (1) intimal fibroplasia, (2) medial hyperplasia, (3) medial fibroplasia, and (4) perimedial dysplasia. The first two are considered distinctly different pathologic processes, whereas the last two are believed to represent a continuum of disease. Certain clinical, morphologic, and histologic features are characteristic of each dysplastic category.

Intimal fibroplasia affects both sexes equally, and accounts for slightly more than 5% of dysplastic renal artery stenoses. In general, this lesion affects infants and young adults more often than older individuals. Arteriographically, intimal fibroplasia most often involves main arteries as long tubular stenoses in young patients, and as smooth focal stenoses in the older age group (Fig. 1). Less common manifestations of intimal fibroplasia are proximal ostial lesions associated with neurofibromatosis as well as aortic hypoplasia (Fig. 2). Marked intimal

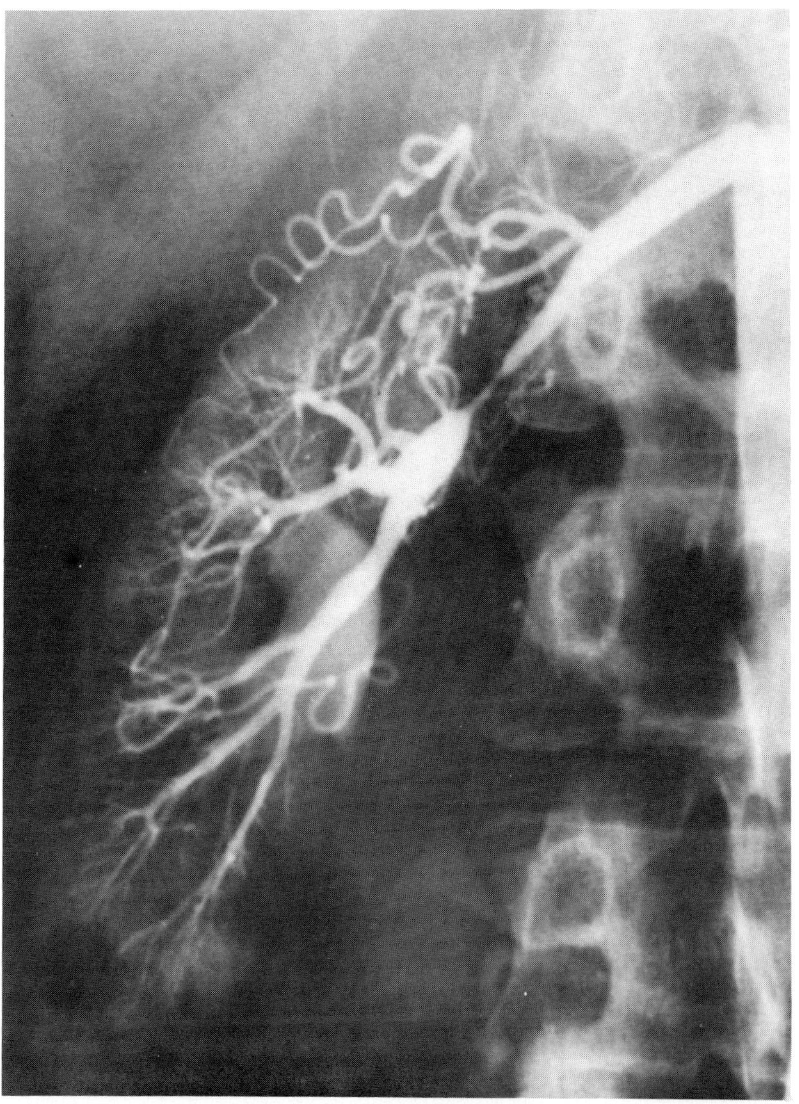

Fig. 1. Intimal fibroplasia producing a midrenal artery focal stenosis.

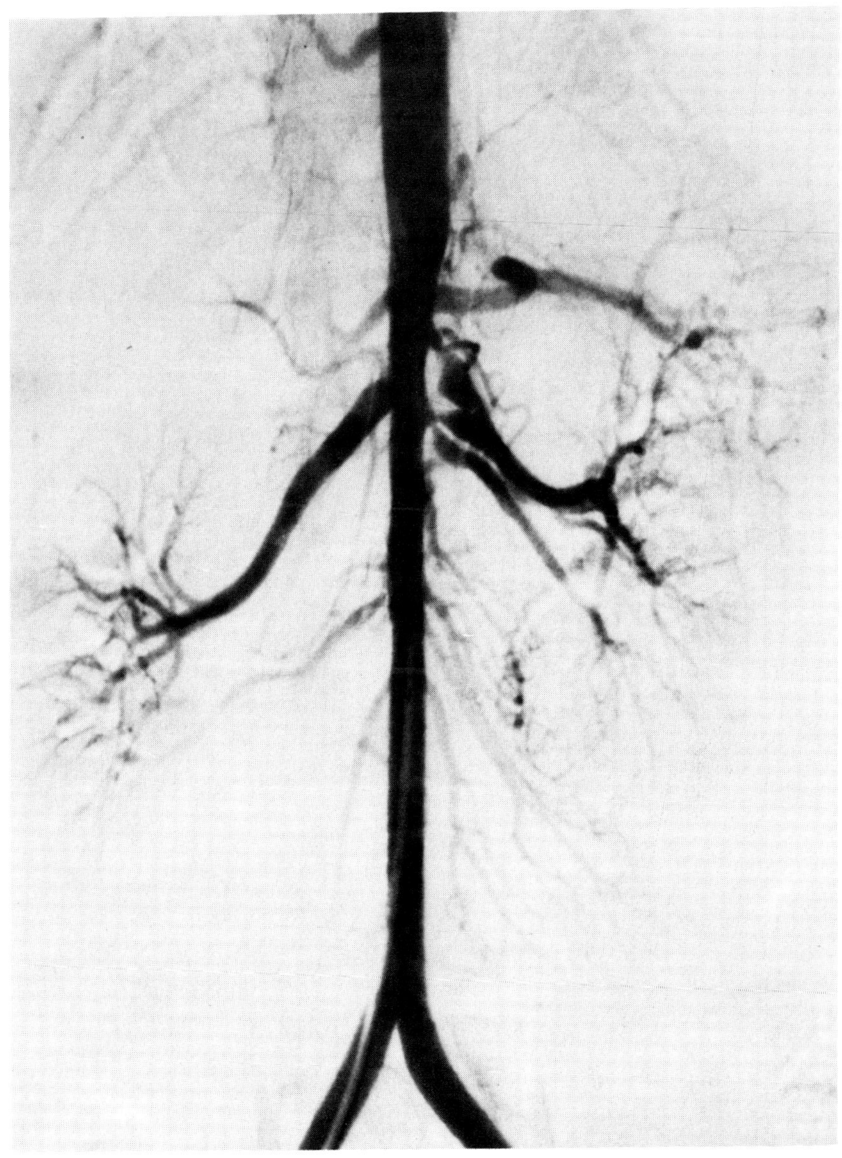

Fig. 2. Intimal fibroplasia of proximal renal arteries in patient with neurofibromatosis and hypoplastic aorta.

thickening has been a constant finding in neurofibromatosis, although medial abnormalities, perhaps representing a developmental defect, are also seen.

This form of dysplasia results from an accumulation of irregularly arranged subendothelial mesenchymal cells within a loose matrix of fibrous connective tissue (Fig. 3). The internal elastic lamina is frequently fragmented, but always identifiable. Medial and adventitial structures are usually normal. Intimal fibroproliferation may appear eccentric and, as such, is similar to musculoelastic cushions seen throughout arteries of neonates and intimal cushions affecting cerebral artery bifurcations in adults. Lipid-containing foam cells and inflammatory cells are not seen within these lesions.

The cause of primary intimal fibroplasia remains an enigma. Secondary intimal fibroplasia is a common result of arterial injury, including external trauma as well as intraluminal insults. Tubular stenoses of infancy may reflect an arteritis. Rubella has been implicated in such instances [14]. Focal lesions encountered in adulthood may represent persistent embryonic intimal cushions [17]. Regardless of the etiology, once intimal fibroplasia has significantly encroached upon the vessel lumen, progression appears likely as a consequence of local blood flow alterations.

Medial hyperplasia, represented by an excess in medial smooth muscle, without demonstrable fibrotic changes, is a rare cause of renal arterial stenosis. This lesion accounts for less than 1% of dysplastic renal artery disease and is usually encountered in females in the fourth and fifth decade of life. Focal stenoses caused by medial hyperplasia are difficult to differentiate roentgenographically from intimal fibroplasia. Increases in smooth muscle cells exhibiting minimal disorganization, without abnormal ground substances, characterize medial hyperplasia (Fig. 4). Intimal and adventitial structures are usually normal.

Medial hyperplasia, like intimal disease, is not associated with an easily identifiable cause. Isolated hyperplasia of smooth muscle within the circulatory system is a very unusual phenomenon. The very existence of this particular dysplastic lesion is subject to question. The unusually high frequencies of medial hyperplasia alluded to in earlier reports [1, 6] included diseased vessels currently classified as medial fibroplasia.

Medial fibroplasia is the most common dysplastic renovascular disease, accounting for nearly 85% of these renal artery lesions. Ninety percent of patients with medial fibroplasia are female. The usual age at time of recognition is during the fourth decade. This entity is also encountered in the extracranial internal carotid, superior mesenteric, common hepatic, and external iliac vessels. Medial fibroplasia provides a spectrum of morphologic and histologic findings [13]. Its appearance varies from a focal stenosis to series of stenoses with intervening aneurysmal outpouchings (Fig. 5). Medial fibroplasia usually affects the distal part of the main renal artery, extending to segmental branches in approximately 25% of cases.

Two histologic extremes occur as part of this dysplastic lesion. Fibrodysplasia is grossly limited to the outer media of some specimens (peripheral form),

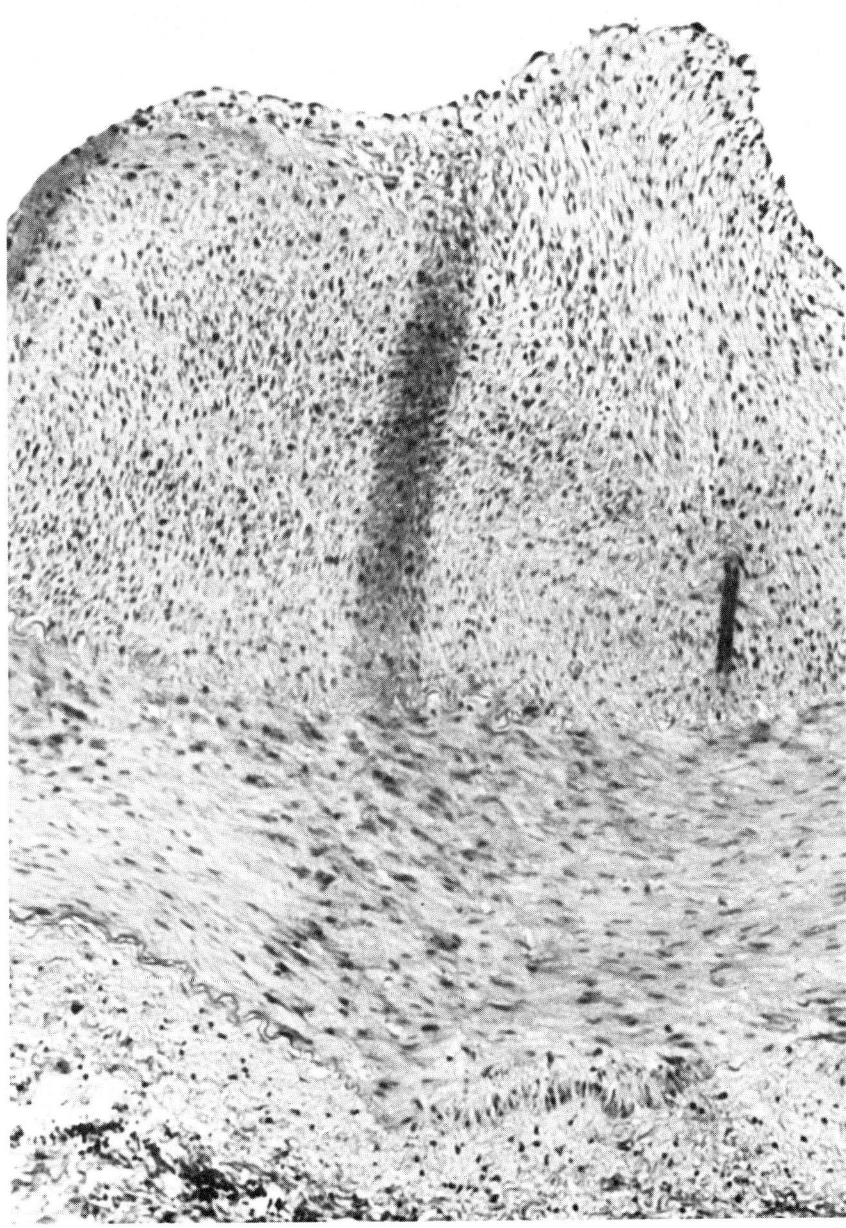

Fig. 3. Intimal fibroplasia manifested by irregularly arranged subendothelial mesenchymal cells. Medial and adventitial structures are normal. × 80. Hematoxylin and eosin.

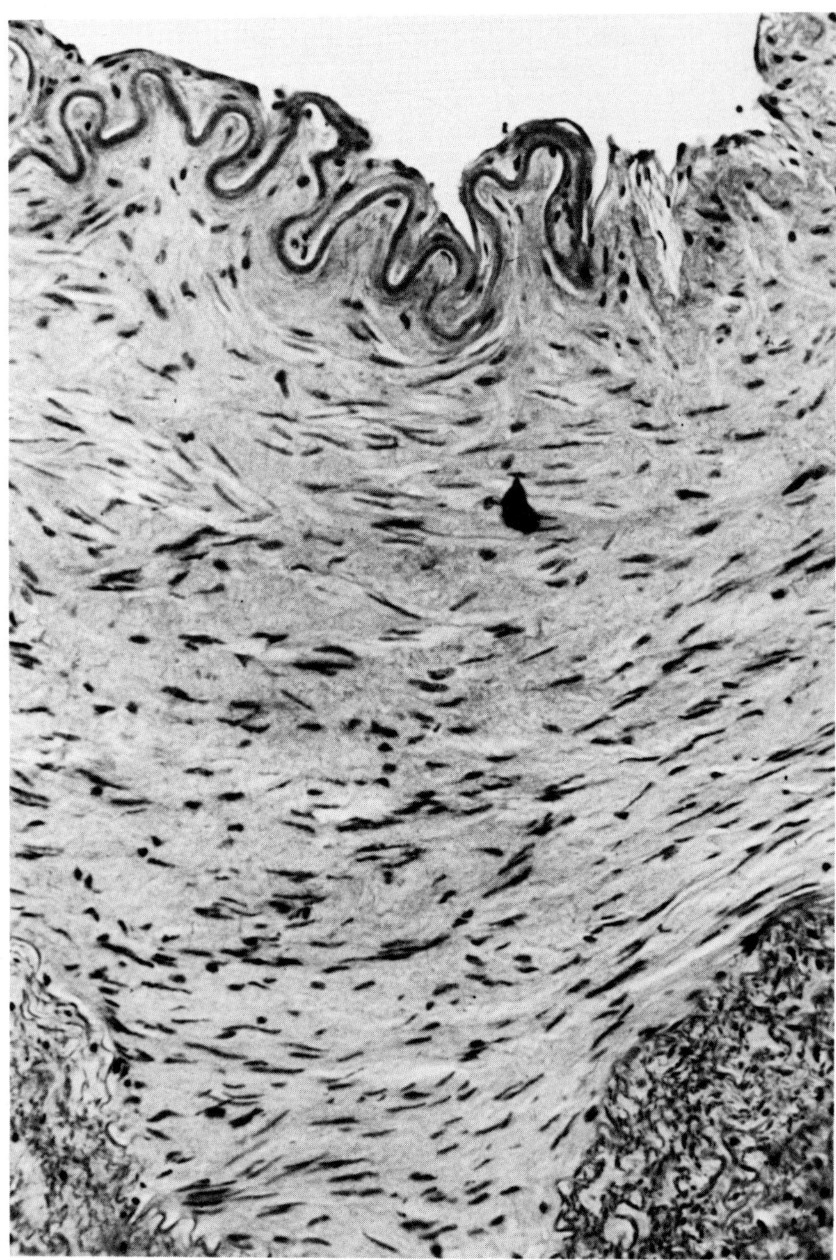

Fig. 4. Medial hyperplasia exhibiting increased numbers of smooth muscle cells with minimal derangement of their orientation. × 120. H & E.

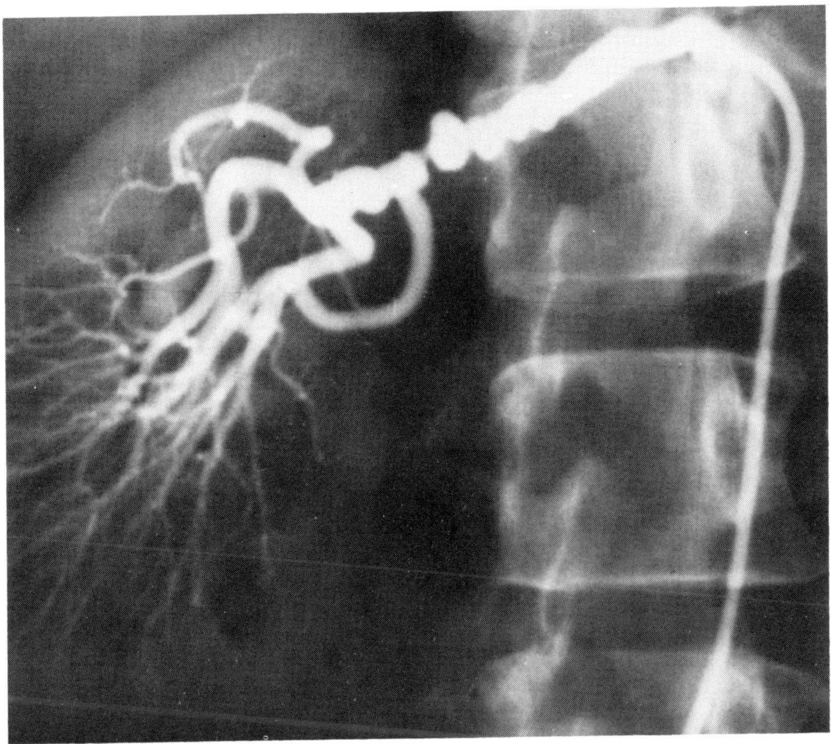

Fig. 5. Medial fibroplasia with a series of constricting lesions and intervening aneurysmal outpouchings of distal renal artery extending beyond segmental branching.

whereas in others the entire media is diseased (diffuse form). Gradations between these two types may be encountered in the same vessel.

The most prominent histologic feature of peripheral medial fibroplasia is compact fibrous connective tissue replacing smooth muscle peripherally (Fig. 6). The inner media exhibits moderate accumulations of collagen and ground substance separating minimally disorganized smooth muscle cells. Intimal tissue and the internal elastic lamina are usually unaffected, although continuity of the external elastic lamina was frequently lost. Prior reports have classified some of these lesions as subadventitial in location [5].

Diffuse medial fibrodysplasia is characterized by more severe medial disruption with replacement of smooth muscle by haphazard arrangements of myofibroblasts and collagen (Fig. 7). Medial thinning, alternating with dysplastic accumulations of fibrous tissue, accounts for the mural dilations and microaneurysms accompanying medial fibroplasia (Fig. 8). Internal elastic lamina fragmentation and subendothelial fibrosis are common in advanced lesions but are considered secondary events.

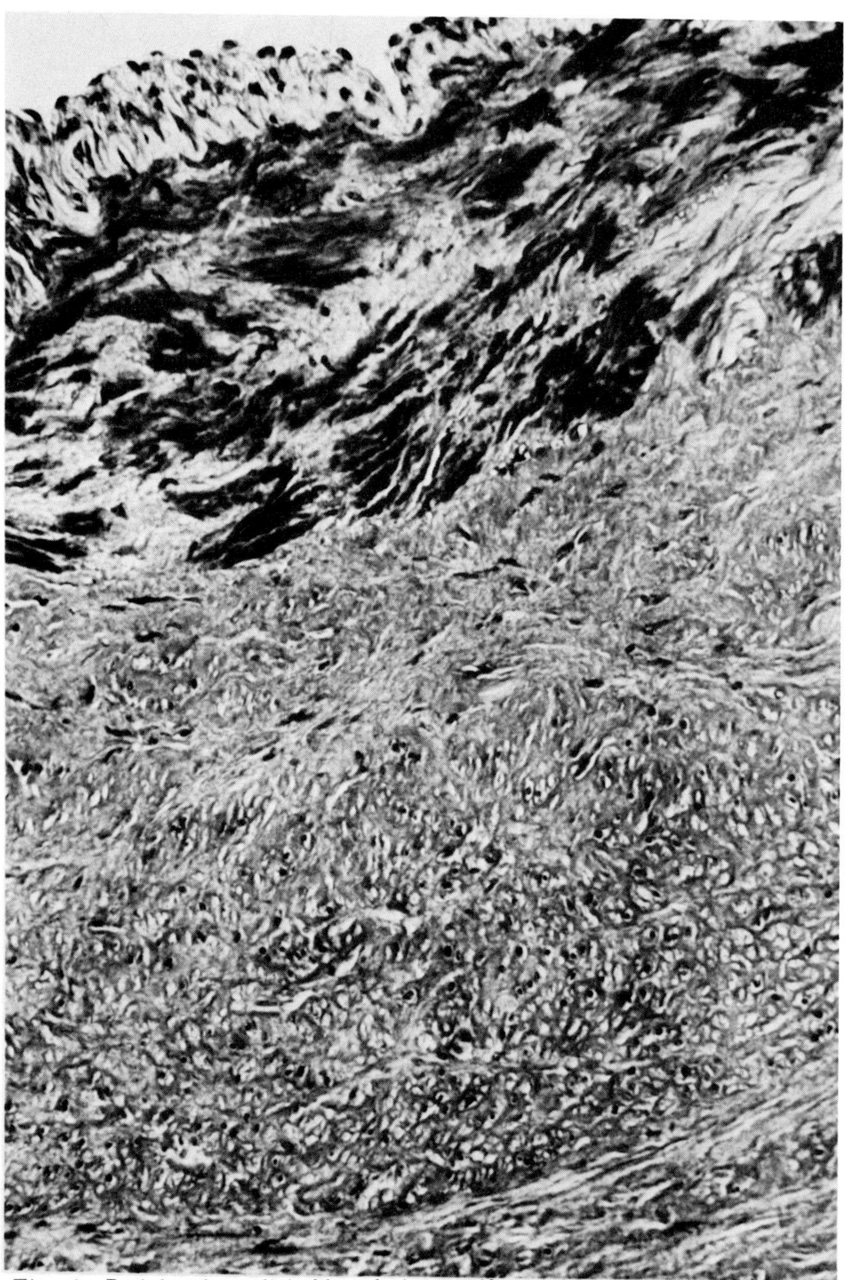

Fig. 6. Peripheral medial fibroplasia manifested by dense fibroproliferative process and loss of recognizable smooth muscle in outer media. Intimal structures are normal. × 120. Masson stain.

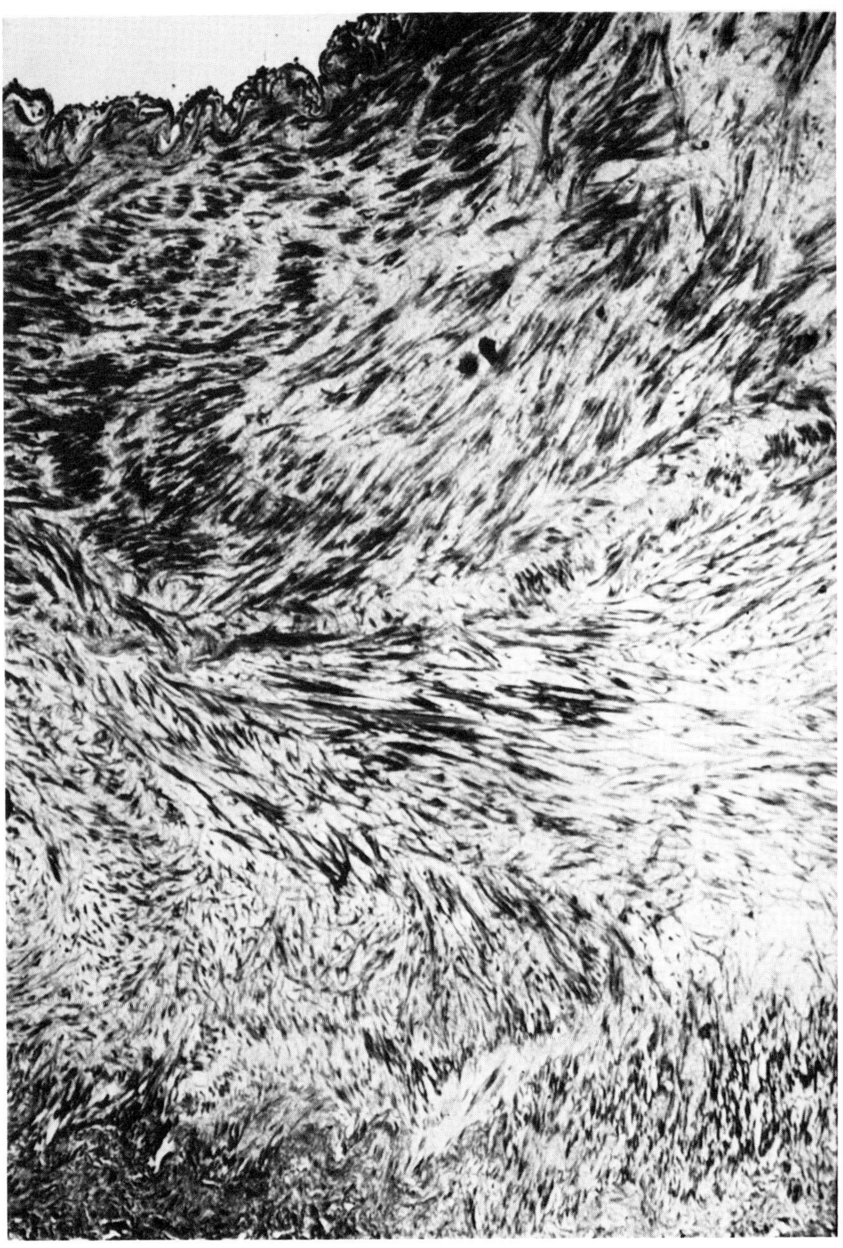

Fig. 7. Diffuse medial fibroplasia with extensive medial fibroproliferation and loss of normal smooth muscle throughout media. × 120. Masson stain.

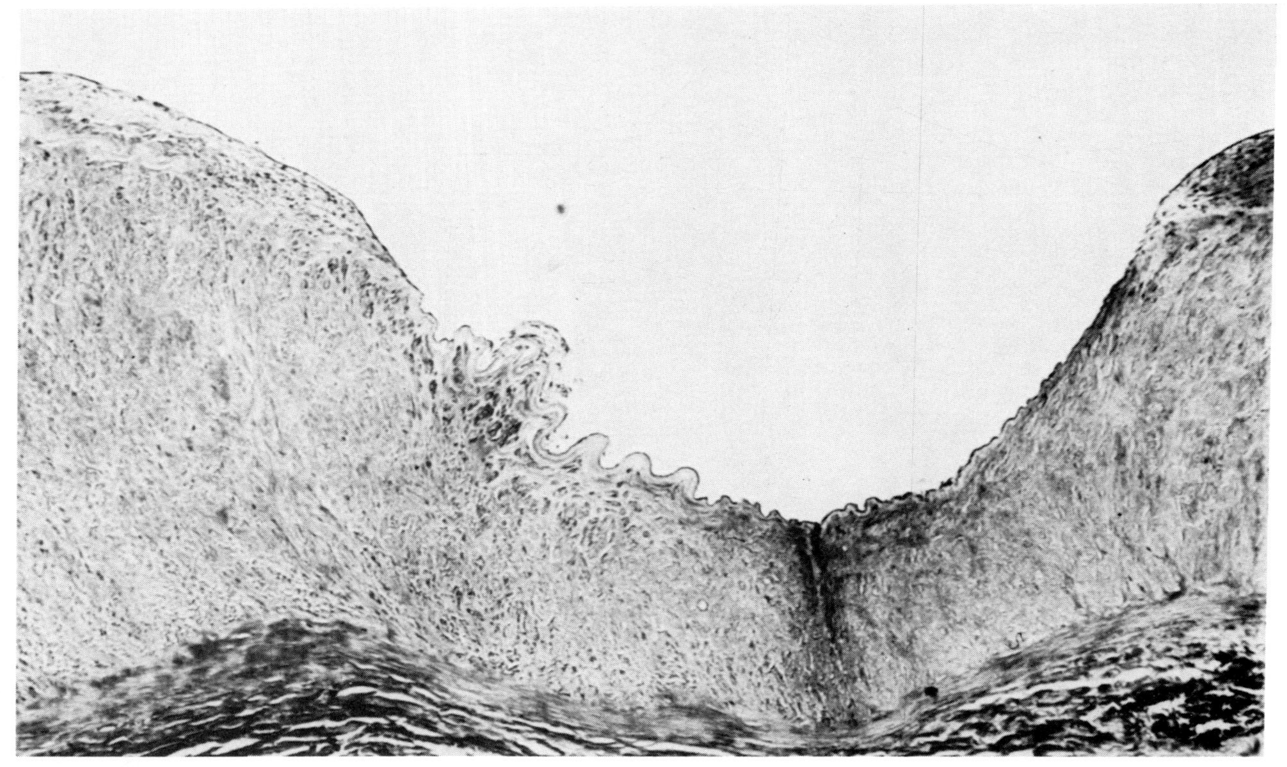

Fig. 8. Diffuse medial fibroplasia (longitudinal section) exhibiting medial thinning adjacent to regions of excessive fibroplasia accounting for mural aneurysms and stenoses, respectively. × 40. Masson stain.

The unusual predilection for females raises certain questions, including (1) possible effects of pregnancy on evolution of this disease, (2) the role of antiovulant medications in dysplastic processes, and (3) the obvious consideration that normal hormonal (progestin-estrogen) substances may contribute to the genesis of fibrodysplastic disease. Pregnancy may be responsible for rather profound vascular wall alterations involving medial structures and elastic tissue in particular. Although gestational changes may affect vessels that manifest fibrodysplastic disease, the reproductive histories of patients in a previous report did not reveal gravity or parity rates different from the general population [13]. Likewise, antiovulants may produce arterial wall alterations, yet use of these drugs by less than half of the former study's adult female patients does not support any obvious cause and effect association to fibrodysplasia. Certain smooth muscle cells and fibroblasts respond to various stimuli, including estrogen with an increased synthesis of proteinaceous substances, including collagen [8, 9]. Physiologic preconditioning of medial smooth muscle to a secretory state by agents such as estrogens may account for the more frequent occurrence of dysplastic lesions in females. Progression of this lesion has been verified in 12% of cases, and probably occurs more often [13]. Premenopausal patients are most likely to demonstrate these changes.

Unusual stretch forces are associated with most arteries exhibiting fibrodysplastic changes. Renal artery traction due to ptotic kidneys (the right greater than the left), and internal carotid artery stretching over the upper cervical vertebrae with neck hyperextension, may represent important factors in development of these lesions. Renal ptosis is common among patients with renovascular dysplasia. Larger degrees of ptosis of the right kidney may explain the greater severity of right-sided disease in the majority of adults having bilateral lesions and the fact that nearly 80% of unilateral lesions affect the right renal artery.

Stretch-traction stresses may predispose to fibroplasia by directly altering vessel wall tissues. Repeated stretching of smooth muscle cells in culture has been shown to cause increased synthesis of collagen and certain acid mucopolysaccharides [4]. Although the exact mechanisms are unknown, the predilection for dysplastic lesions to occur in vessels where peculiar mechanical forces exist cannot easily be discounted.

Vasa vasorum of muscular arteries usually arise from branchings of the parent vessel [3]. Renal, extracranial internal carotid, and external iliac arteries have relatively few branches compared to other vessels of similar caliber. This fact raises the possibility of insufficient vessel wall nourishment as a cause of fibrodysplasia. Such a concept is supported by observation of dysplasia limited to the outer media. Ischemia predictably would be greatest in this area if vasa vasorum blood flow were to be inadequate [15]. Fibrodysplasia limited to the inner part of the media has not been encountered. Experimental studies lend credence to the theory that mural ischemia might play a role in the evolution of renal artery fibrodysplasia [7, 11].

Perimedial dysplasia accounts for approximately 10% of dysplastic renal arteries. Almost all patients with this lesion have been female, usually in their fourth and fifth decades. Arteriographic manifestations include focal stenoses and, occasionally, multiple constrictions without mural aneurysms involving the midportion of the renal artery (Fig. 9). Excessive elastic tissue at the junction of the media and adventitia is a dominant feature of this lesion. Special stains document the circumferential aggregations of elastic tissue along the outer medial border (Fig. 10). Intimal elastic lamina and elastic fibrils within the media are usually normal. Noticeable increases in medial ground substance

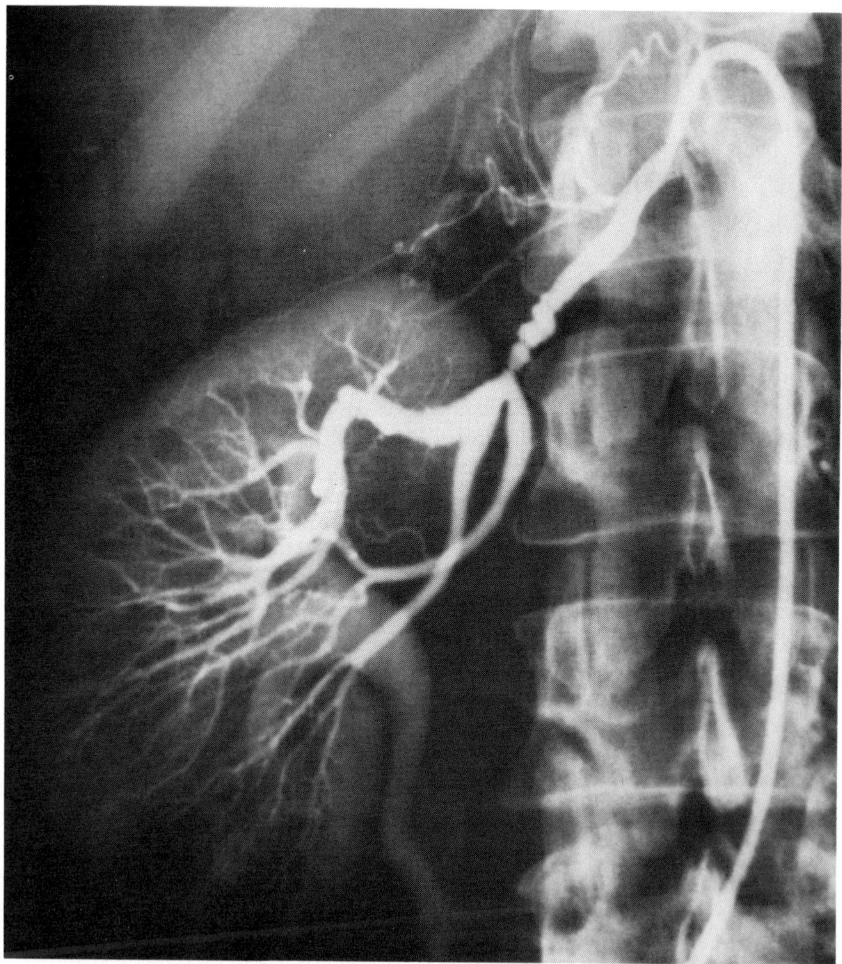

Fig. 9. Perimedial dysplasia exhibiting multiple stenoses in series *without* intervening mural dilations.

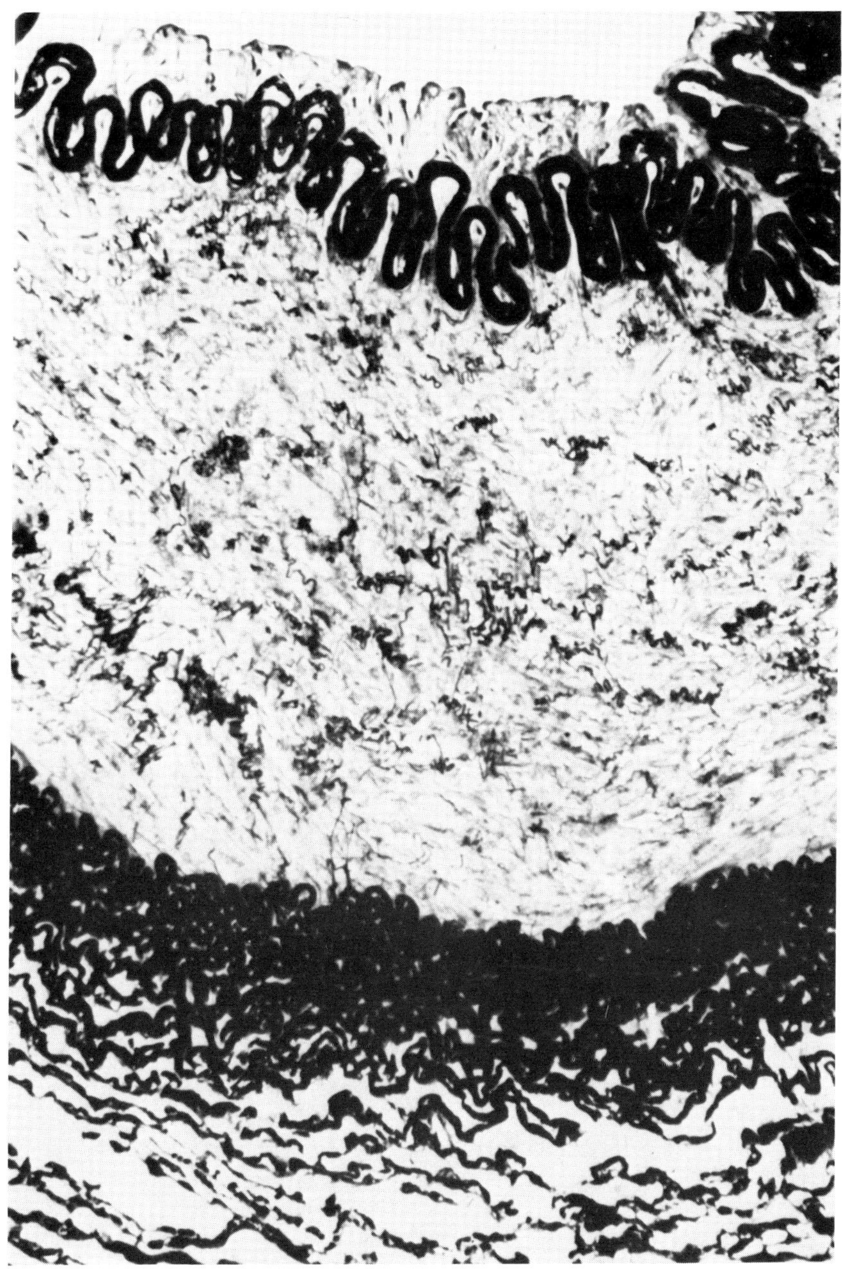

Fig. 10. Perimedial dysplasia manifested by excessive elastic tissue adjacent to outer media. × 120. Verhoeff stain.

surrounding intact smooth muscle cells, with little alteration of normal intimal structures, characterize the remainder of the vessel wall (Fig. 11).

Evidence to date, including the occurrence of these lesions in the midrenal artery rather than distally, supports segregation of perimedial dysplasia to a distinct pathologic group dissimilar to other fibrodysplastic processes. Mechanisms responsible for this elastic tissue must be unique to this form of dysplasia. Effects of physical stresses on arterial wall connective tissue, causing elastic tissue fragmentation and excessive replication with repair, are perhaps most important in the pathogenesis of perimedial dysplasia.

Certain ultrastructural features are common to medial fibroplasia and perimedial dysplasia [12]. Both are characterized by accumulations of homogenous ground substances and fibrous elements and by a spectrum of changes in medial smooth muscle cells ranging from near-normal to myofibroblasts.

Earliest recognizable modifications of smooth muscle ultrastructure are confined to subcellular organelles and myofilaments. These cells, usually the most distant from the dysplastic process, exhibit focal myofilament reductions as well as particular sublemmal and cytoplasmic vacuolations. In distinct contrast to minimally affected smooth muscle have been noticeable derangements occurring in areas of advanced dysplasia. Certain smooth muscle cells are transformed to fibroblastlike cells, whereas others exhibit extreme cell deterioration (Fig. 12). The latter are invariably isolated from surrounding cells by excessive amounts of ground substances. Long slender cytoplasmic processes with obvious reductions in the cytoplasmic to nuclear volume are common. The nucleus, often appearing pyknotic, contains dense chromatin material. Cell membranes are often indistinct, confluences of micropinocytotic vesicles are frequently observed, and subcellular organelles are sparse.

Modification of smooth muscle cells to fibroblastlike cells presents a continuum within the dysplastic media. Alterations in nuclear contour, loss of myofilaments, and increasing subcellular organelles including free ribosomes, rough endoplasmic reticulum, Golgi complexes, and mitochondria seemingly parallel altered function from one of contractility to one of secretion. More complete transformations result in myofibroblasts (Fig. 13). These cells have a convoluted nucleus with numerous indentations and evaginations. Major increases of subcellular organelles in a juxtanuclear location and peripheral cytoplasmic filaments characterize myofibroblasts. Myofilaments are scant and ill-defined. Active deposition of proteinaceous matter by exopinocytosis has been observed in these cells. Although myofibroblasts have obvious features depicting their fibroblastlike function, cells typical of fibroblasts do not normally exist within the media.

Vasa vasorum in the media of diseased arteries are usually widely separated from adjacent cellular elements by either collagen fibrous tissue, homogeneous mucoid substances, or both. The type of surrounding connective tissue is related to the category of arterial dysplasia. Vasa vasorum within medial fibroplasia are

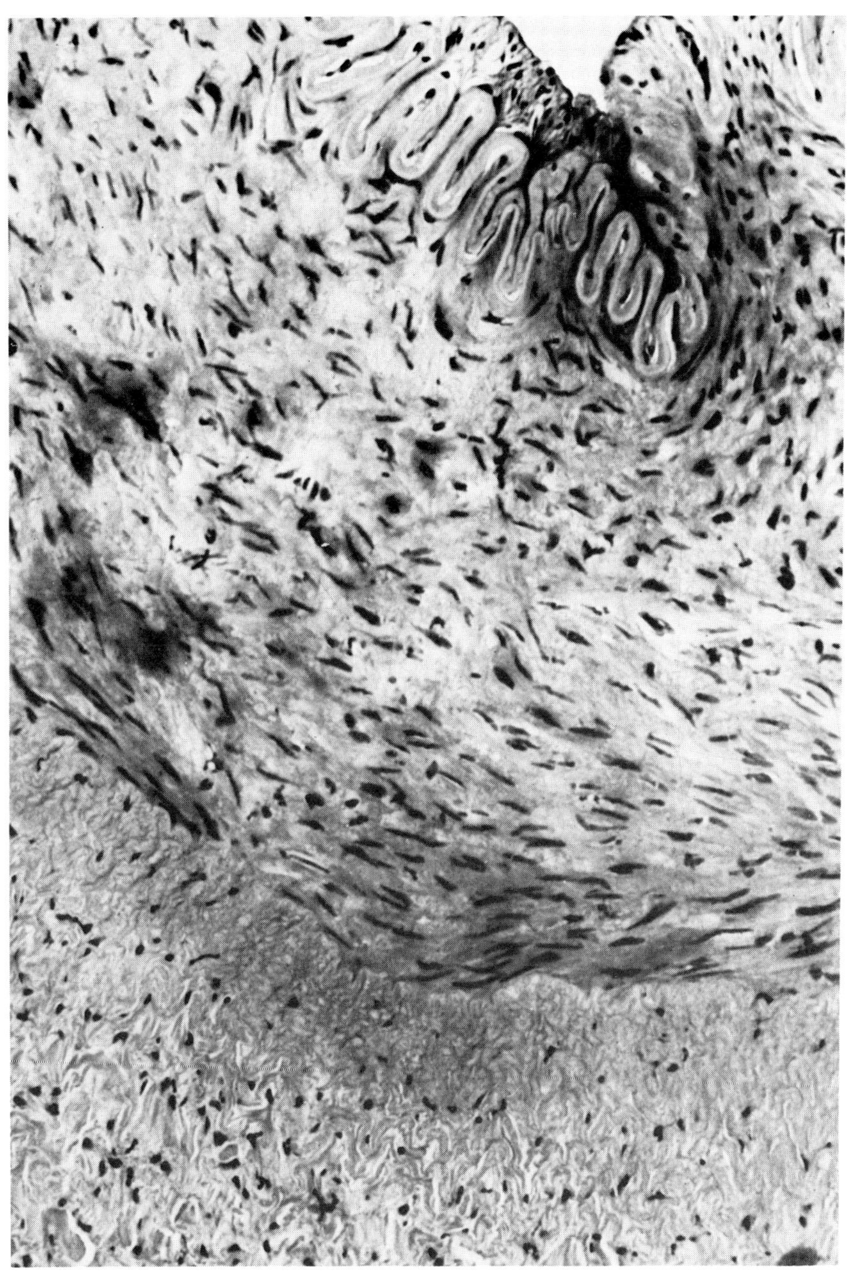

Fig. 11. Perimedial dysplasia exhibiting relatively homogeneous collar of elastic tissue at junction of media and adventitia. Abnormal medial smooth muscle surrounded by increased amounts of ground substance is evident. × 120. H & E.

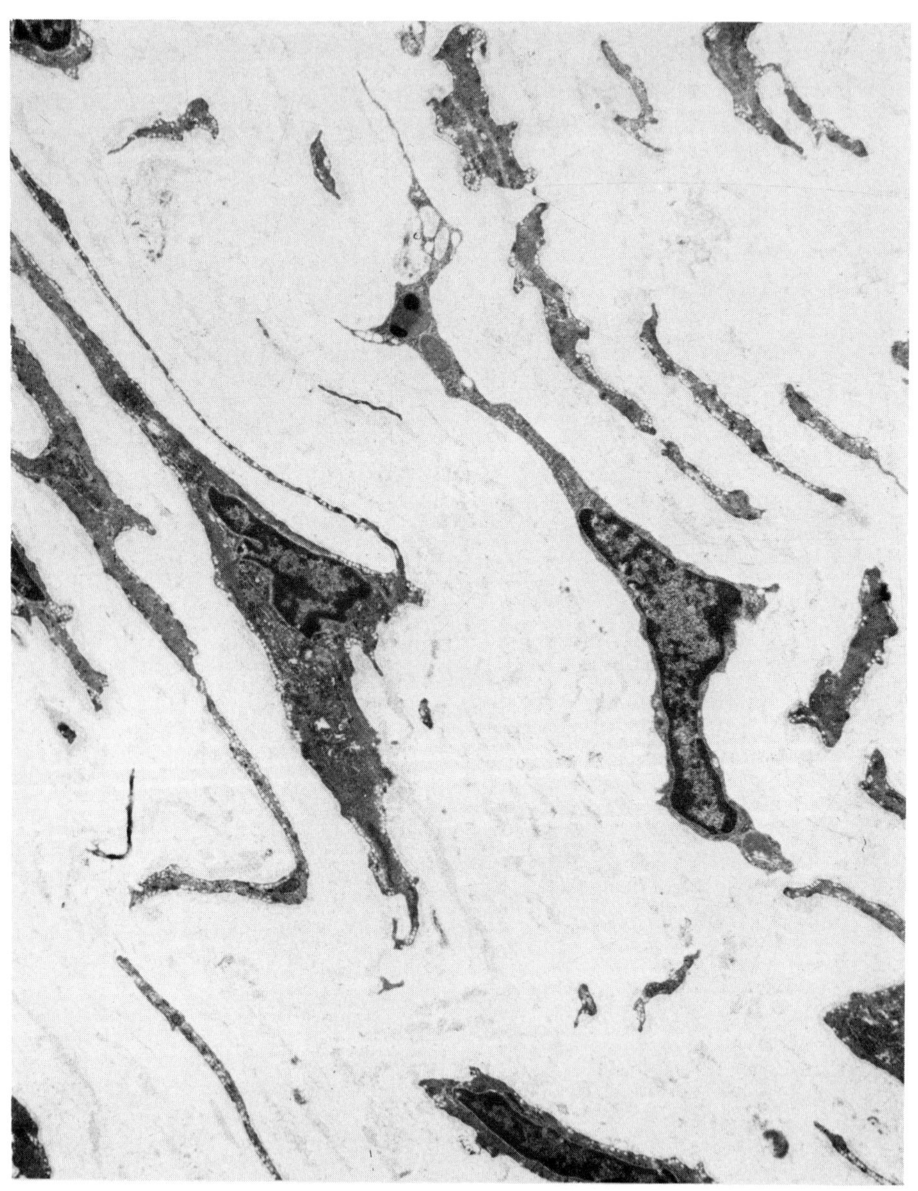

surrounded predominantly by collagen fibrous bundles, whereas those in perimedial dysplasia are more often surrounded by amorphous mucoid substances. The most striking observation regarding vasa vasorum is their constant intramedial isolation. Reduction in numbers of vasa vasorum, or their insufficient medial distribution, has yet to be demonstrated in human arterial dysplasia.

ARTERIOSCLEROSIS

Arteriosclerotic renovascular disease is a relatively common entity. Males are affected with arteriosclerotic stenoses twice as often as females, a finding consistent with observations of arteriosclerosis affecting the remainder of the arterial circulation. Sex differences tend to be less apparent in elderly individuals. The prevalence of renovascular arteriosclerosis is age-dependent [10]. Risk factors including hyperlipoproteinemic disorders, diabetes mellitus, smoking, and hypertension occur with the same frequency in patients having renal artery arteriosclerosis as extrarenal arteriosclerotic disease. In an earlier necropsy study, moderate or severe disease was documented in 49% of normotensive cases and 77% of hypertensive individuals [2]. Despite the high frequency of renovascular arteriosclerosis in the general population, arterial fibrodysplasia may be a more common cause of secondary hypertension.

Renovascular arteriosclerosis usually affects the aortic orifice or proximal portion of the main renal artery. Eccentric or concentric focal stenoses result in typical arteriographic appearances of this lesion in approximately 80% of patients (Fig. 14). Early plaques most often originate on the inferior and posterior aspects of the vessel, extending occasionally along the posterior vessel wall into segmental branches. Arteriosclerotic lesions isolated to segments of the distal renal artery are observed in less than 5% of patients. Slightly more than 50% of patients presenting with hemodynamically important stenoses exhibit bilateral lesions. Right- and left-sided stenotic disease in the remaining patients exist with equal frequencies.

Subendothelial and medial accumulation of cholesterol-laden cells, accumulation of fibrous tissue, and loss of smooth muscle typify arteriosclerosis; evidence of plaque necrosis, hemorrhage, and calcification are encountered in most stenoses responsible for secondary hypertension (Fig. 15). Clinically overt arteriosclerosis of the aorta and its major branches is apparent in approximately 85% of patients having advanced renal artery arteriosclerotic occlusive disease. The remaining patients, without evidence of distinct arteriosclerotic cardio-

---

Fig. 12. Medial smooth muscle in area of medial fibroplasia exhibiting pyknotic-appearing nuclei, decreased cytoplasmic volume with dense myofilaments, and isolation by abnormal amounts of ground substance. Transmission electron microscopy × 5400.

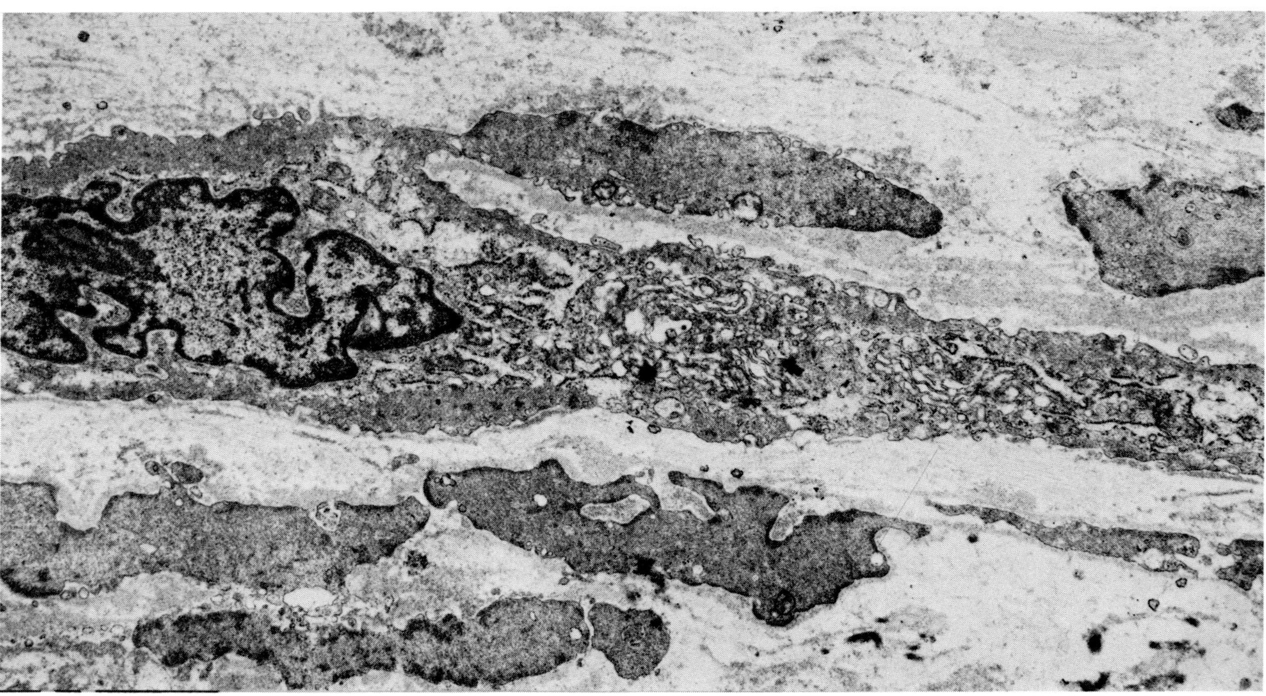

Fig. 13. Myofibroblast in area of fibrodysplasia. Nuclear contour is similar to convoluted smooth muscle cell nucleus. Central organelles are representative of active secretory state. Transmission electron microscopy × 8000.

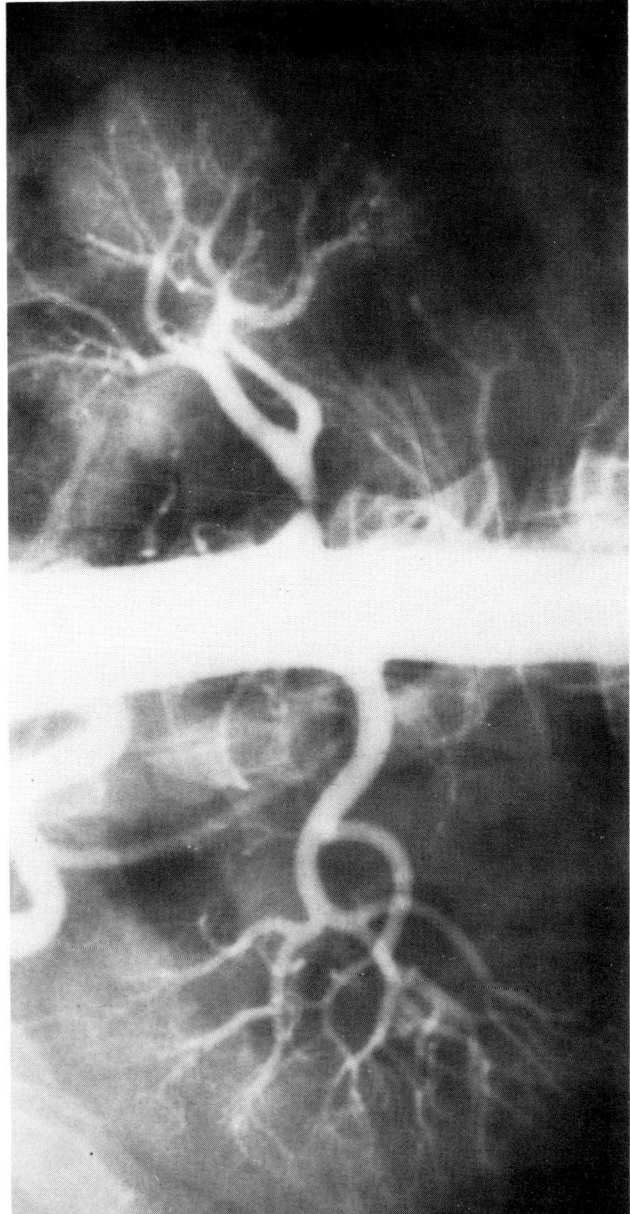

Fig. 14. Arteriosclerosis resulting in a concentric stenosis of the proximal renal artery.

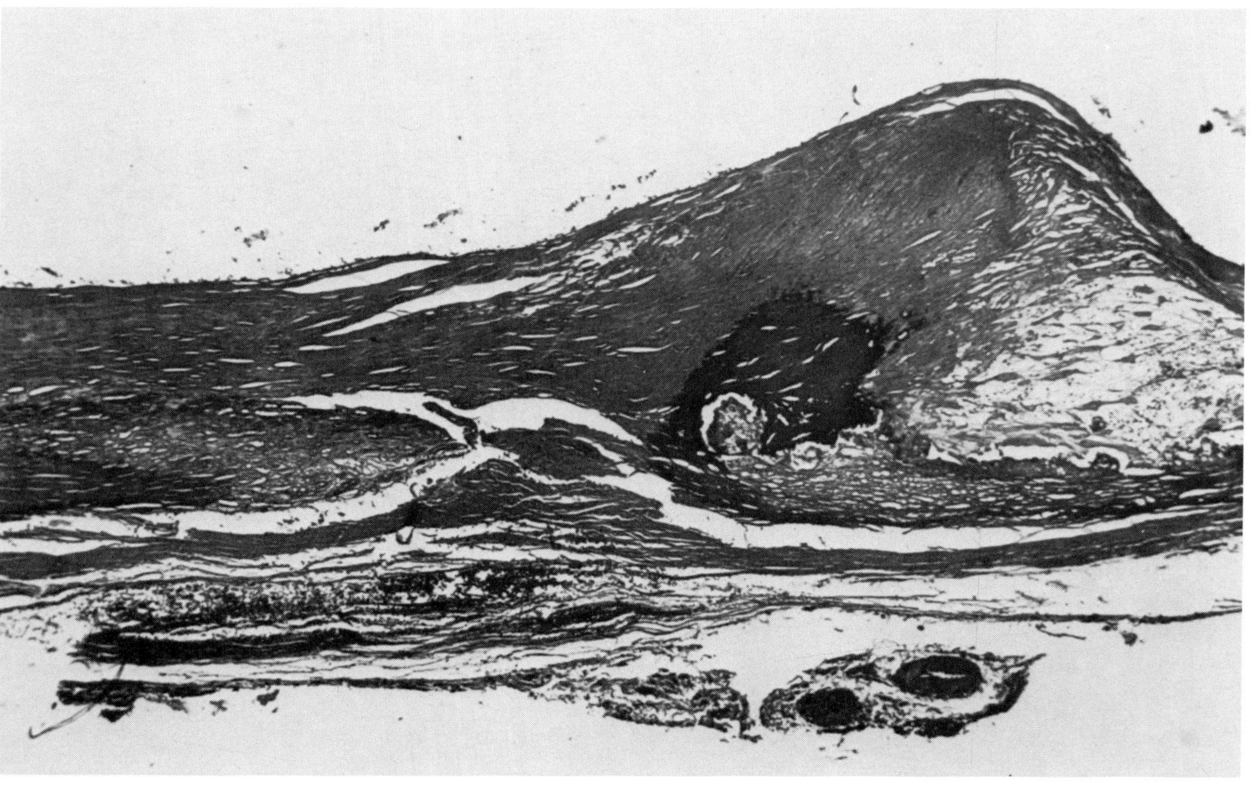

Fig. 15. Arteriosclerosis manifested by plaque formation exhibiting collections of cholesterol, extensive fibrosis, and calcification. × 120. H & E.

vascular disease, may have had developmental or nonarteriosclerotic constrictions of the renal artery preceding secondary arteriosclerotic changes. Progression of renal artery arteriosclerosis occurs with an unusually high frequency [16]. In this regard it is representative of the inexorable progression of arteriosclerotic disease as observed in other areas of the arterial circulation.

REFERENCES

1. Harrison EG, McCormack LJ: Pathologic classification of renal artery disease in renovascular hypertension. Mayo Clin. Proc. 46:161-167, 1971
2. Holley KE, Hunt JC, Brown AL Jr, et al: Renal artery stenosis: A clinical-pathologic study in normotensive and hypertensive patients. Am. J. Med. 37:14-22, 1964
3. Lang J: Mikroskopische anatomie der arterien. Angiologica 2:225-284, 1965
4. Leung DYM, Glagov S, Mathews MB: Cyclic stretching stimulates synthesis of matrix components by arterial smooth muscle cells in vitro. Science 191:475-477, 1976
5. McCormack LJ, Noto TJ Jr, Meaney TF, et al: Subadventitial fibroplasia of the renal artery: A disease of young women. Am. Heart J. 73:602-614, 1967
6. McCormack LJ, Poutasse EF, Meaney TF, et al: A pathologic-arteriographic correlation of renal arterial disease. Am. Heart J. 72:188-198, 1966
7. Paule WJ, Zemplenyi TK, Rounds DE, et al: Light- and electron-microscopic characteristics of arterial smooth muscle cell cultures subjected to hypoxia or carbon monoxide. Atherosclerosis 25:111-123, 1976
8. Ross R: The smooth muscle cell: II. Growth of smooth muscle in culture and formation of elastic fibers. J. Cell Biol. 50:172-186, 1971
9. Ross R, Klebanoff SJ: The smooth muscle cell: I. In vivo synthesis of connective tissue proteins. J. Cell Biol. 50:159-167, 1967
10. Schwartz CJ, White TA: Stenosis of renal artery. Br. Med. J. 2:1415-1421, 1964
11. Sottiurai VS, Fry WJ, Stanley JC: Ultrastructural characteristics of experimental arterial medial fibrodysplasia induced by vasa vasorum occlusion. J. Surg. Res. 24:169-177, 1978
12. Sottiurai VS, Fry WJ, Stanley JC: Ultrastructure of medial smooth muscle and myofibroblasts in human arterial dysplasia. Arch. Surg. 113:1280-1288, 1978
13. Stanley JC, Gewertz BC, Bove EL, et al: Arterial fibrodysplasia. Histopathologic character and current etiologic concepts. Arch. Surg. 110:561-566, 1975
14. Stewart DR, Price RA, Nebesar R, et al: Progressing peripheral fibromuscular hyperplasia in an infant. A possible manifestation of the rubella syndrome. Surgery 73:374-380, 1973

15. Wolinsky H, Glagov S: Nature of species differences in the medial distribution of aortic vasa vasorum in mammals. Circ. Res. 20:409-421, 1967
16. Wollenweber J, Sheps SG, Davis GD: Clinical course of arteriosclerotic renovascular disease. Am. J. Cardiol. 21:60-71, 1968

Richard H. Dean, M.D.

Operative Management of Renovascular Hypertension

Disease of the renal artery may take many forms. Occasionally, renal artery aneurysms, arteriovenous fistulae, renal artery emboli, and trauma to the renal vasculature may all require operation. Nevertheless, occlusive disease of the renal artery causing secondary hypertension is, by far, the most common entity requiring surgical management. The incidence of such secondary renovascular hypertension (RVH) is difficult to define. It probably accounts for 5%-10% of all causes of significant hypertension (diastolic BP > 105 mm Hg). If there are 30 million hypertensive individuals in the United States alone, as some have suggested, then it is a common disorder. Nevertheless, interest in RVH varies widely from one center to another. While some centers routinely identify and treat patients with RVH, others seldom investigate and rarely operate upon individuals with RVH. The reasons for this disparity in interest among different centers stems from the past results of the operative management as well as recent improvements in antihypertensive therapy. Considerable controversy still surrounds the methods of recognition and the merits of operative management of this disease.

HISTORICAL LANDMARKS

Richard Bright of Guy's Hospital, London [3] called attention to the association of hypertension and renal disease in 1836. He observed the apparent association between hardness of the pulse, "dropsy," albuminuria, and granular

Supported in part by NHL Grant 5-P17-HL14192.

shrunken kidneys. This is especially remarkable since the modern sphygmomanometer was not described until 1896. Although Bright's observation stimulated much interest in the kidney, 70 years passed before Tigerstedt and Bergman [39], in 1897, discovered a renal pressor substance in the rabbit. They called this crude extract "renin." Confirmation of a renovascular source of hypertension, however, awaited Goldblatt's classic experiment [19]. In 1934, he and co-workers showed that constriction of the renal artery produced atrophy of the kidney and hypertension in the dog. Following this documentation of a renovascular origin for hypertension, many patients were treated by nephrectomy on the basis of hypertension and a small kidney on intravenous pyelography. Curiously, there was rarely any interest in documenting a renal artery occlusive lesion in any of these patients. Dissatisfaction with the results of this form of treatment prompted Smith [36], in 1956, to review 575 cases. He found only a 26% cure of hypertension by nephrectomy using these criteria. This led him to suggest that nephrectomy be limited to strict urological indications. Two years previously, however, Freeman and his associates [15] performed an aortic and bilateral renal artery thromboendarterectomy on a hypertensive patient with resultant resolution of hypertension. This was the first cure of hypertension by renal revascularization.

DeCamp [10], Morris [32], and others [24, 29] soon followed with additional descriptions of relief of hypertension by renal revascularization. Concomitant with these reports, aortography began to be widely utilized. During the late 1950s, many centers were demonstrating renal artery stenosis in hypertensive patients by aortography and then performing either aortorenal bypass or thromboendarterectomy. Nevertheless, by 1960, it became apparent that revascularization in hypertensive individuals with renal artery stenosis was associated with reduction of blood pressure in less than 50%. General pessimism followed regarding the merits of operative treatment of hypertension.

As this experience pointed out, the coexistence of renal artery stenosis and hypertension does not establish a causal relationship. Many normotensive patients, especially those past the age of 50, have renal artery stenosis. Obviously, special studies are required to establish the functional significance of renal artery lesions. The most recent era in the history of the operative treatment of renovascular hypertension began with the introduction of meaningful tests of split renal function by Howard [21] and by Stamey [37]. Further, the work of Page and Helmes [35] and others [2, 27, 40] in the identification of the renin-angiotensin system of blood pressure control added a new dimension to our understanding of renovascular hypertension. With the later addition of accurate methods of measuring plasma renin activity, the physician now can accurately predict which renal artery lesion is producing renovascular hypertension. Our experience had shown that if the split renal function studies or renal vein renin assays are positive, one can expect a good response in blood pressure following successful operation in over 95% of the cases.

PATHOLOGY

Occlusive lesions of the renal artery can be divided into two groups, atherosclerotic and fibromuscular dysplasia. There is nothing peculiar to atherosclerosis of the renal artery. The pathogenesis parallels atherosclerotic lesions elsewhere with cholesterol-rich lipid deposition and intimal thickening. Later, this "atheroma" may undergo central degeneration and even calcification. They typically occur at or near the renal artery ostium (Fig. 1), are most commonly found on the left, and account for about 65% of patients with renovascular hypertension. Often, there is arteriographic evidence of asymptomatic simultaneous involvement of the abdominal aorta and its bifurcation. Occasionally, the renal artery stenosis is only one manifestation of severe end stage generalized atherosclerosis.

Fibromuscular dysplasia of the renal artery encompasses a variety of hyperplastic and fibrosing lesions of the intima, media, and/or adventitia. They are most frequently seen in young women. This is of no predictive value, however, for fibrodysplastic lesions can be found at any age and in either sex. The right

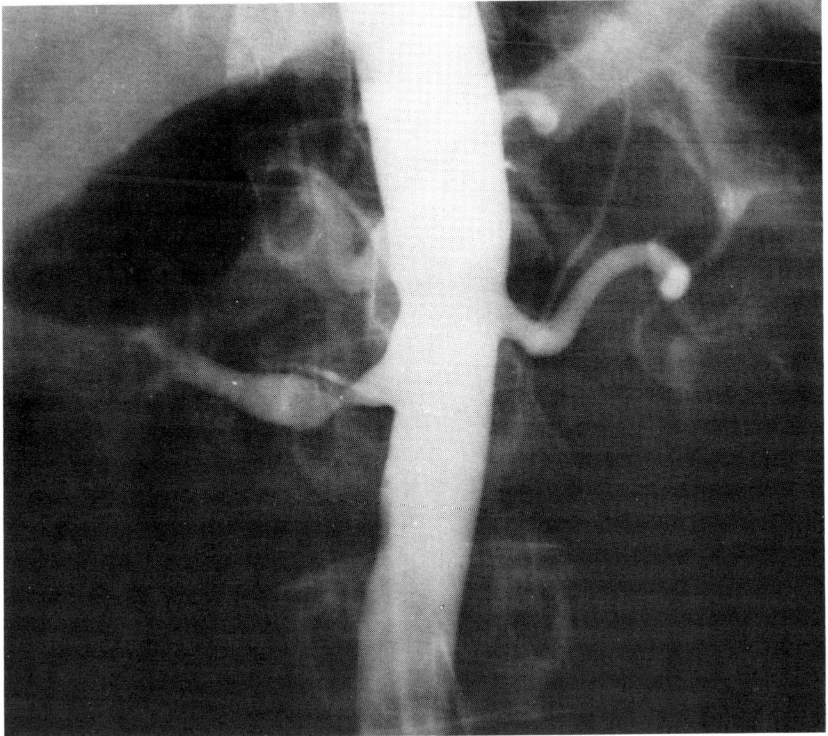

Fig. 1. Arteriogram showing the typical appearance of atherosclerotic stenosis of the right renal artery. Note its proximity to the aorta.

renal artery is more commonly affected than the left, but bilateral involvement is present in the vast majority of patients. The basic cause of fibromuscular dysplasia remains unknown but its frequent occurrence in multiple arteries suggests a common etiologic agent. Embryologic variations, hormonal influences, autoimmune mechanisms, and even recurrent trauma during youth have been suggested as possible etiologic factors. None of these explanations are adequate, however, and the evidence in their support remains mostly conjectural.

Based on the angiographic appearance of fibromuscular disease, several methods of categorization have been suggested. To establish a uniform terminology, Harrison and McCormack [20] combined their experience and developed a classification of these lesions correlating the morphologic and angiographic appearance. Depending on the layer predominantly involved, lesions may either be intimal, medial, or adventitial (Table 1). Clinically, however, it may be difficult to segregate individual lesions into one of their respective categories. The most common variety of fibromuscular dysplasia is medial fibroplasia with mural aneurysms (Fig. 2). This variety accounts for about 70% of all renal artery dysplasias. It often involves long segments of the renal artery and its branches, producing a characteristic "string of beads" appearance angiographically. Less commonly, the dysplastic lesion may be a single mural stenosis (Fig. 3) which may be an intimal or subadventitial variety.

PATHOPHYSIOLOGY

The pathophysiology of renovascular hypertension has been the object of continued investigations for the past 40 years. Whether secondary to atherosclerosis or fibromuscular dysplasia, severe stenosis of the renal artery (greater than 75%) is required to activate the pressor mechanism which ultimately produces systemic hypertension. Knowledge of the mechanism whereby renal artery stenosis causes this hypertension is still somewhat fragmentary. Two intrarenal sites are important in the regulation of blood pressure. These are the macula densa and the juxtaglomerular apparatus. The macula densa is the intrarenal sensor of sodium concentration and thereby exerts a control on renin

Table 1
Classification of Idiopathic Fibrous and Fibromuscular Stenosis of the Renal Artery

Layer	Type of Lesion
Intima	Intimal fibroplasia
Media	Fibroplasia with mural aneurysm; Medial hyperplasia; Perimedial fibroplasia; Medial dissection
Adventitia	Periarterial fibroplasia

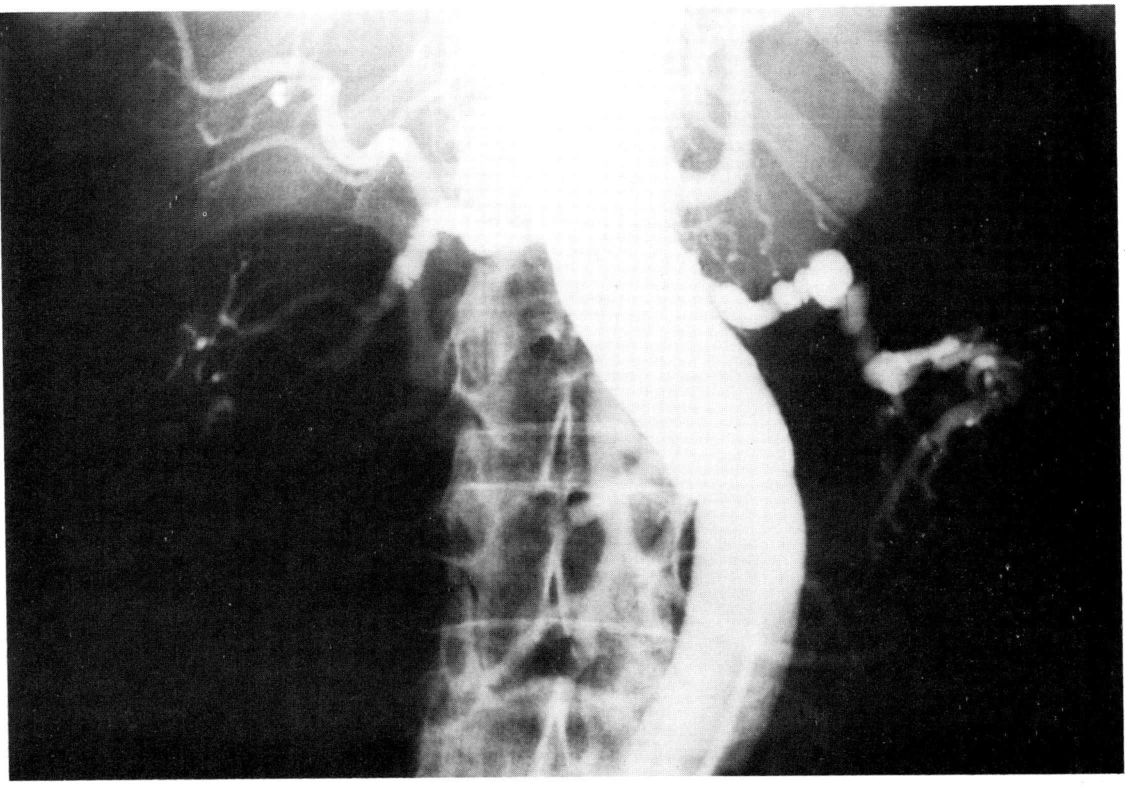

Fig. 2. Fibromuscular dysplasia with medial fibroplasia. The arteriogram shows bilateral multifocal stenoses with multiple aneurysms, several of which have enlarged beyond the perimuscular wall to become saccular aneurysms.

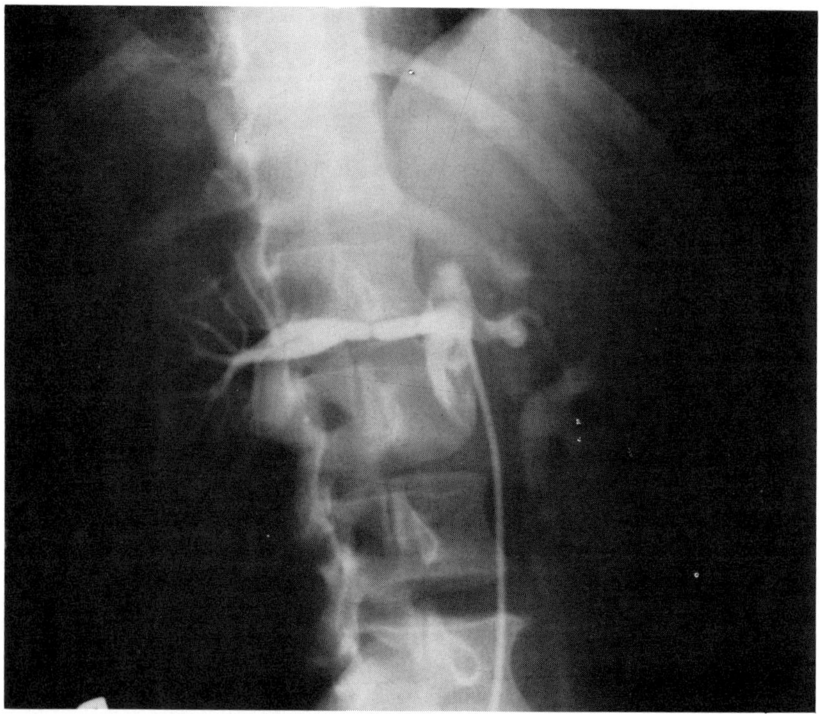

Fig. 3. Arteriogram showing single mural right renal artery a fibrodysplastic lesion in a 24 year old female.

production in the juxtaglomerular apparatus. Although this intrarenal monitor of renin production is important in the normal control of blood pressure, it probably has little influence in the production of renovascular hypertension.

The juxtaglomerular cells are modified smooth muscle cells of the juxtaglomerular afferent arteriole. These richly innervated cells are sensors of intra-arteriolar perfusion pressure. Reduced perfusion pressure causes an increased release of renin by these cells. This increase in the release of renin, a proteolytic enzyme, acts to convert angiotensinogen to angiotensin I. This, in turn, is then converted to the active vasoconstrictor agent angiotensin II by a plasmolytic converting enzyme, predominantly in the pulmonary circulation. This scheme is a simplistic representation of a very complex mechanism. Many intermediate steps remain unknown. The role of the prostaglandins in the regulation of renin release remains speculative. Their action in blood pressure control and specifically the part they play in renovascular hypertension is the source of intensive investigation. The medullary intestinal cells are normally rich in prostaglandin content. A reduction in their prostaglandin content is seen in experimental renovascular hypertension. This may suggest a loss of some intrarenal inhibitory feedback mechanism of renin production or release as a result of the reduction in prostaglandin content. This is highly speculative and much more investigation is required before the exact interactions between the intrarenal content of prostaglandin and renin release can be identified.

HISTORY AND PHYSICAL EXAMINATION

Several features of the history suggest the presence of RVH in the hypertensive patient. Young age, recent onset or accelerated hypertension, and no family history of hypertension all suggest a remediable cause. The absence of these clues, however, does not preclude the presence of RVH. Virtually all patients with hypertension in the first 5 years of life have RVH [26]. Nevertheless, the second most frequent age group with RVH is between the ages of 60 and 69 years; 33% of the hypertensive patients in this latter group have RVH. Whereas RVH from atherosclerosis most frequently affects men, fibromuscular dysplasia occurs more often in women. In a review of 122 patients with RVH, Foster [14] found the mean duration of hypertension to be in excess of 4 years (range, 2 months to 20 years), 43% of patients to be over 50 years old, and 55% to have a family history of hypertension. Only blacks rarely have renovascular hypertension. Although they accounted for 33% of 1070 patients evaluated in Foster's series, only 5 (1%) had RVH.

On physical examination, the presence of an abdominal bruit is said to suggest RVH. Hunt [23] has shown that a continuous systolic-diastolic bruit heard in the epigastrium is highly indicative of renal artery stenosis, although it was only present in 50% of his cases. Therefore there are no features of the history or physical examination which can effectively screen patients for the presence of RVH.

DIAGNOSTIC EVALUATION

The general evaluation of all hypertensive patients is shown in Table 2. Electrocardiography is important to gauge the extent of secondary myocardial hypertrophy or associated ischemic heart disease. Serum electrolytes and serial serum potassium determinations can effectively exclude patients with primary aldosteronism if potassium levels are greater than 3.0 mg/dl. One must remember, however, that hypokalemia is most often due to salt depleting diets and previous diuretic therapy. Estimation of renal function is mandatory. Preexisting renal disease may reduce renal function and cause hypertension. Further, hypertension from any cause may produce intrarenal arteriolar nephrosclerosis and subsequent depression of renal function. Finally, assessment of the urinary 17-hydroxy and ketosteroid and VMA levels will effectively identify the rare patient with a pheochromocytoma or functioning adrenal cortical tumor.

Table 2
General Evaluation of Patients with Hypertension

History and physical examination
Hemogram, SMA-12, urinalysis, urine culture, serum K × 3
Electrocardiogram and chest x-ray
Analysis of 24-hour urine collection for creatinine clearance, electrolytes, catecholamines, VMA, and 17-OH steroids and ketosteroids
Rapid sequence intravenous pyelogram
Renal arteriography

Rapid Sequence Intravenous Pyelogram

This is a simple study employed by many as a screening test for RVH. The patient, having been dehydrated, receives a rapid infusion of contrast medium. Roentgenograms are obtained at 1, 2, 3, 4, 5, 10, 15 and 30 minutes. Findings suggestive of RVH include (1) unilateral delay in appearance of contrast medium, (2) decrease in renal length greater than 1.5 cm as compared to the contralateral side, (3) ureteral notching from enlarged collateral ureteral arteries, (4) late unilateral hyperconcentration of the medium, and (5) defects in the renal outline suggesting segmental infarction. Besides these indicators of renal artery disease, the rapid sequence IVP gives valuable information regarding renal parenchymal disease. This study will effectively screen approximately 70% of patients with RVH. Since its interpretation is largely a comparison between the two sides, it is less accurate in patients with bilateral disease. The fact that it has a 30% incidence of false negative results severely limits its use as the sole screening test for RVH.

Radioisotope Renography

Isotope renography using ^{131}I iodohippurate has been employed for 15 years to evaluate renal disease. Of particular interest has been its use as a screening test for renovascular hypertension. By monitoring the rate of radioactivity appearance and transit through the two kidneys, a comparative assessment of renal perfusion can be obtained. Maxwell et al. [30, 31] reviewed the literature pertinent to renovascular hypertension, however, and found a range of false positive results of 1%-53% and a false negative range of 0%-46%. Nevertheless, recent improvements in radiopharmaceuticals and the introduction of the Anger gamma-ray scintillation camera have increased the sensitivity and reliability of this test. Further, ^{99}Tc chelated diethytriamine pentaacetic acid (DPTA) has the advantage of increased single pass renal extraction and therefore better image production. The exact incidence of false interpretations with the newer techniques of isotope renography are unknown, however, and further comparative studies of its use will be necessary before its role as a screening test in renovascular hypertension will be established.

Renal Arteriography

There continues to be controversy over the use of aortography and renal arteriography in the routine screening of hypertensive individuals. Some feel it should be reserved to a select group of patients. There are no points of the history or physical examination which can effectively screen patients. As stated, isotope renography and the rapid sequence intravenous pyelogram are associated with a 20%-30% false negative interpretation. Renal arteriography is the only test that can definitively exclude the presence of renovascular hypertension. Further, the risk of renal angiography is negligible. Lang [25] reported only seven deaths (0.06%) and 81 (0.7%) serious complications in a series of 11,402 retrograde percutaneous aortograms. Therefore we employ arteriography in all hypertensive patients who would be operative candidates if a functionally significant lesion were found. This excludes the patient with mild hypertension or the patient who is an unacceptable surgical risk.

Both aortography and selective renal arteriography using multiple projections are necessary to adequately examine the entire renal artery. Orifaceal lesions are best seen with aortography. Since the renal artery often arises from a posterolateral site, oblique projections are required to visualize this portion of the vessel. Finally, multiple renal arteries are seen in about 25% of hypertensive patients, and each of these must be scrutinized for hidden areas of stenosis.

Split Renal Function Studies and Renal Vein Renin Assays

When an obstructive lesion is found by renal arteriography, its functional significance is evaluated with renal vein renin assays (RVRA) and split renal function studies (SRFS). Classically, a 1.5 to 1 ratio of the renal vein renin activity from the involved versus the uninvolved side has been considered a positive RVRA. Recent data, by Ernst and his colleagues, suggest that this can be liberalized to a 1.4 to 1 ratio as the index of positivity [11]. In performing these studies using simultaneous bilateral renal venous sampling techniques, however, we still find the most reliable criteria for interpretation to be a 1.5 to 1 ratio.

With the advent of renal vein renin assays, many centers have stopped using split renal function studies because of the associated discomfort, possible complications, and confusing results. Valuable information can be obtained from SRFS that is not obtained from RVRA. Information regarding the likelihood of viability of a severely ischemic kidney and data suggesting the most severely affected side in bilaterally stenotic kidneys are among the benefits of using SRFS. Classically, a positive test shows a 40% reduction in urine volume, a 50% increase in creatinine concentration, and a 100% increase in paraaminohippuric acid concentration on the involved side. Further experience with this test, however, shows that these criteria are much too rigid [5]. We now feel that this test is positive if there is consistent lateralization in each of three samples with a decrease in urine volume and an increase in paraaminohippuric acid and creatinine concentration. When either the renal vein renin assay or the split renal function study is positive, the diagnosis of renovascular hypertension is established.

INDICATIONS FOR OPERATION

The criteria for employing operative management in the treatment of renovascular hypertension vary in many centers. The main controversy stems from conflicting reports of operative risk, success rate of revascularization, and frequency of blood pressure response to successful operation. Much of this controversy, however, originates from the results of poorly performed operations on poorly selected patients. Using modern techniques, operation can be undertaken with minimal risks and a high probability of technical success.

Our indications for operative management of RVH have been outlined in detail elsewhere [4]. Nevertheless, in brief, all patients with severe, difficult to control hypertension should be considered for operation. This includes patients with complicating factors such as branch lesions, extrarenal vascular disease, and patients with associated cardiovascular disease which would be improved by blood pressure reduction. There is substantial evidence which supports the operative management of severely hypertensive patients [16, 17]. Hunt et al. [22] recently compared the results of operative treatment in 100 patients with the results of drug therapy in 114 similar patients. After 7-14 years of followup, 84% of the operated group were alive as compared to 66% in the drug therapy group. Furthermore, of the 84 patients alive in the operated group, 93% were cured or significantly improved, while 16 (21%) of the patients alive in the drug therapy group had required operation for uncontrollable hypertension. Another 7 patients remained uncontrolled without operation. Death during followup was twice as common in the medically treated group. These differences were statistically significant ($p<0.01$) both in patients with atherosclerotic lesions and those with fibromuscular lesions of the renal artery.

Young patients with moderate hypertension and no complaining diseases who have an easily correctable arteriosclerotic or fibromuscular main renal artery stenosis also are candidates for operation. The chance for cure of moderate hypertension is quite good in such patients who have no complicating factors. It remains to be proven that drug control is ever as good as the complete cure of hypertension. In fact, some would argue that reduction in the driving pressure of blood flow across the stenosis by successful drug therapy might accelerate deterioration in renal function by further reducing renal perfusion.

Finally, there is no clear evidence that age (at least under 60 years), type of lesion (whether atherosclerotic or fibromuscular), duration of hypertension, or the presence of bilateral lesions by themselves have proven value as determinants of operative risk or likelihood of successful operative management. Therefore they should not be used as deterrents to such management.

PREOPERATIVE PREPARATION

Antihypertensive medications are reduced during the preoperative period to the minimum necessary for blood pressure control. Frequently patients requiring large doses of multiple medications for control will have significantly reduced requirements while hospitalized. If continued therapy is required, then alpha-methyldopa is the drug of choice. There is little effect on hemodynamics when this agent is combined with anesthesia. We have also commonly continued low dose propranolol therapy as well without any adverse effects. If the patient's diastolic blood pressure is 120-140 mm Hg, it is essential that the pressure be brought under control and that operative treatment be postponed until this is accomplished. It is also important that the anesthesiologist be aware that the patient has been receiving antihypertensive medications and thereby be prepared to provide appropriate support during the operative and postoperative period. This is especially true if reserpine or guanethidine have been employed.

Approximately one-third of patients with RVH have a significant deficit in blood volume ranging from 500 to 1500 ml. Such deficits should be replaced preoperatively; failure to do so can lead to operative hypotensive episodes and further embarrassment of an already compromised renal perfusion.

OPERATIVE TECHNIQUES

A variety of operative techniques have been used to correct renal artery stenoses. From a practical standpoint, two basic operations have been most frequently utilized: aortorenal bypass and thromboendarterectomy. Other procedures such as splenorenal anastomosis and segmental renal artery resection have been discarded following inferior results. We favor aortorenal bypass, preferably with saphenous vein and limit endarterectomy to orifaceal lesions of accessory renal arteries or in an occasional case with severe bilateral orifaceal stenoses. Uncommonly the renal artery will be redundant after it has been circumferentially mobilized. In such patients with orifaceal lesions, renal artery reimplantation also has been used with gratifying results (Fig. 4).

Certain measures and maneuvers are applicable in almost all renal arterial operations. Mannitol 12.5 g is administered intravenously early in the operation. Just prior to renal artery cross-clamping, heparin 50 mg or 5000 units is given intravenously. Protamine is almost never required for reversal of the heparin at the end of the reconstruction.

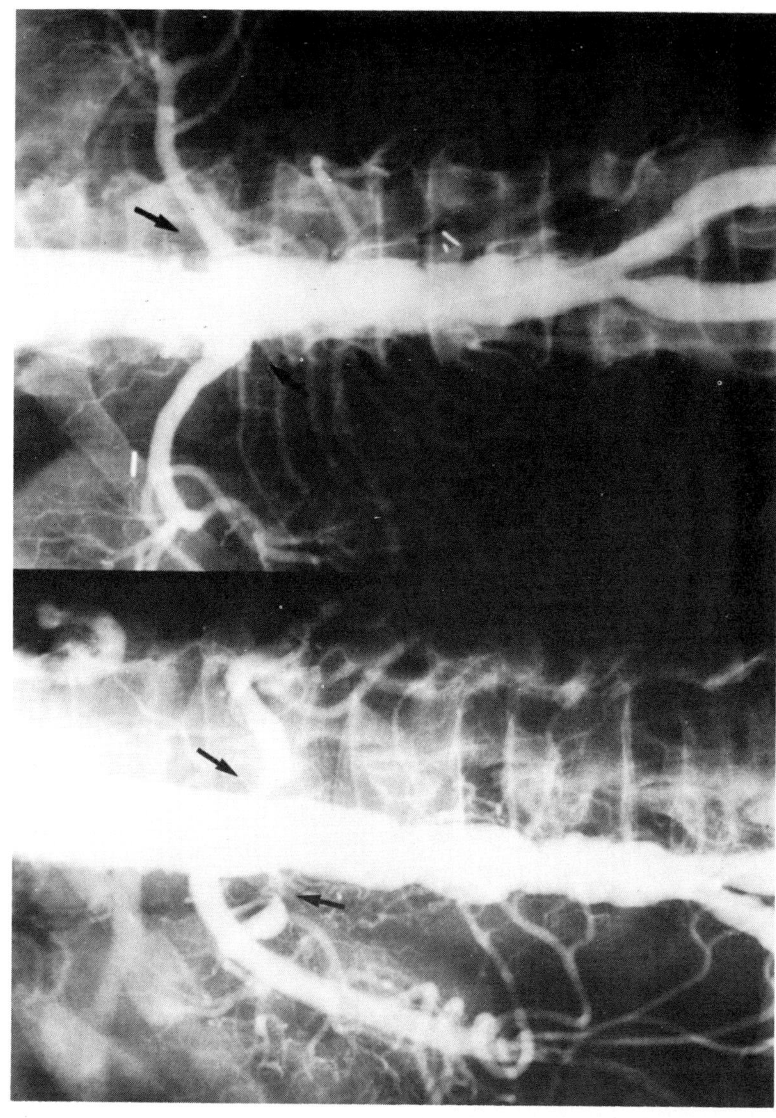

Fig. 4. Preoperative arteriogram (left) and 1 week postoperative arteriogram (right) in a patient submitted to simultaneous bilateral renal artery reimplantations for treatment of bilateral atherosclerotic renal artery stenoses and secondary RVH.

Exposure of the renal arteries is the most difficult aspect of renal artery surgery. A midline xiphoid to pubis incision provides excellent access to either renal artery. To expose the left renal artery, the posterior peritoneum overlying the aorta is incised longitudinally, the duodenum is mobilized to the patient's right, and the left renal vein dissected out and mobilized (Fig. 5). By extending the posterior peritoneal incision to the left along the inferior border of the pancreas, an avascular plane behind the pancreas can be entered. The inferior mesenteric vein courses obliquely through the left retroperitoneal area. This vein is often ligated and divided to facilitate this exposure. When this is done one must be certain that an ascending branch of the inferior mesenteric artery is not accompanying the vein. Ligation of such an ascending arterial branch may compromise colonic perfusion if visceral artery atherosclerotic occlusions are present. This allows excellent exposure of the entire renal hilum on the left and is of special significance when distal lesions are to be managed. The artery lies behind the left renal vein. In some cases, it is easier to retract the vein cephalad in order to expose the artery. In others, caudal retraction of the vein provides better access. Usually, the gonadal vein and adrenal vein which enter the renal vein have to be ligated and divided to facilitate exposure of the artery. Another frequent tributary is a lumbar vein which enters the posterior wall of the left renal vein and is easily avulsed unless special care is taken in mobilizing the renal vein. Similarly, the proximal right renal artery can be exposed through the base

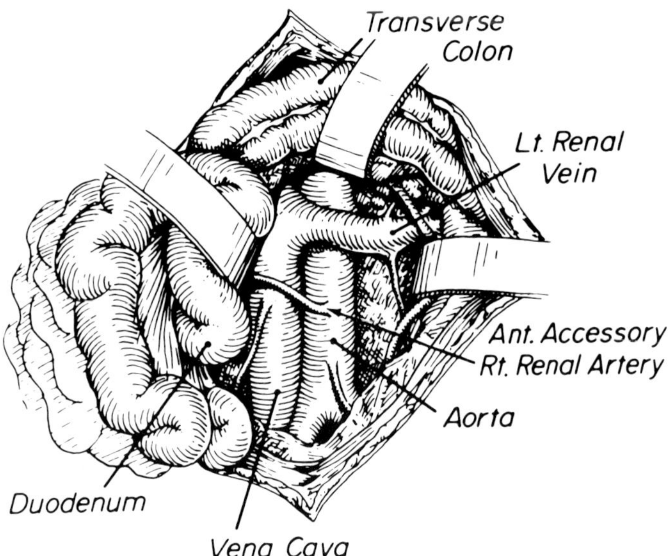

Fig. 5. Drawing depicting limits of posterior peritoneal incision and resulting exposure of the left renal hilum.

of the mesentery by ligating two or more pairs of lumbar veins and retracting the vena cava to the patient's right and the left renal vein cephalad. Usually, however, the right renal artery is best exposed by mobilizing the duodenum and right colon medially. The right renal vein is mobilized and usually retracted cephalad in order to expose the artery. In some patients, there is an accessory right renal artery which arises from the anterior wall of the aorta about 1 inch above the origin of the inferior mesenteric artery. This artery is unusual in that its course is anterior to the vena cava and then over to the lower pole of the right kidney instead of the retrocaval course of the right renal artery. It can easily be injured if one is unaware of its presence.

Aortorenal Bypass Graft

Three types of graft are usually available for aortorenal bypass: (1) autologous saphenous vein, (2) autologous hypogastric artery, and (3) a Dacron prosthesis. The decision as to which graft should be used depends on a number of factors. We use the saphenous vein preferentially. However, if it is small – less than 4 mm in diameter – the hypogastric artery or a Dacron prosthesis may be preferable. A 6 mm Dacron graft is quite satisfactory if the distal renal artery is of large caliber, as is often the case in atherosclerotic renal artery stenosis. Similarly, it may even be useful in children in whom the saphenous vein is too small and immature for use as a renal artery graft (Fig. 6). If the distal renal artery is of small caliber, as is usual in fibromuscular disease, then saphenous vein or hypogastric artery should be used.

The anastomosis between the renal artery and graft is done first. Silastic slings can be used to occlude the renal artery distally. This method of vessel occlusion is especially applicable to this procedure. In contrast to vascular clamps, these slings are essentially atraumatic to the delicate distal renal artery. The absence of clamps in the operative field is also advantageous. Further, when tension is applied to the slings, they lift the vessel out of the retroperitoneal soft tissue for more accurate visualization.

The length of the arteriotomy should be at least three times the diameter of the renal artery to guard against late suture line stenosis. A 6.0 or 7.0 monofilament polypropylene (Prolene) suture material is employed with loop magnification.

After the renal artery anastomosis is completed, the occluding clamps and slings are removed from the renal artery and a small bulldog clamp is placed across the vein graft adjacent to the anastomosis. The aortic anastomosis is then done. First, an ellipse of the anterolateral aortic wall is removed, and then the anastomosis is performed. If the length of the graft is too long, it may result in kinking of the vein and subsequent thrombosis. If there is any element of kinking or twisting of the graft after both anastomoses are completed, the aortic anastomosis should be taken down and redone after appropriate shortening or reorientation of the graft. In certain instances, an end-to-end anastomosis

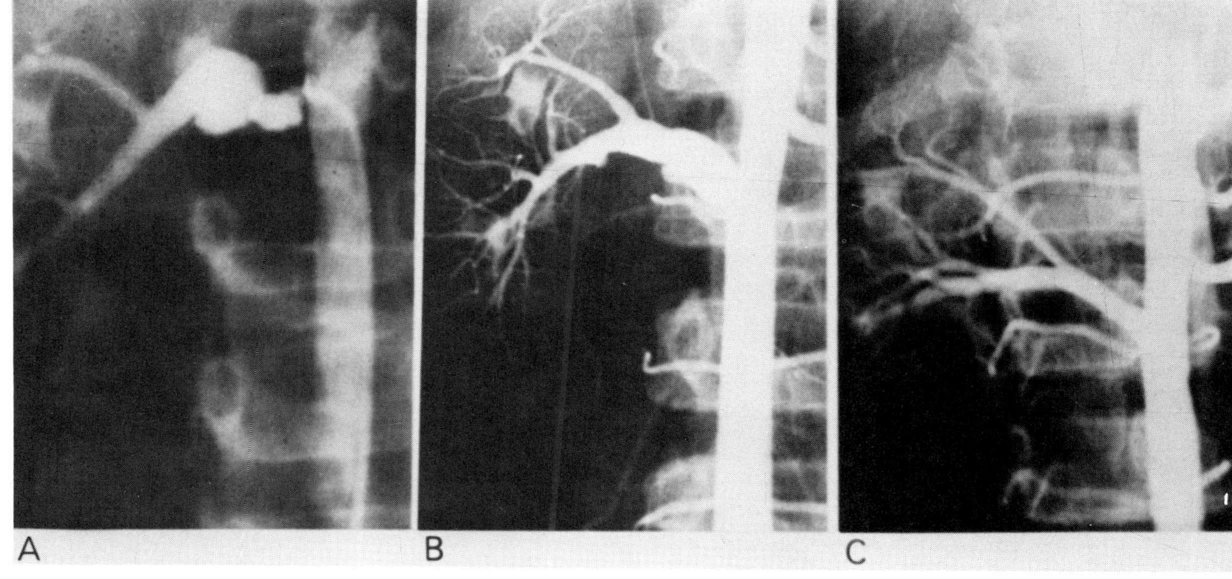

Fig. 6. Preoperative (A), immediate postoperative (B), and 2 years postoperative (C) arteriograms following an aortorenal bypass using a 6 mm Dacron graft in a 7 year old white male. Note the excellent adaptation of the Dacron graft during followup.

between the graft and the renal artery provides a better reconstruction. Fry et al. [12] prefer the end-to-end anastomosis. We routinely employ an end-to-end renal artery anastomosis when combining aortic replacement with renal revascularization. In this circumstance, the saphenous vein is attached to the Dacron aortic graft prior to its insertion. After the aortic graft is attached and flow restored to the distal extremity, the renal artery can be resected and attached to the end of the saphenous vein graft without interrupting aortic flow (Fig. 7).

Thromboendarterectomy

This procedure is employed only for atherosclerotic renal artery stenosis. It is not applicable in fibromuscular disease. Transaortic endarterectomy of bilateral main renal artery lesions has been strongly advocated by Wylie and Stoney [41]. In this procedure, the proximal aortic clamp must usually be placed above the superior mesenteric artery. If it is placed below this artery, it will seriously compromise the exposure of the orifices of the renal arteries. Visualization of the distal extent of the renal artery endarterectomy, however, is often difficult or impossible with this procedure. Because of this, we currently prefer a transverse aortotomy carrying the incision across the stenoses and into each renal artery. By this method the entire endarterectomy can be performed under direct vision.

Intraluminal Dilatation

Until recently, branch lesions of the renal artery causing RVH could only be managed nonoperatively or by nephrectomy. Since there is often bilateral involvement of branch vessels, nephrectomy is a particularly poor choice. Over the past 5 years, significant advances in operative technique have made even these difficult lesions amenable to revascularization. In 1970, Fry et al. [18] described a method of internal dilatation of fibromuscular lesions of the branch arteries. Late results of this technique are not known. Followup angiograms 3 years postoperatively showed no evidence of restenosis in his group, and the patients have remained normotensive.

To perform this technique, the renal artery is mobilized as previously described. Following the arteriotomy, graduated dilators are cautiously passed across the point of stenosis in the branches (Fig. 8). This is repeated with progressively larger dilators until the area of stenosis accepts a dilator the same diameter as the adjoining normal vessel. After this is completed, main renal artery disease can be bypassed as illustrated earlier.

Ex Vivo Repair

A promising approach to management of branch lesions not amenable to other techniques is ex vivo repair. Ota [34], Lim [28], Belzer [1], and Orcutt [33] have reported excellent results in handling these lesions with their

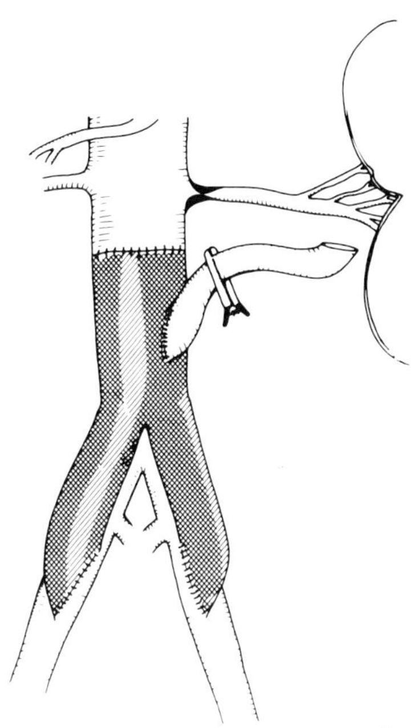

Fig. 7. Drawing showing the method of performing concomitant aortofemoral bypass and renal artery bypass. The saphenous vein graft is attached to the Dacron graft prior to its insertion. With a bulldog clamp occluding the saphenous vein graft the aortic graft is inserted. The renal artery is then transected and an end-to-end anastomosis is performed to the saphenous vein graft.

own variations of the technique. The technique is as follows: Complete mobilization of the kidney, renal artery, renal vein, and the ureter along with its pedicle is performed by blunt and sharp dissection. Following this, the proximal renal artery and vein are divided and the proximal sides closed in the standard fashion. The kidney is then brought out to the abdominal wall with the ureter still intact. The renal artery is perfused with 1000 cc of cold (4°C) modified Collins' solution. Surface cooling is maintained with an ice slush. Continuous perfusion is not necessary. The above process will allow at least several hours of protected ischemia for repair of complicated branch lesions.

Because of the extensive collateral flow through dilated ureteral vessels, a silastic vascular tape is employed on the ureteral pedicle. If this is not done, significant blood loss will occur requiring undesirable amounts of blood replacement. After the microsurgical repair is completed, a saphenous vein graft is anastomosed to the reconstructed renal artery. Autotransplantation of the kidney with anastomosis of the vein graft to the ipsilateral common iliac artery and the renal vein to the accompanying iliac vein can be performed. Recently,

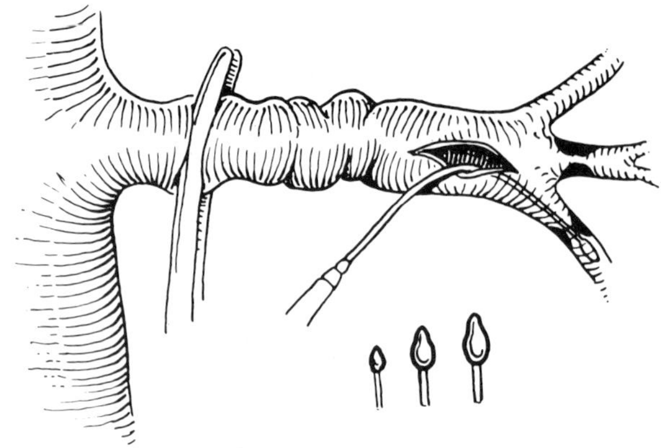

Fig. 8. Graphic demonstration of intraluminal dilatation of branch fibrodysplastic lesions. Proximal lesions can then be managed with an aortorenal bypass graft.

we have simply replaced the kidney in the renal fossa with reattachment of the renal vein at its previous site of transection and connection of the saphenous vein graft to the appropriate site on the aorta. Using this technique, the kidney can be stabilized by the surrounding Gerota's fascia. We believe this allows the greatest latitude for subsequent treatment of aortic iliac disease should it occur during late followup in these patients. Figure 9 is an example of a patient who underwent ex vivo repair of multiple renal artery aneurysms in a single kidney. The postoperative arteriogram shows the position of the kidney after replacement into its original site.

POSTOPERATIVE CARE

The patient is usually kept in the surgical Intensive Care Unit for 2 or 3 days. Body weight is measured daily. Central venous pressure is monitored, as is hourly output. These measurements are used to gauge fluid balance. Longstanding hypertension usually results in some degree of cardiac compromise. Congestive failure or pulmonary edema as the result of fluid overload is a frequent occurrence in the poorly monitored patient. Elastic stockings, leg exercise, and early ambulation are used to avoid thromboembolic complications. Postoperative hypotension is usually the result of inadequate blood replacement. Severe hypertension is commonly encountered and is treated with antihypertensive medications. Fifty percent of the patients who are eventually classified as cured require antihypertensive drugs for several weeks or months postoperatively. If there is rapid acceleration of the hypertension in the postoperative period, thrombosis of the renal artery reconstruction should be suspected and an

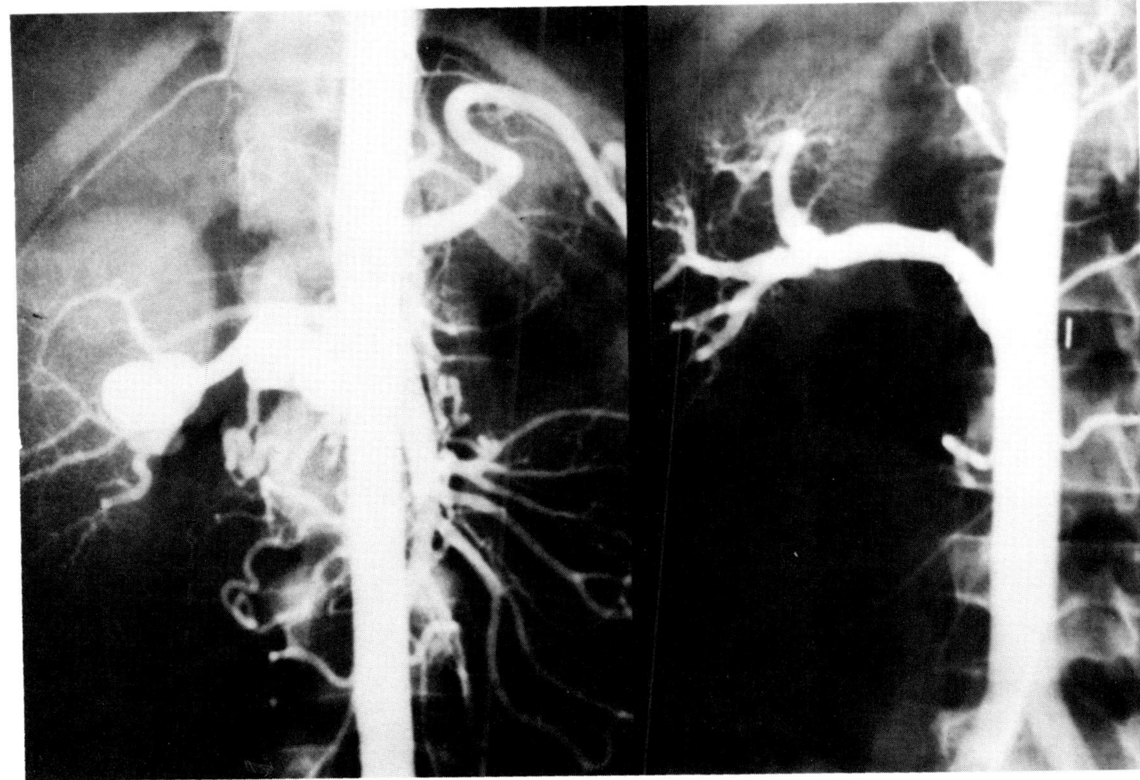

Fig. 9. Preoperative arteriogram (left) in a 25 year old white female showing multiple branch renal artery aneurysms requiring an ex vivo technique for management. Note the congenital absence of the left kidney. The postoperative arteriogram (right) shows the kidney repositioned into its original site following successful operative management.

arteriogram obtained. Even though a bypass graft may have thrombosed, the distal renal artery may remain patent and a second reconstruction may be feasible.

RESULTS OF OPERATIVE TREATMENT

Refinements in patient selection and operative technique have substantially improved the results of renal revascularization in the management of renovascular hypertension. Operation can be performed with minimal risk. In 100 unilateral aortorenal reconstructions, Stanley [38] reported no deaths. We have experienced no operative deaths in the last 200 patients under the age of 65 years.

Although our experience with the operative management of RVH spans 18 years and includes over 400 patients, review of the last 100 patients having had operative management over the past 36 months best demonstrates the current results in our center (Table 3). There was one postoperative mortality. This occurred in a 70 year old white female with associated severe heart disease who died of cardiac decompensation 5 weeks after operation. Of the 100 patients, 96 underwent renal revascularization. Nephrectomy was employed as the primary procedure in only 4 patients. Through the use of routine postoperative angiography successful renal revascularization was documented in 94 of the 95 surviving patients. The single patient who experienced an early graft thrombosis underwent reoperation and repeat renal artery bypass on the fifth postoperative day. Subsequently, he was discharged with a patent graft. Therefore all patients surviving renal revascularization were discharged with a functioning reconstruction.

Postoperative complications in this group were minimal. Three patients had temporary elevation in serum creatinine during the early postoperative period. In

Table 3
Results in Most Recent Experience (100 Patients)

	No. of Patients	Percentage
Operation		
Nephrectomy	4	4
Revascularization	96	96
Revascularization successful	95/96	99
Operative mortality	1	1
Beneficial blood pressure response		
Fibromuscular dysplasia	28/29	96
Atherosclerosis	67/70	96

The single patient who had an early graft thrombosis underwent reoperation on the fifth postoperative day — repeat renal artery bypass — and was discharged with a functioning graft.

each instance, however, these values returned to the preoperative level by the fourth week after operation. None of these instances of mild acute tubular dysfunction required specific therapy. Postoperative bleeding from the aortic suture line (one patient), a ruptured branch renal artery fibromuscular dysplastic microaneurysm (one patient), and an inferior mesenteric vein (one patient) required reoperation for control.

The response to operation has been gratifying in the majority of these patients. Ninety-five of the 99 surviving patients (95%) have had a significant reduction in medication requirements for control of hypertension or cure of hypertension. In this group, 29 patients underwent operation for correction of fibromuscular dysplasia of the renal artery. Seventy-three percent of them were cured of hypertension by operation. Twenty-three percent were improved and four percent had no response in blood pressure control. Although the frequency of a beneficial response (96%) was equally predictable in the 71 patients with atherosclerotic renal artery stenosis, only 24% are cured of hypertension while 72% have residual mild hypertension requiring significantly less medication for control. Interestingly, only one of the four patients receiving no benefit from operation in this group of 100 patients had lateralizing SRFS or RVRA preoperatively. This stresses the importance of these functional studies as predictors of a response to operative management.

Certain aspects of our overall experience with the operative management of RVH in over 400 patients during the past 18 years merit special comments. These areas include the long-term durability of renal artery reconstructions, the management of older patients (> 50 years), patients with bilateral renal artery stenosis and the operative management of patients with poorly functioning kidneys.

Our results of followup angiography from 5 months to 9 years after the operation in 39 patients were published in 1974 [9]. Since that time all patients have had immediate postoperative angiography. By having this as a baseline comparison we have now identified the development of late – 1 year postoperatively – midgraft tubular stenosis from subintimal fibroblastic proliferation in one graft and valvular stenosis of a midsaphenous vein graft venous valve in an additional patient 9 months postoperatively (Fig. 10). Both of these patients had recurrent hypertension that was resolved by reoperation and repeat revascularization. This experience suggests that there is at least a 2% incidence of late failure of saphenous vein bypass grafts secondary to subintimal proliferation of fibrous tissue. Although there has also been a 5% incidence of aneurysmal dilatation of saphenous vein bypass grafts, all of these have stabilized in size and have not required replacement. Interestingly, all of the patients with graft aneurysms remained cured of RVH. The single patient in our operative series who has required replacement of an aneurysmally dilated graft is a child who had an autogenous hypogastric artery used to revascularize the left kidney (Fig. 11). This child also required replacement of the iliac vein graft used to re-

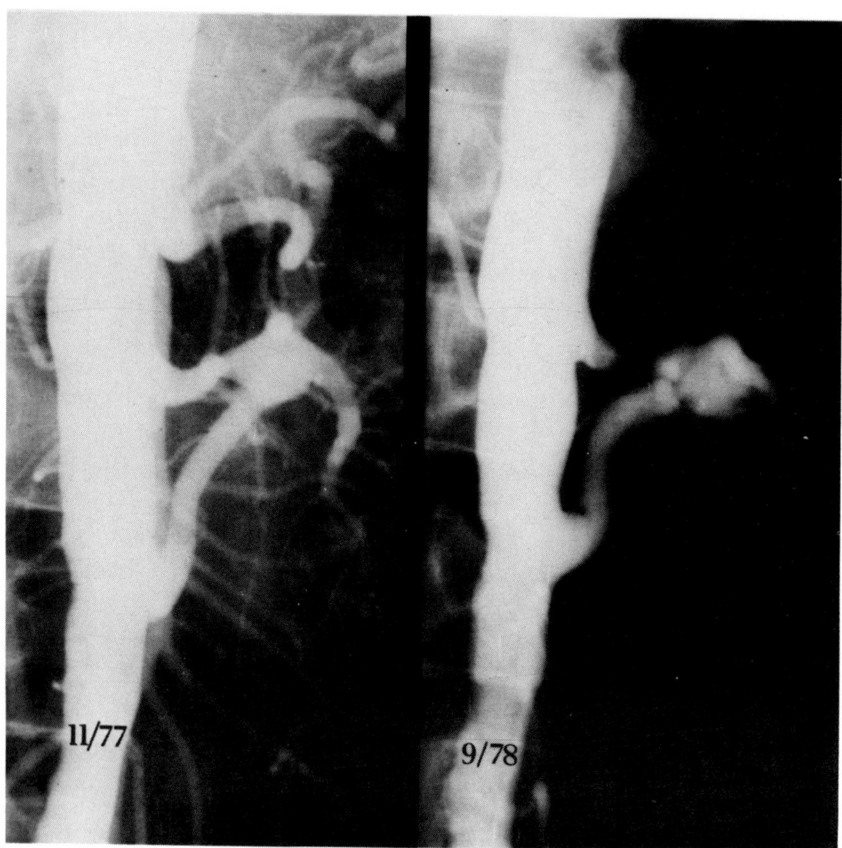

Fig. 10. Arteriograms of a 38 year old white male who developed stenosis of the saphenous vein bypass graft secondary to valvular subintimal thickening secondary to fibroblastic proliferation. Reoperation 10 months later and repeat bypass was required for control of recurrent hypertension.

vascularize the superior mesenteric artery. Unfortunately, followup angiography has shown the development of a branch renal artery aneurysm in the left kidney subsequent to the replacement of these grafts.

Followup angiography also has shown progression of mild to moderate contralateral renovascular disease in 38% of the patients. This is most important in children, where 7 of 15 with fibromuscular dysplasia had bilateral involvement [26]. Only three of these seven children had the contralateral disease demonstrated at the time of the initial evaluation and operation. The remaining four children had documentation of the development and progression of contralateral disease subsequently. Unfortunately, two of four children with no obvious contralateral disease at the time of the initial operation were treated by nephrectomy. This occurrence of subsequent contralateral stenosis has led us to perform nephrectomy in children only if blood pressure is uncontrollable and revascularization is impossible. Since the longest followup in this group is only 10 years, the true incidence of subsequent contralateral disease requires additional longitudinal followup.

Experience with the operative management of RVH in the older atherosclerotic population has been reported by several centers. Ernst et al. [13] reported a low frequency of blood pressure response to operation in 36 patients with diffuse extrarenal atherosclerosis (53%) when compared to 32 patients with isolated atherosclerosis limited to the renal artery lesion (87%). From this experience, they suggested that evidence of diffuse atherosclerosis was a significant prognostic indicator of a poor response to operation. Our experience, however, has not supported this conclusion. We have reported our findings with the operative management of 78 patients over the age of 50 years (mean 58 years) [6]. Seventy-seven patients survived the operation (1.5% operative mortality rate) and 87% had improvement or cure of hypertension. Six of the ten patients not receiving benefit in blood pressure control had early thrombosis of their bypass. Again, the frequency of such early thrombosis of bypass has been significantly reduced in our more recent experience. The more important aspect of this study as it relates to our current interest is that 10 of the 77 surviving patients (13%) died from 2 months to 8 years after the operation. When one considers that the mean followup for the group was only 4 years and that eight of the ten followup deaths occurred within the first 5 years after operation, the frequency of followup death has greater significance. Of greatest importance, however, are the causes of death in this group. Two deaths were unexplained. The remaining eight patients died from progressive atherosclerosis (myocardial infarction, four; congestive heart failure, one; stroke, two; bowel infarction, one). Since all but one of the patients dying during followup in this group had experienced a beneficial response in blood pressure control by operation, this study suggests that evaluation of other risk factors reducing longevity in this group is appropriate. Nevertheless, uncontrolled severe hypertension was present in most of these patients. Without successful management of this risk factor longevity would have been even further reduced.

Our initial review of patients with bilateral renal artery disease and RVH [8] showed that only 50% required bilateral operations for control of hypertension (44 of 86 patients). Thirty-eight of these had bilateral revascularization. The combined use of renal vein renin assay (RVRA) and split renal function studies (SRFS) was particularly helpful in the documentation of functional significance preoperatively in this group, since nonlateralization of RVRA (31%) and SRFS (33%) were frequent. At least one of these studies was positive in 26 of the 28 patients (92%) in whom both studies were performed, however. Technical failure with graft thrombosis occurred in 9 of 42 kidneys (21%) revascularized in 21 patients as simultaneous bilateral procedures. In contrast, 3 of 34 renal revascularizations (9%) performed in 17 patients as staged bilateral procedures throm-

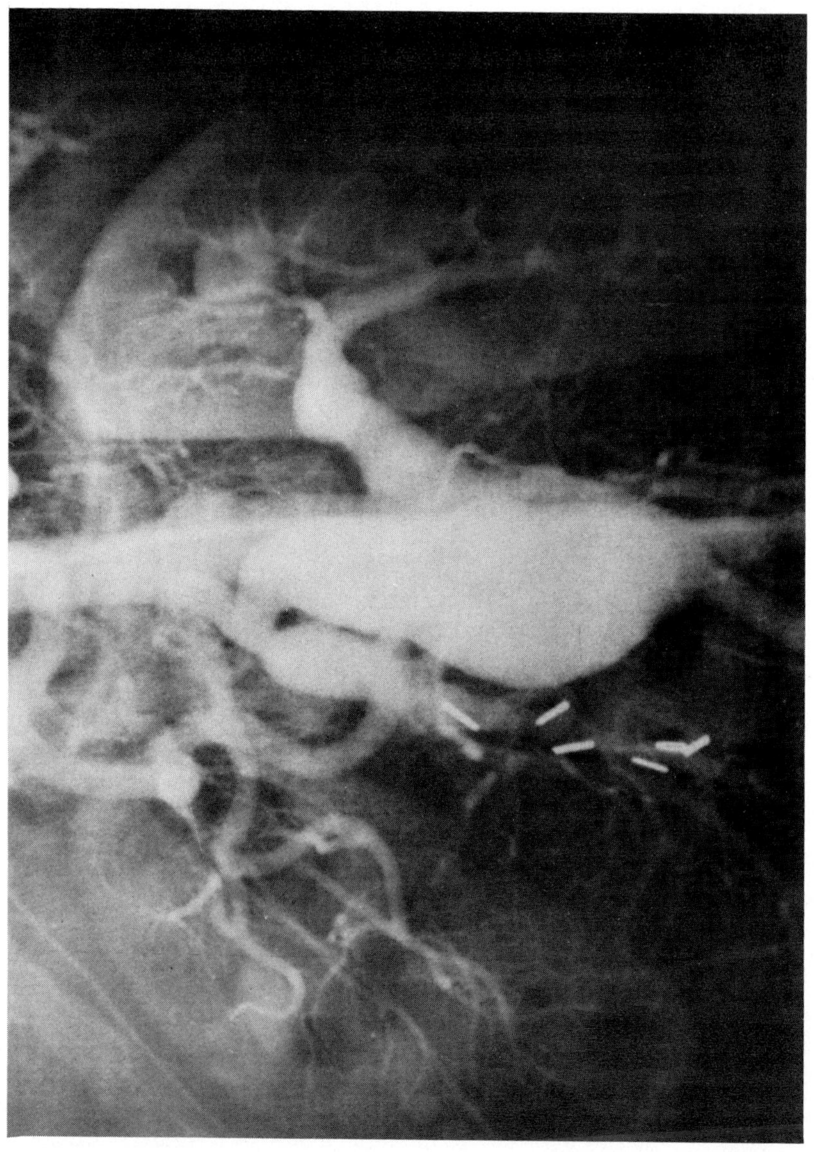

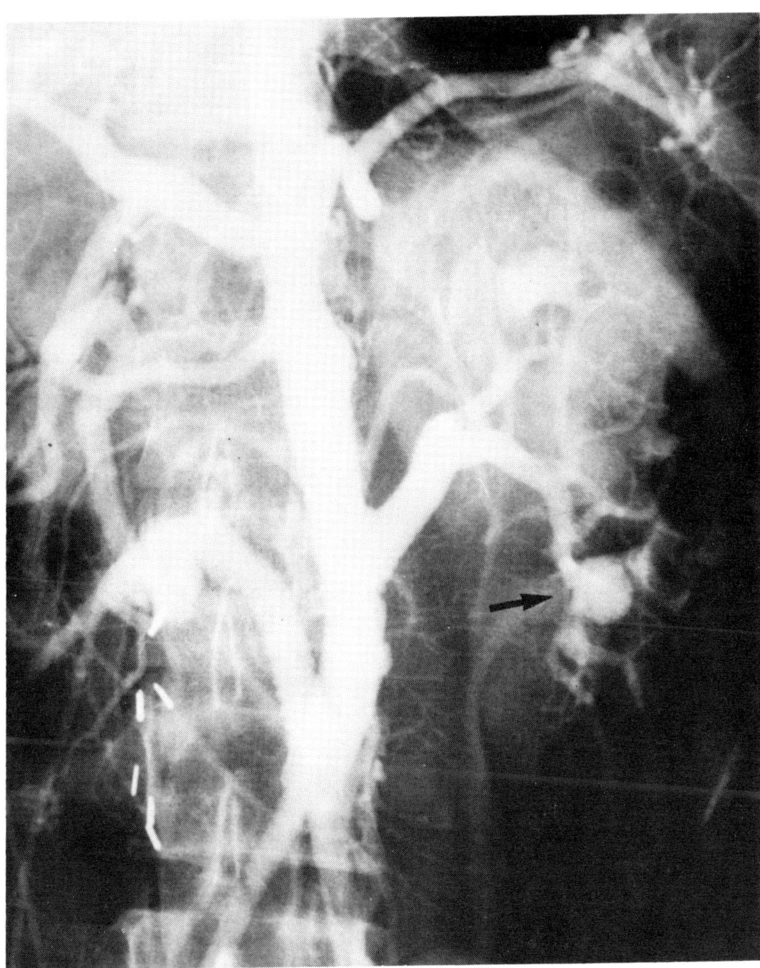

Fig. 11A (left) and B. Arteriograms showing aneurysmal dilatation of a hypogastric artery aortorenal bypass and iliac vein graft for aorta-superior mesenteric bypass. Although these aneurysms appeared stable, replacement with 6 mm Dacron grafts was required. Note the branch left renal artery aneurysm which developed during followup in this 18 year old white male.

bosed. Although this led to our policy of only revascularizing the side to which functional studies lateralized, our more recent experience suggests that this decision requires review. Specifically, although staging bilateral reconstructions decreased the incidence of technical failures, even the 9% failure rate is unacceptable when compared to our current thrombosis rate of 1%. Indeed, if technical success is expected, bilateral simultaneous correction in selected patients may be indicated.

A final area meriting special comment is the effect of renal revascularization on poorly functioning kidneys. In a recent report we summarized the response to revascularization in 25 patients who had preoperative creatinine clearances from the affected kidney of less than 30 cc/min (Fig. 12) [7]. A significant improvement in excretory renal function as determined by repeat postoperative SRFS was seen in patients with less than 20 cc/min creatinine clearance. Even when residual function was negligible (preoperative creatinine clearance < 10 cc/min) a beneficial response in excretory function was seen following revascularization. An example of such a patient is seen in Figs. 13A and 13B. This patient had a chronic total left renal artery occlusion and no urinary output from the kidney during SRFS. The arteriogram showed a patent distal renal artery with normal appearing intrarenal branches. Following saphenous vein aortorenal bypass, repeat SRFS demonstrated a retrieval of 29 cc/min creatinine clearance (Fig. 13C). This experience has led us to employ renal revascularization rather than nephrectomy whenever the distal renal artery is visualized and reasonably free of severe branch artery disease, regardless of the degree of excretory renal function impairment or the status of the contralateral renal artery. Obviously, this approach would have greatest application when contralateral renal function is reduced or contralateral renal artery disease is present. Nevertheless, since progression of apparently insignificant contralateral lesions or the development of new lesions during followup occurs in over 40% of patients undergoing operative management of RVH [9], concern over protection of renal function should not be limited to patients with severe contralateral disease at the time of the initial evaluation. Indeed, if renal function in the poorly functioning kidney is retrievable by revascularization, then nephrectomy would be an inferior choice of operative management, regardless of the status of the contralateral kidney.

Such an aggressive attitude toward the role of revascularization in managing these patients with RVH requires that both operative risk and frequency of graft thrombosis be low. Nevertheless, enthusiasm for revascularization of poorly functioning kidneys in older patients must be weighed against the operative risk when severe associated cardiovascular disease is present. Currently, however, nephrectomy is employed primarily only when intrarenal disease is severe, hypertension is otherwise difficult to control, and residual excretory function in the affected kidney is negligible.

Finally, the role of renal revascularization in severely azotemic patients requires special comment. Obviously, retrieval of renal function by revascularization is of greatest practical importance in this group. Although none of the patients in this study was severely azotemic, all had renovascular hypertension. This was predicted in each instance by the results of RVRA and SRFS and was proven by the response to operation. In this setting severe reductions in excretory function also were improved by revascularization. Therefore if a hypertensive patient with a renal artery stenosis and severe azotemia has positive

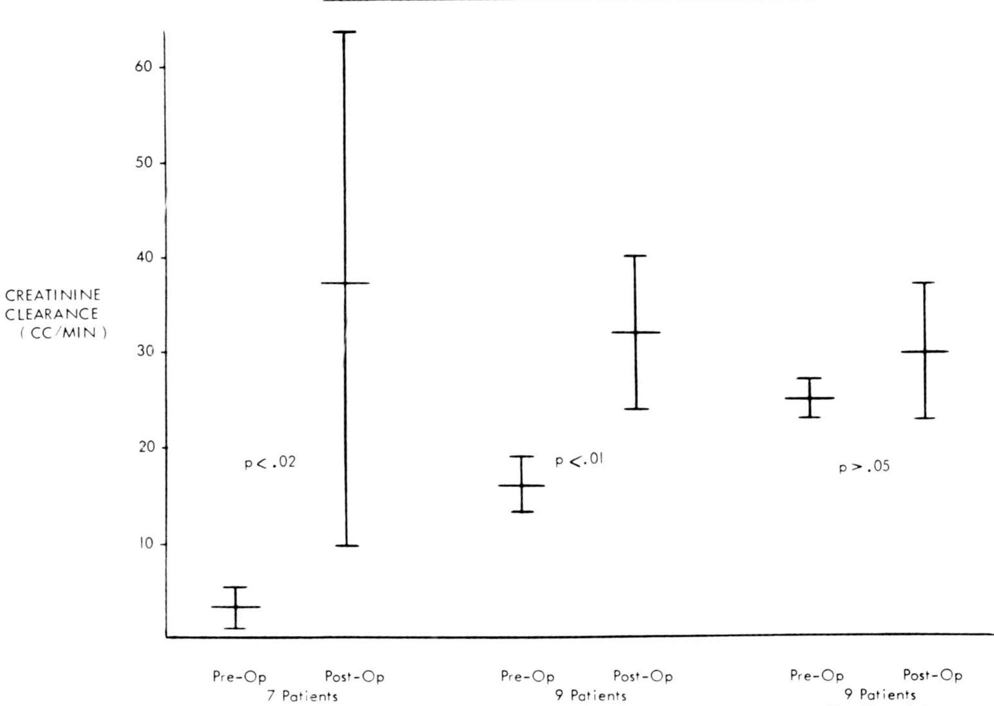

Fig. 12. Creatinine clearances from the affected kidneys are categorized into three groups according to the preoperative value. Values are recorded as the group's mean ± SD creatinine clearance before and after revascularization. Statistically significant improvements were seen in the two groups of kidneys with the poorest excretory function before operation.

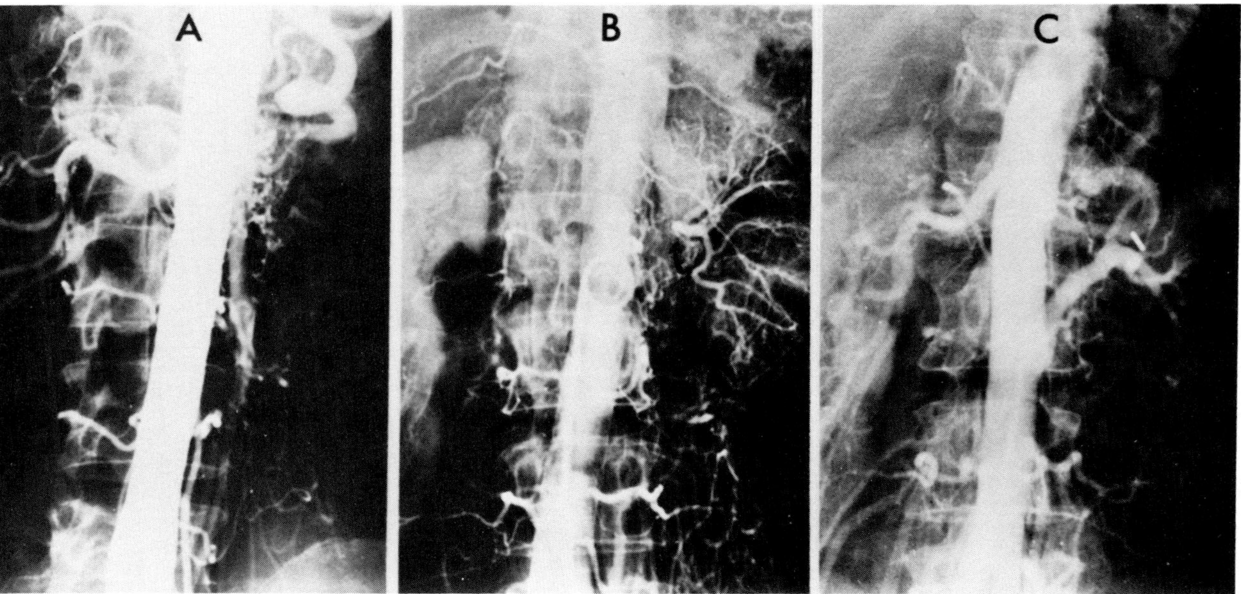

Fig. 13. Preoperative arteriogram (A and B) in a 49 year old white female showing a total occlusion of the left renal artery. No excretory function was demonstrated preoperatively. Following revascularization (C) repeat SRFS revealed the preference of 29 cc/min creatinine clearance from the affected kidney.

RVRA or SRFS a benefit in excretory function should be expected from renal revascularization. Clearly, this beneficial effect would have greatest practical significance if there were bilateral renal artery stenoses to be corrected. The validity of this logic, however, is unproven in the azotemic patient without hypertension. On the contrary, if the patient is normotensive, the renal artery lesion probably is not functionally significant and its correction likely would have no beneficial effect. Similarly, if the azotemic patient with renal artery stenosis had hypertension but RVRA and SRFS were not positive for RVH, a beneficial effect of revascularization also would be less predictable.

In summary, many questions remain unanswered in the field of renovascular surgery. Drug therapy is still preferred in many institutions. Recent experience with the operative management of RVH is encouraging, however, and the theoretical advantages of potential cure of hypertension and retrieval of renal function by operation are obvious. Nevertheless, long-term randomized comparative studies will be required to delineate the respective merits of operative and drug therapy. These studies are now underway, and answers should be forthcoming in the near future.

REFERENCES

1. Belzer FO, Keaveny TV, Reed TW, et al: A new method of renal artery reconstruction. Surgery 68:619, 1970
2. Braun-Menendez E, Fasciolo JC, Leloir LF, et al: La substancia hipertensora de la sangre del rinon, isquemiado. Rev. Soc. Argent. Biol. 15:420, 1939
3. Bright R: Cases and observations illustrative of renal disease accompanied with the secretion of albuminous urine. Guy's Hosp. Rep. 1:388, 1836
4. Dean RH: Indications for operative management of renovascular hypertension. J. South Carolina Med. Assoc. Dec. 1977
5. Dean RH, Foster JH: Criteria for the diagnosis of renovascular hypertension. Surgery 74:926, 1973
6. Dean RH, Foster JH: Surgical management of renovascular hypertension in older patients. Med. Clin. North Am. 61:643, 1977
7. Dean RH, Lawson JD, Hollifield JH, et al: Revascularization of the poorly functioning kidney. Surgery 85:44, 1979
8. Dean RH, Oates JA, Wilson JP, et al: Bilateral renal artery stenosis and renovascular hypertension. Surgery 81:53, 1977
9. Dean RH, Wilson JP, Burko H, et al: Saphenous vein aorto-renal bypass grafts: Serial arteriographic study. Ann. Surg. 180:469, 1974
10. Decamp PT, Birchall R: Recognition and treatment of renal arterial stenosis associated with hypertension. Surgery 43:134, 1958
11. Ernst CB, Bookstein JJ, Montie J, et al: Renal vein renin ratios and collateral vessels in renovascular hypertension. Arch. Surg. 104:496, 1972
12. Ernst CB, Stanley JC, Marshall FF, et al: Autogenous saphenous vein aortorenal grafts. Arch. Surg. 105:855, 1972

13. Ernst CB, Stanley JC, Marshall FF, et al: Renal revascularization for arteriosclerotic renovascular hypertension: Prognostic implications of focal renal arterial vs. overt generalized arteriosclerosis. Surgery 73:859, 1973
14. Foster JH, Dean RH, Pinkerton JA, et al: Ten years experience with the surgical management of renovascular hypertension. Ann. Surg. 177:755, 1973
15. Freeman N: Thromboendarterectomy for hypertension due to renal artery occlusion. JAMA 157:1077, 1954
16. Freis ED: Effects of treatment of morbidity in hypertension. Results in patients with diastolic blood pressure averaging 115 through 129 mm Hg. Veterans Administration Cooperative Study Group on Antihypertensive Agents. JAMA 202:116, 1967
17. Freis ED: Effects of treatment on morbidity in hypertension. II. Results in patients with diastolic blood pressure averaging 90 through 114 mm Hg. Veterans Administration Cooperative Study Group on Antihypertensive Agents. JAMA 213:1143, 1970
18. Fry WJ, Brink BE, Thompson NW: New techniques in the treatment of extensive fibromuscular disease involving the renal arteries. Surgery 68:959, 1970
19. Goldblatt H: Studies on experimental hypertension. J. Exp. Med. 59:347, 1934
20. Harrison EG Jr, McCormack LJ: Pathologic classification of renal arterial disease in renovascular hypertension. Mayo Clin. Proc. 46:161, 1971
21. Howard JE, Conner TB: Use of differential renal function studies in the diagnosis of renovascular hypertension. Am. J. Surg. 107:58, 1964
22. Hunt JC, Strong CG: Renovascular hypertension. Mechanisms, natural history and treatment. Am. J. Cardiol. 32:562, 1973
23. Hunt JC, Strong CG, Harrison EG Jr, et al: Management of hypertension of renal origin. Am. J. Cardiol. 26:280, 1970
24. Hurwitt ES, Seidenburg B, Hainovoco H, et al: Splenorenal arterial anastomosis. Circulation 14:537, 1956
25. Lang EK: A survey of the complications of percutaneous arteriography: Seldinger technique. Radiology 81:257, 1963
26. Lawson JD, Boerth RK, Foster JH, et al: Diagnosis and management of renovascular hypertension in children. Arch. Surg. 112:1307, 1977
27. Lentz KE, Skeggs LT Jr, Woods KR, et al: The amino acid composition of hypertensin II and its biochemical relationship to hypertension I. J. Exp. Med. 104:183, 1956
28. Lim RC Jr, Eastman AB, Blaisdell FW: Renal autotransplantation. Adjunct to repair of renal vascular lesions. Arch. Surg. 105:847, 1972
29. Luke JC, Levitan BA: Revascularization of the kidney in hypertension due to renal artery stenosis. Arch. Surg. 79:269, 1959
30. Maxwell MH, Lupu AN, Taplin GU: Isotope renogram in renal arterial hypertension. J. Urol. 100:376, 1968
31. Maxwell MH, Hayes M: The renogram in hypertension, in Blaufox E (ed): Progress in Nuclear Medicine (vol 2). Baltimore, University Press, 1972, p 248

32. Morris GC Jr, Cooley DA, Crawford ES, et al: Renal revascularization for hypertension. Clinical and physiologic studies in 32 cases. Surgery 48:95, 1960
33. Orcutt TW, Foster JH, Ritchie RE, et al: Bilateral ex vivo renal artery reconstruction with autotransplantation. JAMA 228:493, 1974
34. Ota K, Mori S, Awane Y, et al: Ex situ repair of renal artery for renovascular hypertension. Arch. Surg. 94:370, 1967
35. Page IH, Helmer OM: A crystalline pressor substance (angiotensin) resulting from the reaction between renin and renin-activator. J. Exp. Med. 71:29, 1940
36. Smith HW: Unilateral nephrectomy in hypertensive disease. J. Urol. 76:685, 1956
37. Stamey TA, Nudelman IJ, Good PH, et al: Functional characteristics of renovascular hypertension. Medicine (Baltimore) 40:347, 1961
38. Stanley JC, Ernest CB, Fry WJ: Fate of 100 aorto-renal vein grafts: Characteristics of late graft expansion, aneurysmal dilatation, and stenosis. Surgery 74:931, 1973
39. Tigerstedt R, Bergman PG: Niere und Kreislauf. Skand. Arch. Physiol. 8:223, 1898
40. Tobian L: Relationship of juxtaglomerular apparatus to renin and angiotensin. Circulation 25:189, 1962
41. Wylie EJ, Perloff DL, Stoney RJ: Autogenous tissue revascularization techniques in surgery for renovascular hypertension. Ann. Surg. 170:416, 1969

John H. Isch, M.D.
Donald E. Schwarten, M.D.

Renal Percutaneous Transluminal Angioplasty: An Alternative Approach in the Management of Renovascular Occlusive Disease

It has been estimated that 5%-10% of patients with hypertension have lesions which are surgically correctable [1, 9, 13]. Approximately 90% of these patients have renovascular occlusive disease. With 20 million Americans presently afflicted with hypertension, approximately one to two million individuals in this country have renovascular hypertension.

Renal arterial obstruction generally results from atherosclerotic disease [5] or fibromuscular hyperplasia [14]. These lesions lend themselves to operative treatment, although its necessity remains controversial to some authors. Classical operative approaches to this problem have included aortorenal bypass, transrenal endarterectomy, renal autotransplantation, nephrectomy, and intraoperative transluminal dilatation.

Percutaneous intraluminal dilatation of a renal artery obstruction is an alternative approach to these classical operative procedures. Percutaneous transluminal angioplasty (PTA) is not a new concept. Dotter and Judkins initially described this technique in 1964 by which a rigid coaxial catheter system was used to dilate an arterial obstruction [3]. Eleven patients with various obstructive lesions were presented. While in these authors' experience early results with the technique were acceptable, others have found the immediate complication rate unacceptably high and the long-term success rate less than ideal. In 1973, Gruntzig presented an improved technique of intraarterial dilatation in which a flexible coaxial system was used to percutaneously cannulate the obstructive lesion under fluoroscopic visualization [7]. A balloon catheter inflated in a controlled graduated fashion was used to dilate the obstruction. This simpler, safer, and more effective technique has renewed interest in percutaneous arterial dilatation. Twenty-seven patients have undergone PTA at the St. Vincent Hospital and Health Care Center. This report is a presentation of these data and a preliminary evaluation of early results.

MATERIALS AND METHODS

From May 1, 1978 until June 1, 1979 renal PTA was attempted in 27 patients, 16 female and 11 male. In 25 patients the procedure was successfully performed. In one patient restenosis occurred 6 months following dilatation and PTA was again performed. This series was divided into two groups. Group I consisted of 16 patients who underwent PTA primarily because of difficulty controlling hypertension despite aggressive medical therapy. This group had normal renal function by all clinical parameters. Group II consisted of 11 patients who were also hypertensive but had markedly compromised renal function. These patients underwent dilatation to restore and/or preserve threatened renal function. All patients prior to dilatation were taking at least two antihypertensive medications. Twenty-six patients had atherosclerotic obstructive lesions and one fibromuscular hyperplasia. Further clinical data of this series are presented in Table 1.

Studies prior to consideration for dilatation included serial blood pressure evaluations, serum blood urea nitrogen and creatinine levels, urinalysis, creatinine clearance, hypertensive intravenous pyelography, renal scanning, renal venous renin sampling, and renal arteriography. Early in this series, these studies were not all performed on every patient.

Technique

Renal PTA is performed with local anesthesia using the Seldinger technique to puncture the common femoral artery. The right side is preferably used. A soft "J" guidewire is advanced into the abdominal aorta; over this guidewire a 5 French (1.6 mm O.D.) "cobra" selective catheter is advanced. The guidewire is removed and the catheter advanced to the orifice of the involved renal artery. The renal orifice is engaged and a selective arteriogram performed (Fig. 1). Following the contrast study, a 0.028 inch guidewire is advanced through the catheter beyond the stenotic lesion into the distal main or branch renal vessel. Over this guidewire, a 5 French catheter is advanced through the obstructive lesion. A guidewire exchange is made and a heavy duty 0.35 inch guidewire is advanced into an interlobar branch. Leaving the guidewire in place, the 5 French catheter is removed and exchanged for a 7 French Gruntzig catheter with a balloon segment appropriate to the size of the renal artery to be dilated. The balloon is placed into the stenotic arterial segment and the balloon inflated with dilute contrast medium to 5 atmospheres of pressure. The Gruntzig catheter is then removed, a catheter exchange is made, and a flush catheter placed into the

Table 1
Patient Data

		Group I	Group II
Number Patients:		16	11
Sex:	Male	9	4
	Female	7	7
Age:		57 yrs.	59 yrs.
Arterial Lesions:	Rt.	4	0
	Lt.	12	11
Average B.P.			
Pre-PTA		190/110	205/102
Post-PTA (48 hrs)		135/75	175/66
Last Evaluation		135/76	167/80

abdominal aorta. A contrast examination is carried out to observe the angioplastic result (Fig. 2). Five thousand units of heparin are infused intraarterially at the completion of this study and only partially reversed after catheter removal.

Aspirin 10 grains and Persantin 50 mg were given twice daily beginning 24 hours prior to and resumed immediately after the procedure. These medications were continued for 3 weeks.

Blood pressures were evaluated very frequently for the first few hours following dilatation and then at progressively longer intervals until discharge. Absolute bed rest was maintained for 12 hours in an appropriately monitored bed. An intravenous line was maintained until the threat of hypertension had abated.

Following hospital discharge, serial blood pressure evaluations and medication adjustments were made by either the referring physician or primary investigators at regular intervals. Serial blood urea nitrogen, creatinine, urine, and renal scan studies were performed on consenting patients. Followup evaluations ranged from 1 week to 1 year postdilatation. Six patients were either unavailable or refused late followup evaluation.

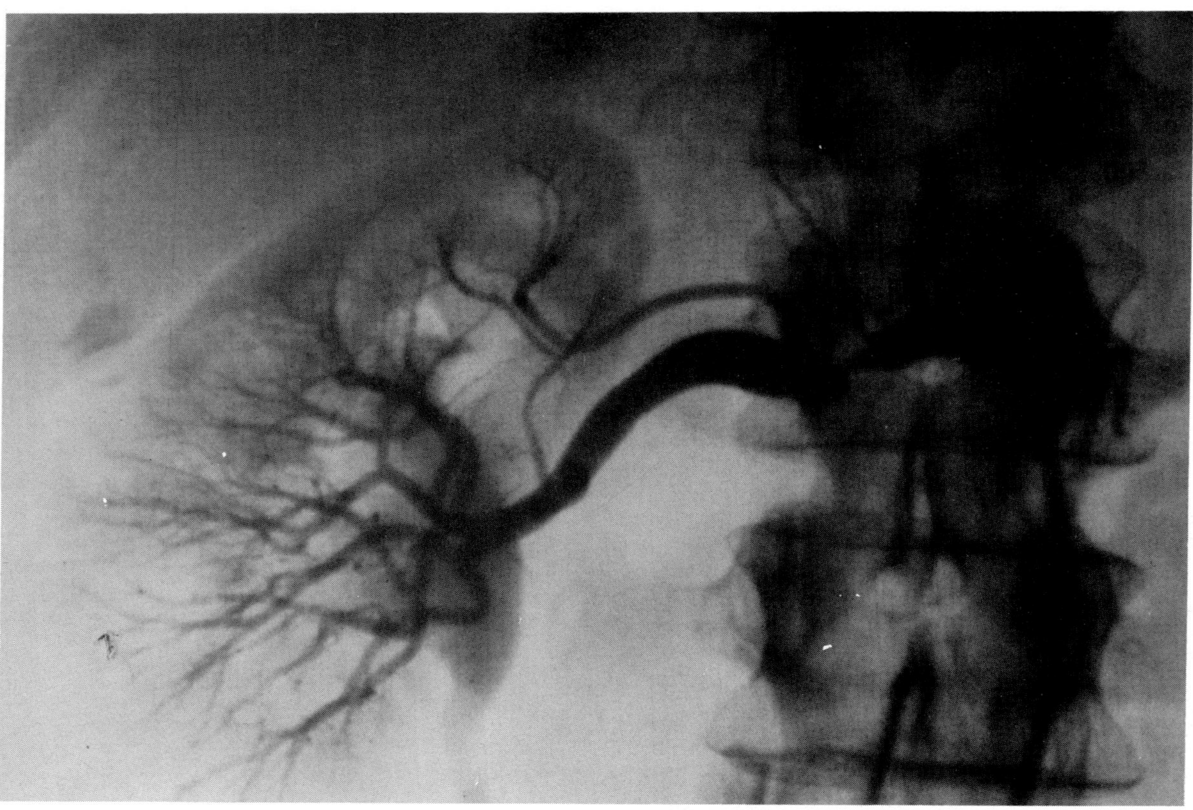

Fig. 1. Right renal arteriogram predilatation.

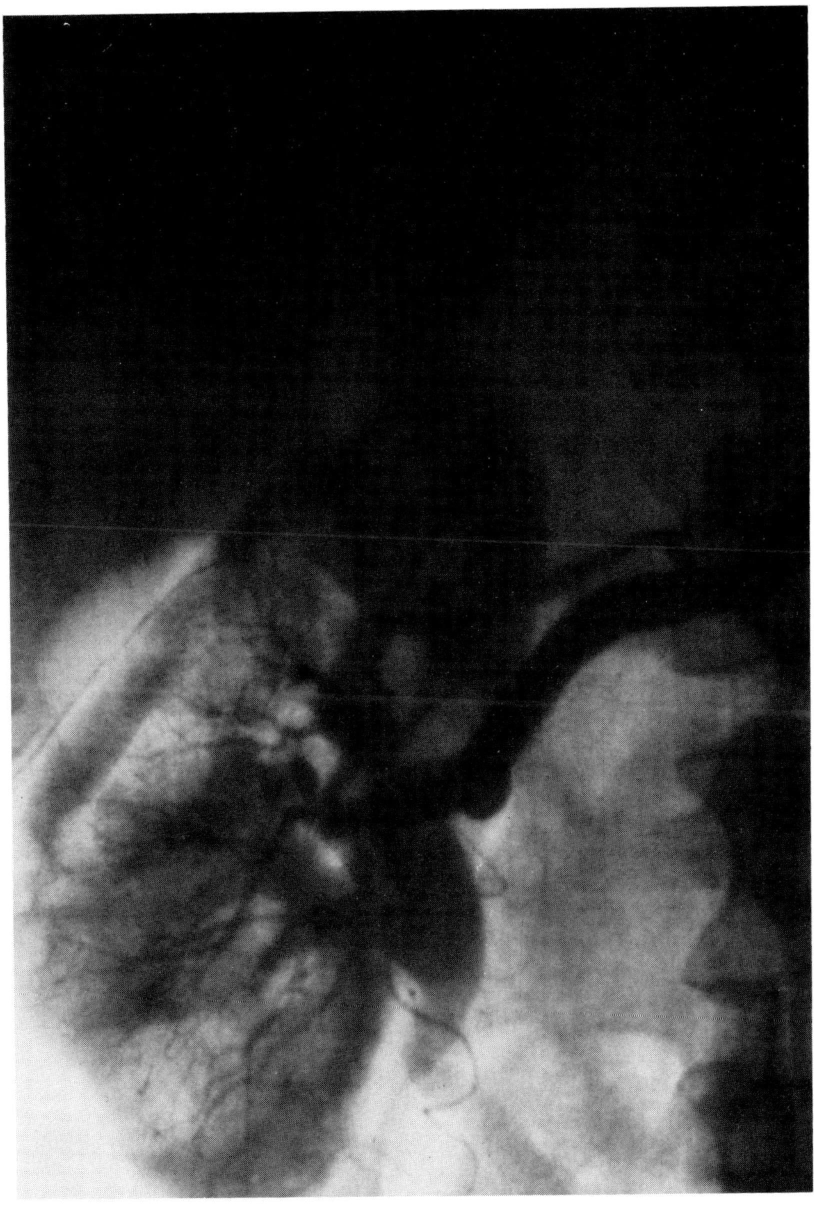

Fig. 2. Right renal arteriogram postdilatation.

RESULTS

Twenty-seven patients underwent 28 angioplasties, and 26 had successful procedures performed. A subintimal dissection occurred in one patient during selective renal arteriography prior to attempted angioplasty. The procedure was aborted without untoward problems and the patient remained hypertensive. The case was included as a procedural failure. In another patient, the selective guidewire and balloon catheter were passed through the obstructed renal segment, but the lesion could not be anatomically dilated. In the remaining 25 patients, successful anatomic dilatation was performed. In one patient, anatomic stenosis recurred 6 months following PTA coinciding with recurrence of clinical hypertension. Angioplasty was again successfully performed.

Beginning promptly after dilatation, brisk fall in both systolic and diastolic blood pressure occurred in all 25 patients. Patients with localizing differential renin values had a more precipitous blood pressure drop and lower terminal blood pressures at 48 hours than patients without localizing differential renin levels (Fig. 3).

In group I (hypertension with normal renal function), the blood pressure in 16 patients averaged 190/110 mm Hg on hospital admission and at 48 hours following dilatation averaged 135/70 mm Hg (Fig. 4). At 1 month following the procedure, this same group had an average blood pressure of 135/80 mm Hg and at 3 months 130/80 mm Hg. Blood pressure in seven patients followed to 6 months rose to 170/90 mm Hg, but the sample size fell off after this point. This

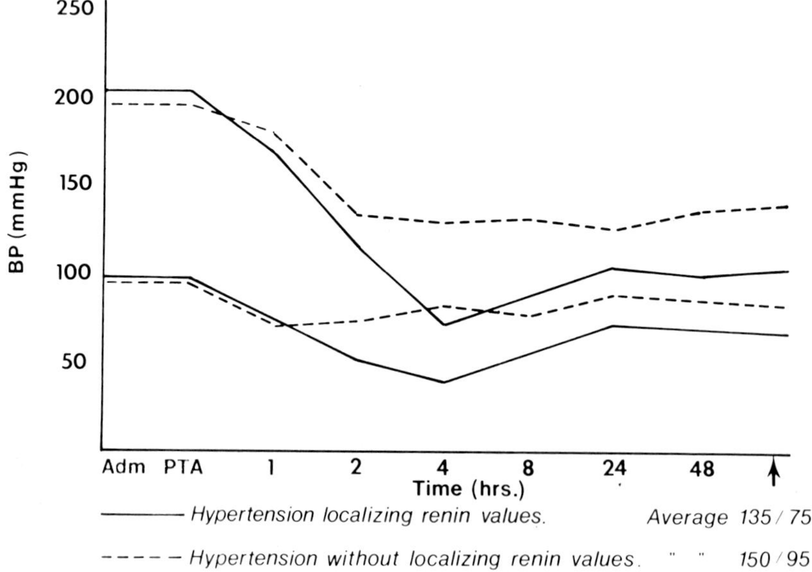

Fig. 3. Hypertensive values.

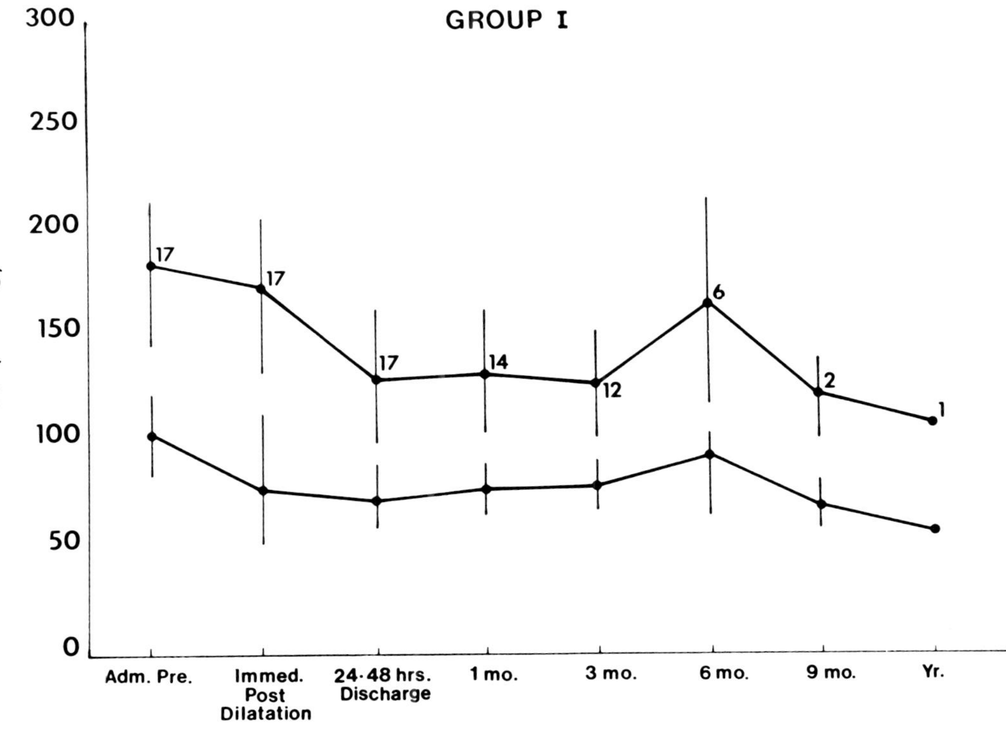

Fig. 4. Blood pressures. Number adjacent to systolic pressure equals total number of patients available for evaluation at that interval.

6 month average blood pressure rise was a consequence of a single patient who became severely hypertensive from restenosis at this interval.

This same hypertensive group (Group I) averaged 3.1 major antihypertensive medications per patient prior to angioplasty, 1.3 drugs per patient at the time of discharge, and 1.6 drugs per patient at last followup from 1 to 12 months following PTA (Fig. 5).

In group II (hypertension with azotemia), 11 patients had an average blood pressure on admission of 205/102 mm Hg. A similar although not as dramatic postangioplasty fall in blood pressure was noted in this group (Fig. 6). Blood pressure at 48 hours following PTA averaged 175/66 mm Hg. Blood pressure remained controlled in seven patients at 1 month, averaging 135/75 mm Hg, but in five of these patients at 3 months the average pressure had risen to 180/80 mm Hg. This same group was taking an average of 2.5 major antihypertensive medications on admission, which progressively rose at discharge and at last followup to 2.6 and 3.3 drugs per patient, respectively (Fig. 5). One patient in

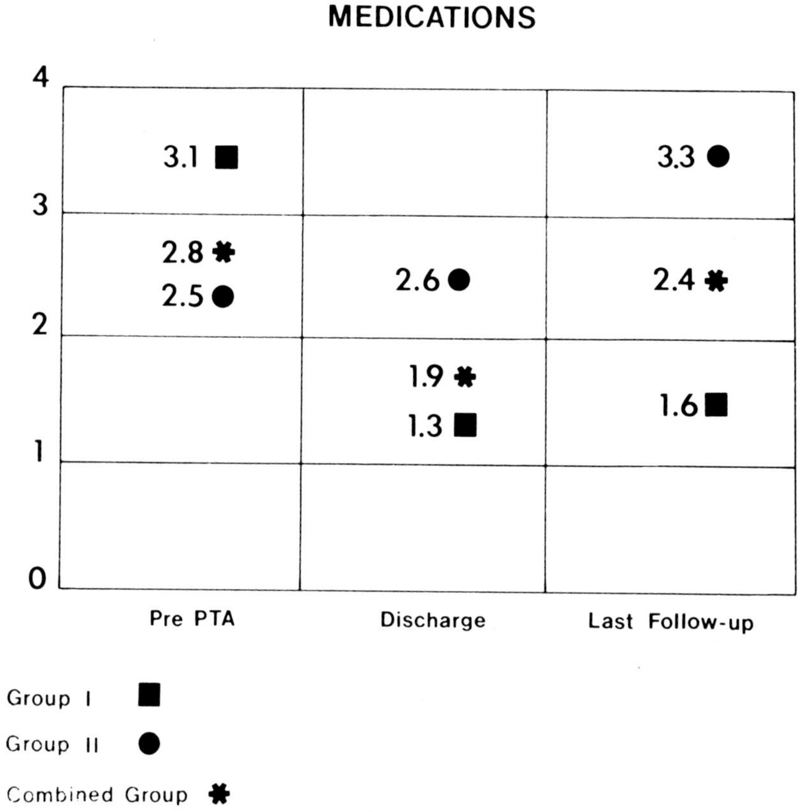

MEDICATIONS

	Pre PTA	Discharge	Last Follow-up
Group I ■	3.1	1.3	1.6
Group II ●	2.5	2.6	3.3
Combined Group ✱	2.8	1.9	2.4

Group I ■
Group II ●
Combined Group ✱

Fig. 5. Medications. Number of major antihypertensive drugs/patient.

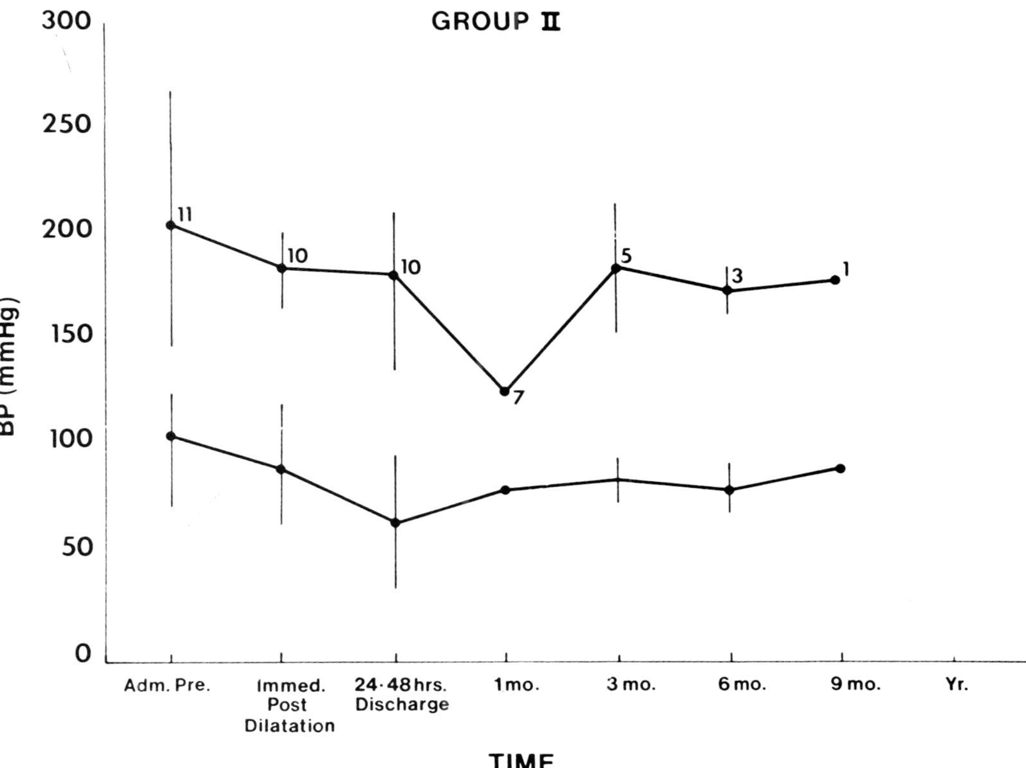

Fig. 6. Blood pressure. Number adjacent to systolic pressure equals total number of patients available for evaluation at that interval.

this group died 2 months following dilatation from the complications of a myocardial infarction.

In group I, renal function which was normal predilatation remained normal in all patients at 48 hours and until last evaluation following angioplasty (Fig. 7). The markedly compromised preangioplasty renal function in group II patients did not significantly improve either early or late following dilatation.

The single patient with fibromuscular hyperplasia included in group I remained controlled with a blood pressure of 110/70 mm Hg at 1 year following dilatation on antihypertensive medications (Figs. 8 and 9).

DISCUSSION

Percutaneous transluminal angioplasty would seem to be an attractive alternative to the more classical, time honored, and proven operative approaches to renovascular hypertension. For this statement to be entirely true, three considerations must be met: the procedure must be simple, safe, and therapeutically effective.

The procedure is without question simple, but only if performed by an experienced, careful angiographer who understands the meticulous techniques that are required with angioplastic procedures. The capability of performing high quality, selective arteriography to accurately define the obstructed lesion must

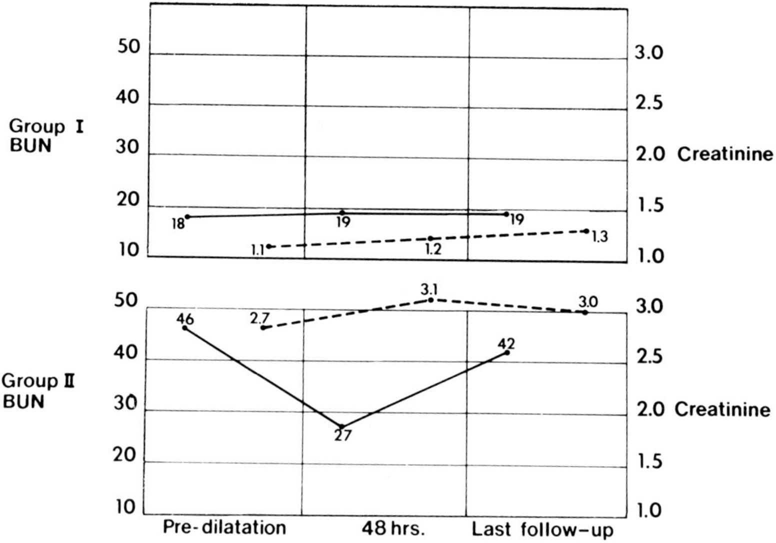

Fig. 7. BUN (solid line) and creatinine (dashed line) levels.

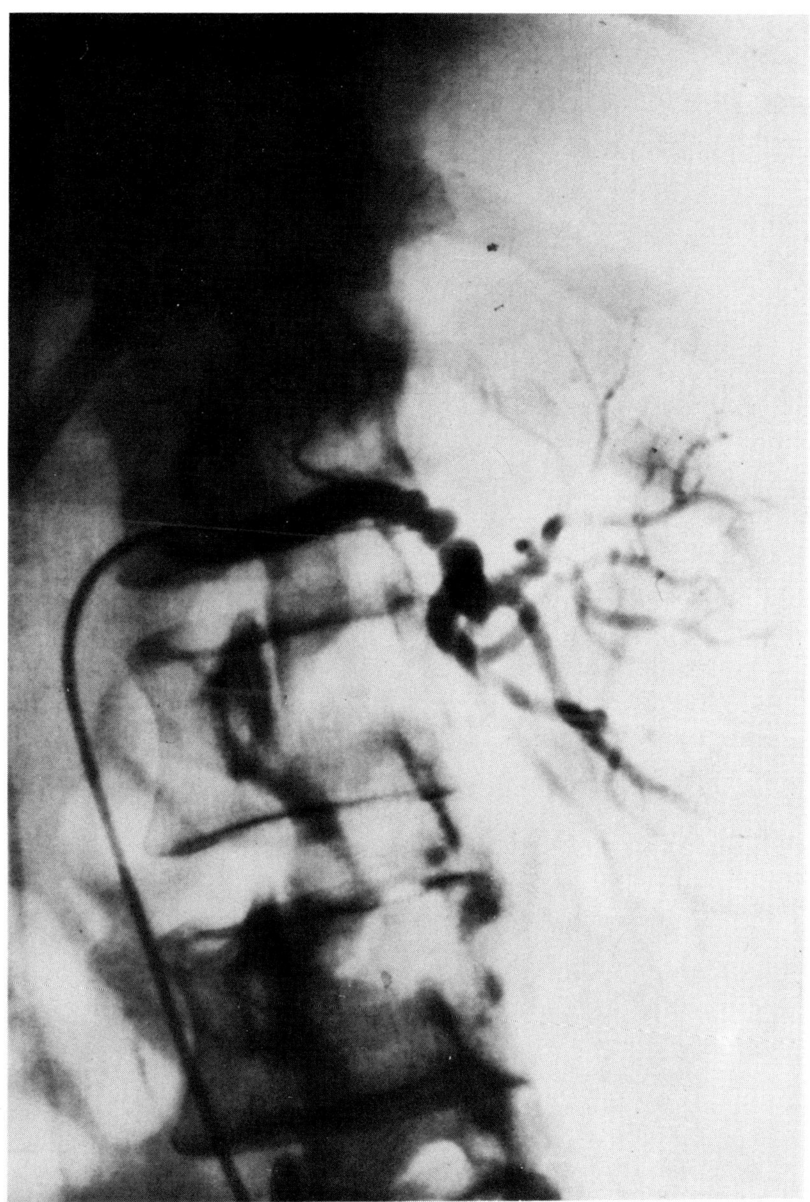

Fig. 8. Left renal arteriogram predilatation in patient with fibromuscular hyperplasia.

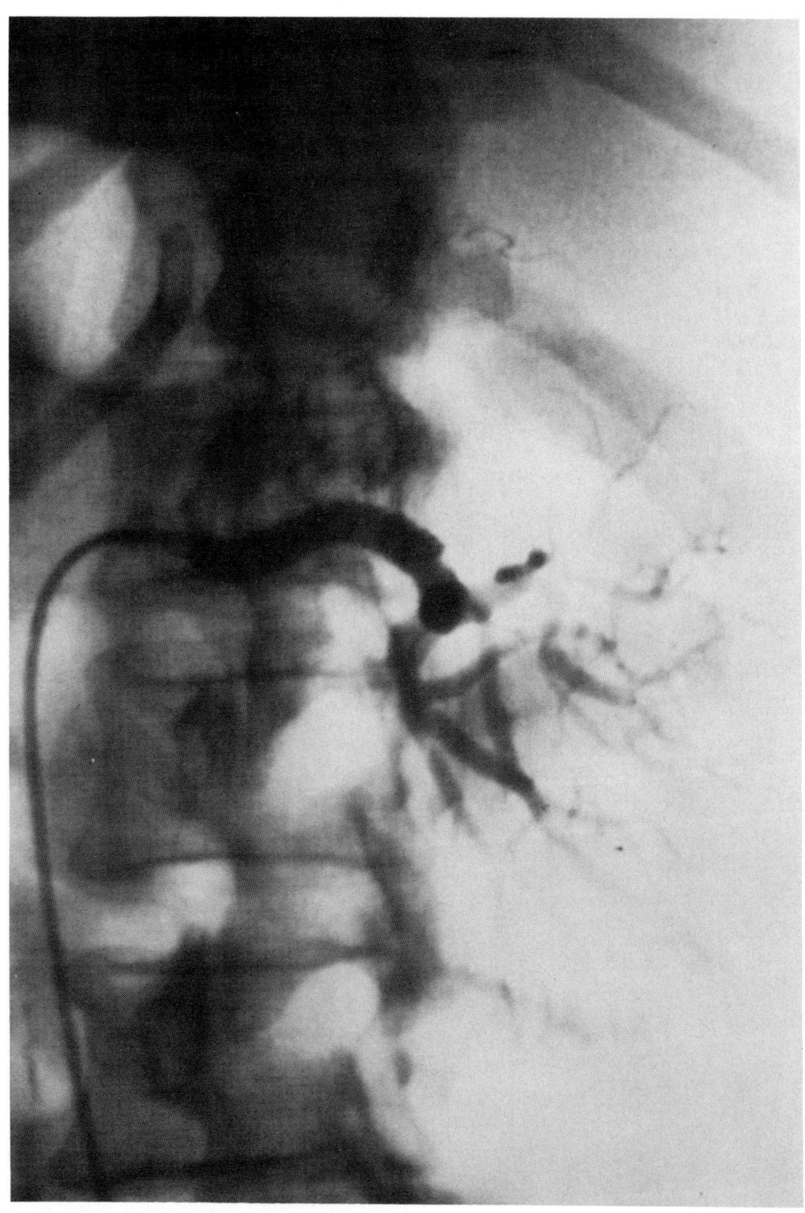

Fig. 9. Left renal arteriogram postdilatation in patient with fibromuscular hyperplasia.

obviously be available so that only appropriate patients can be selected for dilatation.

The procedure can be performed using standard angiographic techniques in any well equipped angiographic laboratory. High quality balloon catheters are now commercially available from multiple manufacturers. The procedure is brief, usually taking less than 90 minutes to perform. The patient's discomfort is minimal and generally related to local catheterization site trauma and the necessity of lying supine and immobile on a firm x-ray table. The usual sensation of a hot flush with dye infusion during angiography does occur, but discomfort from catheter manipulation and inflation during dilatation is unusual. The occurrence of pain during balloon inflation suggests that overdistention of the vessel has occurred with stretching of adventitial perivascular nerve fibers.

Gruntzig has demonstrated histopathologically that dilatation eliminates a local obstructive lesion by dispersing the subintimal obstructive debris into the arterial medial layer while preserving the smooth intimal surface [6]. Overdistention of the vessel with fracture of outer medial layers allows subadventitial extravasation of atherosclerotic debris and likely sets the stage for false aneurysm formation and possible vessel rupture. This problem has not been encountered in this series.

Gradual, steady blood pressure decline over a 48 hour period following PTA is the usual early response. Infrequently, however, precipitous hypotension may immediately follow dilatation; therefore frequent serial blood pressure evaluations are necessary in the early hours following dilatation. Vigorous fluid volume loading is occasionally necessary in managing this brisk pressure drop. In only one patient in our series was transient vasopressor therapy necessary. Figure 10 illustrates this patient's precipitous blood pressure drop. Immediately following carotid thromboendarterectomy, this patient had further acceleration of chronic hypertension. Aggressive systemic antihypertensive therapy with large doses of nitroprusside and hydralazine was unsuccessful in controlling hypertension. Rather significant wound bleeding occurred and it was felt that prompt renal dilatation would be helpful in controlling this malignant hypertensive course. A dilatation was performed uneventfully (Figs. 11 and 12). Fortunately, the patient tolerated the transient hypotensive episode without untoward sequelae. The large amounts of antihypertensive drugs that this patient received immediately predilatation were likely responsible for this dramatic blood pressure fall and obviously should be avoided immediately prior to dilatation to minimize this potentially serious problem.

The patients are kept supine for approximately 12 hours following dilatation to prevent the occurrence of orthostatic hypotension and catheterization site bleeding. The patients are mobilized at 24 hours following the procedure and are usually ready for discharge 48-72 hours later. By this period, blood pressure levels have generally stabilized. Further manipulation of required antihypertensive therapy can usually be managed on an outpatient basis. This brief hospital

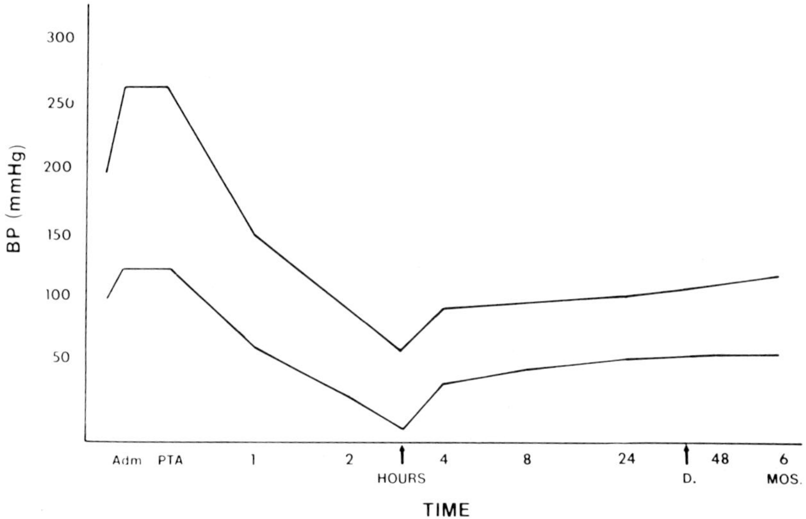

Fig. 10. Postoperatively patient developed dramatic BP rise upon admission to ICU. First arrow notes initiation of vasopressor therapy (continued for 1 hour). Arrow at "D" notes discharge from ICU.

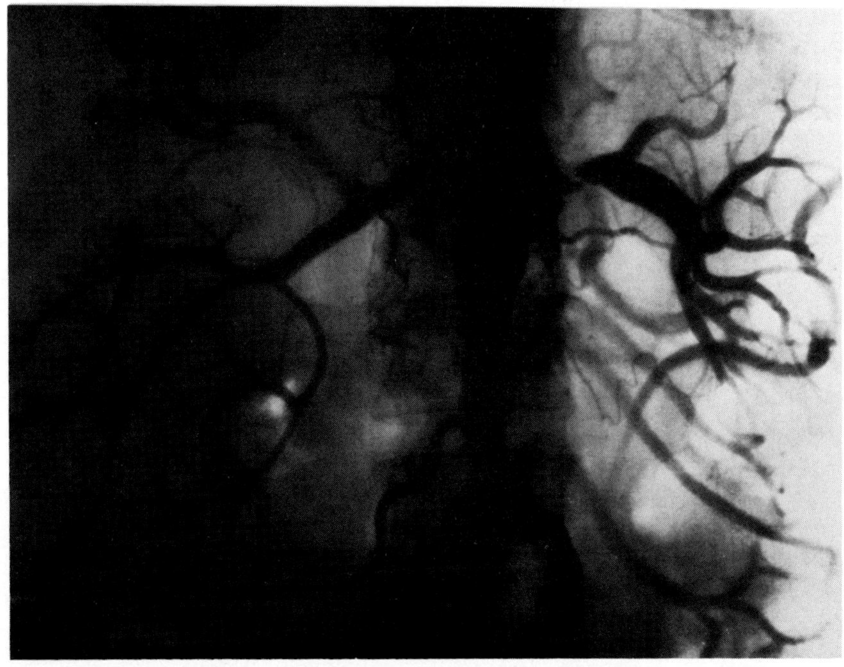

Fig. 11. Left renal arteriogram predilatation.

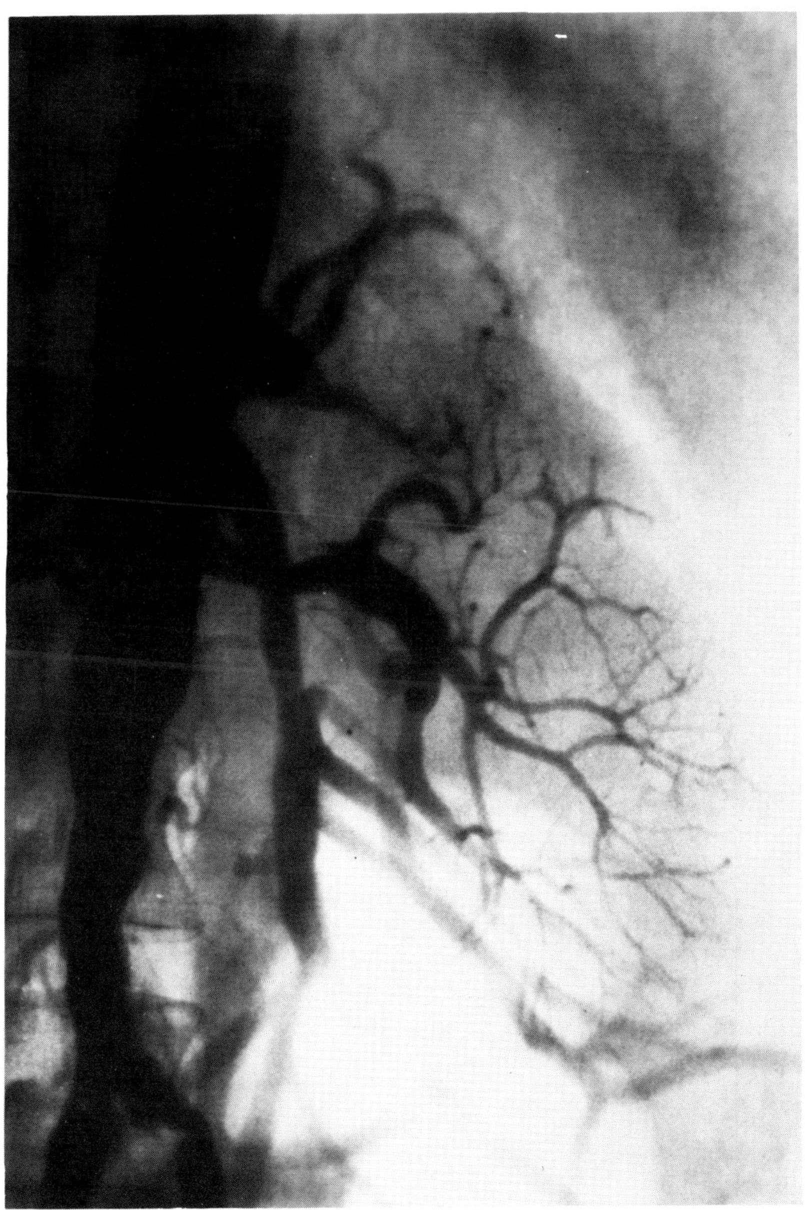

Fig. 12. Left renal arteriogram postdilatation.

stay and relatively inexpensive radiologic procedure compare favorably to the more lengthy hospital stay and higher surgical costs which accompany the more classic operative approaches. The procedure also allows the patient to return very promptly to a functional productive capacity. Both considerations make PTA a cost effective therapeutic approach to renovascular hypertension.

The patient's safety during and following the procedure must also be considered when evaluating this new technique. In our series of 27 patients, only one complication specifically related to PTA occurred. A small subintimal dissection occurred in one patient during selective renal arteriography prior to attempted dilatation. Patency of the renal vessel was maintained and no untoward result developed. Angioplasty, however, was not performed. In another patient, although the selective balloon catheter could be manipulated through a tight renal arterial obstruction, the lesion was so rigid that despite maximal balloon inflation to 5 atmospheres of pressure, dilatation did not occur. Because present catheter design prevents safe inflation above this pressure, nothing further could be done. Therefore the procedure was terminated, again without harmful effect. Because the hemodynamically significant lesion was not altered, this patient, as predicted, did not have the usual hypotensive response and has remained clinically hypertensive requiring aggressive medical therapy. These two patients remain treatment failures, but no harm has resulted.

All misfortunes that can occur with percutaneous angiographic techniques are theoretically possible with selective renal angiography and dilatation. These include local puncture site injury and/or bleeding, overdistention of the renal artery with false aneurysm formation and/or rupture, arterial thrombosis, distal embolization, etc. None of these problems have occurred in this series. Similarly, in a combined series of five patients reported by Gruntzig [8] and Katzen [10], no major complications are described.

Furthermore, in our personal series of over 100 peripheral PTAs the single technical complication that occurred was a postdilatation false aneurysm at an iliac dilatation site. Overzealous dilatation with an inappropriately large balloon may be responsible for medial and adventitial fracture with extravasation leading to false aneurysm formation. Dilatation of an obstructive segment to approximate the size of an adjacent poststenotic dilated arterial lumen is neither wise nor advisable. It is imperative, however, than an obstructive lesion be dilated to a luminal diameter that eliminates the flow limiting lesion. Pressure measurements across the lesion during the study are essential in assessing this adequacy of dilatation.

No recognized problems from peripheral embolization have occurred in either this series or the larger arterial series. Microhematuria, free urinary fat globules, and hyaline cast formation probably represent the best clinical evidence of tissue trauma from embolization. Occasional hyaline casts were noted in post-PTA urine specimens, but no free fat or microscopic hematuria appeared.

Should microembolization occur, it is doubtful that major difficulty would follow unless these fragments showered in large volume. Deliberate segmental renal arterial embolization has been reported in the treatment of both renal hemorrhage [2] and hypertension secondary to peripheral segmental renal artery stenosis [12], both without subsequent hypertension developing.

The procedure is easily performed with local anesthetic techniques; thus the potential risks of general anesthesia are avoided. Likewise, the patient is spared operative trauma with its attendant blood loss and potential complications. If dilatation fails, as it did in two patients in this series, then the classic operative approaches remain available and can be performed without delay.

Does intraluminal dilatation induce adventitial or perivascular inflammation, fibrosis, and scarring? This question is of obvious concern to the surgeon who considers possible future standard operative treatment of dilatation failures. Obviously, these changes would result in increased operative technical difficulties. This consideration remains unanswered. However, one patient in this series underwent aortic thromboendarterectomy and aortobifemoral bypass grafting 4 months following renal dilatation. Extensive dissection of the dilated renal artery revealed the vessel to be soft and pliable without evidence of perivascular inflammatory reaction.

Should stenosis recur following PTA, the possibility of repeat dilatation with secondary therapeutic benefit remains. In this series, one patient remained normotensive (130/75 mm Hg) on minimal medication for 6 months following dilatation (Figs. 13 and 14), and then developed aggressive recurrence of symptoms and hypertension (230/110 mm Hg). Restenosis was documented angiographically (Fig. 15), and redilatation was uneventfully performed (Fig. 16). This dilatation resulted in a more satisfactory angiographic appearance than the initial PTA. The patient's blood pressure remained acceptably controlled at 130/80 mm Hg early postdilatation although yet requiring antihypertensive drugs.

Important factors which may predispose to early restenosis are not yet known but may include patient age, predilatation blood pressure level and duration, anatomy, technical ease of dilatation, postdilatation blood pressure course, etc. Long-term fate of patients who develop restenosis early following angioplasty is not clear. It may be that redilatation will not be effective in achieving sustained control of hypertension in these patients. These patients, like those who are immediate dilatation failures, may need standard operative revascularization procedures performed.

The last and probably most important consideration in evaluating renal PTA concerns its therapeutic effectiveness. Many series have documented that operative revascularization can be performed with minimal risk and very acceptable early and long-term results. In the Foster et al. [4] classic series of 122 patients followed a minimum of 6 months, over 90% of these patients were either cured

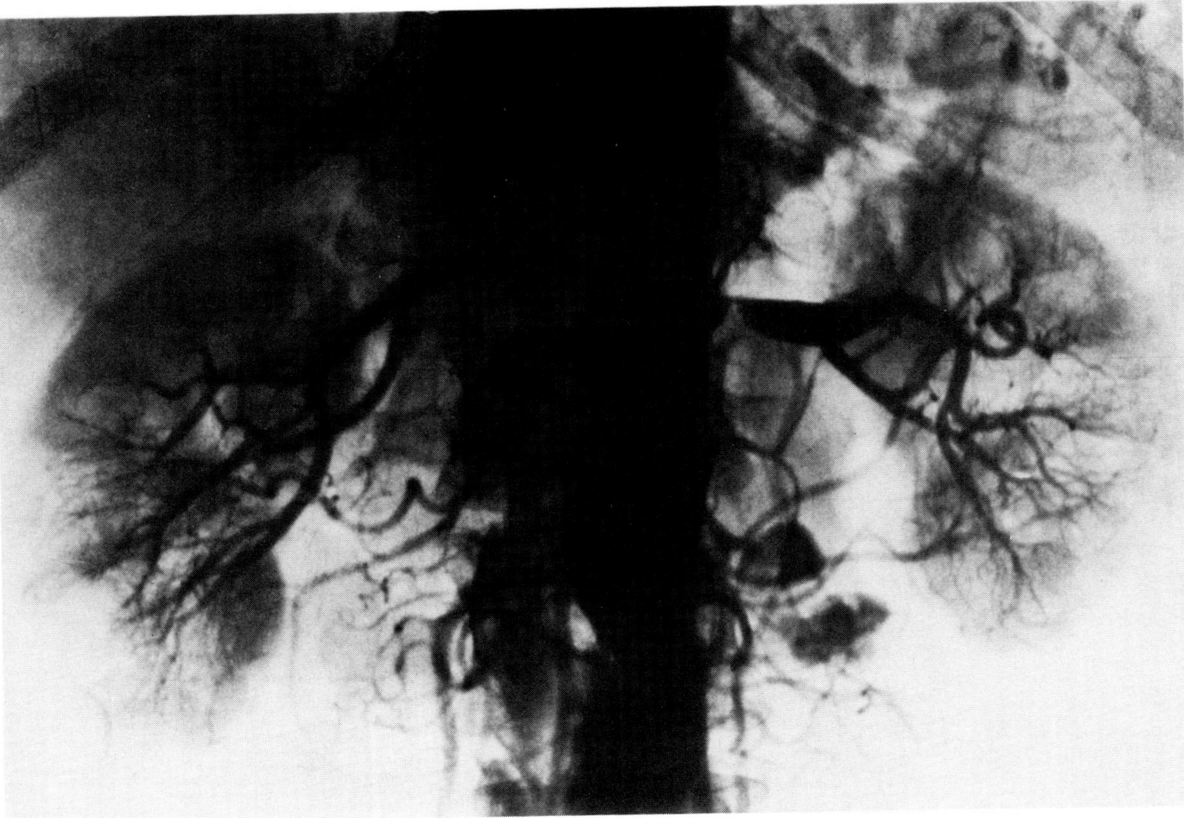

Fig. 13. Left renal arteriogram predilatation.

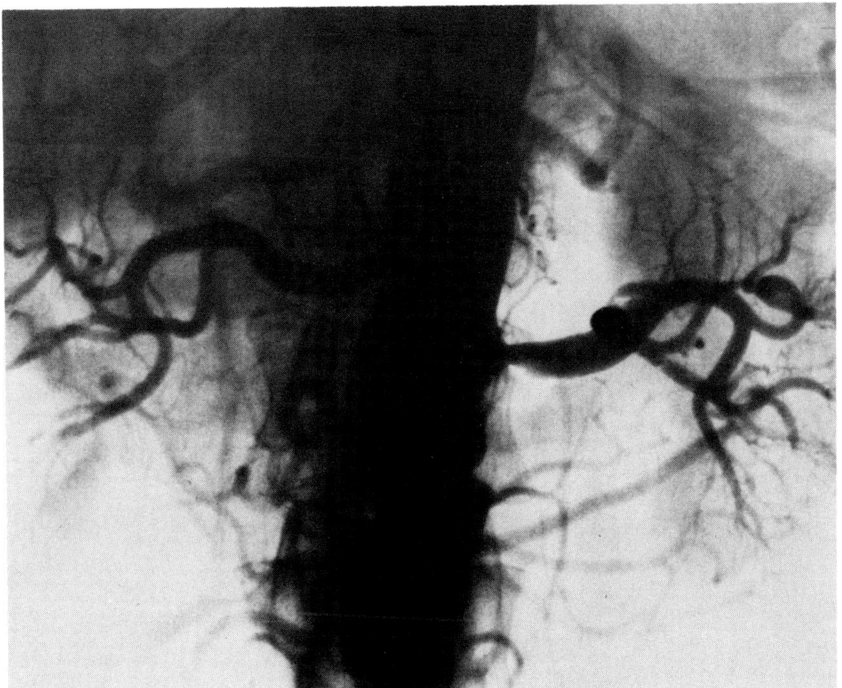

Fig. 14. Left renal arteriogram following initial dilatation.

or improved.* However, death occurred in eight patients (6.6%) and major postoperative complications occured in 34%. McComb reported similar treatment effectiveness with no operative deaths in 38 patients [11]. Major morbidity was not reported. These reports must be considered as the "gold standard" to which renal PTA must be compared in evaluating therapeutic benefit.

In group I (hypertension with normal renal function), all 16 patients had a brisk blood pressure drop immediately following dilatation. This blood pressure control has persisted in all but one patient at last followup ranging from 2 weeks to 1 year following PTA (Fig. 4). Likewise, the need for antihypertensive medication has been significantly reduced (Fig. 5).

Recurrent hypertension developed 6 months following dilatation in one patient and is responsible for the brisk elevation of average blood pressure at the 6 month interval in Fig. 4. This patient, as mentioned earlier, developed

*Cured, normotensive with diastolic blood pressure less than 90 mm Hg; improved, reduction of diastolic blood pressure greater than 20 mm Hg but with diastolic blood pressure remaining 90-100 mm Hg.

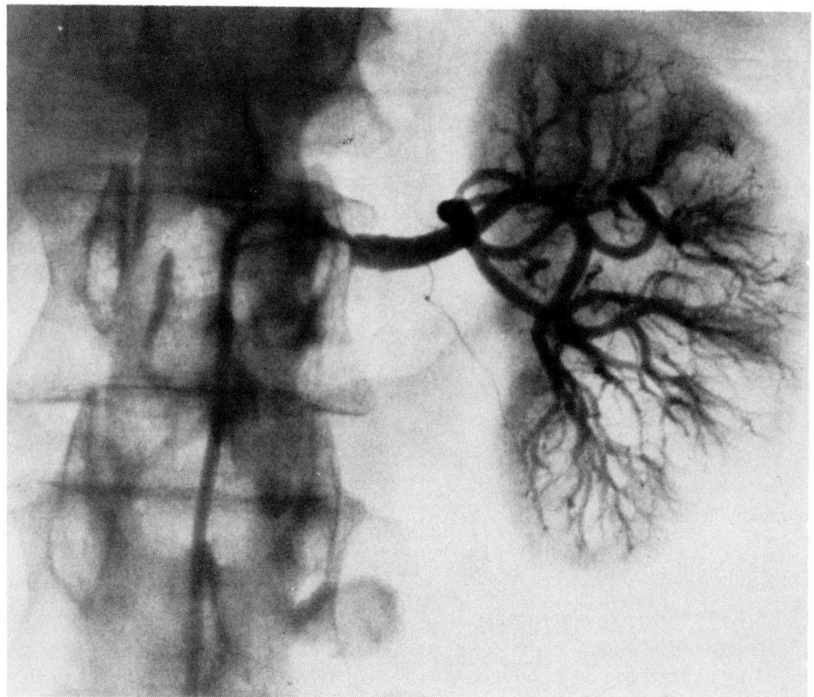

Fig. 15. Six months following initial PTA, with left renal arteriogram demonstrating recurrent stenosis.

recurrent stenosis, was uneventfully redilated, and has remained normotensive since.

Patients with differential localizing renin levels (greater than 2.1 ng/ml/hr) had more abrupt and profound pressure drop following PTA than those without (Fig. 3). Likewise, blood pressure at discharge was substantially lower in patients with localizing renin elevations. From a pathophysiologic standpoint, this result is as expected and is also in keeping with the results in operatively treated series.

In group II (hypertension with azotemia), 11 patients were dilated in an attempt to preserve and/or improve renal function. The first patient in this group and the one with by far the best overall result was a 53 year old woman admitted in renal failure with a blood pressure of 260/120 mm Hg. BUN and creatinine were 146 and 7 mg%, respectively, and the patient was anuric. Hemodialysis was performed three times prior to angiography which subsequently documented a 90% right renal artery obstruction (Fig. 17). The left kidney was not functional secondary to chronic hydronephrosis resulting from an earlier ureteral injury during pelvic surgery. Dilatation was uneventfully performed (Fig. 18) in a salvage effort to avoid a high risk major operative procedure. Four hours following dilatation, urinary output began. Within the

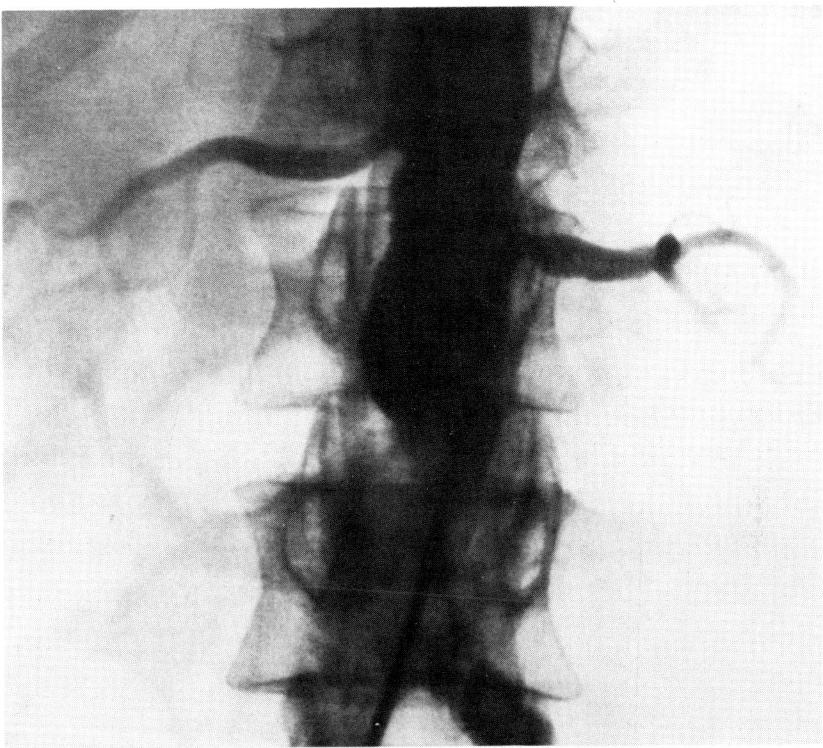

Fig. 16. Left renal arteriogram immediately following redilatation.

next 5 days, progressive improvement in renal function occurred and transient high output renal failure resolved. No further dialysis was required and the patient was discharged 10 days later. Nine months following PTA, blood pressure was 175/90 mm Hg and BUN and creatinine levels were 11 and 1.3 mg%, respectively. The patient has remained on no antihypertensive medications, and repeat arteriogram 9 months following PTA is seen in Fig. 19.

Two other patients in this group were immediate dilatation failures and have remained severely hypertensive. Renal arterial dissection occurred in one during angiography and dilatation was not attempted. Another had very diffuse, aggressive atherosclerotic obstructive disease with a rigid renal artery and dilatation could not be technically accomplished. One other patient developed recurrent hypertension (210/95 mm Hg) 3 months following dilatation.

Long-term blood pressure response was not as dramatic in this group as those patients with normal renal function. Figure 6 illustrates that while diastolic pressures have remained relatively well controlled for up to 9 months, systolic pressures have remained modestly elevated. This group also has continued to require aggressive drug therapy to maintain blood pressure control (Fig. 5). With

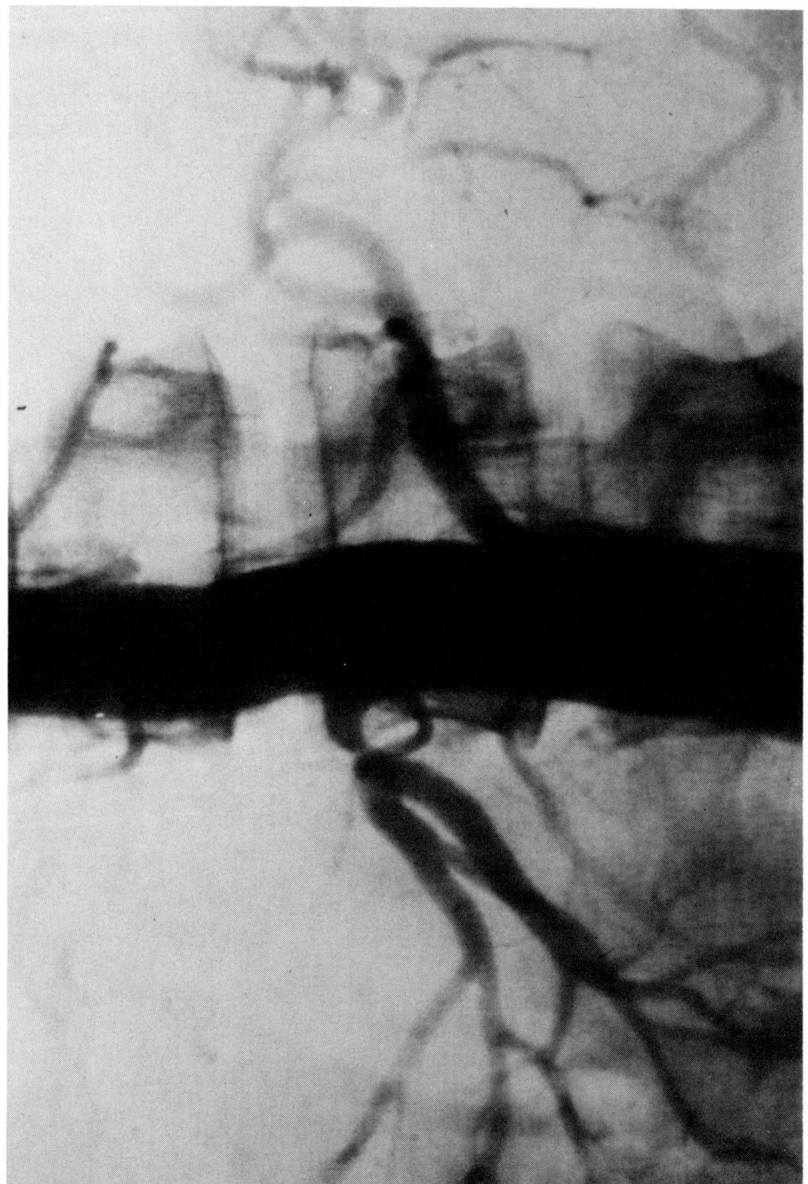

Fig. 17. Right renal arteriogram predilatation.

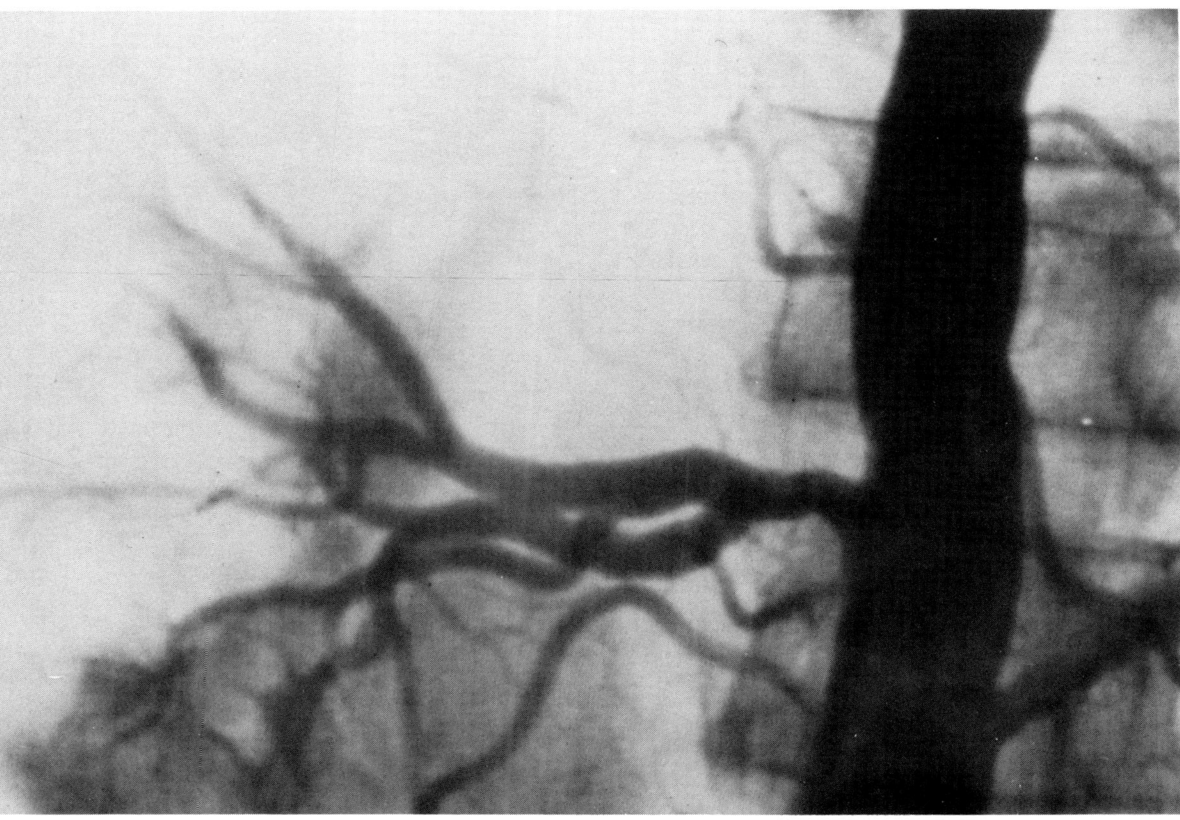

Fig. 18. Right renal arteriogram immediately postdilatation.

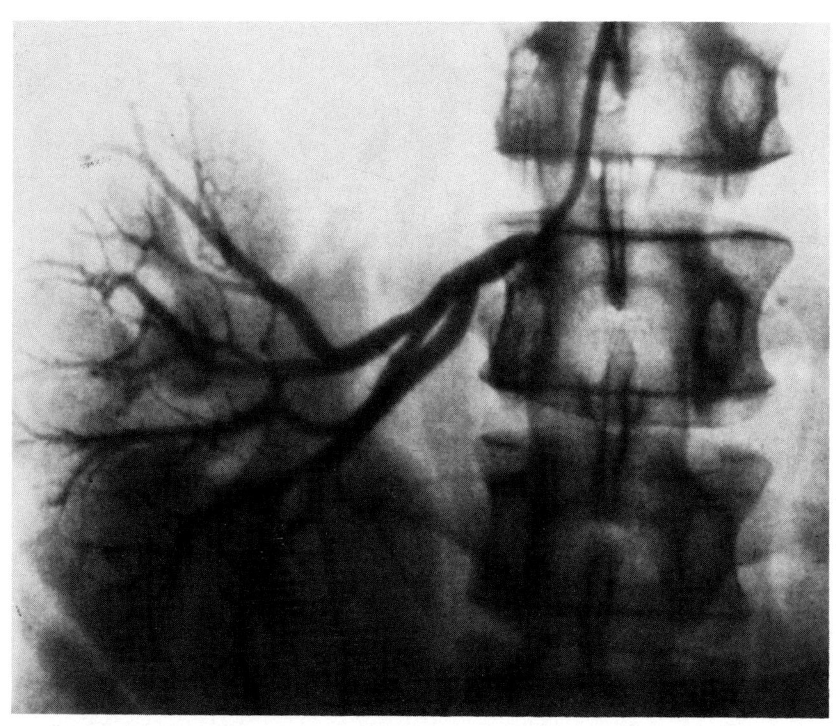

Fig. 19. Right renal arteriogram 9 months following PTA.

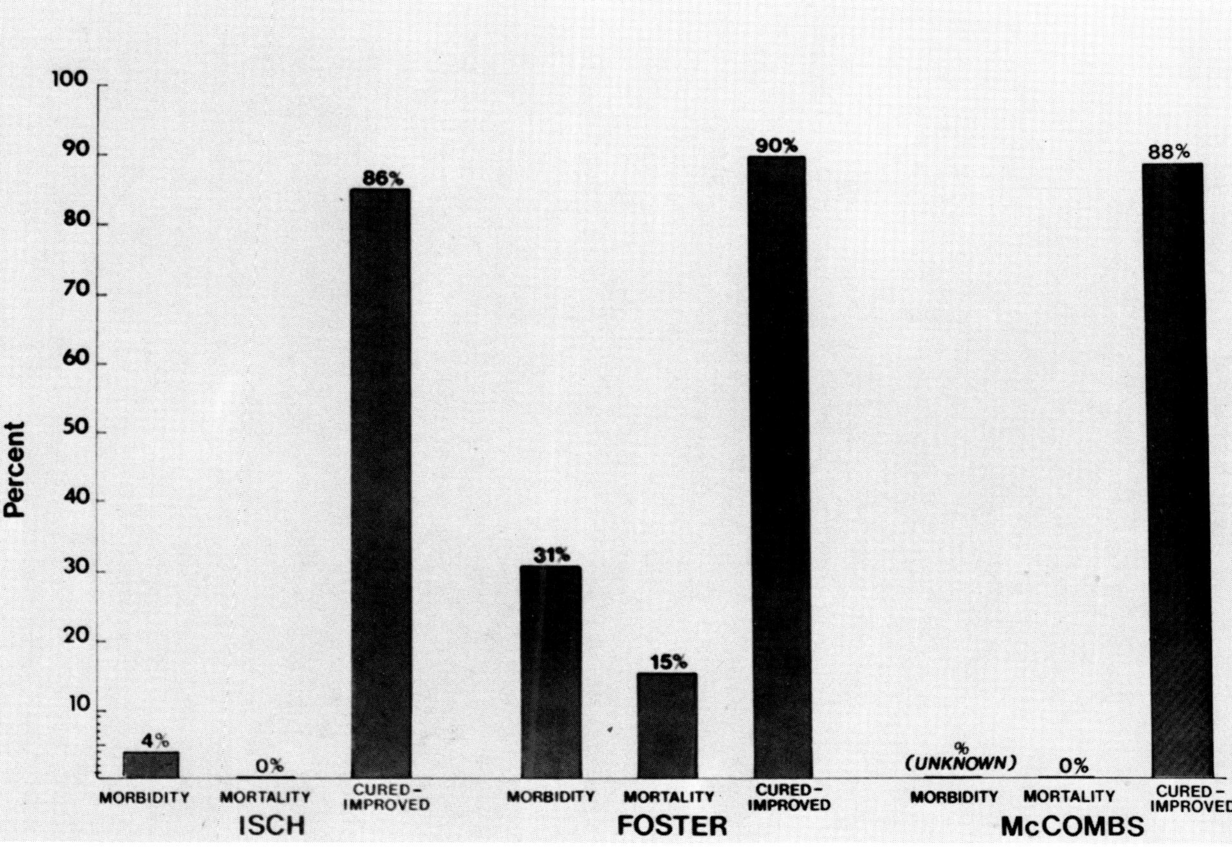

Fig. 20. Results of various studies.

the exception of the rather dramatic case mentioned above, little improvement in renal function has occurred in this group as noted by serial BUN and creatinine levels (Fig. 7).

REFERENCES

1. Bookstein JJ, Abrams HL, Buenger RE: Radiologic aspect of renovascular hypertension. Part 2. The role of urology in unilateral renovascular disease. JAMA 220:1225, 1972
2. Chuang VP, Reuter SR, Walter J, et al: Control of renal hemorrhage by selective arterial embolization. Am. J. Roentgenol. 125:300-306, 1975
3. Dotter CT, Judkins MP: Transluminal treatment of arteriosclerotic obstruction. Circulation 30:654-670, 1964
4. Foster JH, Dean RH, Pinkerton JA, et al: Ten years experience with the surgical management of renovascular hypertension. Ann. Surg. 177:755-766, 1973
5. Foster JH, Rhamy RK, Oates JA, et al: Renovascular hypertension secondary to atherosclerosis. Am. J. Med. 46:741-750, 1969
6. Gruntzig A: Personal communication, 1975
7. Gruntzig A, Bollinger A, Brunner U, et al: Perkutane rekanalisation chronischer arterieller verschlusse nach Dotter – Eine nicht-operative kathetertechnik. Schweiz. Med. Wochenschr. 103:825-831, 1973
8. Gruntzig A, Kuhlmann U, Vetter W, et al: Treatment of renovascular hypertension with percutaneous transluminal dilatation of a renal artery stenosis. Lancet 1:801-802, 1978
9. Kaplan NM: Clinical Hypertension. New York, Medcom Press, 1973
10. Katzen B, Chang J, Lukowsky G, et al: Percutaneous transluminal angioplasty for treatment of renovascular hypertension. Radiology 131:53-58, 1979
11. McCombs PR, Berkowitz HD, Roberts B: Operative management of renovascular hypertension. Ann. Surg. 182:762-766, 1975
12. Reuter SR, Pomeroy PR, Chuang VP, et al: Embolic control of hypertension caused by sequential renal artery stenosis. Am. J. Roentgenol. 127:389-392, 1976
13. Simon N, Franklin SS, Bleifer KH, et al: Clinical characteristic of renovascular hypertension. JAMA 220:1209, 1972
14. Stanley JC, Fry WJ: Renovascular hypertension secondary to arterial fibrodysplasia in adults. Arch. Surg. 110:922-928, 1975

William J. Casarella, M.D.

Percutaneous Transluminal Angioplasty of the Renal and Iliac Arteries

In 1964 Dotter and Judkins [4] introduced the concept of nonoperative dilatation of atherosclerotic arterial stenoses by the passage of catheters through obstructing vascular lesions. Their technique was a logical extension of standard diagnostic angiography. Stiff Teflon catheters were introduced percutaneously with standard Seldinger technique and spring guidewires advanced to the point of obstruction in the superficial femoral artery. In the majority of stenoses and in most total occlusions the guidewire could be passed through the lesion and followed by the stiff 8 French Teflon catheter. In order to further dilate the vessel, the technique then required coaxial passage of a larger 12 French catheter through the lesion. The net effect was radial compression of soft atheromatous material against the arterial wall and effective dilatation of the lesion. In a report of their results in 1968 [5], Dotter et al. claimed a 71% primary success rate in 41 patients with superficial femoral artery stenosis and only a 29% success rate in 112 patients with total occlusion of the superficial femoral artery. In 30 patients being considered for amputation, 12 were successfully dilated and amputation averted. In a later report in 1973, Zeitler [17] reported Dotter's results in 237 patients with a 90% success rate in superficial femoral stenoses, an 80% primary success in lesions less than 2 cm long, a 30% success rate for occlusions of 2-10 cm, and only a 10% success for those longer than 10 cm.

Although Dotter and his co-workers at the University of Oregon did much of the pioneering, innovative early work with percutaneous vascular recanalization, the major advances during the past 10 years have come from several European workers. Zeitler, working at the Agger Talklinik in Engelskirchen, West Germany, accumulated the most experience with catheter dilatation of the superficial femoral artery. In 1975 he reported his primary results [20] in 534 patients with superficial femoral artery lesions. In his series 93% with stenosis had a primary success. In total occlusions, his group achieved successful dilatation in 88% of lesions less than 10 cm long and in 72% of those lesions longer than 10 cm. In his review of the work of Brahme in Malmö, Sweden and Berglund in Karlstad, Sweden, van Andel [15] noted similar results with a 90% success rate in stenoses and a 60% success in occlusions less than 6 cm compared with a 39% success rate in longer occlusions. In van Andel's own series, an 89% success rate was reported in femoral dilatation.

Initial results with catheter dilatation of the superficial femoral arteries in the United States and Europe could probably be summarized as being promising with a high degree of success in stenoses and a considerably lesser chance of success in occlusions. Not unexpectedly, the longer the occlusion, the more likely was the procedure to fail.

ILIAC ARTERY ANGIOPLASTY

In 1974 Grüntzig and Hopff [7] introduced a new catheter which was destined to broaden the applicability of transluminal angioplasty to branches of the aorta other than the superficial femoral artery and to vessels larger than 12 French in caliber. Their design consists of a basic polyethylene catheter of varying sizes and an outer sleeve catheter made of polyvinyl chloride which fits very snugly over it. A segment of the polyvinyl chloride sleeve is prestretched to a desired diameter for varying lengths, and the stretched segment communicates with the catheter hub by means of a groove cut in the surface of the inner catheter. The cylindrical polyvinyl chloride balloon near the catheter tip can then be filled with dilute contrast material to a predetermined length and caliber after the catheter has been positioned at the appropriate site to dilate the lesion. Usually a 7F catheter with a 4-6 mm balloon may be used in the femoral arteries and a 9F catheter with a 7-10 mm balloon used for the iliac vessels. Prior to the introduction of this catheter, Zeitler [16] attempted to dilate iliac artery lesions with a Fogarty-type balloon catheter. Although the precise results were not reported, technical difficulties were encountered because of the spherical shape of the catheter and a tendency of it to overinflate with small increases in pressure applied to the balloon. With simple latex catheters, Zeitler found that the balloon expanded in the path of least resistance and frequently failed to dilate the more resistant diseased portion of the vessel. Porstmann [13] attempted to solve this problem in 1973 with the introduction of the so-called "corset" catheter or "caged-balloon" system. Basically he cut four 1 cm longitudinal strips in an 8F Teflon catheter and advanced a latex balloon through the Teflon catheter to the area of the Teflon strips or cage. When the balloon was inflated, the strips prevented overinflation and allowed greater pressure to be delivered to the arterial stenosis. At the present time, the Grüntzig system has become the method of choice in performing iliac artery angioplasty because of

GRÜNTZIG BALLOON DILATATION CATHETER

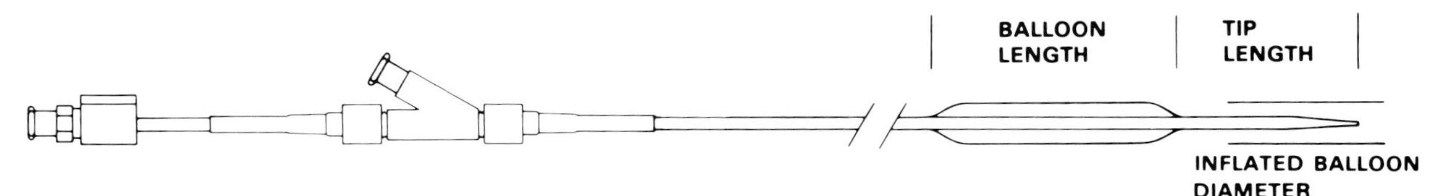

Fig. 1. Diagram of the two-lumen Grüntzig balloon catheter. The polyvinyl chloride outer sleeve of the catheter is fashioned into a cylindrical balloon which can be manufactured in various lengths and calibers for different lesions. The tip length can also be shortened for applications in the renal arteries.

its ease of insertion, relative safety, great flexibility, and the variety of balloons and sizes that can be pretailored to fit the needs of the individual patient.

With the introduction of the Grüntzig balloon catheter, iliac artery angioplasty has become significantly easier to perform. In their compilation of results of iliac angioplasties performed in seven European centers, Grüntzig and Zeitler [19] collected 206 cases of iliac artery stenosis treated by balloon angioplasty. The average age was 58 years, with a 9:1 male to female sex ratio. In five centers most of the lesions were stenoses, although more than 50% of the cases from Munich and Pecs, Hungary were total occlusions. The average success rate was 92%, and in 3% of the failures complications that required surgical intervention were encountered. This compares favorably to a primary success rate of 74% in the femoral artery in association with a 10% complication rate at the same centers. Grüntzig's personal series of iliac artery stenoses includes 50 initial successes in 54 patients [6]. Only six of these patients had total occlusions, and 48 had severe stenoses producing pressure gradients across the lesion. After 2 years, the patency rate of the iliac arteries in the 50 successfully dilated patients was 88%. It is interesting to note that no reocclusions occurred in the second year postdilatation.

Katzen and Chang [10] confirmed Grüntzig's results in reporting a 96% initial success rate in iliac artery lesions. Bachman, Casarella, and Sos [1] utilized the flexibility of the balloon catheter to perform iliac angioplasty in six patients following retrograde puncture of the contralateral common femoral artery and passage of the catheter over the aortic bifurcation. This modification allowed the dilatation of bilateral lesions with only one arterial puncture, facilitated dilatation of the hypogastric artery, allowed the common femoral artery to be safely dilated, and avoided any possible contamination or hematoma on the side of the lesion which might complicate subsequent surgery if necessary.

Percutaneous dilatation of the iliac arteries appears to be an effective relatively safe procedure which has a high probability of success in properly selected cases. There is good evidence that stenoses less than 3 cm in length will respond to dilatation. Short segmental occlusions are probably also amenable to the technique. However, long iliac occlusions (greater than 5 cm) carry a higher risk of failure and should properly be considered unsuited for angioplasty unless surgery is contraindicated.

RENAL ANGIOPLASTY

With the iliac and femoral experience in hand, Grüntzig turned his attention to modifying his balloon catheter system in order to dilate the renal and coronary arteries. The major modifications were to miniaturize the catheters to 4 French in caliber and to develop 9F or 10F Teflon guiding catheters which could serve as a coaxial conduit to the origin of the renal or coronary arteries.

The first case report of a successful renal angioplasty was by Grüntzig et al. in 1978 [9]. The same group expanded their series to six cases in a subsequent abstract [8], and Katzen and Chang reported four successful dilatations in patients with refractory hypertension due to renal artery stenosis [11]. Millan and Madios [12] reported successful dilatation of renal artery stenosis secondary to medial fibroplasia in a 43 year old female. Their patient has remained free of hypertension off all medication for 4 months following the procedure.

Many other groups in the United States and Europe are rapidly gaining experience with renal artery dilatation. Much of this experience is not yet recorded in the literature, since it has been acquired only during the past year. Schwarten has probably the most extensive early experience with the technique [14]. He reported 23 consecutive primary successes in patients with hypertension and renal artery stenoses.

Schwarten, Millan, and Katzen all advocate the use of modified Grüntzig balloon catheters which can be passed over a guidewire into the renal artery. In this technique, the artery is first entered with a curved selective diagnostic catheter and the lesion gently probed with a guidewire. Once the guidewire traverses the lesion, the 5F or 6F diagnostic catheter is passed through it, and the patient is heparinized through the arterial catheter. A somewhat stiffer guide can then safely be passed through the catheter into the renal artery beyond the lesion, and the flexible 5F or 7F balloon catheter advanced over it into the renal artery. It is essential that the balloon be positioned as close as possible to the tip of the catheter, so that the tip does not wedge distally in the renal arterial tree as the balloon crosses the lesion. With constant monitoring of arterial pressure at the catheter tip, an immediate fall in pressure will accompany the catheter's traversing the lesion. After inflation and deflation of the balloon, recording of a normal pressure curve beyond the lesion indicates successful dilatation and allows the angiographer to withdraw the catheter from the renal artery in order to do a diagnostic study.

Aside from atherosclerosis and fibromuscular disease there has been successful experience with renal transplants. One case from our own laboratory [3] has remained normotensive for 1 year since successful dilatation of critical arterial stenosis in a transplanted kidney. We have been unsuccessful in attempting to dilate two renal arteries severely narrowed by neurofibromatosis, but did achieve primary success in a 10 year old girl with Takayasu's arteritis.

A review of the first year's experience in three laboratories, including our own, collected 23 patients [2], with primary success in 20. In the successful cases there was a sustained fall in the blood pressure from a group mean of 212/120 to 130/84. Twelve of the patients are off all medications, and the other eight have had a marked reduction in their antihypertensive requirements. Significant drop in renin production has occurred in all eight of the patients who hade undergone subsequent renin analysis. In this series complications have included one small segmental renal infarct, two cases of transient oliguria

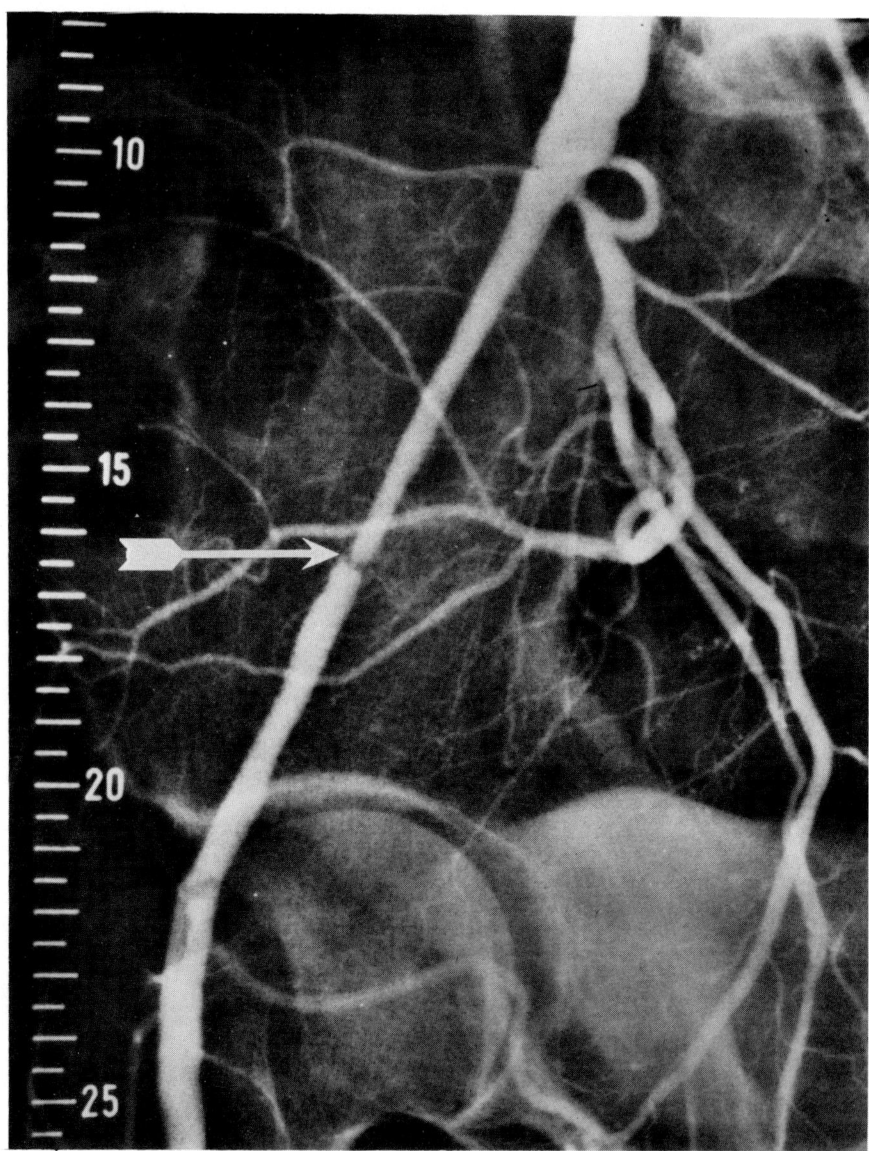

Fig. 2A,B. Right external iliac artery stenosis in a 47 year old man. The lesion appears as a diaphragm (white arrow). After dilatation from the opposite femoral artery and passage of the catheter over the aortic bifurcation, residual of the lesion is identified but the pressure gradient across it was eliminated and thigh claudication relieved. The centimeter ruler is used to assist the angiographer to precisely locate the lesion and the balloon during fluoroscopy.

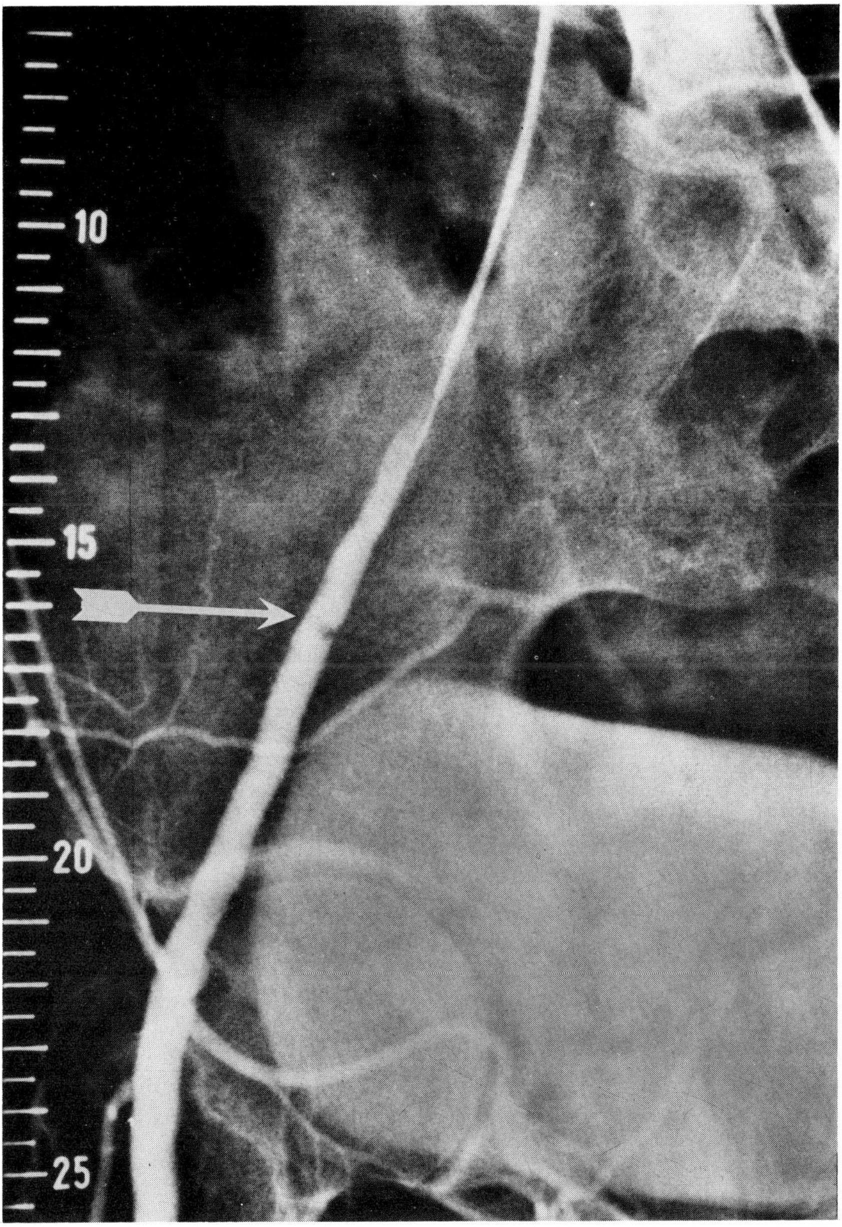

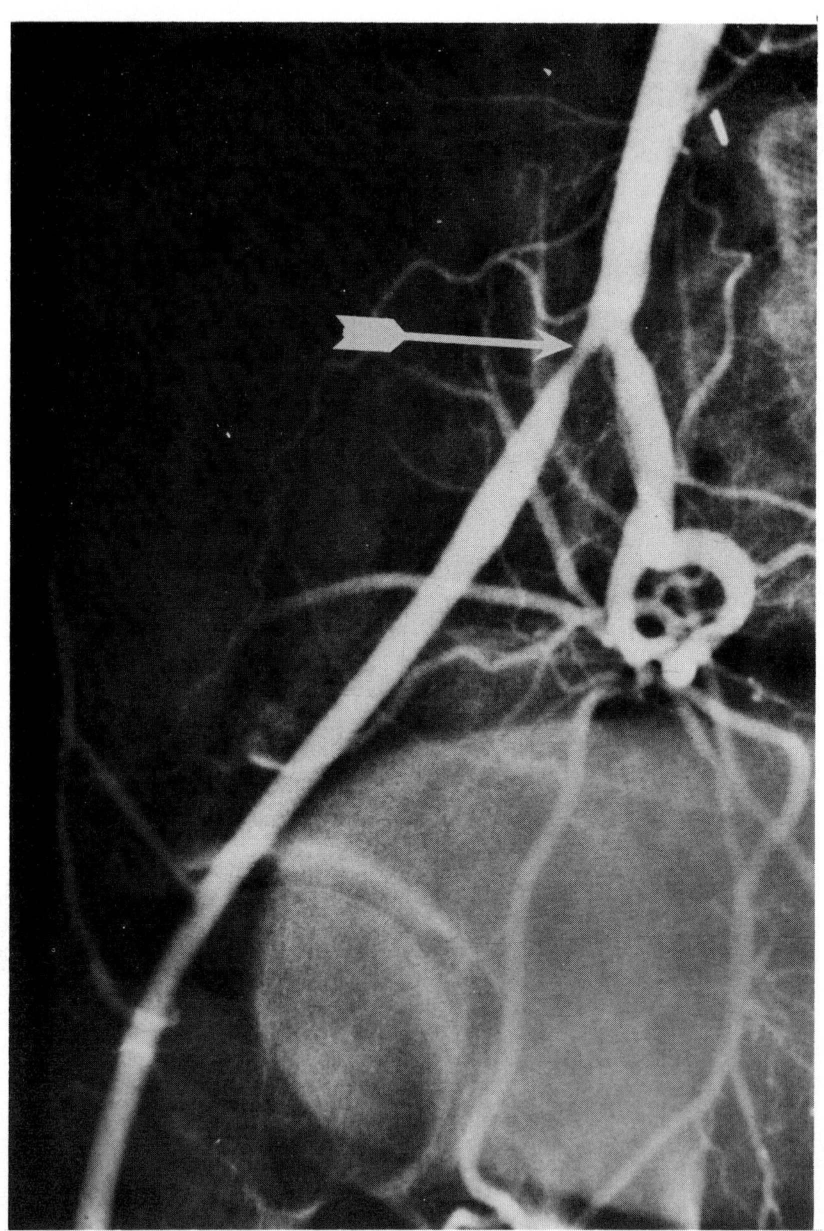

Fig. 3A,B. Cylindrical right external iliac artery lesion before and after dilatation (white arrow). This lesion is ideal for angioplasty since it is a focal, short stenosis without heavy calcification. Elimination of the pressure gradient across the lesion indicates the endpoint for the dilatation procedure.

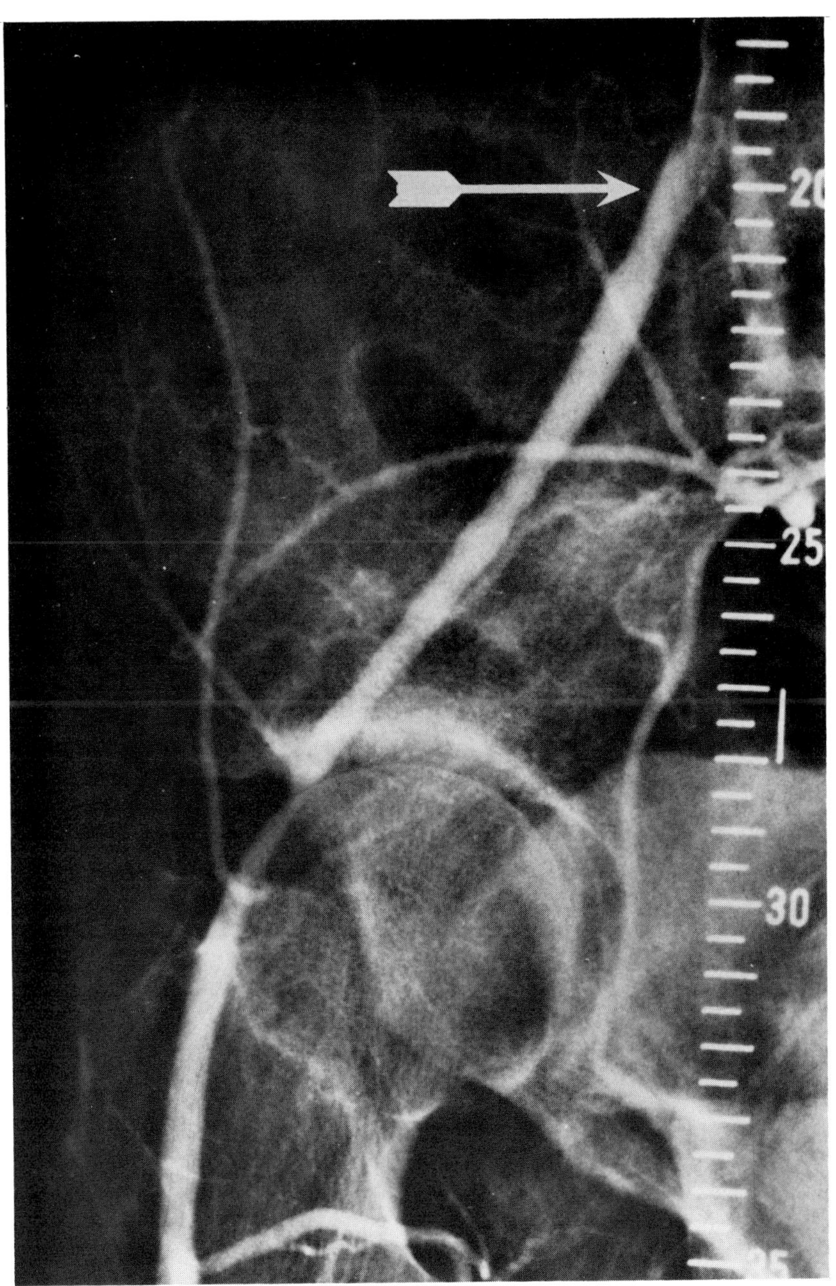
25
30

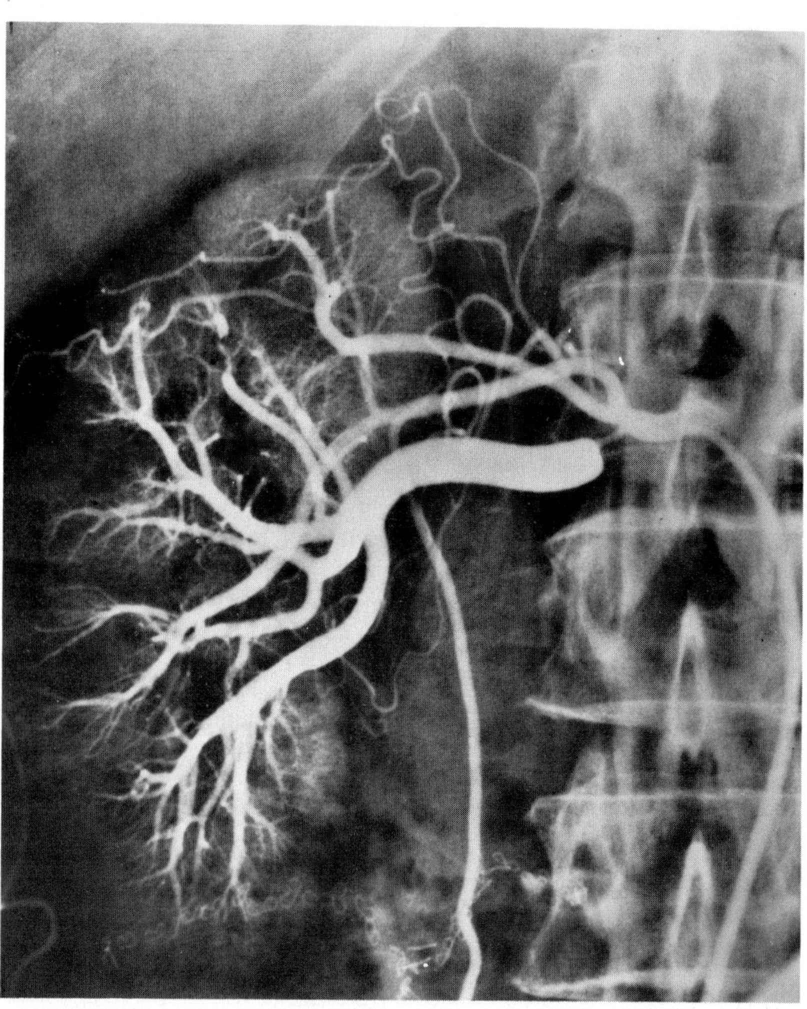

Fig. 4A,B. Renal artery stenosis in a 67 year old man. The short cylindrical lesion (A) is involving the lower pole branch of the right renal artery. Elevated renin production was demonstrated from the lower pole of the right kidney by subselective renin samples. Following dilatation, a 4 mm lumen was established and elevated renin production abolished.

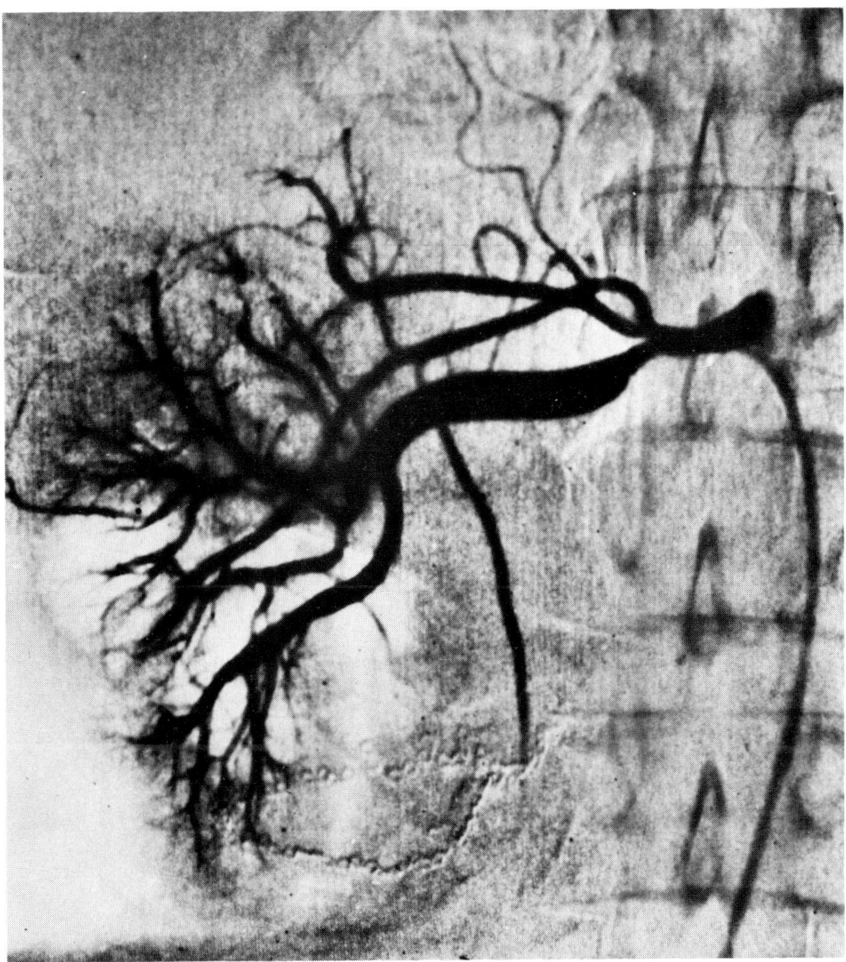

probably related to contrast material, two hematomas at the femoral artery, and one probable incident of distal cholesterol embolization. In no case was there a decrease in renal function and no emergency operations were required. No detectable damage was done to the arteries that could not be dilated. The unsuccessful cases included one case of total occlusion due to atherosclerosis, one case of bilateral neurofibromatosis, and a severely stenotic calcified lesion in a patient with a diffusely diseased aorta. No evident restenosis has occurred, although the followup period is very short.

Zeitler collected data from several centers in Europe and the United States and reported very preliminary results in 115 patients [18]. There was an 88% primary success rate with dilatation and an initial decrease in blood pressure. One renal infarct with loss of a kidney was reported.

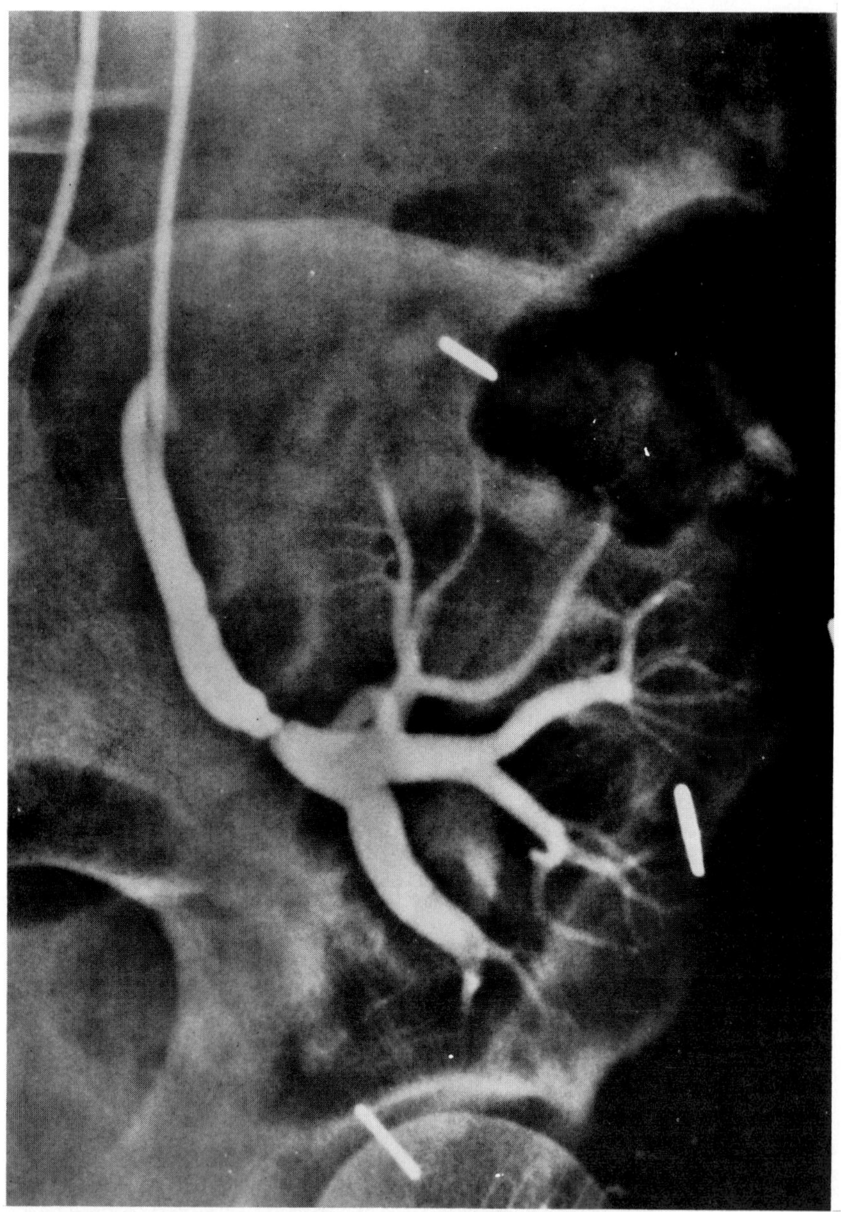

Fig. 5A,B. Renal artery stenosis in a transplanted kidney. The critical diaphragmlike stenosis near the anastomosis resulted in uncontrollable hypertension. The lesion was largely eliminated by dilatation with the catheter advanced from the axillary artery. The patient has remained normotensive for the past year following angioplasty.

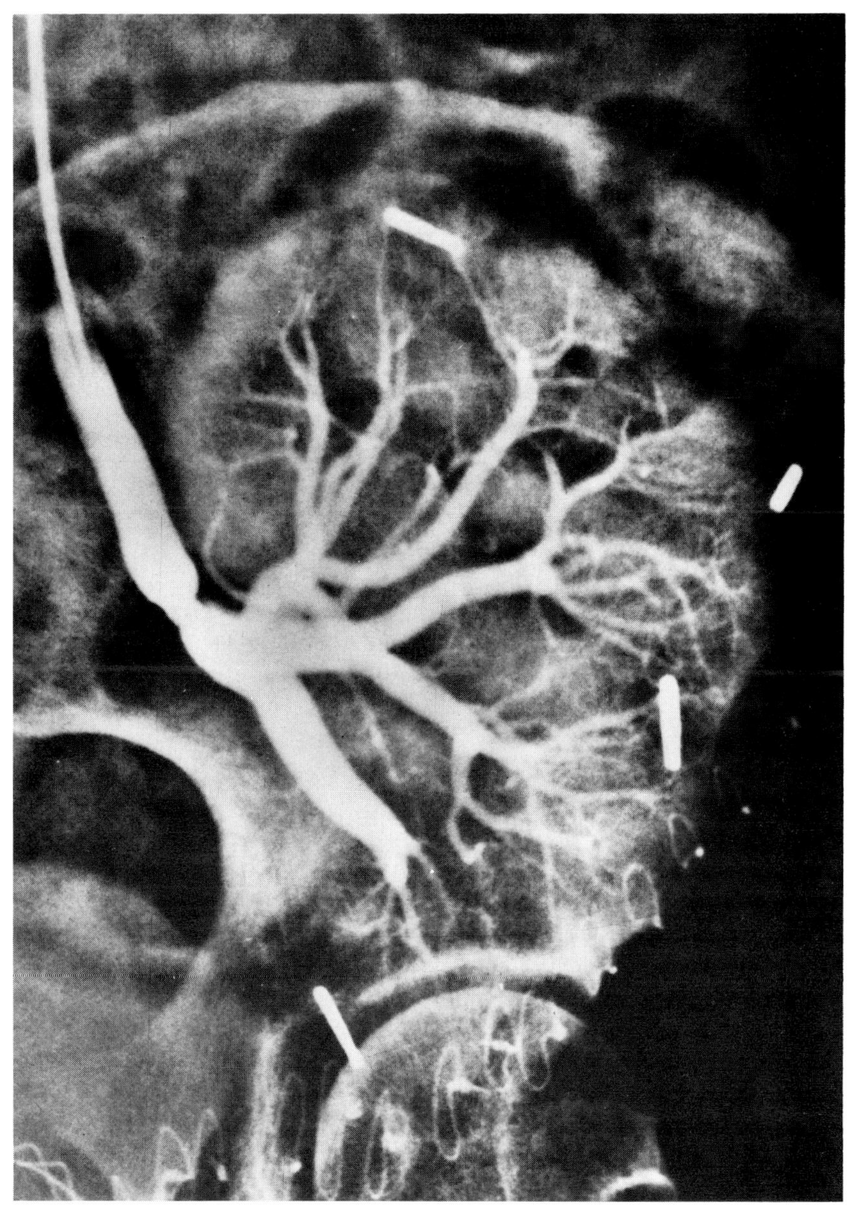

Much of the data on renal artery angioplasty is very preliminary and still anecdotal because the procedure is so new. However, there appears to be a universally high primary success rate of at least 80% in all centers, and the complication rate appears to be acceptably low. The procedure does not obviate the possibility of subsequent surgery if unsuccessful, and the associated morbidity, mortality, and expense are lower than those of major reconstructive surgery.

COMPLICATIONS AND TECHNICAL CONSIDERATIONS

Although complications of angioplasty are fairly low, they can be very serious and require meticulous technique to keep to a minimum. Hematomas at the puncture site occur in approximately 10% of patients. This is higher than in routine angiography because of the use of systemic heparinization and the introduction of larger lumen catheters. The smaller lumen of the balloon catheter is one of its major advantages over the 12F Dotter catheters. Retroperitoneal hemorrhage can occur if the femoral puncture site is above the inguinal ligament. This is particularly hazardous in the antegrade puncture technique for superficial femoral lesions. Zeitler reported an incidence of two instances of retroperitoneal bleeding in 975 cases of angioplasty [21]. False aneurysm at the puncture site has also been reported [21].

Dissection of the femoral or iliac arteries with a guidewire, perforation of the arterial wall with the guidewire, and thrombosis at the puncture site may occur, but the incidence appears to be about the same as in diagnostic angiography.

Peripheral embolism is a very worrisome and feared complication. Grüntzig [6] reported an incidence of 5%. This corresponds to our own experience although the incidence of this complication increases with one's diligence in looking for it. Clinically apparent distal emboli probably occur in about 5% of superficial femoral dilatations, and there is a general feeling that the incidence is higher in total occlusions than in stenoses. Spasm of the popliteal artery appears to be a significant problem in distal femoral lesions and has been successfully treated with vasodilators, especially ATP and xylocaine.

Perforation of the artery at the site of dilatation is an extremely rare complication. Prevention of this calamity is achieved by the design of the balloon catheter which will not dilate beyond a fixed diameter unless extreme pressure is applied to it. Automatic pumps with preselected pressure settings are available. Alternatively, manometers may be attached to the catheters and the balloon inflated manually. Intraluminal pressures of 4-8 atmospheres are usually applied to achieve dilatation. Above 8 atmospheres and following multiple dilatations, the balloons have a tendency to weaken and may rupture. This in itself causes no problem except that it may be difficult to extract the ragged, torn balloon from the femoral artery.

Thrombosis during the procedure is readily reduced by sytemic heparinization. Most authors recommend long term anticoagulation with coumadin to increase patency rates. However, the data supporting this conclusion are scanty. The data of Zeitler and Schmidtke [21] provide the best support for long term anticoagulation. At 36 months 80% of their patients with anticoagulation were still patent, whereas only 33% with no anticoagulation remained patent. This study included only patients with femoral lesions and was not a well controlled prospective analysis. However, these data suggest that femoral dilatation patients do better with anticoagulation. There are no data on its efficacy in renal or iliac lesions. No comparison of coumadin with other anticoagulants or platelet inhibitors has been undertaken.

REFERENCES

1. Bachman DM, Casarella WJ, Sos TA: Percutaneous iliofemoral angioplasty via the contralateral femoral artery. Radiology 130:617-621, 1979
2. Casarella WJ, Katzen BT, Chang J: Percutaneous transluminal angioplasty of the renal arteries: The first year's experience. (Submitted for publication)
3. Diamond NL, Casarella WJ, Appel G, et al: Successful dilatation of renal artery stenosis in a transplanted kidney with percutaneous transluminal angioplasty. Am. J. Roentgenol. (in press)
4. Dotter CT, Judkins MP: Transluminal treatment of arteriosclerotic obstruction. Description of a new technique and a preliminary report of its application. Circulation 30:654-670, 1964
5. Dotter CT, Judkins MP, Rösch J: Night operative, transluminale Behandling der arteriosklerotischen Verschlüss affektionen. Fortschr. Roentgenstr. 109:125-135, 1968
6. Grüntzig A: Percutaneous balloon catheter angioplasty. Presented at the Annual Meeting of the Society of Cardiovascular Radiology, New Orleans, 1978
7. Grüntzig A, Hopff H: Perkutane Rekanalisation chronischer arterieller Verschlüsse mit einem neuen Dilationskatheter Modifikation der Dotter-Technik. Dtsch. Med. Wochenschr. 99:2502-2507, 1974
8. Grüntzig A, Kuhlmann U, Vetter W, et al: Percutaneous transluminal dilatation of atherosclerotic renal artery stenoses. Circulation [Suppl] 58:213, 1978 (Abstr)
9. Grüntzig A, Vetter W, Meier B: Treatment of renovascular hypertension with percutaneous transluminal dilatation of a renal artery stenosis. Lancet 1:801-802, 1978
10. Katzen BT, Chang J: Percutaneous transluminal angioplasty with the Grüntzig balloon catheter. Radiology 130:623-626, 1979
11. Katzen BT, Chang J: Percutaneous transluminal angioplasty for treatment of renovascular hypertension. Radiology 131:53-58, 1979

12. Millan VG, Madias NE: Percutaneous transluminal angioplasty for severe renovascular hypertension due to renal artery medial fibroplasia. Lancet 1:993-995, 1979
13. Porstmann W: Ein neuer Korsett-Ballonkatheter zur transluminalen Rekanalisation nach Dotter unter besanderer Berücksightigung von Obliterationen an den Becken arterien. Radiol. Diagn. (Berlin) 14:239-244, 1973
14. Schwarten D: Percutaneous transluminal angioplasty of the renal artery. Presented at the Annual Meeting of the Radiological Society of North America, Chicago, December 1978
15. van Andel GJ: Percutaneous Transluminal Angioplasty: The Dotter Procedure. Amsterdan-Oxford, Excerpta Medica, New York, American Elsevier, 1976
16. Zeitler E: Transluminale Verschlüss Rekanalisation mit Angiographic Katheter. Herz/Kreisl 4:138-142, 1972
17. Zeitler E: Die percutane Behandlung von arteriellen durch blutungsstoriengen der Extremetäten mit Katheter. Radiologie 13:319-325, 1973
18. Zeitler E: Percutaneous vascular recanalization of the renal artery. Presented at the Annual Meeting of the European College of Angiography, Dublin, June 1979
19. Zeitler E, Grüntzig A, Schoop W: Percutaneous Vascular Recanalization. Berlin, Springer-Verlag, 1978
20. Zeitler E, Schmidtke I, Schoop W, et al: Ergebnisse nach perkutanen translumeniler Angioplastik bei uber 700 Behandlungen. Presented at the Third Congress of the European Association of Radiology, Edinburgh, 1975
21. Zeitler E, Schmidtke I, Schoop W, et al: Ergebnisse der perkutanen transluminalen Angioplastik bei uber 700 Behandlungen. Röntgenpraxis 29:78-98, 1976

Mesenteric Ischemia

Scott J. Boley, M.D.
Lawrence J. Brandt, M.D.

The Pathophysiology of Mesenteric Blood Flow and Nonocclusive Mesenteric Ischemia

The mesenteric circulation can be defined as that portion of the splanchnic circulation supplying the small and large intestines. The major arteries contributing to this intestinal vascular bed are the superior and inferior mesenteric arteries, branches of the celiac axis and the middle and inferior hemorrhoidal branches of the internal iliac artery.

The intestines are protected from ischemia to a great extent by their abundant collateral circulation. Communications between the celiac, superior, and inferior mesenteric beds are numerous, and a general rule that has proved valid over many years is that at least two of these vessels must be compromised to produce symptomatic intestinal ischemia. Moreover, occlusion of two of the vessels occurs frequently without evidence of ischemia and total occlusion of all three vessels has been observed without symptoms.

Collateral pathways around occlusions of smaller mesenteric arterial branches are provided by the primary, secondary, and tertiary arcades in the mesentery of the small bowel, and the marginal arterial complex of Drummond in the mesocolon. Within the bowel wall itself there is a network of communicating submucosal vessels which can maintain the viability of short segments of the intestine whose extramural arterial supply has been lost.

In response to the fall in arterial pressure distal to an obstruction, collateral pathways open immediately when a major vessel is occluded. Increased blood flow through this collateral circulation continues as long as the pressure in the vascular bed distal to the obstruction remains below the systemic pressure. If vasoconstriction develops in this distal bed, arterial pressure is elevated and causes diminution of collateral flow. Similarly, if normal blood flow is reconstituted, flow through collateral channels ceases.

In the resting state the mesenteric circulation receives up to 25% of the cardiac output. This percentage may increase modestly after eating or decrease during exercise. Motor control of the mesenteric circulation is mediated primarily through the sympathetic nervous system; although beta adrenergic receptors are present, alpha adrenergic receptors predominate. Thus increased sympathetic activity produces vasoconstriction which increases resistance and decreases blood flow. Folkow et al. [14] have shown that vasoconstriction induced by sympathetic nervous stimulation can virtually stop blood flow for brief intervals.

The degree of reduction in blood flow that the bowel can tolerate without damage is remarkable. In one of our studies mesenteric arterial flow was reduced to 75% of normal for 12 hours. No morphologic changes could be identified by light microscopy, and there was normal distribution of infused Patent Blue V dye. One reason for these findings is that only one-fifth of the mesenteric blood flow passes through open capillaries at any one moment. Since the uptake of oxygen occurs only from open capillaries, a normal supply of oxygen to intestinal tissues can be maintained with only 20%-25% of normal blood flow if all the blood passes through the capillaries. In animal studies this apparently occurred as extraction of oxygen, reflected by an increased arteriovenous oxygen difference, increased when arterial blood flow was reduced by partially occluding the superior mesenteric artery (SMA).

Intestinal ischemia may result from a reduction in blood flow, from redistribution of blood flow, or from a combination of both. A reduction in blood flow to the intestine may reflect generalized poor perfusion as in shock or with a failing heart, or it may result from either local morphologic or functional changes. Narrowings of the major mesenteric vessels, emboli, vasculitis as part of a systemic disease, or mesenteric vasoconstriction all can lead to inadequate circulation. However, whatever the cause, intestinal ischemia has the same end results – a spectrum ranging from completely reversible functional alterations to total hemorrhagic necrosis of portions or all of the bowel. Two situations that can dramatically produce or sustain diminished intestinal blood flow in the absence of vascular occlusion are bowel distention and systemic conditions producing lowered cardiac output and transient falls in mesenteric arterial blood flow.

EFFECT OF BOWEL DISTENTION ON INTESTINAL BLOOD FLOW

Increased intraluminal pressure can vary in degree and duration, may be sustained or intermittent, and may affect blood flow to the distended segment or to the entire intestine. Observations based on a series of experiments performed on more than 80 anesthetized dogs emphasize the profound influence of bowel distention and increased intraluminal pressure on intestinal blood flow [4].

In each animal a multihole catheter was inserted into the lumen of a segment of ileum 12-18 inches long or colon 6-12 inches long, and umbilical tapes were tied around the segment at both ends. The catheter was attached to a constant pressure regulator that maintained intraluminal pressure with air at selected levels. Systemic and mesenteric arterial pressure were monitored via catheters inserted into the femoral artery and into a small mesenteric arterial branch of the intestinal segment under study, respectively.

Blood flows were measured with electromagnetic flow meters (Biotronex Laboratory Inc., Silver Spring, Md.) and noncannulating flow probes. In studies of the distended bowel this segment was isolated to receive its blood supply from a single artery and the probe placed on this vessel. In studies of the entire small intestine, probes were placed on the superior mesenteric artery (SMA) near its origin from the abdominal aorta and also on the same artery just proximal and just distal to the branches supplying the distended segment. Samples of systemic arterial blood and venous effluent from the intestine being studied were taken to determine arteriovenous oxygen difference during periods of distention and decompression as well as after the final release of pressure.

Silicone rubber (Microfil, Boulder, Colo.) injections of intestinal segments were made in situ through Teflon catheters placed in the artery supplying the segment under study, both during periods of distention and after the final release of pressure. After injection, specimens were removed and cleared in graduated concentrations of glycerin over 5-7 days as described by Reynolds [23].

Blood flows were determined while intraluminal pressure was increased from 0 to 210 mm Hg in 30 mm Hg increments. Each pressure was maintained for 5-10 minutes. No consistent change in blood flow was noted with sustained intraluminal pressures under 30 mm Hg. In both the large and the small bowel, pressures at or above 30-60 mm Hg resulted in a stepwise decrease in intestinal blood flow as the pressure was increased. The maximal diminution in flow occurred when intraluminal pressure had reached 90-120 mm Hg. Further increases in distending pressure did not influence flow; 20%-35% of control flow persisted even at pressures of 210 mm Hg and higher. Blood flow diminished consistently and reproducibly and responded similarly whether or not the bowel was decompressed between increments of pressure.

Of special note was the normal pink external appearance of the bowel at distending pressures of 180 mm Hg or greater, even though total blood flow to the segment was only 20% of control values. This observation is explained by a high oxygen saturation of the venous blood and the continuing flow through the serosal vessels. The oxygen tension (pO_2) in the intestinal venous effluent increased in stepwise fashion as intraluminal pressure was increased and almost reached systemic arterial levels when blood flow had fallen to 20%-35% of control. The resulting drop in arteriovenous oxygen difference (Fig. 1) is indicative of a marked diminution in oxygen extraction in the presence of the diminished blood flow.

Injected specimens of normal undistended bowel showed excellent filling of the vessels of all layers of the intestinal wall, with the villous capillaries clearly demonstrated (Fig. 2A). At pressures at which blood flow fell significantly (60-90 mm Hg) only submucosal and serosal vessels filled, whereas vessels in the mucosa and muscles were almost devoid of the injected silicone rubber (Fig. 2B). At 30 mm Hg a few vessels in the mucosa and muscles were filled although markedly less than in the normal bowel. Filling of the submucosal and serosal vessels was seen at all pressure levels.

In summary, these studies demonstrated that increasing intraluminal pressure diminishes blood flow to the distended intestine until an irreducible level of 20%-35% of control is reached. The injection studies suggest that the remaining blood flows through vessels in the submucosa and serosa. Arteriovenous oxygen difference across the bowel diminishes as intestinal blood flow falls. This shows that oxygen extraction is decreasing while blood flow is declining, which suggests that the remaining blood flow is passing through functional, if not anatomic, arteriovenous communications. The result of this alteration in the distribution of blood flow is that any diminution in intestinal blood flow, because of the associated decrease in oxygen extraction, results in a proportionately greater fall in oxygen utilization. The deleterious effect of bowel distention on the blood flow and oxygen utilization is further exaggerated by a selective ischemia of mucosa and muscle.

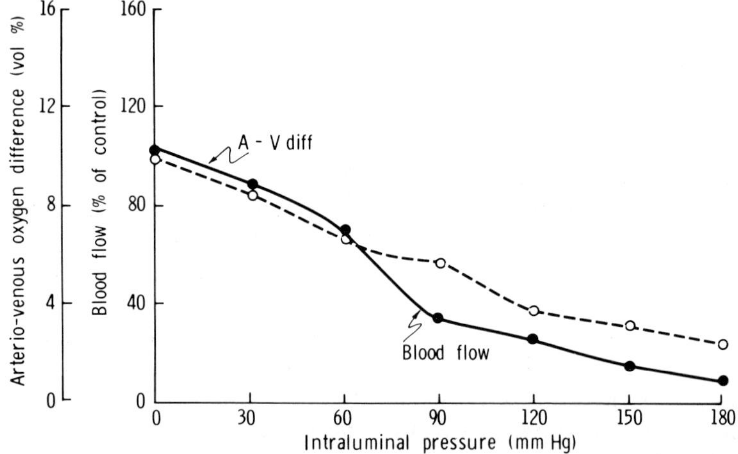

Fig. 1. Effects of bowel distention on blood flow and arteriovenous oxygen difference of intestinal blood. Oxygen extraction diminishes almost to zero as blood flow falls. [From Boley SJ, et al: Pathophysiologic effects of bowel distention on intestinal blood flow. Am. J. Surg. 117:228, 1969, used by permission.]

Of perhaps greater clinical importance than alterations observed with sustained pressure were those noted in other experiments with intermittent distention [27]. Intermittent increases in intraluminal pressure significantly reduced blood flow not only to the distended segment but also to the entire small bowel, and this diminution in flow persisted for hours after relief of distention. Although arteriovenous shunting was not associated with a decrease in blood flow to undistended segments, the pronounced and prolonged ischemia to the entire bowel is itself potentially detrimental. Such generalized and sustained ischemia could interfere with the recovery of decompressed segments of bowel already damaged by ischemia and shunting when they were distended.

The quantitative changes in intestinal blood flow and its distribution during bowel distention were reflected in identifiable alterations in the angiographically visualized intestinal vasculature, including

1. A slowing of blood flow to the distended segments with stasis of contrast material within the moderate-sized arteries;
2. Delayed visualization of vascular arcades supplying the distended bowel;
3. A sudden abnormal tapering and poor peripheral filling of fine arterial branches in the affected loops; and
4. A markedly diminished capillary blush in the intestinal mucosa.

Angiography performed at varying intervals from 15 min to 1 hour following release of the intestinal distention always revealed some degree of persistent vasoconstriction. In several animals "thumbprinting," a radiologic sign of intestinal ischemia, was noted in the bowel loops that had been distended.

SUSTAINED EFFECTS OF TRANSIENT FALLS IN MESENTERIC ARTERIAL FLOW

One of the puzzling characteristics of intestinal necrosis caused by low-flow states is the frequent time lag between correction of the primary systemic problem and the onset of abdominal symptoms and signs. In order to study the delayed or protracted effects of diminished mesenteric blood flow, experiments were performed on more than 200 anesthetized dogs in which the superior mesenteric artery (SMA) flow was decreased 50% with a hydraulic occluder and maintained at this level while alterations in cardiac output, intestinal perfusion, oxygen consumption, systemic and mesenteric arterial pressures, and blood flow through other arteries of the splanchnic circulation were measured.

The following observations are based upon those studies [6, 9, 13]: Following 50% acute diminution in SMA flow, the mesenteric arterial pressure (MAP) in the peripheral bed immediately fell by 48% (mean range 36%-71%), and in several instances the percentage fall in MAP exceeded the percentage fall in blood flow. While the greater fall in mesenteric pressure suggests lowered

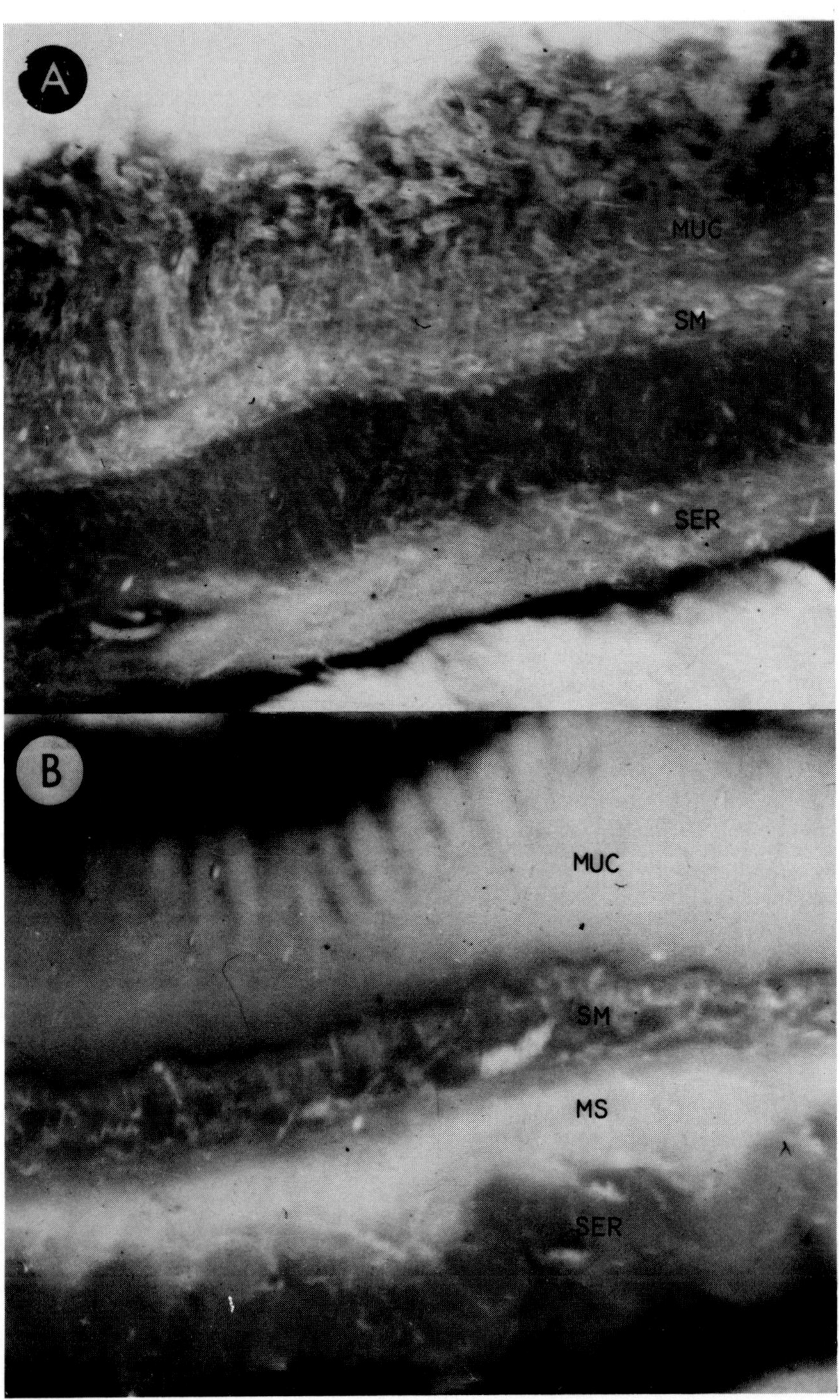
A
MUC
SM
SER
B
MUC
SM
MS
SER

resistance or vasodilation in the mesenteric bed, Selkurt and his coworkers [25] have demonstrated that changes in active resistance cannot be deduced when pressure and flow are changing in the same direction. There was certainly no evidence of any immediate active mesenteric vasoconstriction similar to that seen in response to systemic hypotension or diminished cardiac output.

When SMA flow was maintained at 50%, the MAP returned to control levels within 1-6 hours, while celiac artery flow which initially had increased, returned to normal. If the occluder was released when MAP first returned to control, the SMA flow immediately rose to control levels (Fig. 3). However, if the SMA occlusion was continued for 30 min to 4 hours after MAP had returned to control, SMA flows remained at 30%-53% of control, even after removal of the occluder (Fig. 4). These low SMA flows persisted and were observed for up to 5 hours. In several animals injection of papaverine into the SMA produced an immediate return of normal SMA flow.

If papaverine was infused continuously into the SMA (30-60 mg per hour) when SMA flow was maintained at 50%, then MAP remained down during the entire 4 hours of the experiment, and SMA flow returned to normal promptly upon releasing the occluder (Fig. 5).

Low SMA flow initially produces mesenteric vascular responses that tend to maintain adequate intestinal flow, but if the diminished flow is prolonged active vasoconstriction develops and may persist even after the primary cause of mesenteric ischemia is corrected. Such persistent vasoconstriction appears to violate the principle of autoregulatory escape. A similar potential for persistent vasoconstriction has been described in the kidney in man [17].

The intestinal lesions associated with nonocclusive mesenteric ischemia have mostly been related to congestive heart failure, arrhythmias, and shock and have been attributed to low mesenteric blood flow. While it had been postulated that the bowel was injured during the episode of diminished cardiac output or hypotension, and that with correction of the primary problem mesenteric blood flow returned to normal, this theory did not explain the operative finding of persistent ischemic bowel without venous or arterial occlusion in patients whose cardiovascular problems had been corrected. This paradox can be explained, however, by our experimental observation that an episode of low mesenteric flow of as short as 2 hours duration can produce mesenteric ischemia which may persist for many hours after the primary problem is corrected. Furthermore, the occurrence of persistent vasoconstriction following low SMA flow and its prevention and reversibility with locally administered vasodilators suggested that

Fig. 2. Dog intestine injected with silicone rubber. (A) At normal intraluminal pressure. Vessels in all four layers are filled. (B) With intraluminal pressure of 90 mm Hg. Vessels in submucosa (SM) and serosa (SER) are filled, whereas those of mucosa (MUC) and muscle (MS) are almost empty. [From Boley SJ, et al: Pathophysiologic effects of bowel distention on intestinal blood flow. Am. J. Surg. 117:228, 1969, used by permission.]

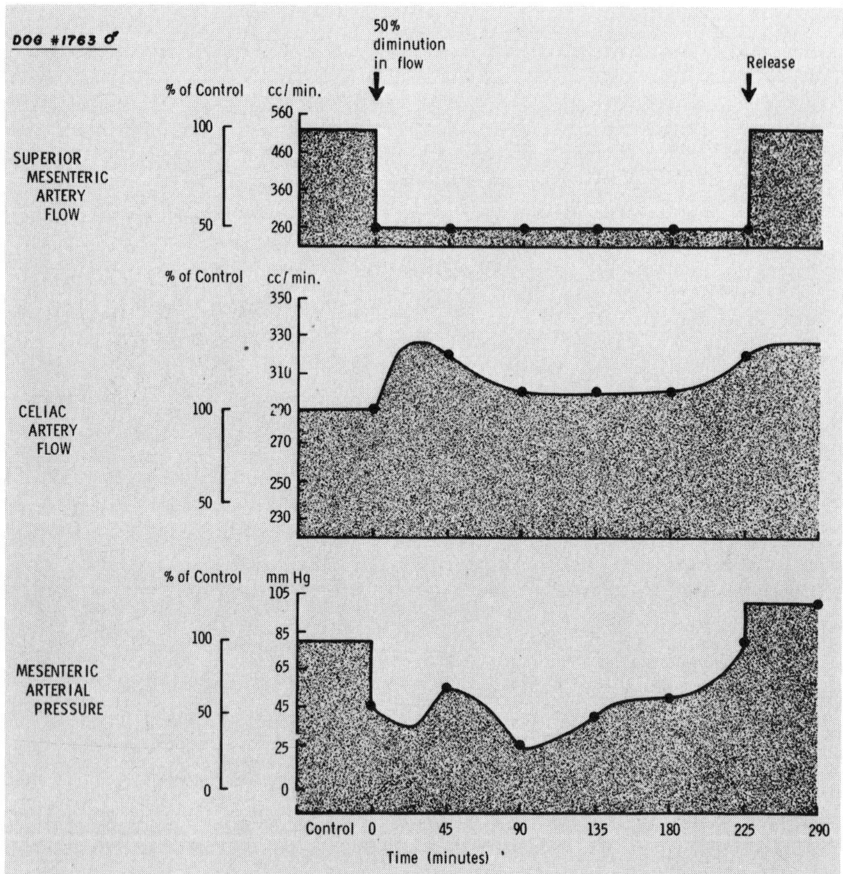

Fig. 3. Effect of low SMA flow on mesenteric vascular bed. Celiac arterial flow rose and mesenteric pressure fell when SMA flow was decreased. SMA occlusion was released as soon as MAP had returned to control levels, and SMA flow rose promptly to its original rate. [From Boley SJ, et al: Persistent vasoconstriction – A major factor in nonocclusive mesenteric ischemia. Curr. Topics Surg. Res. 3:425, 1971, used by permission.]

local intraarterial papaverine be used clinically to treat the vasoconstriction of the low-flow syndrome and that seen after SMA embolus.

Kukovetz and Poch [19] showed that the effectiveness of papaverine was a result of its potent inhibition of the enzyme phosphodiesterase, which is necessary for the degradation of cyclic AMP, the modulator of vascular smooth muscle relaxation. Drugs which stimulate the formation of cyclic AMP, e.g., prostaglandin E_1 and glucagon, also have been recommended either alone or in combination with papaverine to produce maximal vasodilatation [28].

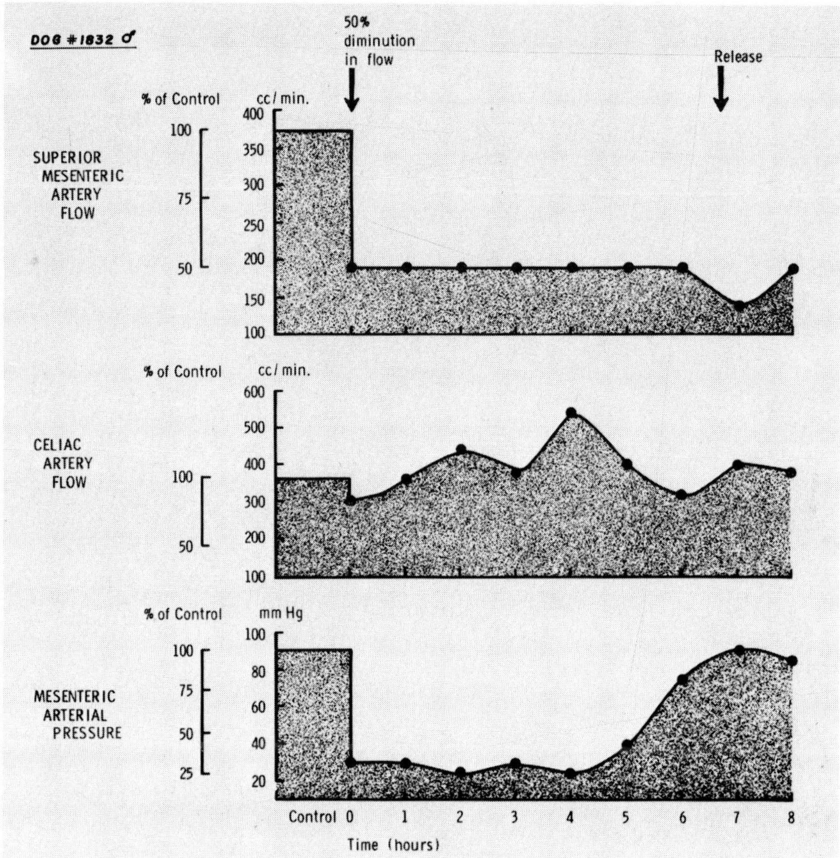

Fig. 4. Effect of low SMA flow on mesenteric vascular bed. Mesenteric arterial pressure had returned to normal for 2 hours before SMA occlusion was removed, and SMA flow remained at 50% of its original flow. [From Boley SJ, et al: Persistent vasoconstriction – A major factor of nonocclusive mesenteric ischemia. Curr. Topics Surg. Res. 3:425, 1971, used by permission.]

ANGIOGRAPHY AND MESENTERIC VASOCONSTRICTION

It rapidly became apparent during our experimental studies that recognition of the occurrence of persistent vasoconstriction would only be of clinical importance if it could be identified angiographically, thus permitting the direct intraarterial infusion of papaverine before tissue necrosis developed. We have studied the roentgenologic criteria of mesenteric arterial vasoconstriction both in dogs and in man and believe that this entity can be identified with reasonable accuracy.

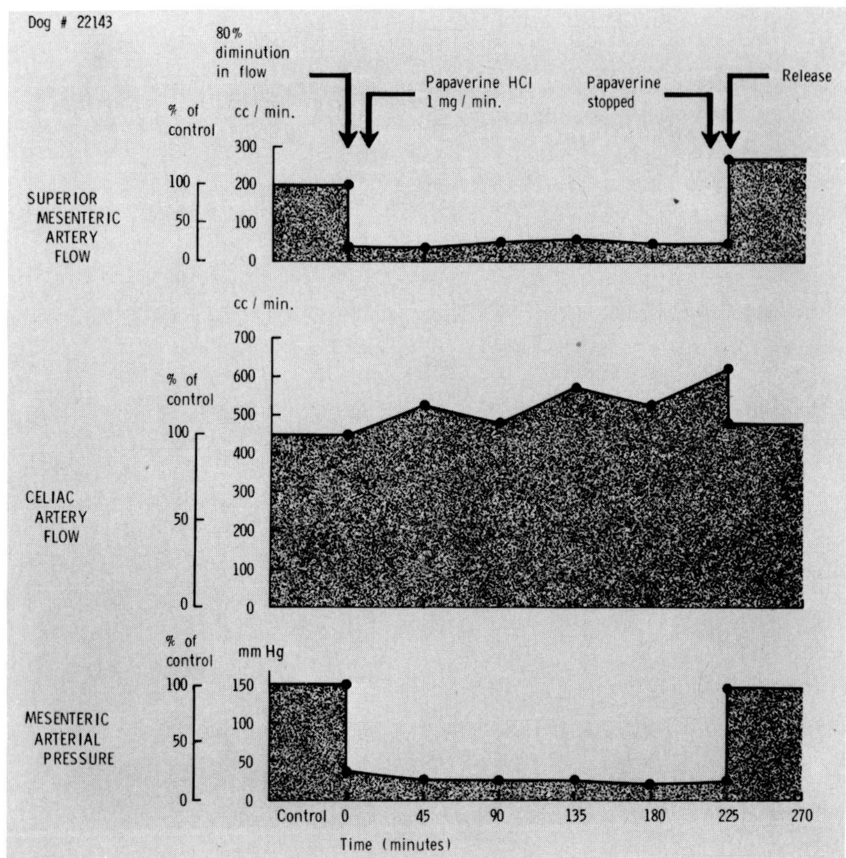

Fig. 5. Effect of papaverine on mesenteric vasoconstriction. Papaverine was infused into the SMA when SMA flow was decreased. MAP remained down throughout the 4-hour period of ischemia and SMA flow returned to normal upon release of the occluder. Papaverine thus prevented the occurrence of vasoconstriction. [From Boley SJ, et al: Persistent vasoconstriction – A major factor in nonocclusive mesenteric ischemia. Curr. Topics Surg. Res. 3:425, 1971, used by permission.]

Angiography has been successfully employed in suspected cases of acute mesenteric ischemia, but until recently its role has been limited to the exclusion of an embolus or acute thrombosis, both of which might be successfully treated by prompt operation. In 1974 we reported on a series of studies [26] whose goal was to establish criteria for the angiographic diagnosis of mesenteric vasoconstriction so that nonocclusive as well as occlusive mesenteric ischemia could be identified and intraarterial papaverine utilized to overcome the vasoconstriction.

Initially, mesenteric vasoconstriction was produced in the dog and the resulting angiographic abnormalities identified (Fig. 6). Subsequently, selective superior mesenteric angiograms were examined in a control group of 65 patients to determine whether any of the observed angiographic abnormalities occurred in the absence of vasoconstriction. The reliability of these angiographic signs of vasoconstriction was then evaluated in patients acutely ill with mesenteric ischemia.

Based upon these studies, four reliable angiographic criteria for the diagnosis of mesenteric vasoconstriction were identified: (1) narrowings at the origins of multiple branches of the SMA, (2) irregularities in intestinal branches, (3) spasm of arcades, and (4) impaired filling of intramural vessels. While mesenteric vasoconstriction occurs with hemorrhage, pancreatitis, and other conditions, its presence in patients with suspected intestinal ischemia who are not in shock or receiving vasopressors is strong evidence for the presence of nonocclusive mesenteric ischemia. Thus if angiography is performed sufficiently early in their course, patients with acute mesenteric ischemia of a nonocclusive origin as well as those with surgically correctable occlusive lesions can be identified before bowel infarction occurs.

NONOCCLUSIVE MESENTERIC ISCHEMIA

Acute mesenteric ischemia has been diagnosed with increasing frequency during the past 25 years, but until recently this intraabdominal catastrophe remained as lethal as in 1933, when Hibbard et al. reported a mortality of 70% [16]. This continuing high mortality can be attributed mainly to three factors: (1) inability to make the diagnosis before intestinal gangrene develops, (2) progression of the bowel infarction after the primary initiating vascular or systemic cause has been corrected, and (3) the increasing frequency of nonocclusive mesenteric ischemia, or the "low flow" syndrome, as a cause of intestinal vascular catastrophies.

Nonocclusive mesenteric ischemia refers to intestinal ischemia and necrosis in the absence of major arterial or venous occlusion. It is now recognized that this entity results from prolonged mesenteric vasoconstriction, a distinctive pathophysiologic state that can be identified by its characteristic clinical and radiologic features. Although isolated colonic ischemia is also usually nonocclusive in nature, it is a different clinical entity from nonocclusive mesenteric ischemia of the small intestine, and most often follows a benign course and has an excellent prognosis. Colonic ischemia should not be included in discussions of nonocclusive mesenteric ischemia of the small intestine, which presents totally different problems in management.

Although several authors had described isolated instances of mesenteric infarction in the absence of major arterial or venous occlusion, Ende [12] in

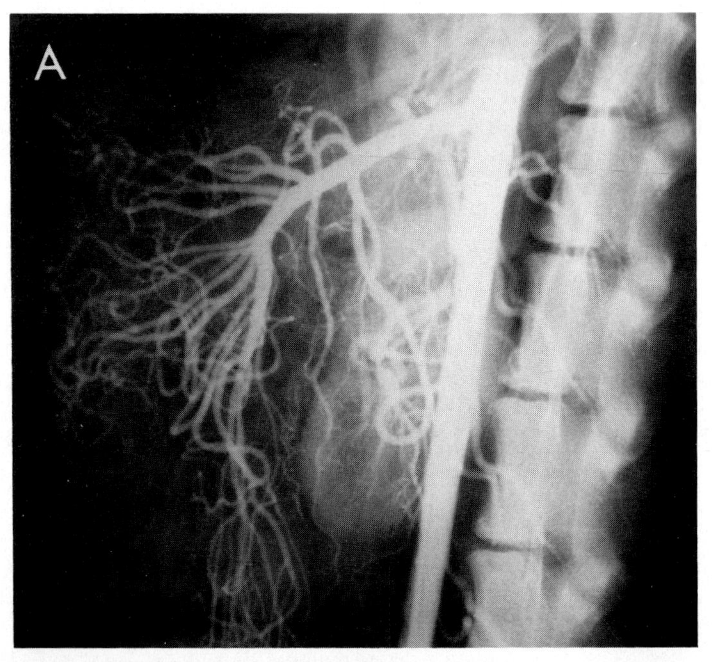
A

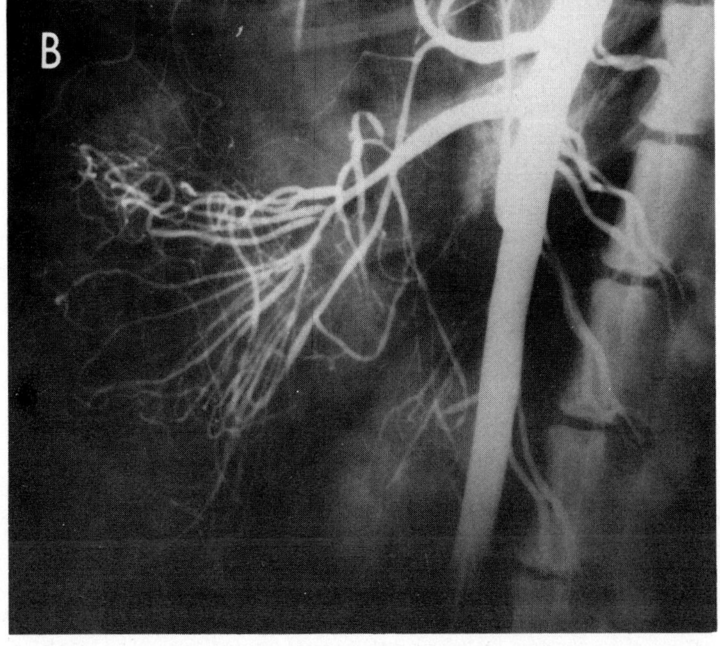
B

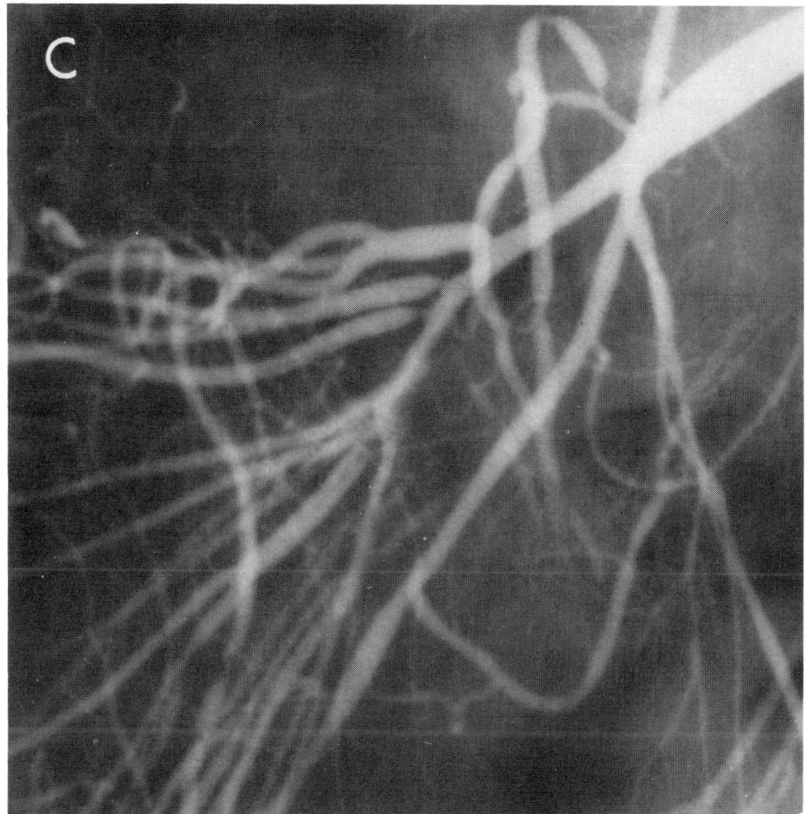

Fig. 6. Experimental production of mesenteric arterial vasoconstriction. (A, left) Baseline angiogram. (B, left) Repeat angiogram during intravenous infusion of 50 μg/min of levarterenol shows extensive vasoconstriction. (C) Closeup of part B showing narrowings at origins of major branches of the superior mesenteric artery with segments of narrowing and abnormal tapering in intestinal branches. [From Siegelman SS, et al: Angiographic diagnosis of mesenteric arterial vasoconstriction. Radiology 112:533, 1974, used by permission.]

1958 first focused attention on nonocclusive mesenteric ischemia as a distinct entity. Since that time the proportion of mesenteric vascular accidents recognized as being due to this cause has risen from 12% to over 50% in recently reported series [18, 22,31]. Treatment of this form of acute mesenteric ischemia has been ineffective in reducing its 90% mortality rate [15]. This is due primarily to the fact that the underlying cause of the inadequate blood flow often is not amenable to surgical correction, and thus the role of operation is limited to resection of already infarcted bowel. The pathogenesis of this entity is presently believed to be splanchnic vasoconstriction which occurs in response to a decrease in cardiac output, hypovolemia, dehydration, vasopressor agents, or hypotension. Predisposing conditions include myocardial infarction, congestive heart failure, renal and hepatic failure, or major abdominal or cardiac operations. In addition, a more immediate precipitating cause such as pulmonary edema, cardiac arrhythmias, or shock is usually present, although the intestinal ischemic episode may not become manifest until hours to days later.

Several investigators have implicated disseminated intravascular coagulation in the pathogenesis of nonocclusive mesenteric ischemia based upon the presence of fibrin thrombi in intestinal specimens from patients with this entity [20, 30]. In a study of infarcted intestine from patients with occlusive and nonocclusive intestinal ischemia we identified significant fibrin thrombi in only 20% of the intestinal sections from patients with nonocclusive mesenteric ischemia, but in 50% of those sections from patients with occlusive mesenteric ischemia [10]. Since fibrin thrombi appear to be a nonspecific feature of intestinal infarctions regardless of etiology, their presence in specimens from patients with nonocclusive mesenteric ischemia should not be the basis for attributing a primary etiologic role to disseminated intravascular coagulation.

Other facts responsible for the poor prognosis of patients with nonocclusive mesenteric ischemia are their advanced age, extreme illness, and the presence of multisystem disease. Many are in Coronary or Intensive Care Units. Hence there has been an understandable reluctance in the past to subject such individuals to aggressive invasive diagnostic studies and therapy. However, despite their critical condition, a significant number of these patients survive their major cardiac insult only to succumb to intestinal infarction.

Clinical Features

The usual clinical setting is that of a patient having or recovering from an episode of one of the precipitating conditions previously enumerated. The predominant symptom is abdominal pain, although it is absent in up to 25% of patients. The pain is most often diffuse and varying in severity, but can be severe and midepigastric as seen with mesenteric arterial embolus. Early in the course of nonocclusive mesenteric ischemia there are a few positive physical findings, but even at this stage the stools are positive for occult blood in 75% of patients. Later, abdominal distention and peritoneal signs may develop along with other symptoms and signs of more advanced ischemic bowel damage (i.e., back pain, nausea, vomiting, or diarrhea).

Leukocytosis, especially out of proportion to the physical findings, an elevated hematocrit, and blood tinged peritoneal fluid obtained by paracentesis are all signs of advanced intestinal necrosis. Other laboratory findings suggestive, but not diagnostic, of intestinal ischemia are unexplained metabolic acidosis, elevated serum amylase or intestinal alkaline phosphatase, and elevations in serum or peritoneal fluid phosphate.

Several potential diagnostic radioisotope techniques have been developed in animal studies but as yet have not been clinically proven. Schimmel and

Moss [24] employed technetium-99m pyrophosphate, which had been shown to localize in acutely infarcted myocardium, but they had only moderate success in detecting intestinal infarcts by external scanning. However, Barth et al. [3], using the same agent, and Ortiz and his colleagues [21], using technetium-99m diphosphonate, have reported successful external scanning of infarcted bowel after intravenous administration of the radioisotopes. We have investigated the use of technetium-99m sulfur colloid labeled leukocytes to diagnose ischemic intestine [2]. In 13 of 15 dogs, external scintigrams showed increased radionuclide uptake corresponding to the ischemic bowel. Radioactivity of the excised ischemic intestine averaged 5.9 times greater than that of normal bowel. This technique, which depends upon the marked inflammatory response to intestinal ischemia, is of potential clinical value since it can be performed in 3-4 hours. In our experiments increased radionuclide uptake was detectable within 2 hours of the onset of ischemia and also was present 24 hours after the onset.

Management

Our clinical and experimental experiences have led us to conclude that

1. The mortality rate of all forms of acute mesenteric ischemia will remain at its present high level unless the diagnosis is established and therapy instituted before intestinal necrosis develops;
2. Early diagnosis only can be accomplished if all patients suspected of having acute mesenteric ischemia are subjected to prompt roentgenologic studies;
3. Reluctance to subject these severely ill patients to the rigors of angiography because of its previously limited value (only to exclude embolus or thrombosis) is no longer valid, as the diagnosis of occlusive *and* nonocclusive mesenteric ischemia is now possible and active therapeutic measures are available for both; and
4. Persistent vasoconstriction is a major factor in both nonocclusive and occlusive mesenteric ischemia and can be relieved or prevented by direct intraarterial infusion of papaverine.

In 1972, based upon these conclusions, we proposed an aggressive approach to the management of acute mesenteric ischemia [8] with the hope of preventing intestinal gangrene and decreasing the extremely high mortality rate reported with this entity. The essential features in this approach are the earlier and more extensive use of angiography to diagnose mesenteric ischemia and to determine its cause, and the intraarterial infusion of papaverine to interrupt the splanchnic vasoconstriction persisting after successful management of the underlying local or systemic cardiovascular etiology. The proper incorporation of these concepts in a comprehensive radiologic and therapeutic plan for the management of patients with suspected acute mesenteric ischemia has resulted in an impressive improvement in both patient survival and salvage of compromised bowel.

General Approach

Patients at risk are considered to be those over 50 years of age with either (1) valvular or arteriosclerotic heart disease, (2) long-standing congestive heart failure, especially with unsatisfactory control by digitalis therapy or prolonged use of diuretics, (3) cardiac arrhythmias of any etiology, (4) hypovolemia or hypotension of any origin such as burns, pancreatitis, or gastrointestinal hemorrhage, or (5) recent myocardial infarctions.

Patients in any of these high-risk categories who develop sudden onset of abdominal pain lasting more than 2 or 3 hours are started on the management protocol outlined in Fig. 7. These broad selection criteria are essential if early diagnosis and treatment are to be achieved because the presence of more extensive and specific signs and symptoms usually signifies irreversible intestinal damage.

Initial treatment is directed toward correction of predisposing or precipitating causes of the mesenteric ischemia. Relief of acute congestive heart failure, reversion of cardiac arrhythmias, and replacement of blood or plasma volume precede any diagnostic studies. Because of their direct vasoconstrictor effect on the SMA, digitalis and vasopressors are discontinued whenever possible.

When intestinal ischemia has progressed far enough that systemic alterations associated with bowel infarction are present, appropriate replacement of plasma volume and fluid loss, gastrointestinal decompression, and parenteral antibiotics are included in the preparation prior to roentgenologic studies. In patients requiring large fluid volumes, a central venous catheter or pulmonary artery wedge catheter is placed to facilitate rapid replacement in the face of a precarious cardiac reserve.

After the initial corrective and supportive measures have been completed, roentgenologic studies are undertaken irrespective of the abdominal physical findings or the surgeon's decision whether or not to operate. Plain film examination of the abdomen is performed not to help in the diagnosis of acute mesenteric ischemia but to exclude other roentgenologically diagnosable causes of abdominal pain, e.g., a perforated viscus or intestinal obstruction. If the plain films do not reveal an acute abdominal condition other than mesenteric ischemia, angiography is performed.

Angiographic examination includes multiple injections of contrast material. An initial flush aortogram is obtained to detect aneurysms, dissections, and emboli or other occlusions of major visceral arteries and to evaluate the collateral circulation between the superior mesenteric and celiac and/or inferior mesenteric arterial systems. Selective angiography is then performed to detect emboli, thrombosis, or mesenteric vasoconstriction in the SMA or its branches. If either an embolus or mesenteric vasoconstriction is found a single bolus of 25 mg of tolazoline is given into the SMA catheter followed by a repeat angiogram. This provides both better visualization of the peripheral circulation and a general idea of the potential effectiveness of a papaverine infusion. However, the response or

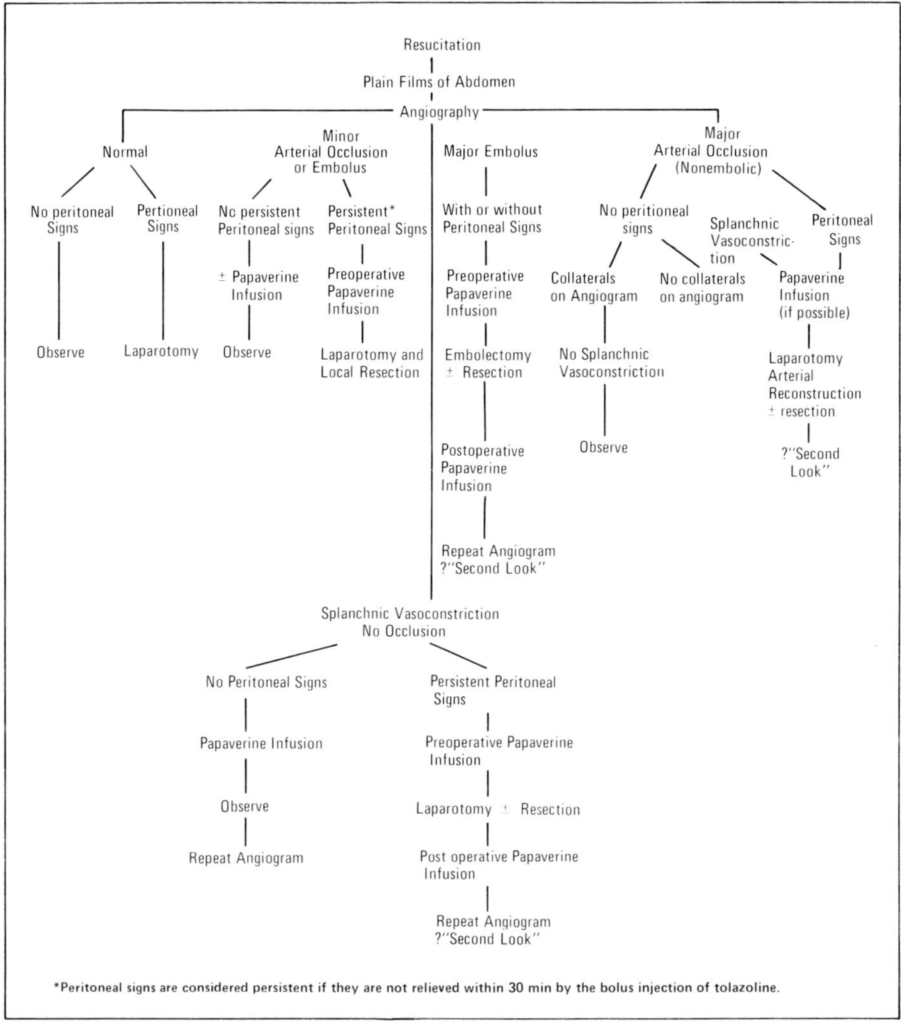

Fig. 7. Scheme of proposed plan for diagnosis and treatment of acute mesenteric ischemia.

lack of response to the bolus injection does not effect the decision to employ a papaverine infusion if indicated. Tolazoline is not used for infusions as it is neither as effective nor as safe as papaverine by this method of administration. One-half the usual volume of contrast material is used in all the selective studies to minimize renal damage.

Based upon the angiographic findings and the presence or absence of persistent signs of peritoneal irritation on physical examination of the abdomen, the patients are treated according to the scheme in Fig. 7. In two of our patients with acute mesenteric ischemia both the abdominal pain and the physical signs of peritonitis disappeared after an injection of tolazoline during angiography. The clinical changes were accompanied by improvement of the mesenteric vasoconstriction on the repeat angiograms. Thus only signs which persist after the bolus of tolazoline are considered indications for operation.

Nonocclusive mesenteric ischemia is diagnosed when the angiographic signs of mesenteric vasoconstriction are seen in a patient with a clinical picture suggestive of intestinal ischemia who is neither in shock nor receiving vasopressors. The angiographic findings may vary from localized spasm to a "pruned" appearance of the entire mesenteric arterial tree (Fig. 8).

A papaverine infusion is begun on all patients with nonocclusive mesenteric ischemia as soon as the diagnosis is made, and in patients with persistent peritoneal signs the infusion is continued during and after laparotomy.

At operation manipulation of the SMA is kept to a minimum. Obviously necrotic bowel is resected and a primary anastomosis performed. If bowel of questionable viability is left behind, a "second look" is scheduled. It is better to leave bowel of doubtful viability than to perform a massive small bowel resection, for in many instances the circulation will have improved by the time of the second exploration.

Whether or not the patient is operated upon, the papaverine infusion is continued for approximately 24 hours and then a repeat angiogram is performed

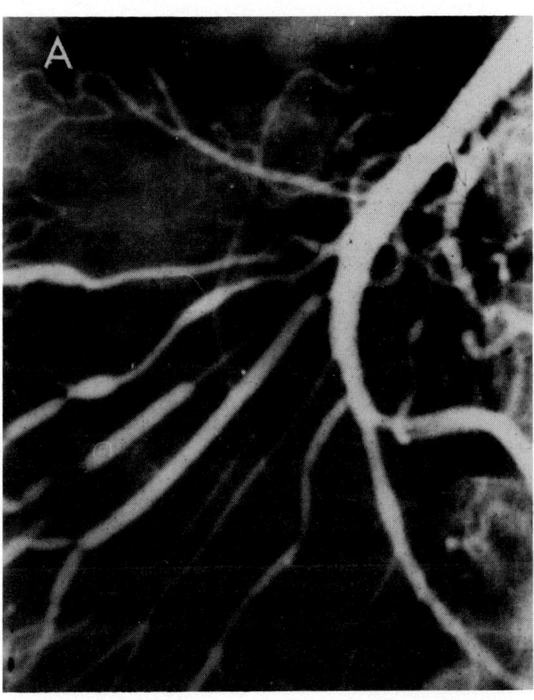

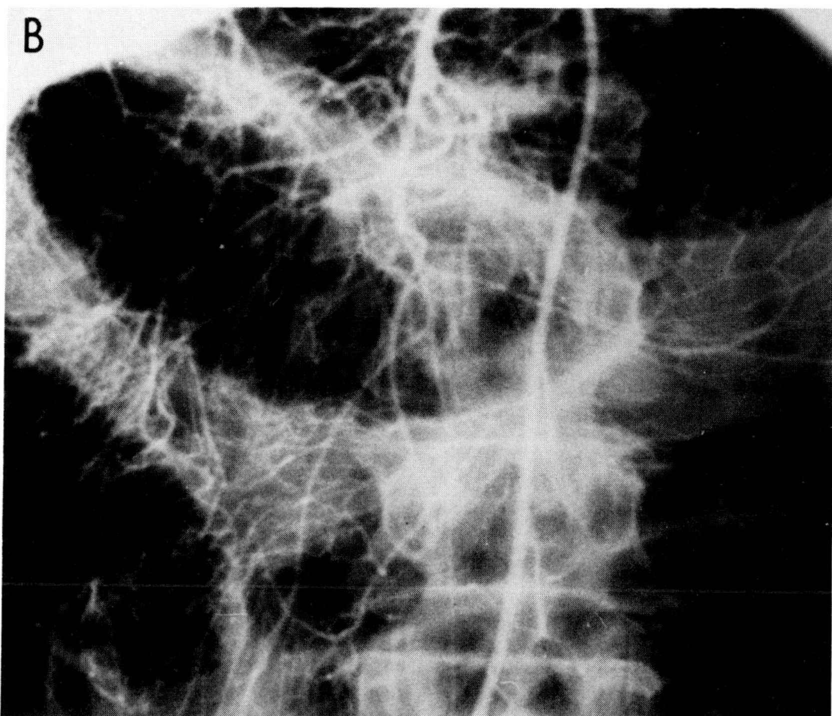

Fig. 8. Angiographic appearance of mesenteric vasoconstriction in patients. (A, left) Spasm at origins of major SMA branches and multiple areas of intermittent spasm and dilatation ("string of sausages"). [Courtesy of S. S. Siegelman, Baltimore, Md.] (B) Typical appearance of marked constriction of entire SMA and its major branches. [Reproduced with permission from Boley SJ, et al: Ischemic disorders of the intestines, in Ravitch MM, et al (eds): Current Problems in Surgery. Copyright © 1978 by Year Book Medical Publishers, Inc., Chicago.]

30 min after changing the infusion to isotonic saline without papaverine. Based upon the clinical course of the patient (e.g., abdominal distention, bowel function, abdominal findings, and evidence of blood in the stools) and the response of the vasoconstriction to therapy as noted on the angiogram, the infusion is discontinued or maintained for another 24 hours; the patient is then reevaluated (Fig. 9). Infusions have been continued for up to 5 days, but usually can be stopped after 24 hours. When papaverine is used in conjunction with laparotomy for nonocclusive disease, a "second look" is frequently necessary. In such cases the infusion is continued until the "second look" operation and afterwards if necessary. The papaverine infusion is discontinued when no signs of vasoconstriction remain on an angiogram which is obtained 30 min after the vasodilator infusion is temporarily replaced by saline alone. The SMA catheter is removed promptly when the intraarterial infusion is stopped.

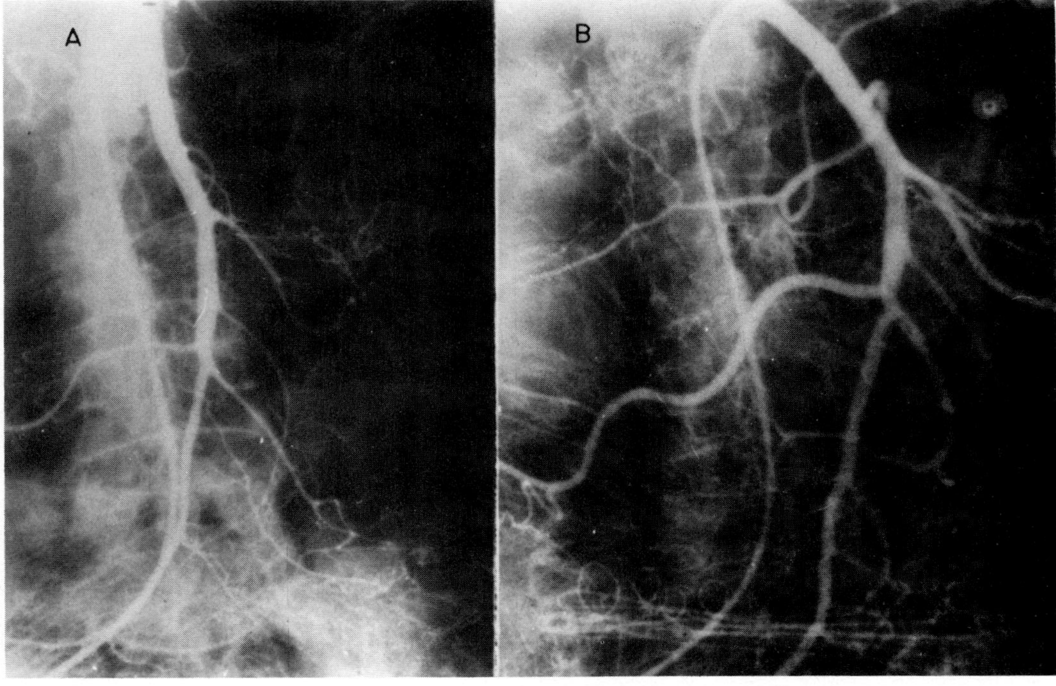

Fig. 9. Patient with nonocclusive mesenteric ischemia managed with papaverine infusion for 3 days. (A) Initial angiogram showing spasm of main SMA, origins of branches, and intestinal arcades. (B) Angiogram after 36 hours of papaverine infusion. Study was obtained 30 min after papaverine was replaced with saline. At this time the patient's abdominal symptoms and signs were gone. [Reproduced with permission from Boley SJ, et al: Ischemic disorders of the intestines, in Ravitch MM, et al (eds): Current Problems in Surgery. Copyright © 1978 by Year Book Medical Publishers, Inc., Chicago.]

Supportive Therapy

An essential aspect of the supportive therapy of patients with acute mesenteric ischemia is the maintenance of an adequate plasma volume. Just as massive losses of protein-rich fluids occur with early bowel infarction, so may they occur following revascularization of ischemic bowel. Hence it is important to continually correct for losses preparatory to undertaking therapy, during papaverine infusions, and following surgical relief of arterial occlusions. The use of low molecular weight dextran may serve a dual purpose because of its effect as a plasma expander and because of its potential value in decreasing sludging in the microcirculation.

The value of both systemic and locally instilled antibiotics in improving the viability of compromised bowel is well accepted. For this reason, and because of the high incidence of positive blood cultures with acute mesenteric ischemia, systemic antibiotics are started as soon as the diagnosis is established. Antibiotics also can be locally instilled into the intestine by means of a fine catheter inserted at the time of operation, as described by Delany et al. [11].

Intestinal decompression by nasogastric suction, the use of furosemide and mannitol to maintain urinary output, and specific therapy for the cardiac problems all play a role in the management of most patients. Digitalis, as previously mentioned, must be used cautiously, and vasopressors should be avoided. Anticoagulant therapy is specifically avoided except in venous thrombosis because of the danger of intestinal hemorrhage. Early in our experience we had two patients who bled massively as a result of heparin administered after successful embolectomy.

Prognosis

The reported mortality of nonocclusive mesenteric ischemia treated by traditional methods have varied from 70% to 100% [1, 22, 29]. Authors reporting better results have included in their series patients with isolated colonic ischemia, which as previously mentioned is a distinctly different problem with an excellent prognosis. In the initial series of 50 patients managed by our aggressive approach [7], 35 (70%) proved to have acute mesenteric ischemia, 15 of whom had nonocclusive mesenteric ischemia. Five patients with nonocclusive mesenteric ischemia had no peritoneal signs and all survived without operation. Seven of the ten patients with peritoneal signs were operated upon, and all had gangrenous bowel. In two of these the involvement was too extensive for resection. The five others underwent resection, and two survived. Of the three patients with peritoneal signs who were not operated upon, one died before an operation could be performed, and in the other two the pain and abdominal findings subsided after a vasodilator was infused into the SMA.

Nine of the fifteen patients (60%) with nonocclusive mesenteric ischemia survived. However, only two of the eight patients in whom intestinal necrosis occurred survived, emphasizing the contribution of early diagnosis and treatment to our improved results.

CONCLUSIONS

The response of the mesenteric vascular bed to systemic and local cardiovascular disturbances is often severe vasoconstriction, which may persist after the primary problem has been corrected. Nonocclusive mesenteric ischemia is the primary example and result of this sequence of events.

Our aggressive approach to acute mesenteric ischemia offers promise of a markedly improved prognosis for patients with either the nonocclusive or occlusive forms of these vascular catastrophies. We believe that the results of earlier application of the diagnostic and therapeutic methods included in this approach justify the risks and will ultimately increase both the number of survivors and the quality of their survival. An increased awareness and acceptance of the need for early angiographic study in patients "at risk" must be the first step in wider adoption of these concepts.

REFERENCES

1. Aldrete JS, Han SY, Laws HL, et al: Intestinal infarction complicating lower cardiac output states. Surg. Gynecol. Obstet. 144:371, 1977
2. Bardfeld PA, Boley SJ, Sammartano RJ, et al: Scintographic diagnosis of ischemic intestine with Technetium 99m sulfur colloid labelled leukocytes. Radiology 112:553, 1974
3. Barth KH, Alderson PO, Stroudberg JD, et al: ^{99m}Tc pyrophosphate imaging experimental mesenteric infarction: Relationship of tracer uptake to the degree of ischemic injury. Radiology 129:491, 1978
4. Boley SJ, Agrawal GP, Warren AR, et al: Pathophysiologic effects of bowel distention on intestinal blood flow. Am. J. Surg. 117:228, 1969
5. Boley SJ, Brandt LJ, Veith FJ: Ischemic disorders of the intestines, in Ravitch MM, et al (eds): Current Problems in Surgery. Chicago, Year Book Medical, 1978
6. Boley SJ, Regan JA, Tunick PA, et al: Persistent vasoconstriction – A major factor in nonocclusive mesenteric ischemia. Curr. Topics Surg. Res. 3:425, 1971
7. Boley SJ, Sprayregen S, Siegelman SS, et al: Initial results from an aggressive approach to acute mesenteric ischemia. Surgery 82:848, 1977
8. Boley SJ, Sprayregen S, Veith FJ, et al: An aggressive roentgenologic and surgical approach to acute mesenteric ischemia, in Nyhus LM (ed): Surgery Annual. New York, Appleton-Century-Crofts, 1973, p 355

9. Boley SJ, Treiber W, Winslow PR, et al: Circulatory responses to acute reduction of superior mesenteric arterial blood flow. Physiologist 12:180, 1969
10. Brandt LJ, Gomery P, Mitsudo SM, et al: Disseminated intravascular coagulation in nonocclusive mesenteric ischemia: The lack of specificity of fibrin thrombi in intestinal infarction. Gastroenterology 7:954, 1976
11. Delany HM, Carnevale NJ, Garvey JM: Jejunostomy by a needle catheter technique. Surgery 73:786, 1973
12. Ende N: Infarction of the bowel in cardiac failure. N. Engl. J. Med. 258:879, 1958
13. Everhard ME, Regan JA, Veith FJ, et al: Mesenteric vasomotor response to reduced mesenteric blood flow. Physiologist 13:191, 1970
14. Folkow B, Lewis D, Lundgran O, et al: The effect of the sympathetic vasoconstrictor fibers on the distribution of the capillary blood flow in the intestine. Acta Physiol. Scand. 61:458, 1964
15. Herr FW, Silen W, French SW: Intestinal gangrene without apparent vascular occlusion. Am. J. Surg. 110:231, 1965
16. Hibbard JS, Swenson JC, Levin AG: Roentgenology of experimental mesenteric vascular occlusion. Arch. Surg. 26:20, 1933
17. Holenberg NK, Epstein M, Rosen SM, et al: Acute oliguric renal failure in man: Evidence of preferential renal cortical ischemia. Medicine (Baltimore) 45:455, 1968
18. Jackson BB: Occlusion of the superior mesenteric artery, in: Monograph in American Lectures in Surgery. Springfield, Ill., Charles C. Thomas, 1963, pp 1-141
19. Kukovetz WR, Poch G: Inhibition of cyclic-3′,5′ nucleotide-phosphodiesterase as a possible mode of action of papaverine and similarly acting drugs. Naunyn-Schmiedebergs Arch. Pharmacol. 267:189, 1970
20. Margaretten W, McKay DG: Thrombotic ulcerations of the gastrointestinal tract. Arch. Intern. Med. 12:250, 1971
21. Ortiz VN, Sfakinakis G, Haase GM, et al: The value of radionuclide scanning in early diagnosis of intestinal infarction. J. Pediatr. Surg. 13:616, 1978
22. Ottinger LW, Austen WG: A study of 136 patients with mesenteric infarction. Surg. Gynecol. Obstet. 124:251, 1967
23. Reynolds DG: Silicone rubber technique for microvascular studies. Lab. Management 6:24, 1968
24. Schimmel DH, Moss AA, Hoffer PB: Radionuclide imaging of intestinal infarction in dogs. Invest. Radiol. 11:277, 1976
25. Selkurt EE, Scibetta MP, Cull TE: Haemodynamics of intestinal circulation. Circ. Res. 6:92, 1958
26. Siegelman SS, Sprayregen S, Boley SJ: Angiographic diagnosis of mesenteric arterial vasoconstriction. Radiology 112:553, 1974
27. Tunik P, Treiber WF, Frank M, et al: Pathophysiologic effects of bowel distention on intestinal blood flow II. Curr. Topics Surg. Res. 2:59, 1970
28. Ulano HB, Treat E, Shanbour LL, et al: Selective dilatation of the constricted superior mesenteric artery. Gastroenterology 62:39, 1972

29. Veller ID, Doyle JC: Acute mesenteric ischemia. Aust. N. Z. J. Surg. 47:54, 1977
30. Whitehead R: Ischemic enterocolitis: An expression of the intravascular coagulation syndrome. Gut 12:912, 1971
31. Williams LF, Wittenberg J: Vascular insufficiency of the intestine. Viewpoints Digest. Dis. March 1973

John J. Bergan, M.D.

Acute Mesenteric Ischemia

Recently, a 68 year old woman with polycythemia rubra vera treated by venisection was admitted for diagnosis of postprandial abdominal pain and severe weight loss. The entire evaluation was normal except for an enlarged spleen and liver and an abnormal volume response to secretin administration, so she was discharged home. A possible diagnosis of pancreatic carcinoma was entertained. The ultrasound examination of the pancreas and small bowel and colon roentgenograms were normal.

Within a month, she was readmitted for exploratory laparotomy because of worsening symptoms. Postprandial pain was lasting so long that the abdominal discomfort was almost continuous. The abdominal viscera were normal, including the entire pancreas. A salpingo-oophorectomy was done.

Within another month, cramping abdominal pain persisted and the patient was again readmitted with a suspected bowel obstruction. During this admission, her white blood count was 67,000, which was twice her normal value. Later, her temperature rose to 101°F, and her white blood count became 90,000. Although the patient felt fairly comfortable, the white count continued to increase to levels of 100,000 and 105,000.

Ultimately, an exploratory laparotomy revealed small bowel infarcted from the ligament of Treitz to the cecum with additional involvement of the ascending, transverse, and part of the descending colon. Resection was done, an anastomotic leak occurred, and the patient died on the tenth postoperative day.

The object of setting forth this case is that it exactly typifies the development of mesenteric infarction as we know it today. The case shows an insidious onset of intestinal thrombosis heralded by abdominal pain and weight loss. It illustrates an adequate opportunity for appropriate diagnosis by angiography before the mesenteric arterial circulation occludes. It depicts the suspected diagnosis of malignancy in such patients and shows the futility of intestinal resection as therapy of mesenteric infarction. Management of this case was consistent with traditional surgical teaching, but such teaching regarding vascular disease of the intestine has been confusing. Only during this last decade of surgical experience has it been possible for us to look at syndromes of intestinal ischemia in new ways so that specific diagnosis is emphasized and so that reconstructive vascular surgery can be applied in treatment. Fortunately, the acute syndromes which demand urgent surgical care are those which are best understood. By applying the lessons learned in treatment of acute ischemia of the limbs, surgeons can treat acute ischemia of the intestine so that mortality of mesenteric infarction can be decreased.

PHILOSOPHY OF TREATMENT

As detailed below, accurate diagnosis can be made in the three major syndromes of acute intestinal infarction. Thereafter, specific reconstructive vascular surgery can be performed with an expectation of survival of the patient. However, many patients with acute intestinal infarction are aged, sometimes senile, often residents of custodial care institutions, and are admitted to general hospitals for surgical evaluation late in the progress of their disease. They arrive dehydrated, hypovolemic, acidotic, hypotensive, and hemoconcentrated. In this situation, facing vigorous diagnostic manipulation and rigorous surgical therapy, the patient may be in no condition to survive the contemplated procedures. It may be that the kindest treatment for the patient and the surrounding family members is to do nothing except to support mildly the patient's vital signs. This is a personal philosophy for each surgeon. One must be aware of this because one should not automatically initiate invasive diagnostic manipulations and plan surgery of the magnitude which the condition dictates without understanding what is liable to happen. Swift death may be preferable to agonizing and slow, expensive deterioration.

On the other hand, many patients with intestinal infarction have a prospect of productive longevity. It is these persons in whom the following lessons can be applied with vigor.

SYNDROMES OF PRESENTATION

Although there are many rare cases of intestinal necrosis due to small artery occlusion [2, 22], the major causes of acute intestinal infarction relate to acute occlusion of the mesenteric artery itself.

Superior Mesenteric Artery Embolization

Embolic occlusion of the superior mesenteric artery was realized as being the most common cause of surgically treated intestinal infarction some years ago [4, 19]. More recently, this point of view has been supported again.

Ottinger's series from the Massachusetts General Hospital [24] cited 55% of patients with embolic occlusion of the superior mesenteric artery. It is clear that the syndrome of mesenteric artery embolization can be recognized by the onset of catastrophic abdominal pain in a patient with a cardiac lesion which might produce embolization. The sudden onset of pain is followed by gut emptying, vomiting, and diarrhea. A history of a previous embolic event is present in one-third of patients, and severe leukocytosis is present in more than two-thirds of such patients. Marston [20] disagrees with this point of view and states that "the terms mesenteric embolus, mesenteric thrombosis and non-occlusive infarction have to an extent lost their value and acute intestinal failure is preferred."

While atherosclerotic heart disease is the most common cause of embolization to the mesenteric artery and rheumatic heart disease is the next most frequent, it is important to understand that iatrogenic causes of embolization from the heart are becoming increasingly common. Such lesions include embolization from cardiac valves and after electrical conversion of rhythm.

One should remember that patients with acute occlusion of a relatively normal mesenteric artery will have no prodromal symptomatology of weight loss or postprandial abdominal pain.

Thrombotic Mesenteric Infarction

In 1936, Dunphy [11] noted that half the cases of intestinal infarction studied by him at the autopsy table had gastrointestinal symptoms which preceded the fatal bowel infarction. Now it is recognized that patients with mesenteric artery thrombosis may have such symptoms preceding bowel infarction, while patients with acute mesenteric embolization do not. The syndrome of thrombotic occlusion of the mesenteric artery is very much as that stated in the introduction to this paper. The syndrome develops insidiously and is progressive. There is steady, sometimes colicky abdominal pain caused by intestinal spasm. The patient may or may not bring a history of weight loss, postprandial pain, and altered bowel habits. Following the establishment of the constant abdominal pain, the syndrome progresses. It is characterized by bowel emptying, systemic hypovolemia, hemoconcentration, and intestinal fluid extravasation. As the bowel dies, there is abdominal distention, vomiting, and late bloody diarrhea. Profound leukocytosis is almost uniformly present, and fever will also be seen if sepsis and peritonitis occur.

The astute clinician will note that the patient is subject to great pain and prostration, appears ill out of proportion to his physical findings, and has evidence of other atherosclerotic occlusive disease in the periphery, in the limbs, the heart, or the brain. These findings should suggest the presence of thrombotic bowel infarction.

Nonorganic Intestinal Infarction

Strictly speaking, nonorganic mesenteric infarction is not a surgical condition. It must be differentiated from the mesenteric infarction caused by organic occlusion for two reasons. One is the opportunity to treat the nonorganic occlusive condition by intraarterial vasodilator administration. Another is the necessity for recognizing coincidental intestinal artery atheromatous narrowings which may be precipitating events to the nonocclusive intestinal infarction syndrome.

From whatever cause, in nonorganic bowel infarction a vicious cycle appears in which there is a constriction of the mesenteric arterial bed. It is usually induced by remote stimulus. Such a stimulus may be cardiac failure, systemic shock, head injury, or digitalis manipulation. The resultant bowel ischemia allows bacterial penetration of the mucosa and subsequent sepsis. The systemic response to such sepsis is sympathetic stimulation, which perpetuates the worsening cycle of intestinal ischemia.

The clinical presentation is much like that of other intestinal infarction and includes abdominal pain due to gut spasm, gut emptying, and leukocytosis. Late in this condition, as in mesenteric thrombosis and mesenteric embolization, melena and hematemesis are seen. Similar to the situation in mesenteric thrombosis, the patient appears ill out of proportion to the physical findings and is usually under treatment for a primary cardiac condition.

PATHOPHYSIOLOGY OF INTESTINAL INFARCTION

Experience in intestinal revascularization has shown that the pathophysiologic changes affect the mucosa of the bowel more than seromuscular layers. The appearance of the bowel therefore may be entirely deceptive; the bowel may appear to be irreversibly dead even though revascularization will allow return of viability and eventual regeneration of mucosa [10].

Experimentally, one can find early mitochondrial changes, clumping of nuclear chromatin and dilation of endoplasmic reticulum as the first signs of damage due to intestinal ischemia. Later, breakage of microvilli and swelling of mitochondria are observed. Within 2 hours, junctional complexes between many cells broaden, cells tend to detach from each other through cell membrane disruption, and changes in intracellular organelles progress. Within 4 hours, lethal changes become apparent [1]. Normally, the mitochondria are the prime organelles in the intestine responsible for efficient production of ATP through the aerobic cycle. When ischemia occurs, conversion from aerobic to anaerobic metabolism occurs. As the mechanical separation between cells and basement membrane develops, a fluid block modifies the transport of oxygen and substrate to epithelial cells. Lesser degrees of ischemic insult are reversible, while greater degrees of insult produce permanent damage [9].

DIAGNOSIS BY ANGIOGRAPHY

In the past, it was thought that patients with acute intestinal infarction were too ill to withstand angiography. However, this is not true [14]. Actually, a clinical diagnosis of embolus to the intestinal arteries can be made by an experienced surgeon. Nevertheless, confirmation by angiography is desirable. In a situation of insidious onset of intestinal infarction due to thrombosis, aortography must be performed to confirm the diagnosis. In the situation of nonorganic intestinal occlusion, emergency aortoarteriography must be done so that the diagnosis can be made and treatment initiated by intraarterial instillation of vasodilators.

Boley [6] has reported the results of an aggressive angiographic approach to intestinal infarction. Of the first 50 patients studied, 70% had acute mesenteric artery occlusion. Ultimately, 19 of these 35 patients survived, including 9 of 15 with nonocclusive mesenteric ischemia, 7 of 16 with severe mesenteric artery embolus, and 2 of 3 patients with superior mesenteric artery thrombosis.

The emergency aortoarteriogram is done by placing an intraaortic catheter at the level of the first lumbar vertebra and making an injection near the origin of the superior mesenteric artery. Embolic occlusion will appear as an obstructing lesion with a meniscuslike marin near the origin of the midcolic artery. This mercury meniscus sign should be looked for, as it is frequently observed. When the embolus lodges in this location, a number of proximal collateral channels will be patent. It is these proximal jejunal arteries which occasionally allow spontaneous resolution of the acute ischemia [13] and differentiate embolic from thrombotic occlusion.

Mesenteric thrombosis will be shown on angiography as a sharp cutoff of the contrast medium near the origin of the superior mesenteric artery. This will best be seen on the lateral films. The celiac axis may or may not be occluded. Similarly, the inferior mesenteric artery may not be visualized.

If sharp cutoffs or mercury meniscus signs near the origin of the mesenteric artery are not seen, the clinician should look for segmental spasm of the peripheral mesenteric vessels. This segmental spasm seen throughout the intestinal arborization may be the only indication that a diagnosis of nonorganic intestinal infarction can be made. Alteration of caliber of arcade vessels, smooth margins, or symmetrical lesions involving these vessels indicate spasm. In contrast, irregular margins and sharp cutoffs at bifurcations are characteristic of thrombotic, atherosclerotic occlusions.

It is now recognized that proximal mesenteric artery constriction may be an important component of nonocclusive mesenteric infarction [27]. Such a lesion can produce intestinal ischemia, which heals by scarring and stricture formation, or may produce segmental infarction. Therefore particular attention should be paid to the geometry of the proximal mesenteric artery.

SURGICAL TREATMENT OF MESENTERIC INFARCTION

"Since pure resectional therapy for intestinal infarction results in disastrously high mortality, attempts at revascularization are now being made. A limited degree of success is reported." [5] That conservative statement of the situation in 1976 has been verified and expanded in the subsequent 3 years of experience.

The first step in effective surgical therapy consists of accurate observation of the state of the intestines after these have been exposed at laparotomy. At this time, confirmation of the diagnosis must be made. The proximal jejunum in the region of the ligament of Treitz will be found to be normal and pulsatile arcade vessels will be seen if the diagnosis is superior mesenteric artery embolization. Distal to these pulsatile vessels will be variable lengths of intestine showing various ischemic changes. When these are seen, the mesenteric artery should be palpated in the mesentery and the point of cessation of pulsation determined.

Gross findings of the intestine will be dependent upon the time interval between mesenteric artery occlusion and surgical exploration. Immediately following occlusion of the mesenteric artery, the bowel will exhibit accordion pleating and bluish-white rippling of the seromuscular surface. Later, as the bowel relaxes, it will become increasingly pale, with a bluish tinge. The peritoneal coverings will lose their shiny appearance and peristalsis will be absent. Later, gross signs of hemorrhage into the mesentery will be seen. The bowel will become swollen, infiltrated with blood, and the mucosa becomes necrotic. When purulent peritonitis occurs, the picture will be one of hemorrhagic necrosis. At this time, with advanced intestinal changes, there will be permeability to bacteria and fluid, and bidirectional fluid flow will cause massive intraluminal loss of plasma and fluid. All of these changes will be evident at laparotomy.

Embolectomy

If mesenteric artery embolization is confirmed as the cause of intestinal artery occlusion, the mesenteric artery should be skeletonized in the mesentery through a transverse incision made through the peritoneum. A transverse arteriotomy should be done between atraumatic artery occluders. A No. 3 Fogarty thromboembolectomy catheter should be used to clear as much of the distal arterial tree as possible. The arteriotomy should be closed with interrupted or running sutures.

Following restoration of blood flow, pulsations will be seen to return to marginal vessels. After an appropriate period of time, judgment should be made whether or not intestinal resection should be performed. Similarly, it is at this time that a second look procedure should be decided upon.

Bypass for Thrombosis

If initial inspection of the intestinal wall shows that the area of ischemic necrosis or compromised viability of intestine extends to the ligament of Treitz, the diagnosis of mesenteric artery thrombosis is confirmed. Since death from intestinal fistula is now acknowledged to be the most important cause of mortality in patients surviving massive intestinal resection, it is logical to practice revascularization of the intestine prior to resection.

Thromboendarterectomy has been shown to be too massive a surgical insult for patients who are desperately ill with intestinal infarction. Therefore aortomesenteric grafting is now utilized for intestinal revascularization. Simple thrombectomy using a Fogarty catheter should not be done.

Vessels to be revascularized are exposed by standard arterial surgical techniques. The infrarenal lumbar aorta is skeletonized, the mesenteric artery exposed for an adequate length, and saphenous vein used as the graft material. The short graft from the infrarenal lumbar aorta to the mesenteric artery is made end of vein to side of artery in both instances. Although preoperative angiography may show celiac axis occlusion as well as superior mesenteric artery occlusion, only one of these vessels need be revascularized during this acute surgical event.

Following revascularization, the surgeon should decide for or against intestinal resection. Similarly, the surgeon must decide for or against a second look procedure to follow 24 hours later.

THE SECOND LOOK PROCEDURE

Unfortunately, none of the clinical signs following an exploratory laparotomy will allow judgment for or against a second look procedure within the first postoperative 24 hours. Also, it should be recognized that second look procedures are not mandatory following mesenteric embolectomy or grafting for thrombosis. In a review of 49 successful cases, it was found that only 7 required a second look procedure, and in only 2 of these was intestinal resection required. On the other hand, the presence of dead bowel within the abdomen is so dangerous that negative second look explorations are certainly warranted.

In Ottinger's recent series of 36 patients who might be possible candidates for elective reexploration, 15 actually underwent a planned operation between 12 and 36 hours after the initial procedure. Of these 15 patients undergoing a second look, 8 required a bowel resection, and such operation enhanced their chance of survival [24]. Ottinger's summary of the situation was that the decision to perform a second look operation was usually correct when the indication for such second visualization of the intestine was the question of intestinal viability. Interestingly, of 17 patients who did not have a second look, 4 would have benefitted by such exploration.

SPECIAL PROBLEMS OF NONOCCLUSIVE MESENTERIC INFARCTION

Many conditions result in decreased cardiac output and mesenteric vasospasm. These may include digitalis intoxication, hypovolemia, cardiac and septic shock, hemoconcentration, and vasopressor therapy [12, 15, 21, 23]. The importance of these is indicated by the fact that nonocclusive vascular disease accounts for 20%-50% of all cases of mesenteric infarction [8, 17, 25]. Recently, emphasis in teaching about nonocclusive mesenteric infarction was that no organic intestinal lesions were present. Nevertheless, several reports have indicated that significant stenosis of the superior mesenteric artery may be demonstrated in such conditions [12, 15, 18]. While we do not know in what proportion of cases such stenosis exists, we do know that it is mandatory to detect such lesions.

The pathophysiology of nonocclusive mesenteric infarction indicates that proximal superior mesenteric artery narrowing may be important. In situations of low cardiac output, there is a selective distribution of blood flow away from the mesenteric circulation to more vital organs. As the law of La Place is satisfied, intraarterial perfusion pressure decreases below the tension of the vessel wall and the vessel closes. Resultant ischemia leads to submucosal hemorrhage, mucosal slough, bloody diarrhea, infarction of the entire bowel wall, and final perforation. Knowledge of such pathophysiology allows specific nonoperative therapy to alleviate mesenteric vasospasm. Specific treatment includes supportive care, aortoarteriography to differentiate occlusive from nonocclusive ischemia, direct infusion of intraarterial vasodilators such as isoproterenol, phenoxybenzamine, tolazoline, papaverine, and glucagon. All of these have been utilized [4, 23], as has epidural anesthesia [16].

If superior mesenteric artery stenosis is present, an elective repair of the lesion can be done.

Although nonocclusive mesenteric ischemia is thought to be a nonsurgical condition, surgery may in fact have to be performed for general surgical indications. Whenever necrotic bowel is present, peritonitis or intestinal perforation is suspected, laparotomy will reveal the exact pathophysiologic process. Specific treatment by segmental resection of intestine can be done. Nevertheless, maximum vascularization of residual intestinal ends must be assured before anastomosis is created.

REFERENCES

1. Aho AJ, Arstila AI, Ahonen J, et al: Ultrastructural alterations in ischaemic lesion of small intestinal mucosa in experimental superior mesenteric artery occlusion. Effect of oxygen breathing. Scand. J. Gastroenterol. 8:439, 1973

2. Anderson WR, Richards A MacD, Weiss L: Hemorrhage and necrosis of the stomach and bowel due to atheroembolism. Am. J. Clin. Pathol. 48:30, 1967
3. Barnett SM, Davidson ED, Bradley EL III: Intestinal alkaline phosphatase and base deficit in mesenteric occlusion. J. Surg. Res. 20:243, 1976
4. Bergan JJ: Recognition and treatment of intestinal ischemia. Surg. Clin. North Am. 47:109, 1967
5. Bergan JJ, Yao JST: Visceral ischemic syndromes: Obstruction of the superior mesenteric artery, celiac axis and inferior mesenteric artery, in Sabiston DC Jr (ed): Davis-Christopher Textbook of Surgery. Philadelphia, W. B. Saunders, 1977, p 1987
6. Boley SJ, Sprayregan S, Siegelman S, Veith FJ: Initial results from an aggressive roentgenological and surgical approach to acute mesenteric ischemia. Surgery 82:848, 1977
7. Bonakdarpour A, Ming S, Lynch PR, et al: Superior mesenteric artery occlusion in dogs: A model to produce the spectrum of intestinal ischemia. J. Surg. Res. 19:251, 1975
8. Britt LG, Cheek RC: Nonocclusive mesenteric vascular disease: Clinical and experimental observations. Ann. Surg. 169:704, 1969
9. Brown RA, Chiu C-J, Scott HJ, et al: Ultrastructural changes in the canine ileal mucosal cell after mesenteric arterial occlusion. Arch. Surg. 101:290, 1970
10. Dumont AE, Tice DA, Mulholland JH: Arteriosclerotic occlusion of the superior mesenteric artery. Ann. Surg. 154:833, 1961
11. Dunphy JE: Abdominal pain of vascular origin. Am. J. Med. Sci. 192:109, 1936
12. Fogarty TJ, Fletcher WS: Genesis of nonocclusive mesenteric ischemia. Am. J. Surg. 111:130, 1966
13. Gusberg R, Gump FE: Combined surgical and nutritional management of patients with acute mesenteric vascular occlusion. Ann. Surg. 179:358, 1974
14. Harper DR, Buist TAS: Selective angiography in acute mid-gut ischemia. Gut 19:132, 1978
15. Heer FE, Silen W, French SW: Intestinal gangrene without apparent vascular occlusion. Am. J. Surg. 110:231, 1965
16. Jackson BB, Lykins R: Serial epidural analgesia in mesenteric arterial failure. Arch. Surg. 90:177, 1965
17. Jenson CB, Smith GA: A clinical study of 51 cases of mesenteric infarction. Surgery 40:930, 1956
18. Jordan PH, Boulafendis D, Guinn GA: Factors other than major vascular occlusion that contribute to intestinal infarction. Ann. Surg. 171:189, 1970
19. Liavag I: Acute mesenteric vascular insufficiency. A five-year material, including a case of successful superior mesenteric artery embolectomy. Acta Chir. Scand. 133:631, 1967
20. Marston A: Intestinal Ischaemia. Chicago, Year Book Medical, 1977
21. Ming SC: Hemorrhagic necrosis of the gastrointestinal tract and its relation to cardiovascular status. Circulation 32:332, 1965

22. Nygaard K, Flatmark A: Mesenteric arteritis with extensive intestinal gangrene. Acta Chir. Scand. 139:470, 1973
23. Ottinger LW: Nonocclusive mesenteric infarction. Surg. Clin. North Am. 54:689, 1974
24. Ottinger LW: The surgical management of acute occlusion of the superior mesenteric artery. Ann. Surg. 188:721, 1978
25. Ottinger LW, Austen WG: A study of 136 patients with mesenteric infarction. Surg. Gynecol. Obstet. 124:251, 1967
26. Robertson GS, Lyall AD, Macrae JGC: Acid-base disturbances in mesenteric occlusion. Surg. Gynecol. Obstet. 129:15, 1969
27. Russ JE, Haid SP, Yao JST, et al: Surgical treatment of nonocclusive mesenteric infarction. Am. J. Surg. 134:638, 1977
28. Vyden JK, Nagasawa K, Corday E: Hemodynamic consequences of acute occlusion of the superior mesenteric artery. Am. J. Cardiol. 34:687, 1974

Special Problems in Aortic Surgery

Jonathan B. Towne, M.D.

Revascularization of the Ischemic Kidney

Following acute renal artery obstruction, the viability of the nephron may be maintained by collateral blood flow from the capsular and periureteric vessels. However, this flow is at a subfiltration pressure and results in anuric renal failure if both kidneys or a solitary kidney are involved. This blood flow maintains the viability of the glomerulus, but the renal tubule cells atrophy. If renal artery blood flow is restored, filtration is resumed and the renal tubular cells regenerate. Occasionally, if extensive collateral flow develops, renal function will return spontaneously several months after renal artery obstruction [2]. Our experience with renal failure secondary to acute renal artery obstruction demonstrated that this is often a surgically remedial lesion.

CASE REPORTS

Case 1. A 64-year-old hypertensive woman was transferred to our hospital 3 days following elective resection of an abdominal aortic aneurysm. The patient had been anuric since surgery. During the aneurysm resection, the aorta was cross-clamped above the renal arteries for 2 min to control bleeding at the proximal suture line. On admission to our hospital on the third postoperative day, her BUN level was 83 mg/100 ml and her serum potassium level was 6 meq/liter. An aortogram demonstrated a patent graft; however, both renal arteries were occluded at their origin.

At celiotomy, backbleeding was obtained from both renal arteries following thrombectomy. Bilateral aortorenal bypass was constructed utilizing 8-mm knitted Dacron prostheses. The cyanotic, flaccid kidneys distended and became pink following restoration of arterial flow. Examination of biopsy specimens revealed patchy areas of cortical necrosis, as well as acute tubular necrosis. Abdominal aortography on the second postoperative day demonstrated functioning aortorenal grafts. In the early postoperative period, the patient required hemodialysis five times until diuresis began on the 12th postoperative day. Convalescence was prolonged by pulmonary and cardiac complications, but the patient was discharged on the 46th postoperative day. An intravenous pyelogram at the time of discharge revealed function in the right kidney, but nonvisualization of the left.

The patient did well postoperatively, with blood pressures ranging from 160 to 180 mm Hg systolic and 90 to 110 mm Hg diastolic on moderate doses of chlorothiazide and reserpine. The BUN level ranged from 48 to 70 mg/100 ml and the serum creatinine from 3 to 5 mg/100 ml. Intravenous pyelograms 2 years postoperatively demonstrated bilateral function, although there was considerable cortical thinning of the left kidney. The patient died of pneumonia and pulmonary emboli 4 years postoperatively.

Case 2. A 72-year-old man was admitted to the vascular service with a 36-hour history of left flank pain, nausea, and vomiting. He had been anuric for 18 hours prior to admission. An arteriogram performed at the referring hospital demonstrated total occlusion of the abdominal aorta extending proximally to the origin of the renal arteries.

The patient's cardiac function was stable at this time, although he had had four previous myocardial infarctions with congestive heart failure. His serum potassium level on admission was 6.2 meq/liter. At celiotomy, thromboendarterectomy of the perirenal aorta and the right renal artery, as well as thrombectomy of the left renal artery, was performed. There was backbleeding from both renal arteries. Following restoration of blood flow, both kidneys became distended and pink. An aortofemoral bypass restored circulation to the lower extremities. At the completion of the procedure, a Schribner shunt was inserted. Postoperatively, the patient required hemodialysis four times until diuresis commenced on the 18th postoperative day. An aortogram on the fifth postoperative day demonstrated patent renal arteries, with a filling defect in the dorsal division branch of the left kidney causing subtotal obstruction of that branch (Fig. 1).

The patient was discharged on the 40th postoperative day. He has remained well for the past 20 months, with a blood pressure of 152/94 mm Hg without medication. His serum creatinine level is 3 mg/100 ml and his BUN level is 39 mg/100 ml.

Case 3. A 65-year-old man was admitted to the medical service with congestive heart failure. The patient had previously had two myocardial infarctions, and he had a long history of chronic atrial fibrillation treated with digitalis and quinidine sulfate. He had undergone a left nephrectomy in 1968 for chronic pyelonephritis.

He was noted to be anuric shortly after admission. An arteriogram done 12 hours after admission revealed an occlusion of the right renal artery 3.5 cm distal to its origin from the aorta. Eighteen hours after admission, a renal artery embolectomy was performed and a Schribner shunt inserted. Arteriogram obtained on the second postoperative day demonstrated a patent renal artery with a residual filling defect in the right lower pole branch (Fig. 2).

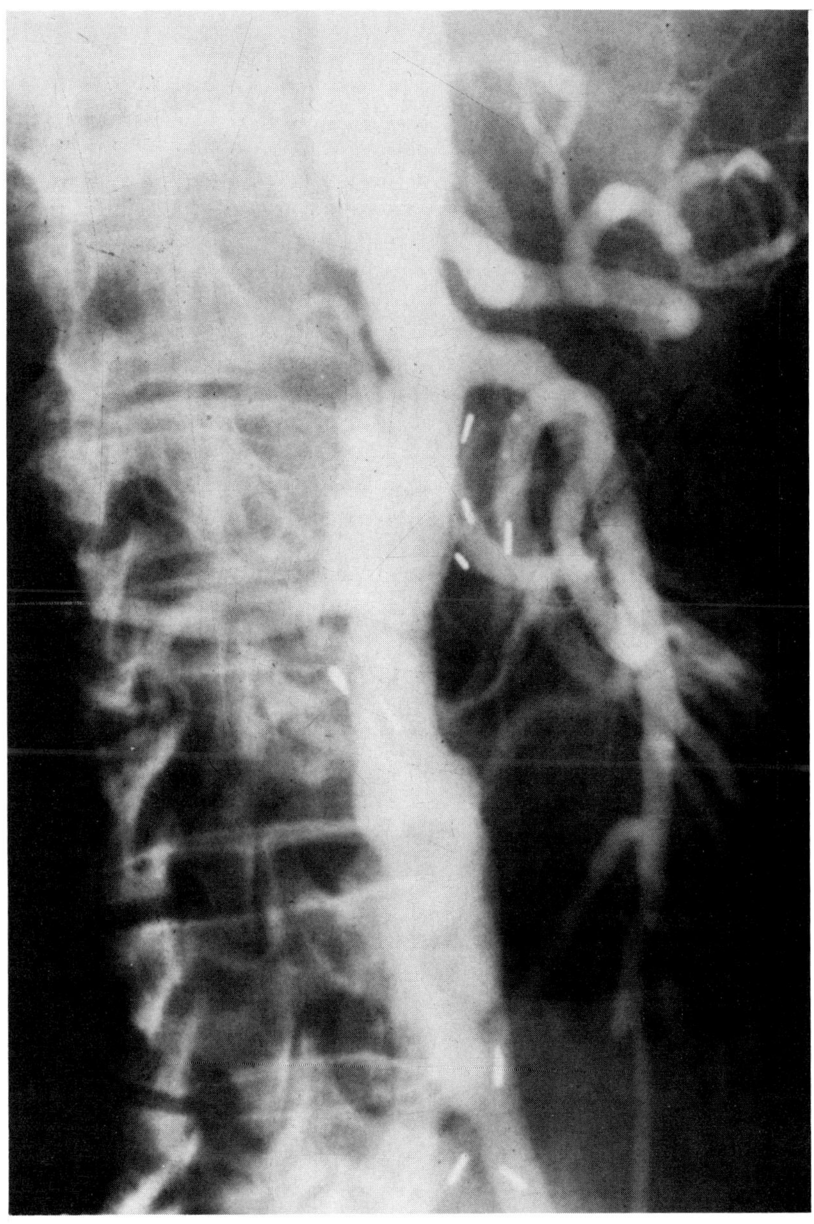

Fig. 1. Case 2. Postoperative arteriogram demonstrating patent renal arteries. [Reproduced from Towne JB, Bernhard VM: Revascularization of the ischemic kidney. Arch. Surg. 113:216-218, 1978. Copyright 1978, American Medical Association.]

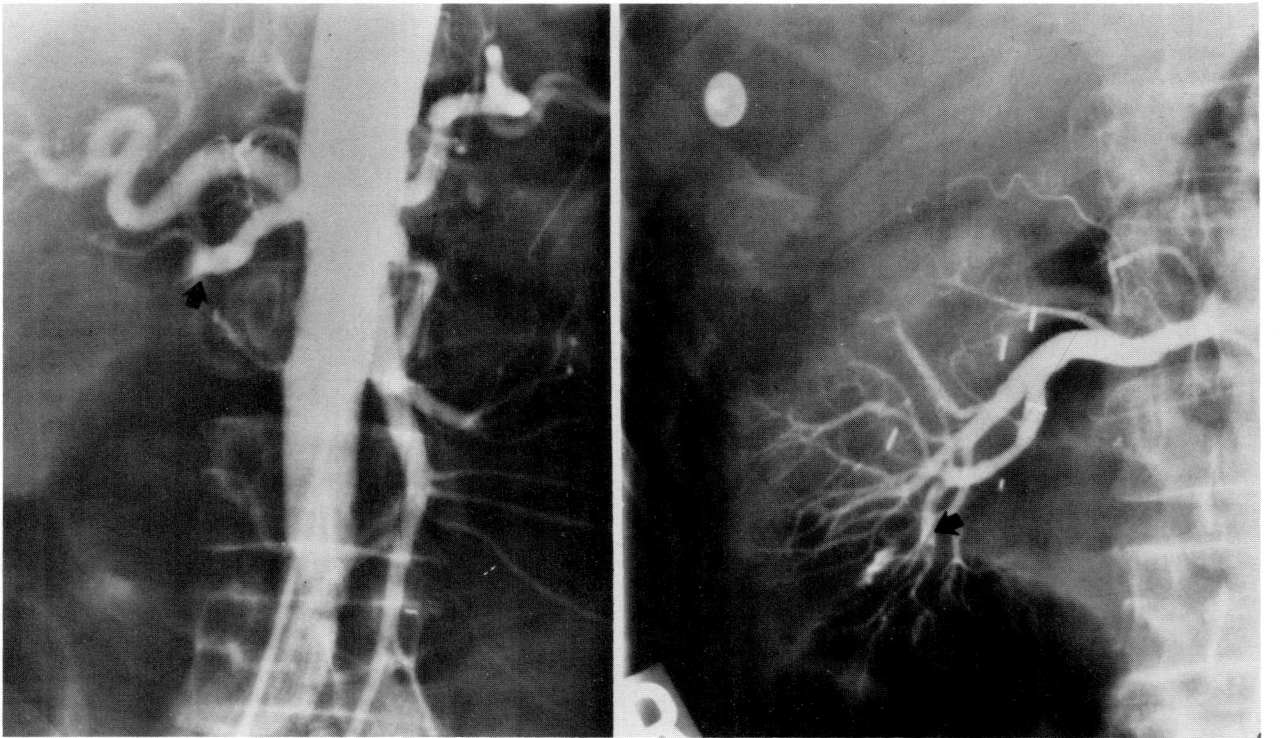

Fig. 2. Case 3. Left, preoperative abdominal aortogram. Arrow indicates occlusion of right renal artery. Right, postoperative right selective renal arteriogram. Arrow indicates residual embolus in lower pole branch artery. [Reproduced from Towne JB, Bernhard VM: Revascularization of the ischemic kidney. Arch. Surg. 113:216-218, 1978. Copyright 1978, American Medical Association.]

Postoperatively, the patient required repeated hemodialysis. On the 14th postoperative day, the urine output increased to 2 liters/day. However, he sustained another myocardial infarction with pulmonary edema and hypotension on the 25th postoperative day. Thereafter, renal function deteriorated and further hemodialysis was required. His subsequent hospital course was marked by pulmonary insufficiency and congestive heart failure, and he died on the 40th postoperative day of progressive cardiorespiratory problems. At postmortem examination, the renal artery was patent. Sections of the kidney showed healthy parenchyma as well as multiple areas of necrosis and hemorrhage. Thrombus was found in the peripheral renal arteries adjacent to the areas of necrosis.

Case 4. A 71-year-old man with long-standing history of poorly controlled hypertension was admitted to a local hospital with hypertensive encephalopathy. He had known mild chronic renal failure with BUN ranging from 30 to 35 mg/100 ml. He also was known to have had a nonfunctioning left kidney for many years. Blood pressure on admission ranged from 250/150 to 300/150 mm Hg. Blood pressure was controlled with a sodium nitroprusside intravenous drip and parenteral reserpine and propranolol. The patient had no urinary output for the next 48 hours. Angiograms at that time demonstrated a totally obstructed right renal artery with collateral filling of the distal renal artery. No vascularity could be seen in the left renal artery distribution.

Following transfer to our hospital, the patient's BUN was 100 mg/ml and serum creatinine was 9 mg/100 ml. The night of transfer he underwent a right iliac to right renal artery bypass using a reversed saphenous vein. A Schribner shunt was inserted at the conclusion of the operative procedure.

The patient required hemodialysis on the first and third postoperative days. He produced 1120 cc urine for the first 24 hours following surgery. Subsequent urine output varied between 1 and 2 liters per day. He was discharged on the 23rd postoperative day with a BUN of 56 mg/100 ml and a serum creatinine of 3.0 mg/100 ml. Two months postoperatively his BUN was 33 mg/100 ml and serum creatinine was 3.7 mg/100 ml. The patient died of a myocardial infarction complicated by severe congestive heart failure 4 months postoperatively. At autopsy, the bypass graft was patent and histologically normal nephron architecture was demonstrated on sections of the right kidney (Fig. 3).

DISCUSSION

In the presence of acute renal artery obstruction, the kidney can be resistant to ischemic necrosis because the viability of the nephron is often maintained by collateral flow. Since the collateral blood flow is not sufficient to maintain filtration of the glomerulus, the presence of anuria gives no indication of viability of the kidney. There are no reliable roentgenographic criteria for the reversibility of renal artery ischemia, since arteriography in the immediate postocclusive period usually will not demonstrate the collateral flow.

The duration of the ischemia also does not correlate with the reversibility and salvage potential of the kidney. In our patients, the duration of ischemia

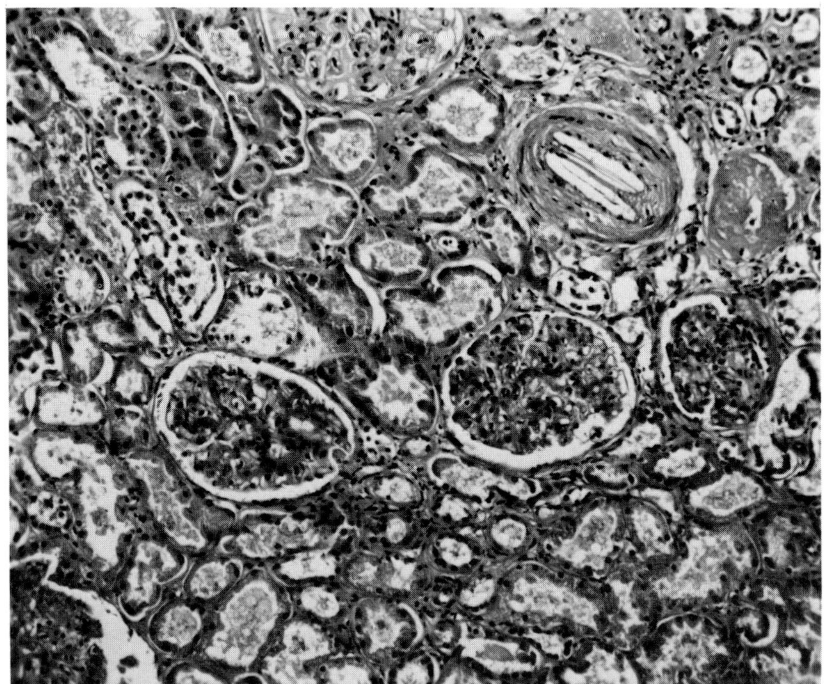

Fig. 3. Photomicrograph of autopsy specimen of patient 4 obtained 4 months postrevascularization demonstrating intact nephron architecture.

ranged from 18 hours to 3 days, and all kidneys functioned in the postoperative period. Although renal function was not normal in the three survivors, it was sufficient to maintain life without hemodialysis. Several authors [3, 5, 6] have reported successful renal embolectomy more than 30 days after renal artery occlusion.

Renal size does not correlate with the reversibility of the renal ischemia. Morgan et al. [4] reported revascularization of chronically occluded renal arteries in kidneys measuring 7.5 and 8 cm long. Satisfactory function was obtained in both, with the former increasing to 13 cm in length 2 years postoperatively and the latter increasing to 10 cm in length at 1 year. In patients with long-term, poorly controlled hypertension and an atrophic kidney secondary to renal artery occlusive disease, the good kidney may be the atrophic kidney, since the renal artery stenosis has protected it from the ravages of renal hypertension, while the contralateral unobstructed kidney has been virtually destroyed, demonstrating severe arterionephrosclerosis. In some of these patients, the renal artery stenosis is the cause of the hypertension.

The potential salvage rate of acute renal artery obstruction can only be determined by the presence of backbleeding from the kidney once the occluding debris is cleared from the distal renal artery. If the kidney becomes distended and pink following revascularization, some renal function will be retrieved [8]. Similar conclusions were obtained by Magilligan et al., who feel that exploration with direct examination is the only sure way of determining the viability of a kidney which is nonfunctioning on intravenous pyelography and does not demonstrate a vascular pattern on angiography [3].

The recovery of renal function was demonstrated by Dean et al. in patients undergoing renal artery repair for renal vascular hypertension [1]. The improvement in renal function was quantitated by comparing pre- and postoperative split renal functions. They found the greatest improvement in renal function in those patients with the least renal function preoperatively. This supports the thesis that the ischemic kidney may have sufficient blood supply to maintain viability but not the function of the nephron.

Because acute tubular necrosis frequently develops in these patients following successful revascularization, a Schribner shunt should be inserted at the conclusion of renal revascularization. Occasionally, a patient who is too critically ill to tolerate a major abdominal procedure can be maintained on hemodialysis until his clinical status improves. Perkins et al. [5] reported successful aortic thrombectomy 35 days after renal artery occlusion secondary to abdominal aortic thrombosis involving the renal arteries in a patient with severe rheumatic heart disease. Their patient was maintained on hemodialysis during this interval, allowing time to get her into optimal condition.

The potential for renal artery emboli following surgical manipulation of the abdominal aorta was clearly documented by Thurlbeck and Castleman [7]. They reported acute renal artery emboli in 17 of 22 patients who died following aortic operations. Their patients included 11 with ruptured aneurysms, 6 with unruptured aneurysms, and 5 with aortic occlusive disease. When anuria develops following aortic reconstruction, an arteriogram should be obtained to determine if embolism is the underlying cause. A curable lesion, if found, should be immediately corrected.

Thrombosis of the abdominal aorta involving the renal arteries frequently indicates severe preexisting renal artery occlusive disease, since normal renal artery blood flow is generally sufficient to prevent thrombosis of the perirenal aorta. Renal artery stenosis should be identified and corrected by endarterectomy or bypass graft to provide adequate renal perfusion. Since surgical correction of acute renal artery occlusion can salvage sufficient renal function to maintain life without hemodialysis, prompt arteriography and surgical intervention is indicated.

REFERENCES

1. Dean RH, Lawson JD, Hollifield JW, et al: Revascularization of the poorly functioning kidney. Surgery 85:44-52, 1979

2. Dobrzinsky SJ, Voegeli E, Grant HA, et al: Spontaneous reestablishment of renal function after complete occlusion of a renal artery. Arch. Intern. Med. 128:266-268, 1971
3. Magilligan DS, DeWeese SA, May AG, et al: The occluded renal artery. Surgery 78:730-738, 1975
4. Morgan T, Wilson T, Johnston W: Restoration of renal function by arterial surgery. Lancet 1:653-656, 1974
5. Perkins RP, Jacobsen DS, Feder FP, et al: Return of renal function after late embolectomy. N. Engl. J. Med. 276:1194-1196, 1967
6. Peterson NE, McDonald DF: Renal embolization. J. Urol. 100:140-145, 1968
7. Thurlbeck WM, Castleman B: Atheromatous emboli to the kidneys after aortic surgery. N. Engl. J. Med. 257:442-447, 1957
8. Towne JB, Bernhard VM: Revascularization of the ischemic kidney. Arch. Surg. 113:216-218, 1978

James C. Stanley, M.D.
Walter M. Whitehouse, Jr., M.D.

Aneurysms of Splanchnic and Renal Arteries

Aneurysmal disease of the major visceral branches of the abdominal aorta has become recognized with increasing frequency. More than 2400 splanchnic and renal aneurysms have been described in the literature. The cumulative experience as reported suggests the frequency of splanchnic aneurysms to be approximately twice that of renal aneurysms. These aneurysms are best addressed separately because of the marked variability in their biologic character.

SPLANCHNIC ARTERY ANEURYSMS

Visceral artery aneurysms affecting splanchnic vessels have been discovered with increasing regularity as a consequence of more common arteriographic studies for both vascular and nonvascular disease [5, 29]. A review of this subject documents that our understanding of certain aneurysms is anecdotal, whereas for others their natural history and optimal mode of treatment have been well defined.

Celiac artery aneurysms account for 4% of all splanchnic aneurysms (Fig. 1). Males are affected twice as often as females. Arteriosclerosis and medial degeneration are the most common pathologic findings observed in these lesions. In many instances arteriosclerotic changes are considered a secondary event, rather than a primary etiologic factor. Traumatic aneurysms are uncommon. Mycotic aneurysms are rare, and luetic lesions have not recently been reported.

Few celiac artery aneurysms are symptomatic. Vague epigastric discomfort is common when symptoms do occur. Intestinal angina occasionally accompanies these aneurysms when associated with functionally significant occlusive disease of the other mesenteric vessels. Pulsatile masses rarely are evident with these lesions. Rupture is the most dramatic clinical presentation of celiac artery

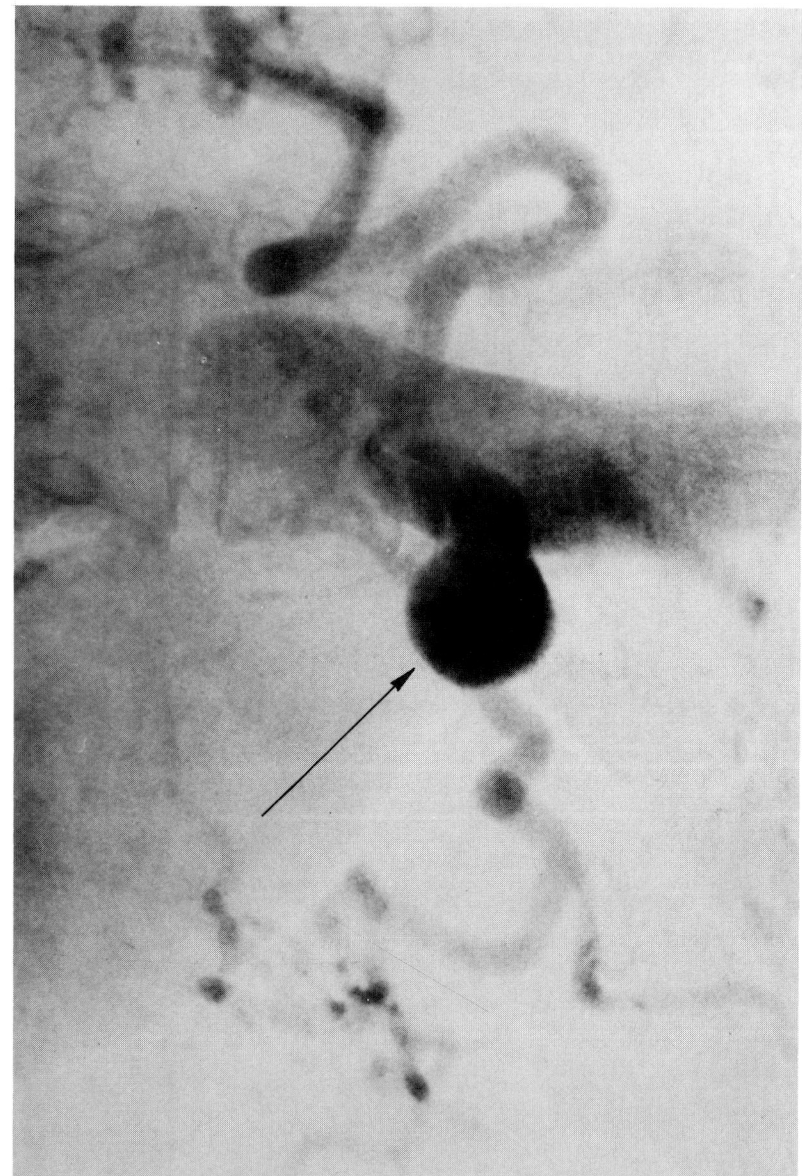

Fig. 1. Celiac artery aneurysm associated with medial degeneration.

aneurysmal disease. Although nearly 80% of previously reported lesions ruptured, most recent experience suggests a rupture rate of less than 20%. The true risk of rupture is probably less than this figure. Both intraperitoneal hemorrhage and bleeding into the gastrointestinal tract occur with rupture. The former has been most frequently described. Intense pain often radiating to the back, with nausea and vomiting, has been attributed to expanding aneurysms.

Incidental recognition of celiac artery aneurysms during angiography or abdominal operation for unrelated disease is currently the most common means of diagnosing these lesions [13]. Although antemortem diagnosis is increasing, preoperative recognition as recently as a decade ago had been made only seven times [29]. Calcification of aneurysmal walls is uncommon, but displacement of contiguous gastrointestinal structures is a frequent radiographic finding.

Operative intervention is recommended for all celiac artery aneurysms [10, 26]. Satisfactory results in more than 90% of cases during the past two decades supports such an approach. Ligation of the celiac artery may be adequate therapy in certain cases, provided hepatic blood flow is not severely compromised. Aneurysmectomy is appropriate therapy for most celiac artery aneurysms. The use of autologous vein or prosthetic grafts is favored over aortic implantation of the artery or its branches when reconstructing the foregut circulation. Aneurysmorrhaphy is not favored in managing these lesions. Celiac artery aneurysms frequently are associated with other aneurysmal or occlusive lesions. Complex arterial reconstructions involving the aorta as well as vessels to the extremities and abdominal viscera may be necessary in treating patients with these lesions.

Gastric or gastroepiploic artery aneurysms account for approximately 5% of splanchnic aneurysmal disease (Fig. 2). Males are affected three times more often than females. Arteriosclerotic changes in many aneurysms support the belief that such represent an important etiologic factor [17]. However, in many others medial degeneration or periarterial inflammation may predispose the aneurysm to secondary arteriosclerosis. Gastric artery aneurysms are nine times more common than those of gastroepiploic arteries. Most lesions are solitary.

All but a few gastric or gastroepiploic artery aneurysms have ruptured at the time of diagnosis. Of these, 70% are associated with serious gastrointestinal bleeding manifested by massive hematemesis [16]. Chronic gastrointestinal bleeding occurs less often. A few patients have experienced antecedent dyspeptic epigastric discomfort. Most have had no abdominal pain prior to aneurysmal rupture. Rupture of gastric and gastroepiploic artery aneurysms results in life-threatening intraperitoneal bleeding in approximately 30% of cases [30]. Antemortem diagnosis of these lesions usually is established during urgent operations for gastrointestinal or intraperitoneal bleeding. Arteriographic studies for unexplained gastrointestinal bleeding have occasionally provided preoperative recognition of these aneurysms. Mucosal changes with these lesions are minor, and endoscopic recognition is usually difficult.

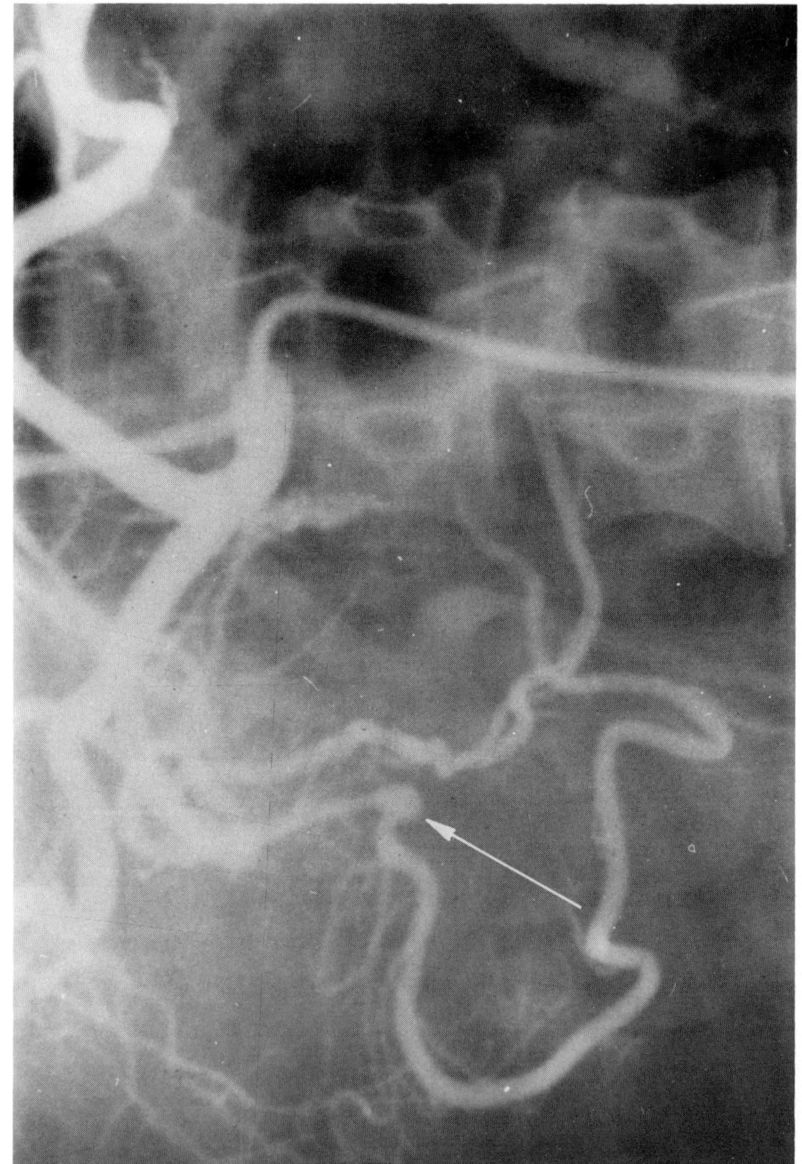

Fig. 2. Gastroepiploic artery aneurysm associated with traumatic pancreatitis.

Treatment of gastric and gastroepiploic aneurysms is directed at life-threatening hemorrhage. Approximately 70% of patients reported before 1970 succumbed following rupture [29]. Aneurysmal ligation, with or without excision, is appropriate treatment for extraintestinal lesions. Intramural aneurysms, and those associated with gastrointestinal tract hemorrhage, are best excised with adjacent gastric tissue.

Gastroduodenal, pancreaticoduodenal, and pancreatic artery aneurysms are uncommon. Gastroduodenal artery aneurysms account for 1.5% of splanchnic aneurysmal disease (Fig. 3), all having been encountered during the past two decades. Pancreaticoduodenal and pancreatic artery aneurysms account for 3% of splanchnic aneurysms. Periarterial inflammation associated with acute or chronic pancreatitis, often with pseudocyst formation, may cause most of these aneurysms [11]. Arteriosclerosis has been alleged to be the most common cause of both aneurysms, but such is usually a secondary event [29]. Males are affected four times more often than females.

Gastroduodenal, pancreaticoduodenal, or pancreatic artery aneurysms are often symptomatic when recognized. Epigastric pain with radiation to the back is common and is often difficult to distinguish from that due to pancreatitis. Approximately 65% of these aneurysms rupture into the intestinal tract and cause massive bleeding. This occurs even more frequently with lesions developing as a consequence of pancreatitis. Hemoperitoneum is an unusual complication of these aneurysms. Duodenal displacement or indentation by an extrinsic mass exhibiting vascular calcifications in a patient with gastrointestinal bleeding of undetermined source should lead to a suspicion of such an aneurysm.

Rupture of gastroduodenal or pancreaticoduodenal artery aneurysms entails a mortality approaching 50%. Operative intervention is appropriate in all but the poorest risk patient [31]. Elective gastroduodenal artery aneurysmectomy usually can be performed without great risks. Aneurysmal ligation from within the sac is more appropriate than aneurysm excision if it is within the pancreas. Pancreaticoduodenal and pancreatic artery aneurysms are more difficult to manage [27, 34]. Multiple vessels communicate with these aneurysms and limit the usefulness of simple ligature. Pancreatic resections, including pancreaticoduodenectomy, may be required in certain instances. Good results have been reported in more than 50% of surgically treated pancreaticoduodenal artery aneurysms.

Hepatic artery aneurysms comprise 19% of aneurysms affecting splanchnic vessels (Fig. 4). Etiologic factors are varied and include arteriosclerosis (32%), medial degeneration (24%), trauma (22%), and infection (10%) [26]. Mycotic aneurysms were more common in the past [7]. Arteriosclerosis is a common histologic finding but may represent a secondary, rather than primary, event in such lesions. True aneurysms and pseudoaneurysms as a direct result of trauma are being encountered with increasing frequency. Central hepatic rupture and deep parenchymal fractures following blunt abdominal injury underlie the

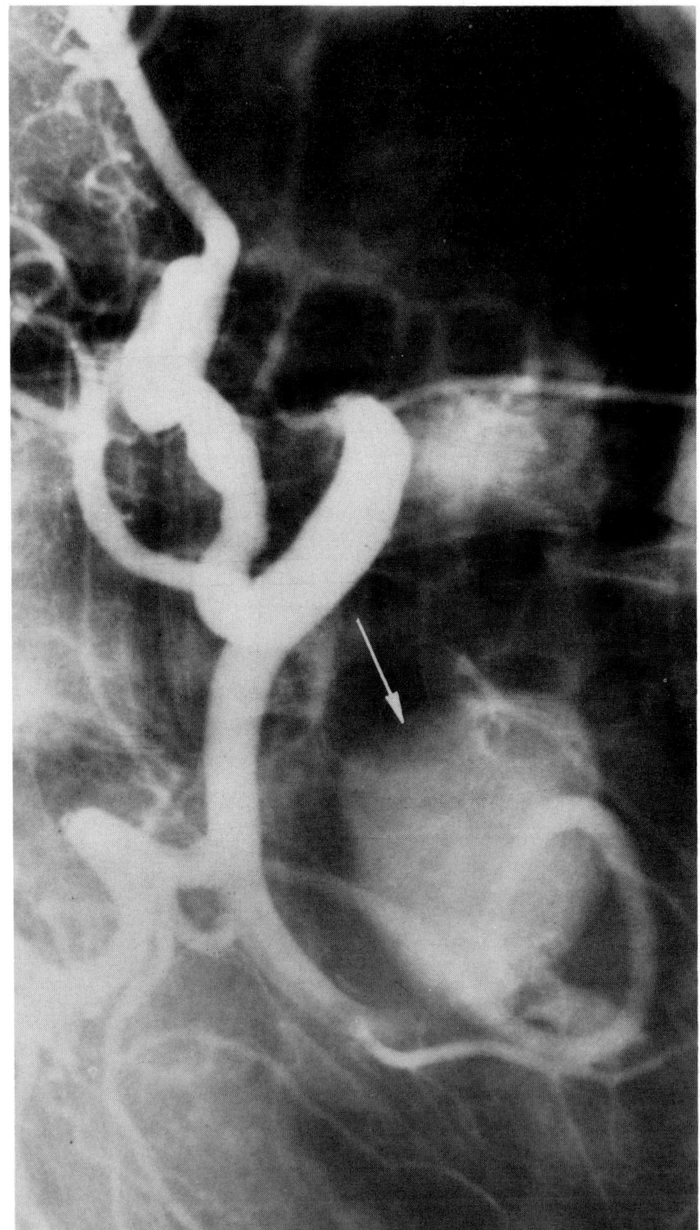

Fig. 3. Gastroduodenal artery aneurysm associated with pancreatitis and periarterial inflammation.

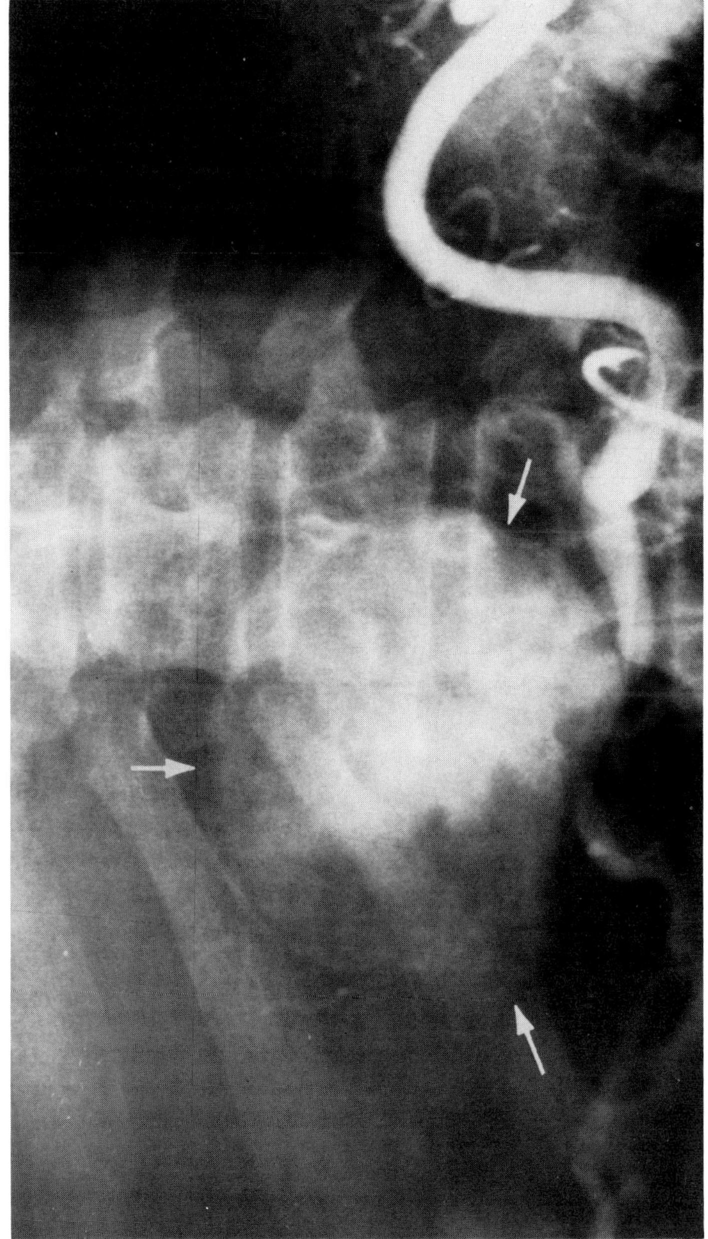

Fig. 4. Hepatic artery aneurysm.

majority of traumatic aneurysms. Periarteritis nodosa, cystic medial necrosis, and periarterial inflammation with cholecystitis or pancreatitis are less common causes of hepatic artery aneurysms. Males are affected by hepatic artery aneurysms twice as often as females. The majority of aneurysms, excluding those due to trauma, are encountered in patients who have entered their sixth decade.

Hepatic artery aneurysms larger than 2 cm in size tend to be saccular. Eighty percent involve the extrahepatic vessels. Twenty percent are within the liver parenchyma. A review of 163 aneurysms revealed the following locations: common hepatic, 63%; right hepatic, 28%; left hepatic, 5%; and both right and left hepatic arteries, 4% [29]. Excluding small microaneurysms associated with systemic arteritis, most hepatic artery aneurysms are solitary.

Symptomatic aneurysms are often associated with right upper quadrant or epigastric pain frequently attributed to cholecystitis. Large aneurysms may result in extrahepatic biliary obstruction. Expanding hepatic artery aneurysms produce severe abdominal discomfort, often with radiation to the back. Pulsatile masses and abdominal bruit are uncommon with bland aneurysms.

Hepatic artery aneurysms rupture with equal frequency into the hepatobiliary tract and the peritoneal cavity. The former often presents with characteristic findings of hemobilia, including intermittent pain similar to biliary colic, massive gastrointestinal bleeding with periodic hematemesis, and jaundice. Most of these patients are febrile. Chronic anemia associated with a history of melena is a less common manifestation of hemobilia. Intraperitoneal bleeding and exsanguinating hemorrhage often accompany extrahepatic aneurysmal rupture.

Vascular calcifications in the upper abdomen and displacement of contiguous structures evidenced on barium studies or cholecystocholangiography may reveal the presence of hepatic artery aneurysms. Arteriographic studies in cases of gastrointestinal hemorrhage and major abdominal trauma have resulted in increased recognition of these aneurysms. Hepatic scans, ultrasonography, and computerized axial tomography in select instances may prove useful for noninvasive diagnosis of hepatic artery aneurysms.

Operative intervention for hepatic artery aneurysms is recommended unless very unusual risks are identified. Rupture affected 44% of those lesions reported from 1960 to 1970 [29]. The actual risk of rupture may be less. Mortality with rupture is approximately 35%. Aneurysmectomy or aneurysm exclusion by proximal and distal ligation, without reconstruction of the involved vessel, comprised nearly 50% of procedures previously described for these lesions. The latter is most applicable to common hepatic artery aneurysms proximal to gastroduodenal and right gastric vessels. Any preexisting disorder compromising hepatic blood flow makes ligation of the proximal hepatic artery less advisable. Aneurysmorrhaphy or direct arterial reconstructions using autogenous or prosthetic grafts are favored in such a situation. Restoration of hepatic blood flow is also important in treating aneurysms of the proper hepatic artery. Intrahepatic arterial aneurysms may require resection of the involved hepatic territory. In a minority of patients, control of bleeding intrahepatic aneurysms by simple ligation of the proximal vessel may be preferable to undertaking a major liver resection. Preoperative arteriographic studies are essential in determining the best surgical management for hepatic artery aneurysms [33].

Jejunal, ileal, and colic artery aneurysms are uncommon (Fig. 5) [12, 22]. They account for approximately 3.5% of all splanchnic aneurysms. No sex predilection has been observed for these lesions. The etiology of most mesenteric branch aneurysms remains unknown. Arteriosclerosis is a dominant feature of some lesions, whereas others appear the result of congenital or acquired medial defects. These aneurysms are usually solitary, although those associated with arteritis are most often multiple.

Symptomatic intact aneurysms are rare. Earlier, aneurysms were usually recognized at operation for rupture into the mesentery, intestinal lumen, or peritoneal cavity. Rarely, a tender mass due to contained rupture or abdominal apoplexy following uncontained hemorrhage have been the initial manifestations of these aneurysms. Bleeding into colonic diverticula has occasionally been

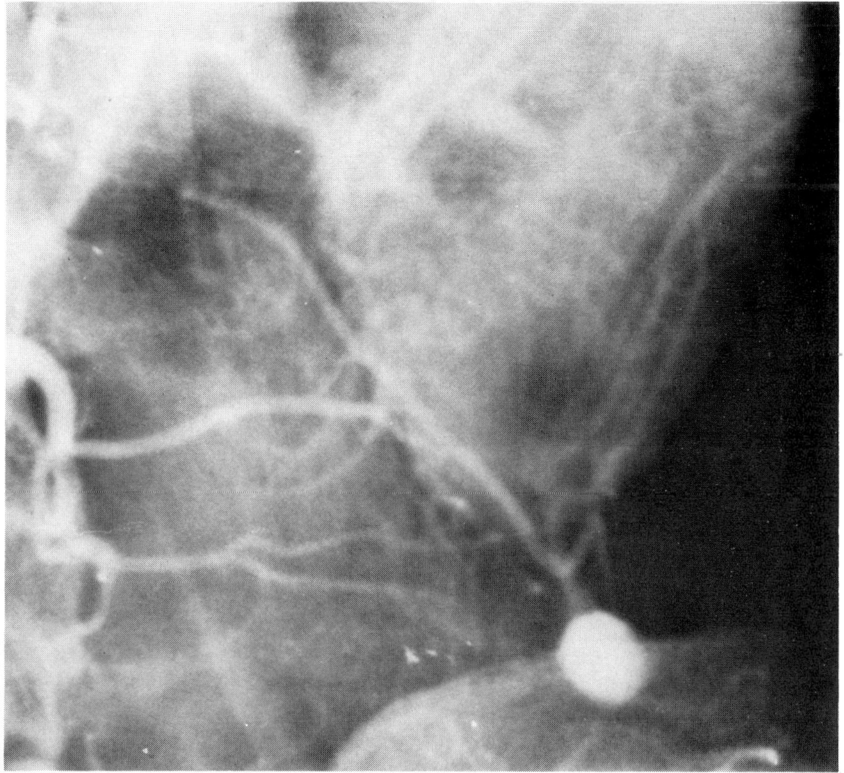

Fig. 5. Ileal artery aneurysm.

misdiagnosed as a colic artery aneurysm. Bland mesenteric branch aneurysms are being recognized more often with increased use of abdominal arteriography for unrelated disease including gastrointestinal bleeding.

Surgical treatment of intestinal aneurysms entails arterial ligation, aneurysmectomy, or bowel resection for mural lesions. It is recommended that most of these lesions be removed once their existence is known. Aneurysms of the inferior mesenteric artery and its branches are exceedingly rare, their existence being somewhat noteworthy [6]. Their cause and natural history have not been defined.

Splenic artery aneurysms are the most common abdominal visceral aneurysms, accounting for 56% of splanchnic aneurysms (Fig. 6). There have been few large clinical experiences reported from a single institution [19, 27]. The incidence of these aneurysms has been reported to range from 0.098% in a collection of nearly 195,000 necropsies to 10.4% in a select autopsy study of elderly patients [1, 18]. Incidental arteriographic demonstration of splenic aneurysms in 0.78% of cases at the University of Michigan may be a more accurate representation of their true frequency in the general population [27]. In the past a bimodal distribution was noted. Diagnosis was most often established in the third and seventh decades, the former associated with rupture during

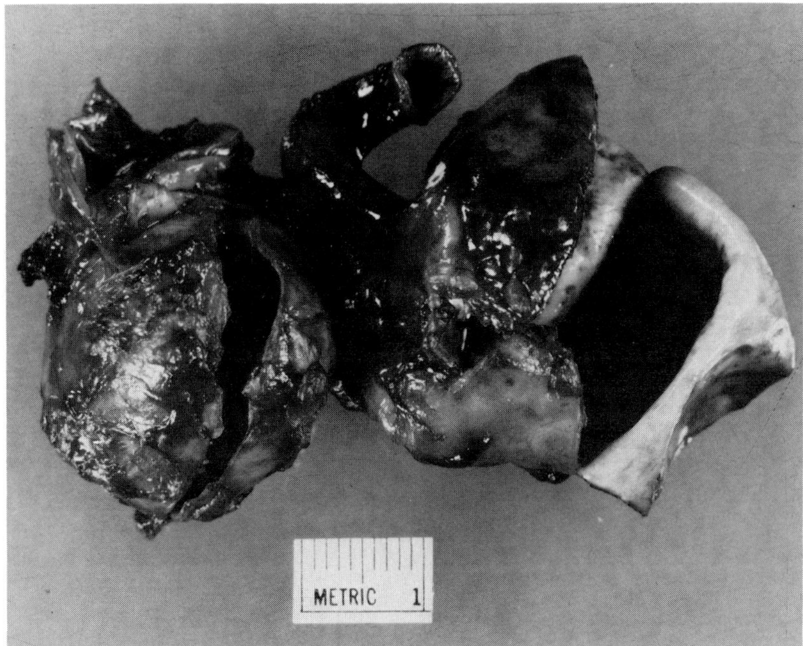

Fig. 6. Splenic artery aneurysms occurring at a bifurcation in a grand multiparous female.

pregnancy, the latter with necropsy studies. In recent times a simple peak incidence has been identified during the sixth decade. An unusual sex predilection is seen with this entity, with females affected four times more often than males. These aneurysms are usually saccular and occur at bifurcations of the main splenic vessel in the hilus. The average size is somewhat greater than 1.5 cm. Multiple aneurysms occur in approximately 20% of cases.

Abnormalities of the media, including elastic fiber fragmentation, loss of smooth muscle, and internal elastic lamina disruption, are considered the cause of most splenic artery aneurysms (Fig. 7). Three distinct conditions associated with medial degeneration have been related to the evolution of these lesions. Four percent of patients having renal artery medial fibrodysplasia exhibit splenic artery aneurysms (Fig. 8). Compromise of vessel integrity with fibrodysplasia is a logical forerunner of aneurysmal development. Portal hypertension with splenomegaly may be a second etiologic factor in certain splenic artery aneurysms [2, 20, 23, 29]. In this situation, aneurysms may result from the same process that causes increased splenic artery diameters in portal hypertension. Seven percent of portal hypertensives studied at the University of Michigan exhibited splenic artery macroaneurysms. Vascular effects of repeated pregnancy are a third factor related to these aneurysms. Forty percent of female patients described in a recent report, without other obvious etiologic factors present, had completed six or more pregnancies [27]. Furthermore, 45% of female patients with splenic artery aneurysms collected from the 1960 to 1970 English literature, in whom parity was stated, were grand multiparas [29]. Gestational alterations, due to hormonal and local hemodynamic events, may cause medial defects and enhance aneurysm formation in these patients.

Occasional aneurysms are a direct result of arteriosclerosis of the splenic vessel (Fig. 9). Frequent localization of calcific arteriosclerotic changes to aneurysms, without involvement of adjacent vessels, suggests that arteriosclerosis often is a secondary process rather than a primary etiologic event. Inflammatory processes affecting tissues adjacent to the splenic artery, particularly pancreatitis with pseudocysts, are a known cause of aneurysms. Penetrating and blunt trauma may also precipitate aneurysmal development. Other uncommon causes include mycotic lesions and those associated with systemic arteritis. Systemic arterial hypertension affects slightly less than half of patients with these aneurysms and may be contributory to their development.

Splenic artery aneurysms usually are asymptomatic. Their clinical importance has been a subject of controversy [14, 27]. Vague left upper quadrant or epigastric discomfort is the most common complaint in those 20% of cases alleged to be symptomatic. Abdominal bruits are considered to be more often due to turbulent blood flow through tortuous splenic vessels than to aneurysmal disease. Most splenic artery aneurysms, being less than 2 cm in size, are not palpable.

Aneurysmal rupture represents the most serious complication of these lesions. Some patients bleed massively and others bleed more slowly into the

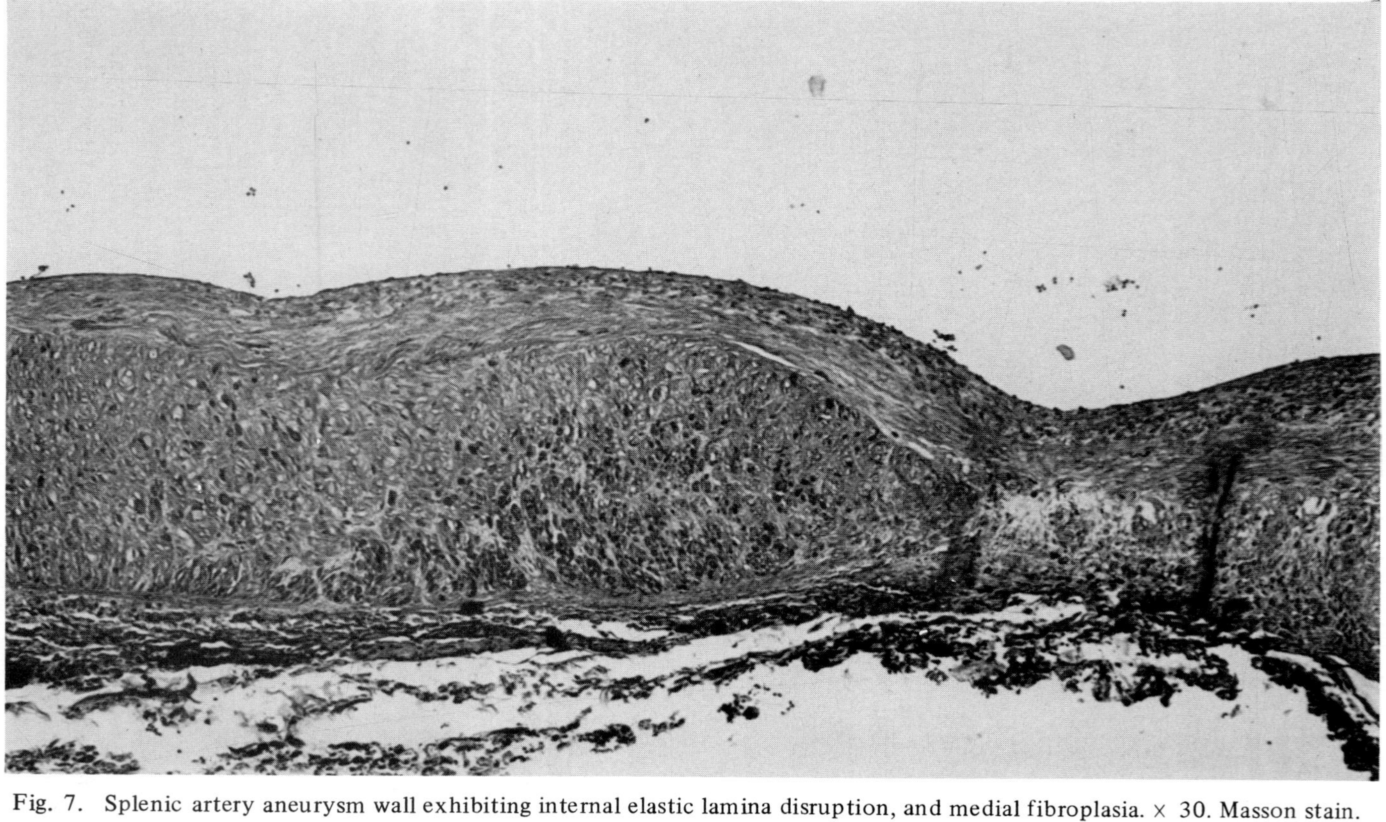

Fig. 7. Splenic artery aneurysm wall exhibiting internal elastic lamina disruption, and medial fibroplasia. × 30. Masson stain.

retrogastric area. Frank intraperitoneal bleeding occurs as the lesser sac containment is lost. Such a double rupture phenomenon often allows treatment before fatal hemorrhage develops. Intermittent gastrointestinal bleeding may reflect a more occult form of rupture. In these instances aneurysms are usually associated with penetrating gastric ulcers or pancreatitis. Rupture with splenic arteriovenous fistula formation and portal hypertension is a rare complication.

Splenic artery aneurysms currently are most often recognized as incidental findings of arteriographic studies. Diagnosis may be considered with curvilinear, "signet ring"-like calcifications in the left upper quadrant noted on abdominal radiographs (Fig. 10). Approximately 30% of aneurysms recognized in recent years have been calcified. Arteriographic studies are necessary to establish the diagnosis. Ultrasonography and computerized axial tomography may prove useful in differentiating aneurysms from other lesions.

Life-threatening splenic artery aneurysm rupture affects fewer than 2% of cases [27]. Disruption of bland lesions occurs less often than previously projected [25, 29]. Clinical experience does not support the contention that rupture is less likely to occur in calcified aneurysms, normotensive patients, or those 60 or more years of age [27]. Aneurysmal rupture during pregnancy is common, with more than 95% having ruptured in such a setting [15, 27].

Operative intervention is recommended for all symptomatic splenic artery aneurysms, as well as bland lesions encountered in pregnant patients or in females of childbearing age. Mortality of aneurysmal rupture during pregnancy is greater than 65% [27]. In nonpregnant patients, death following operation for aneurysmal rupture occurs in fewer than 25% of cases [29]. In view of less than a 2% incidence of rupture, elective operations for bland splenic artery aneurysms appear justified only if the risk of operation is around 0.5%.

Surgical therapy for splenic artery aneurysms usually entails splenectomy. Exclusion of certain proximal splenic aneurysms by ligation of all contributing vessels may be preferred to excision. Such is certainly the case if excessive dissection of adjacent structures, such as within the body of the pancreas, would otherwise be required. Proximal splenic artery aneurysms may be treated by aneurysmectomy and ligation, with avoidance of splenectomy. Operative mortality following elective aneurysmectomy continues to be unreported among cases described in the recent literature.

Superior mesenteric artery aneurysms are the third most common splanchnic artery aneurysms, comprising 8% of these lesions (Fig. 11). Females predominated in earlier series, but more recently the sexes are equally affected. The mean age of patients with these lesions has been in the sixth decade. Mycotic aneurysms continue to be the most common cause [29]. A variety of pathogens associated with endocarditis as well as noncardiac sepsis have been encountered. Nonhemolytic streptococcus has been the most common causative organism. Medial degenerative processes, often with dissections [8], arteriosclerosis, and trauma, are less common causes of superior mesenteric artery aneurysms.

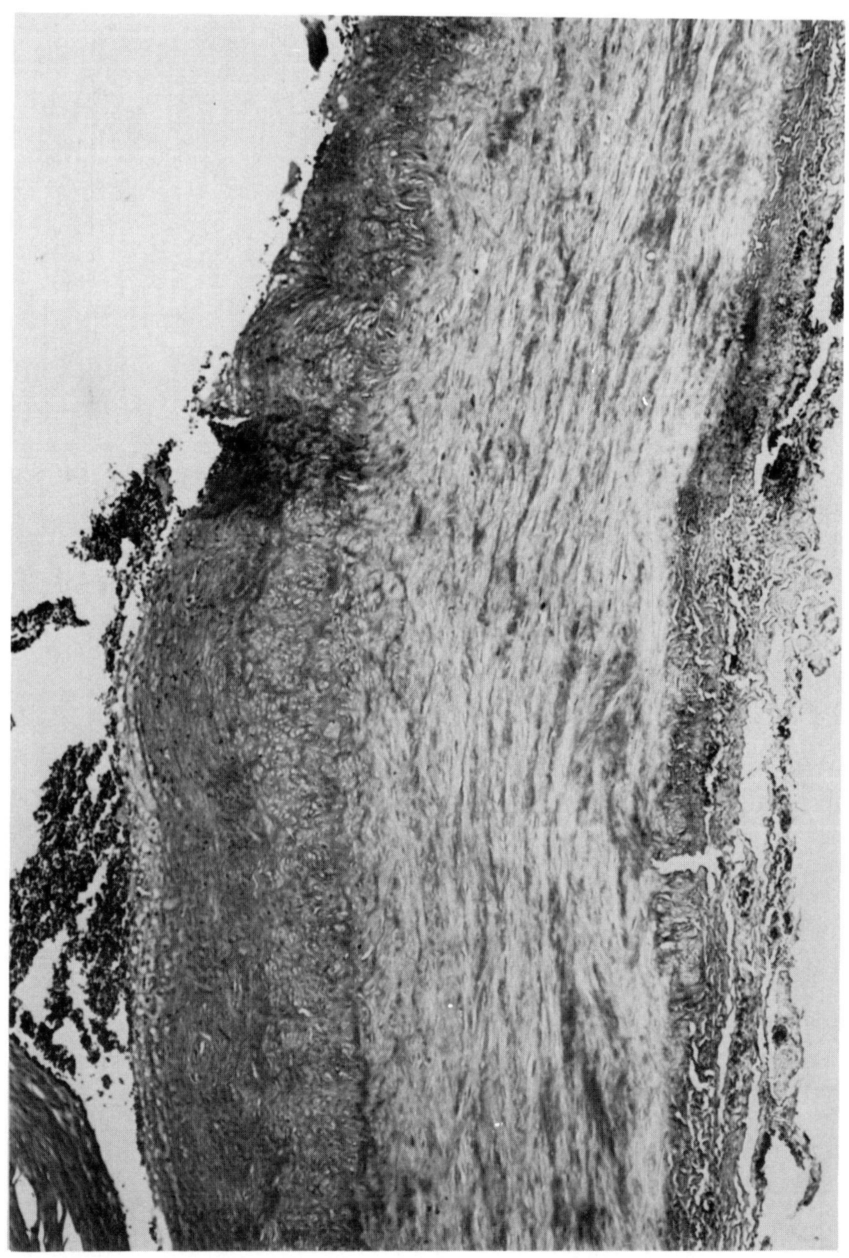

Upper abdominal discomfort that becomes persistent, severe, epigastric pain is often the first manifestation of a symptomatic mycotic superior mesenteric artery aneurysm. Early manifestations of these lesions often represent reductions of midgut blood flow. Aneurysmal expansion, dissection, or propagation of intraluminal thrombus beyond the inferior pancreaticoduodenal or middle colic vessels effectively isolates the superior mesenteric arterial circulation. Any compromise of blood flow through such a diseased artery may cause intestinal angina. Most symptomatic aneurysms expand. A tender, mobile, pulsatile abdominal mass makes such a lesion suspect. However, antemortem recognition of intact superior mesenteric artery aneurysms is unusual.

Operative treatment for most superior mesenteric artery aneurysms appears justified. Following the first successful surgical treatment of superior mesenteric artery aneurysm reported more than three decades ago [3], the most common procedures attempted have been ligation and aneurysmorrhaphy. Ligation of certain aneurysms without arterial reconstruction has proved a reasonable means of treatment. Preexisting collaterals due to coexisting occlusive disease make this direct approach feasible. However, resection of bowel for ischemia after ligation of the superior mesenteric artery may become necessary if the collateral prove insufficient. Aneurysmectomy is unattractive because of the lesion's close proximity to important neighboring structures. Arterial reconstruction after aneurysmal exclusion or excision rarely has been accomplished [32]. Treatment of mycotic superior mesenteric artery aneurysms includes a realization that multiple vessel involvement is common.

RENAL ARTERY ANEURYSMS

The clinical importance of renal artery macroaneurysms remains controversial [9, 26, 28]. In particular, their relation to arterial hypertension continues to be a subject of debate. The actual incidence of renal artery macroaneurysms is not known, since data from existing autopsy studies and arteriographic assessments are highly selected and unrepresentative of the general population. Aneurysms were verified in 2.5% of patients undergoing arteriography as part of a hypertensive evaluation at the University of Michigan. Incidental arteriographic demonstration of aneurysms occurred in 8 of approximately 8500 patients subjected to studies for nonrenal disease at the same institution. The approximate frequency of 0.09% derived from this experience may approach the true incidence of these aneurysms in the normal population recognizable by current diagnostic methods [28]. Marked differences in sex distribution do not exist,

---

Fig. 8. Splenic artery adjacent to aneurysm exhibiting fragmentation of internal elastic lamina, subendothelial and media fibroplasia, and increases in ground substances about abnormal medial smooth muscle cells. × 30. Abul Haj stain.

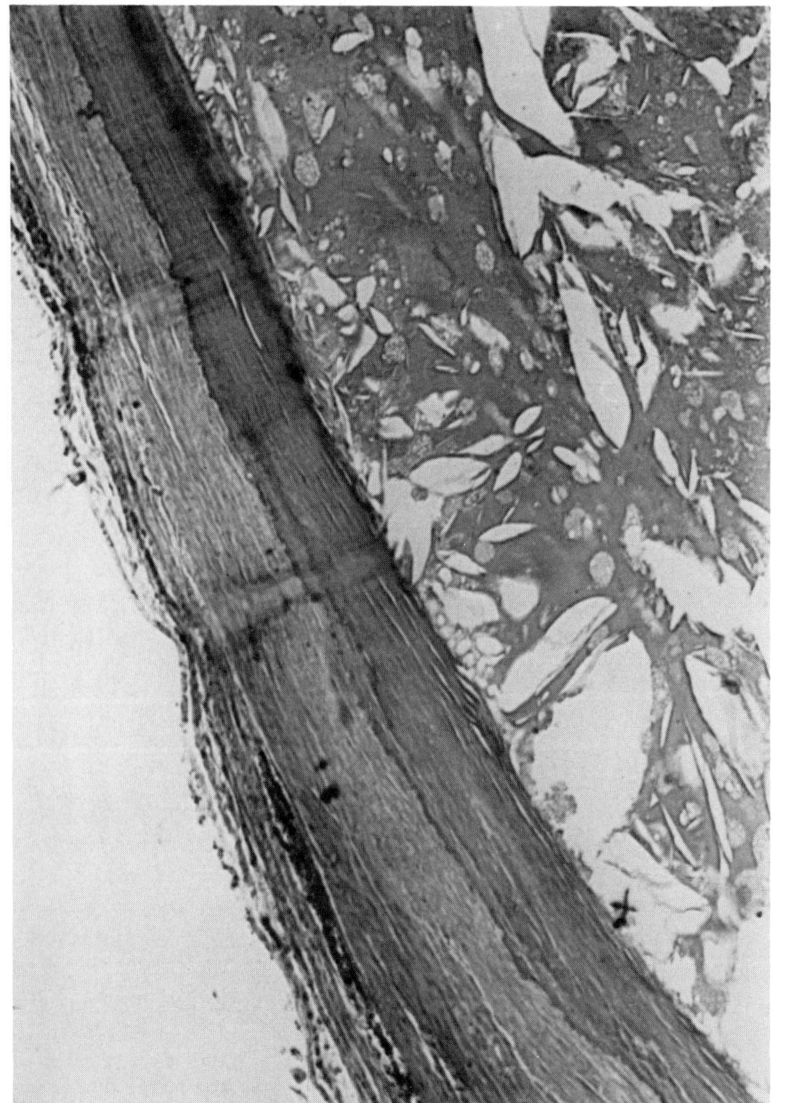

Fig. 9. Splenic artery aneurysm wall exhibiting advanced arteriosclerosis with fibrosis, cholesterol clefts, and calcification. × 30. Hematoxylin and eosin.

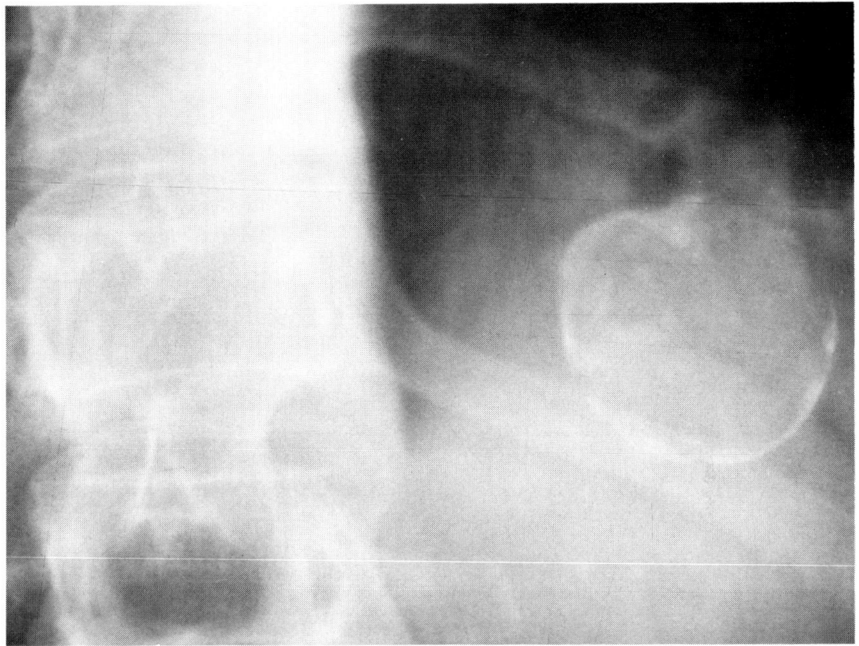

Fig. 10. Splenic artery aneurysm evident by "signet ring"-like calcification.

although females are affected slightly more often than males. The most common causes of renal artery aneurysms are related to arteriosclerosis and medial degeneration. Infection, trauma, and differing arteritides are less common etiologies of these lesions.

Most renal artery aneurysms are saccular, the average size of such lesions being 1.3 cm [28]. Seventy-five percent of saccular aneurysms are located at primary or secondary renal artery bifurcations (Fig. 12). Intraparenchymal locations occur in less than 10% of cases. Fusiform aneurysms do not usually involve bifurcations and are equally distributed throughout the renal artery.

Microscopic changes within the aneurysmal walls facilitate categorization of these lesions into two distinct types. The first, and most common, represents a medial degenerative process. Histologic changes in this group appear similar to those occurring in fusiform mural dilations associated with arterial fibrodysplasia. Excessive collagen and ground substance, scarcity of elastic tissue, and loss of smooth muscle characterize these lesions. This type of aneurysm tends to affect right-sided renal arteries more than the left-sided vessels [28]. The second group of aneurysms exhibits severe arteriosclerosis with calcium deposits and cholesterol clefts within a matrix of fibrous tissue. Advanced arteriosclerosis of the adjacent renal artery is rare. Laminated thrombus within aneurysms is uncommon, and complete thrombotic occlusion is very unusual.

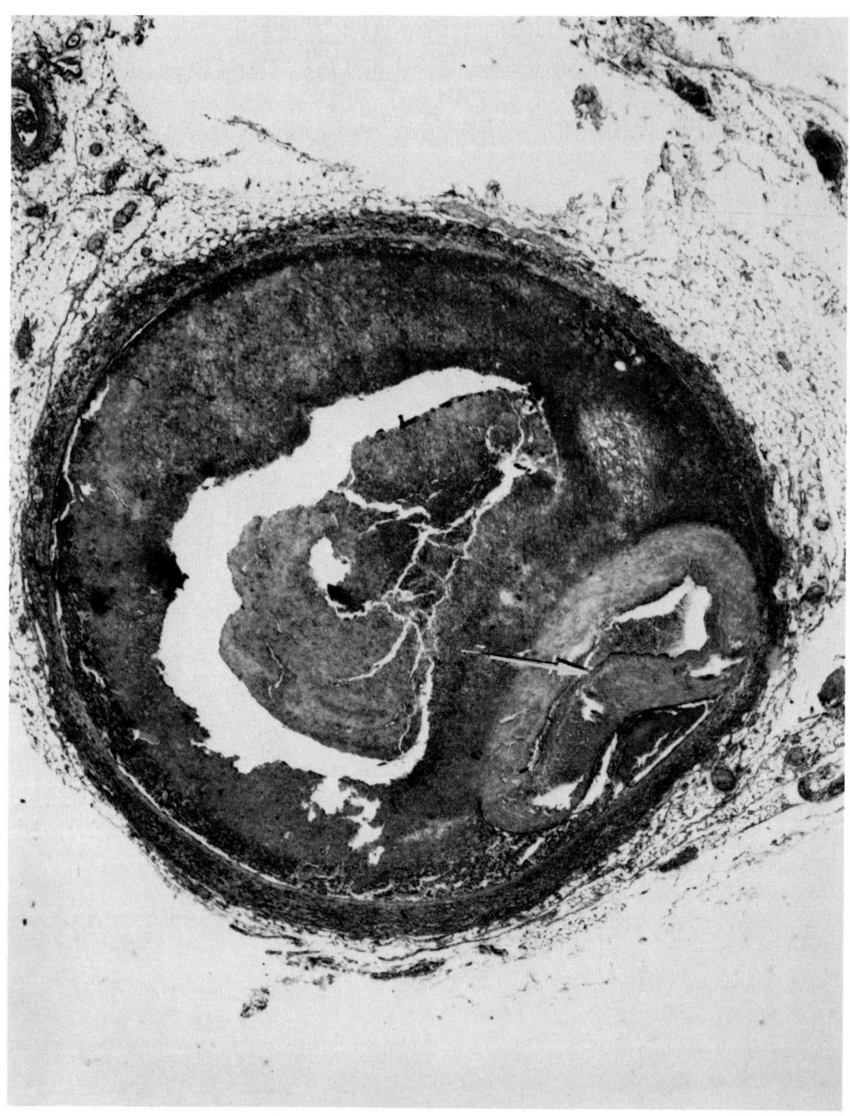

Fig. 11. Dissecting superior mesenteric artery aneurysm exhibiting compression of vessel lumen (arrow) by expanding intramural hematoma. × 16. Hematoxylin and eosin.

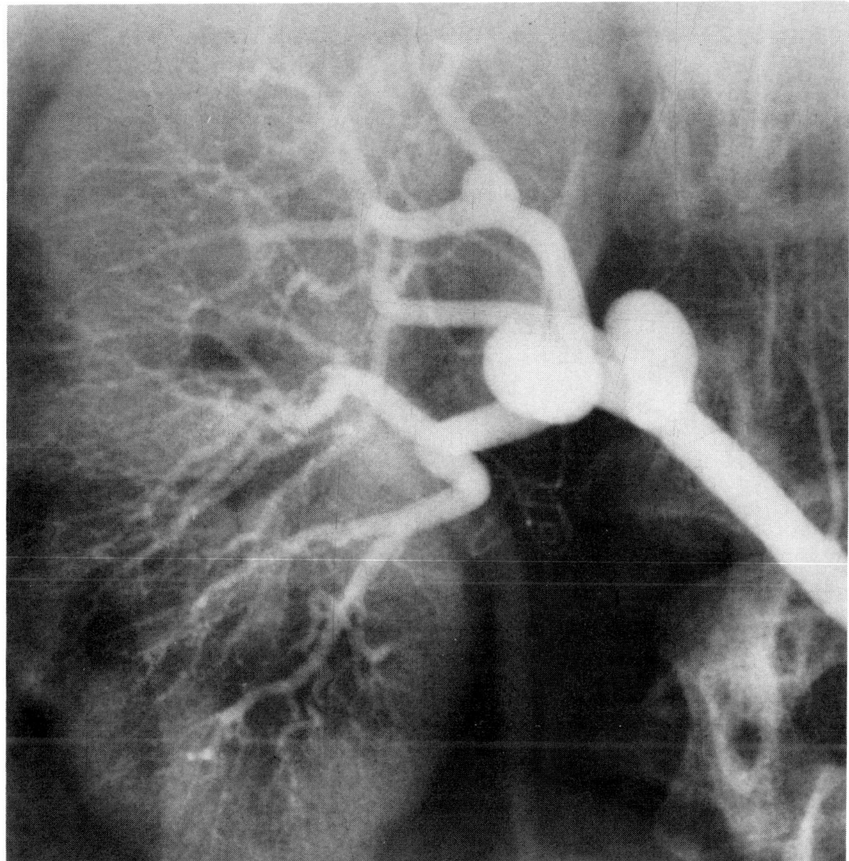

Fig. 12. Renal artery aneurysms (× 3) occurring at primary and secondary branch bifurcations.

Congenital and acquired factors appear important in the pathogenesis of renal artery aneurysms. Preexisting defects in the internal elastic lamina and deficiencies of smooth muscle cells at arterial branchings may be prerequisites to the evolution of these lesions. An unusually high incidence of renal artery aneurysms, approaching 10%, associated with medial fibrodysplasia may be more than coincidence (Fig. 13). Fragmentation and disruption of elastic tissue with loss of smooth muscle in this entity leaves only collagenous connective tissue to restrain arterial pressures. The relation of elevated blood pressure to the evolution of renal artery aneurysms is poorly understood. Effects of increased mural tension and flow on the structural integrity of the renal artery cannot be unequivocally related to aneurysmal development. On the other hand, these forces, especially in the presence of preexisting medial defects, may enhance development of renal aneurysms.

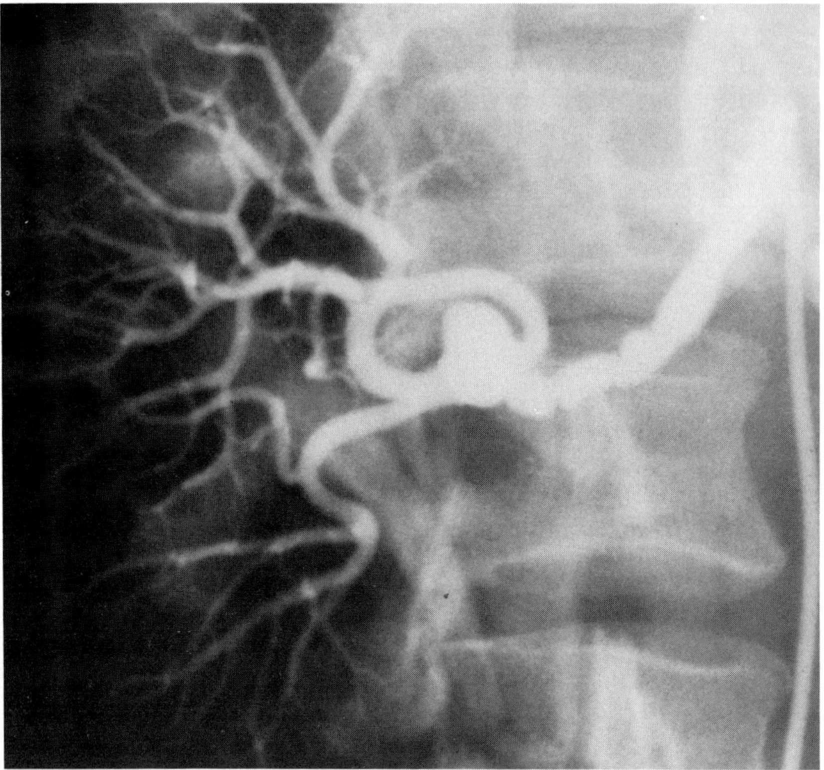

Fig. 13. Renal artery aneurysm occurring at the primary bifurcation of a main renal artery exhibiting fibrodysplastic disease.

Arteriosclerosis appears to be a secondary process rather than an inciting cause of most renal artery macroaneurysms. Arteriosclerotic changes have been noted in some but not all aneurysms of patients having multiple lesions. Arteriosclerotic renal artery aneurysms often occur in young, premenopausal females without distant arteriosclerosis. This supports the concept that arteriosclerosis is a secondary event in many of these cases.

The clinical importance of renal artery aneurysms lies in establishing the morbidity attributable to intact aneurysms, their relation to arterial hypertension, and the risk of catastrophic rupture. The majority of renal artery aneurysms are asymptomatic. Approximately 12% of patients with these lesions have pain compatible with renal origin [28]. Aneurysmal expansion, compression of nearby structures, or renal infarction from dislodged thrombus could account for this symptom. Hematuria and abdominal bruits are often attributed to these lesions. Like abdominal discomfort, these findings are not always associated with aneurysmal disease.

A cause-effect association of renal artery aneurysms to hypertension is subject to speculation. Although uncommon, the potential exists for propagation or embolization of aneurysmal thrombus with occlusion of a distal artery resulting in renal ischemia and renovascular hypertension. Compression of adjacent arteries and changes in the pulsatile character of blood flow beyond an aneurysm have been proposed as causes of renovascular hypertension. Attempts at verification of such phenomena have received little attention or support. Stenotic lesions may occur in the vicinity of an aneurysm which are not apparent on preoperative arteriograms. Because of this possibility, caution is advised in casually discounting existence of occult occlusive lesions in hypertensive patients with aneurysms. Renin studies are appropriate in these patients to document the existence of a renal component to their elevated blood pressure.

Rupture of renal artery aneurysms represents their most serious complication. Rupture causing exsanguinating hemorrhage and loss of life does not appear to be as common as previously implied. Loss of a kidney is perhaps a more likely but less often cited sequela of rupture. Renal artery macro-aneurysms ruptured in 5.6% of 72 patients harboring 94 aneurysms encountered at the University of Michigan [28]. Considering the increasing frequency with which these lesions are being discovered arteriographically, the actual risk for rupture of bland aneurysms must be considerably lower. Increased risk of rupture of aneurysms greater than 1.5 cm in diameter, those associated with calcification, and those in elderly patients is a logical but unproved contention. During pregnancy the risk of rupture and subsequent mortality is considered greater than otherwise predicted.

Indications for surgical intervention do not lend themselves to rigid definition. Symptomatic patients with suspected aneurysmal expansion are obvious operative candidates. Also, aneurysms associated with functionally important renal artery stenoses should be treated operatively. Excision of aneurysms is recommended when they are known to harbor thrombus. Because of catastrophic rupture during pregnancy, operative intervention in all women of childbearing age is recommended. Patients not subjected to operation must be followed carefully.

The objective of therapy is removal of the aneurysm without loss of renal tissue or compromise of normal renal blood flow [4, 9, 13, 28]. Nephrectomy is an untenable primary operation. Many large aneurysms may be excised with primary arterial closure. Excision of small aneurysms usually entails an angioplastic closure of the involved vessel. Renal artery reconstructions with autogenous saphenous vein for bifurcation aneurysms or lesions associated with functionally important stenoses are preferred over segmental resections or complex arterioplastic reconstructions. Occasionally, ex vivo repairs are required. Intraparenchymal aneurysms may necessitate partial nephrectomy. Cautious surgical intervention in properly selected patients with renal artery aneurysms is recommended because of the unpredictable incidence of rupture and the frequent association with functionally important renal artery occlusive disease [9, 28].

REFERENCES

1. Bedford PD, Lodge B: Aneurysm of the splenic artery. Gut 1:312-320, 1960
2. Boijsen E, Efsing HO: Aneurysm of the splenic artery. Acta Radiol. [Diagn.] (Stockh.) 8:29-41, 1969
3. DeBakey ME, Cooley DA: Successful resection of mycotic aneurysm of superior mesenteric artery: Case report and review of the literature. Am. Surgeon 19:202-212, 1953
4. DeBakey ME, Lefrak EA, Garcia-Rinaldi R, et al: Aneurysm of the renal artery: A vascular reconstructive approach. Arch. Surg. 106:438-443, 1973
5. Deterling RA: Aneurysm of the visceral arteries. J. Cardiovasc. Surg. 12:209-232, 1971
6. Duke LJ, Lamberth WC Jr, Wright CB: Inferior mesenteric artery aneurysm: Case report and discussion. Surgery 85:385-387, 1979
7. Guida PM, Moore SW: Aneurysm of the hepatic artery. Report of five cases with a brief review of the previously reported cases. Surgery 60:299-310, 1966
8. Guthrie W, Maclean H: Dissecting aneurysms of arteries other than the aorta. J. Pathol. 108:219-235, 1972
9. Hageman JH, Smith RF, Szilagyi DE, et al: Aneurysms of the renal artery: Problems of prognosis and surgical management. Surgery 84:563-572, 1978
10. Haimovici H, Sprayregen S, Eckstein P, et al: Celiac artery aneurysmectomy: Case report with review of the literature. Surgery 79:592-596, 1976
11. Harris RD, Anderson JE, Coel MN: Aneurysms of the small pancreatic arteries: A cause of upper abdominal pain and intestinal bleeding. Radiology 115:17-20, 1975
12. Hoehn JG, Bartholomew LG, Osmundson PJ, Wallace RB: Aneurysms of the mesenteric artery. Am. J. Surg. 115:832-834, 1968
13. Kraft RO, Fry WJ: Aneurysms of the celiac artery. Surg. Gynecol. Obstet. 117:563-566, 1963
14. Kreel L: The recognition and incidence of splenic artery aneurysms. A historical review. Australas. Radiol. 16:126-136, 1972
15. MacFarlane JR, Thorbjarnason B: Rupture of splenic artery aneurysm during pregnancy. Am. J. Obstet. Gynecol. 95:1025-1037, 1966
16. Mandelbaum I, Kaiser GD, Lempke RE: Gastric intramural aneurysm as a cause for massive gastrointestinal hemorrhage. Ann. Surg. 155:199-203, 1962
17. Milliard M: Fatal rupture of gastric aneurysm. Arch. Pathol. 59:363-371, 1955

18. Moore SW, Guida PM, Schumacher HW: Splenic artery aneurysm. Bull. Soc. Int. Chir. 29:210-218, 1970
19. Moore SW, Lewis RJ: Splenic artery aneurysm. Ann. Surg. 153:1033-1046, 1961
20. Owens JC, Coffey RJ: Aneurysm of the splenic artery including a report of six additional cases. Int. Abstr. Surg. 97:313-328, 1953
21. Poutasse EF: Renal artery aneurysms. J. Urol. 113:443-449, 1975
22. Reuter SR, Fry WJ, Bookstein JJ: Mesenteric artery branch aneurysms. Arch. Surg. 97:497-499, 1968
23. Scheinin TM, Vanttinen E: Aneurysms of the splenic artery in portal hypertension. Ann. Clin. Res. 1:165-168, 1969
24. Spanos PK, Kloppedal EA, Murray CA: Aneurysms of the gastroduodenal and pancreaticoduodenal arteries. Am. J. Surg. 127:345-348, 1974
25. Spittell JA, Fairbairn JF, Kincaid OW, ReMine WH: Aneurysm of the splenic artery. JAMA 175:452-456, 1961
26. Stanley JC: Splanchnic artery aneurysms, in Rutherford RB (ed): Vascular Surgery. Philadelphia, W. B. Saunders, 1977, pp 673-685
27. Stanley JC, Fry WJ: Pathogenesis and clinical significance of splenic artery aneurysms. Surgery 76:898-909, 1974
28. Stanley JC, Rhodes EL, Gewertz BL, et al: Renal artery aneurysms. Significance of macroaneurysms exclusive of dissections and fibrodysplastic mural dilations. Arch. Surg. 110:1327-1333, 1975
29. Stanley JC, Thompson NW, Fry WJ: Splanchnic artery aneurysms. Arch. Surg. 101:689-697, 1970
30. Thomford MR, Yurko JE, Smith EJ: Aneurysm of gastric arteries as a cause of intraperitoneal hemorrhage: Review of literature. Ann. Surg. 168:294-297, 1968
31. Verta MJ Jr, Dean RH, Yao JST, et al: Pancreaticoduodenal artery aneurysms. Ann. Surg. 186:111-114, 1977
32. Violago FC, Downs AR: Ruptured atherosclerotic aneurysm of the superior mesenteric artery with celiac axis occlusion. Ann. Surg. 174:207-210, 1971
33. Weaver DH, Fleming RJ, Barnes WA: Aneurysm of the hepatic artery: The value of arteriography in surgical management. Surgery 64:891-896, 1968
34. West JE, Bernhardt H, Bowers RF: Aneurysms of the pancreaticoduodenal artery. Am. J. Surg. 115:835-839, 1968

Frank J. Veith, M.D.

Surgery of the Infected Aortic Graft

Infection involving a vascular reconstructive operation on the aorta is one of the most catastrophic complications in surgery. With full knowledge of the natural history of this complication and by employing appropriate principles in its treatment, it is possible to salvage the life and limbs of some patients that are stricken with it. In this report we will consider infections that involve prosthetic grafts that have at least one anastomosis with the infrarenal abdominal aorta, although the principles of management can also generally be applied to the rare infections which complicate aortic thromboendarterectomy or operations elsewhere on the aorta.

INCIDENCE AND PREVENTION

Fortunately the incidence of infection involving aortic prosthetic grafts is low, even though it will vary somewhat in different population groups and different institutions. A reasonably representative appraisal of incidence is provided by Szilagyi and his colleagues in their important analysis of infections in arterial reconstructions with synthetic grafts [19]. They found the incidence of serious infection in aortic reconstructive operations performed solely through an abdominal incision to be 0.7%, while there was a 1.6% incidence of infection in aortofemoral operations. Szilagyi and his associates were also the first to point out that superficial wound infections that did not involve the prosthesis were of little consequence after arterial reconstructions [19]. However, it must be recognized that even a superficial infection in a femoral wound must be a serious

Supported in part by a grant from the John Hilton Manning and Emma Austin Manning Foundation.

concern because of the possibility that the superficial infection will spread to involve the nearby vascular prosthetic graft and the arterial suture line.

Although the incidence of infection should be higher after aortic operations for ruptured aneurysm than after elective procedures because of the requirement for haste, the probability of shock, and the inevitable hematoma, this is difficult to prove conclusively. However, the frequency of positive intraoperative cultures has been significantly greater from ruptured than from nonruptured aneurysms [9]. In addition, even in elective aortic procedures, it is probable that poor surgical technique, the presence of wound hematoma, and the need for reexploration will increase the hazard of graft contamination and septic complications. Thus to minimize the incidence of aortic graft sepsis, these surgical errors should, if at all possible, be avoided.

Because of the serious consequences of infections in operations on the arterial tree, many vascular surgeons have long advocated the use of so-called prophylactic antibiotics in conjunction with aortic surgery. Despite experimental evidence that supported their use [1, 4, 16], the efficacy of prophylactic antibiotics in surgery on the aorta in man remained unproven until the prospective, randomized, double blind controlled study of Kaiser, Dale, and their colleagues clearly demonstrated a diminished incidence of infection in reconstructive arterial surgery if appropriate doses of cefazolin were given immediately before and 24 hours after operation [13]. Although the number of serious graft infections in this study was small, they were all in the placebo group; on this basis it can be considered that the appropriate use of prophylactic antibiotics *is* indicated to minimize the incidence of infections involving aortic prosthetic grafts.

ETIOLOGY

Staphylococci have been the predominant organism responsible for aortofemoral prosthetic infection, while gram-negative coliform bacteria have predominated in aortiliac infection [19]. It is probable that the organisms responsible for most infections involving aortic prosthetic grafts are introduced from the operating room environment or the patient's skin at the time of operation, as is the case with most infections that involve clean surgical procedures. In addition, there are other possible sources for bacterial infection that involve aortic prostheses. These include any transient bacteremia which can innoculate a vascular prosthetic, particularly before it is well healed [3, 14, 15, 17]. Furthermore, bacteria that transgress the intestinal wall can occasionally be cultured from the fluid that exudes from the bowel that is frequently eviscerated to gain exposure during aortic operations [9, 10], and positive bacterial cultures have been obtained from the clot that is contained within the lumen of most aortic aneurysms [9]. The frequency of positive bacterial cultures from these sources make it somewhat surprising that the incidence of true infection in aortic procedures is as low as it is and provide further justification for the use of prophylactic antibiotics.

In addition to these sources of bacterial contamination which are generally present, there are three other specific sources which may be present in some instances. These include, first, cases in which the jejunoileum or the duodenum may be injured in gaining aortic exposure. If this is detected, serious consideration must be given to postponing the aortic operation or avoiding the insertion of any prosthetic graft material in the contaminated area. The latter requirement may necessitate the performance of an extraanatomic axillofemoral procedure to revascularize the lower extremities. Second, if the presence of localized or generalized cloudy peritoneal fluid raises the question of preexisting bacterial contamination of the operative field, the surgeon can obtain an immediate smear and Gram stain examination for bacteria. The absence of organisms helps to justify cautious continuation of the operation, whereas the presence of bacteria mandates termination of the operation or, if this is not possible, the performance of an axillofemoral bypass with elimination of the need for placing any foreign vascular prosthetic material in the known contaminated field. The third specific source of contamination, a preoperatively infected abdominal aortic aneurysm [12], can be suspected from a septic course or the presence of retroperitoneal pus. If suspected, this entity can be confirmed by Gram stain examination of smears and is best managed by control of the aneurysm by proximal and distal ligation, excision of all infected tissue, and performance of an axillofemoral bypass.

NATURAL HISTORY AND DIAGNOSIS

The presence of serious infectious involvement of an aortic prosthetic may be a simple matter to detect in some cases. In others, it may be extremely difficult to diagnose, particularly in the early stages. To understand this apparent contradiction, one must have insight into the variable natural history of infections involving aortic prosthetic grafts. This variable natural history is represented by the many different ways that such infections can be classified, as shown in Table 1.

Infections may present at any time within the first postoperative month or they may be extremely delayed in their presentation, with their first signs or symptoms not appearing until several years after the initial operation. Whether this means that the infecting organisms have been lying dormant since their introduction at operation or whether it means they have been newly introduced is not known. However, it is known that some infections can have a rapid course with serious local and systemic manifestations and rapid progression to catastrophic endpoints, whereas others can have an indolent course with minimal

Table 1
Classifications of Infections Involving Aortic Prosthetic Grafts

By time of onset	Early: 0-30 days after operation Late: 1 month to 5 years after operation
By localization	Groin involvement Intraabdominal involvement Total involvement
By severity	Superficial wound: grade I and grade II of Szilagyi [19] Deep wound — perigraft Bacteria in graft interstices Breakdown of anastomosis } grade III of Szilagyi [19]
By manifestation	Systemic — fever, leukocytosis, bacteremia, septicemia Back pain, ureteral obstruction Abscess, sinus Thrombosis False aneurysm, enteric fistula (especially aortoduodenal), hemorrhage

consequences being manifest for a long time before the lethal end phases of the infection occur.

Groin infection. One of the reasons for this variability in course is the intrinsic virulence of the infecting organism in a given patient; another, more important reason is localization of the infection. Whether or not the infection is present in a groin incision is important in determining its presentation and behavior. Many infected aortofemoral prosthetic grafts present only with an abscess or persistent draining sinus in the groin incision. This alone, no matter at what time after the original operation it occurs and no matter whether or not it is accompanied by fever or leukocytosis, must be regarded as an ominous sign. The graft itself may or may not be involved, and other parts of the graft may or may not be infected. If the abscess cavity or the sinus communicates with the prosthetic graft and if the treatment is expectant or conservative, one of two dire consequences will occur even if the infection is initially restricted to the groin incision. One consequence is that the involved limb of the graft will thrombose with spread of the infection to involve the entirety of the thrombosed portion of the graft. Persistent local evidence of infection will continue until all of the infected foreign material is removed. The second and even more serious consequence of unaggressive management of infection in the distal end of an aortofemoral prosthesis is disruption of the graft to artery suture line with formation of an anastomotic false aneurysm or bleeding to the exterior via a previously noted sinus tract. This bleeding often is small in amount at first and may appear of little consequence. However, if the nature and origin of this "sentinel bleeding" is not recognized and managed aggressively, it can lead to exsanguination and death.

Once an arterial prosthetic infection has progressed to the point where bleeding occurs, it means that the artery at the level of the anastomosis is also infected and no attempt to preserve the continuity of that vessel will succeed. The prosthetic graft must be removed and the involved vessel ligated or oversewn with or without a prior or subsequent extraanatomic bypass in a clean field to maintain extremity viability.

It has been thought that infection in a wound surrounding a functioning prosthetic graft, even without anastomotic bleeding, also required similar treatment. This is still true if the aortic end of a prosthetic graft is involved in the septic process. Recently, however, we have observed five patients with purulent wound infections at the site of prosthetic arterial graft origins or insertions. In two cases the grafts were of woven Dacron. In three the graft material was expanded polytetrafluoroethylene. In all five, one graft to artery suture line was visible in the infected wound and obviously bathed in pus. In these 5 cases, surgical debridement or excision of the wound in the operating room, daily packing with povidone-iodine, and intensive appropriate antibiotics resulted in healing of the wound and preservation of graft and artery patency, which have persisted 1-5 years. In two similarly managed cases, graft to artery anastomotic disruption occurred and required the radical treatment already outlined. Nevertheless, our recent experience, supported by the previous observations of Carter, Cohen, and Whalen [5], would appear to justify cautious use of aggressive surgical management *without* graft removal in selected prosthetic infections which are restricted to the groin and in which the graft to artery suture line remains intact.

Intraabdominal infection. In patients whose aortic operation does not have a groin incision and in those whose aortofemoral prosthesis is primarily infected at the proximal end, the infection usually presents differently and may be more difficult to diagnose. Otherwise unexplained fever or leukocytosis with or without back pain that occurs at any time after an aortic procedure should be enough to arouse suspicion. Otherwise unexplained gas bubbles in the retroperitoneal area surrounding the graft and absence of the left psoas shadow may also be noted. Performance of an intravenous pyelogram may show hydronephrosis [18]. In fact, this finding may be the first evidence of an infected aortic graft. Other diagnostic modalities that may be helpful include abdominal sonography, which can reveal an echolucent mass surrounding the aortic graft (Fig. 1), and computerized axial tomography, which can reveal an abnormal water density mass in the retroperitoneal area surrounding the graft. If the patient has a septic course, positive blood cultures obtained by arterial puncture downstream to the graft are persuasive evidence that there is bacterial involvement of the luminal aspect of the prosthesis and that radical treatment is

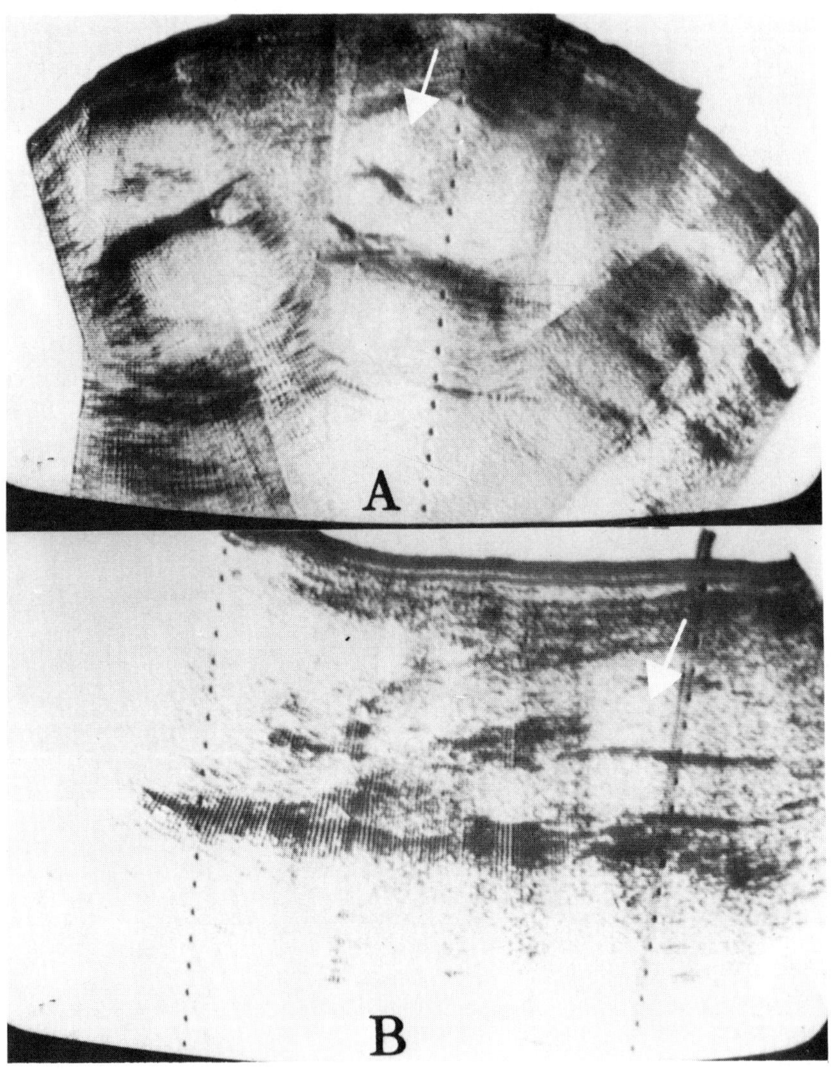

Fig. 1. Transverse (A) and sagittal (B) sonographic cuts demonstrating an echolucent area (arrows) anterior and lateral to an infected aortic prosthesis following operation for ruptured abdominal aortic aneurysm. [Courtesy of Dr. Ruth Rosenblatt.]

required. In the early phases of such an infection, angiography may not be helpful and will probably show intact anastomotic lines and absence of luminal irregularities.

If the proximal end of an aortofemoral prosthesis or either end of a totally intraabdominal prosthesis becomes infected and radical surgical treatment with removal of the graft is not undertaken, disruption of the involved suture line will occur. This may lead to prompt exsanguination, although more commonly it presents as a pulsatile abdominal mass which represents a false aneurysm. If untreated, this can produce pressure effects on adjacent viscera and ultimately exsanguination. If time permits, angiography is the most helpful diagnostic procedure and localizes the involved anastomosis if two or more are at risk. Another possible presentation of an infected aortic or iliac artery anastomosis is by fistulization with the gut. Aortoduodenal fistulas are most common in this regard and are best diagnosed by fiberoptic endoscopy.

It should be noted that other causes of disruption of the proximal aortic suture line and other graft to artery anastomoses exist. False aneurysms unassociated with sepsis may occur from a variety of other causes including a weakened artery wall, loss of suture tensile strength, excessive graft tension, or improper surgical technique. Fistulas between the proximal aortic suture line and the adherent duodenum can occur without initiating sepsis and can be prevented by the interposition of soft tissue or the onlay of a patch of graft material between the anastomosis and the duodenum. Absence of systemic or local evidence of infection and negative smears for bacteria, cultures, and histological examination should permit the surgeon to differentiate these noninfectious complications from those due to infection so that treatment may be appropriate. Graft to artery anastomotic problems unassociated with the presence of bacteria do not require extraanatomic bypass in a clean field.

TREATMENT

Effective management of infected aortic reconstructions must be based on a clear knowledge and understanding of their variable natural history and the classifications by localization, severity, and manifestation listed in Table 1. Infections that are established as being superficial require only good local treatment and appropriate antibiotics to prevent spread. They are not of serious import and will not be considered further in this discussion.

Infections restricted to the groin wound. When these do not involve the interstices of the prosthesis or the femoral artery at the distal anastomosis, they may be treated by radical local debridement or excision of the involved wound followed by povidone-iodine packing and high-dose intravenous antibiotics as dictated by wound cultures and sensitivity. It must be recognized that this is a relatively new and unproven approach to such infections based largely on our own limited experience and that it is associated with the risk that infection may progress in extent with disruption of the anastomosis and serious arterial hemorrhage. If this approach is chosen, appropriate precautions to permit immediate control of bleeding by direct pressure and rapid operation must be taken until the wound is fully healed. Furthermore, if there is any evidence of even minor "sentinel" bleeding, the management should parallel the following classic treatment for infection restricted to the groin incision of an aortofemoral prosthesis. The principles of this treatment were first enunciated by Shaw and Baue [18] and mandate removal of the prosthetic graft to the extent that it is involved in the infectious process, ligation of the involved artery proximal and distal to the infected anastomosis, and if necessary and possible salvage of the involved limb by an extraanatomic bypass in a totally separate, clean operative field. This method of treatment is still clearly the one of choice when an infection localized to the groin is or becomes associated with hemorrhage, false aneurysm, graft thrombosis, or persistent septicemia.

In such circumstances, the operation can best be carried out in two stages. One stage is designed to remove the infected limb of the graft and to control bleeding by ligature or oversewing of the artery or arteries proximal and distal to the infected anastomosis. The other stage provides extraanatomic revascularization of the afflicted limb. Both stages can be performed at one operation through totally separate surgical fields, or either stage can be performed first at a separate operation depending on the preference of the surgeon and the urgency of the situation with regard to bleeding or limb ischemia.

One approach is to perform first, through abdominal and distal thigh incisions, an obturator bypass from the uninfected aortic graft or its opposite iliac limb to the uninvolved distal superficial femoral, deep femoral, or popliteal artery. The technique of obturator bypass has been well described and illustrated elsewhere [11, 18]. Then, through the abdominal incision, the involved limb of the graft can be ligated and divided in an area proximal to any evident infection, and the external iliac artery can be ligated as far distally as possible. After all the wounds are closed and sealed, or possibly at a second operation, the second phase is performed. This consists of removal of the previously divided graft and proximal and distal oversewing or preferably ligation of the common femoral artery and sometimes its branches in the region of the infected anastomosis. Dissection of the arteries in this infected, scarred wound can be extremely difficult and dangerous. It is facilitated by the previous proximal control and may require further temporary intraluminal control by balloon catheters.

Another, simpler approach is the one that we favor. The first phase of this consists of gaining access to the retroperitoneum through an oblique or transverse abdominal incision well above the infected groin. Through this clean field, the limb of the graft is ligated and divided and the external iliac artery is ligated as far distally as possible. An axillopopliteal bypass is performed using an expanded polytetrafluoroethylene graft which is tunneled lateral to the infected

groin wound and diagonally across the anterior surface of the thigh below it to enter the popliteal fossa [22]. After closing and sealing all these clean incisions, the infected graft and groin wound is managed as already described.

A third, albeit somewhat different and less well accepted approach to the infected prosthetic graft has been recommended by Wylie [24] and Ehrenfeld and his associates [8]. This approach uses endarterectomy with or without a vein autograft to permit removal of all infected prosthetic material or employs a clean incision to obtain a segment of the patient's own artery. Either the opposite external iliac artery, which is replaced by a graft, or the endarterectomized superficial femoral artery may be harvested. After closure and sealing of the clean wound, the arterial autograft is then used to replace the infected graft limb. This approach is limited by the requirement that an arterial anastomosis be performed in an infected field. Although autologous arterial suture lines can heal in this circumstance and although the approach can be used successfully [8, 24], it is not recommended for general use.

Infections of an entire aortoiliac graft or restricted to the aortic end of an aortofemoral bypass. Once diagnosed, such infections must be treated aggressively with removal of the infected prosthetic graft, wide drainage, appropriate systemic antibiotics, and restoration of distal flow by extraanatomic bypass through separate clean operative fields. Although restoration of distal flow may not always be required, to our knowledge there are no reported instances when otherwise less radical management was effective for aortic prosthetic grafts infected in this area. Therefore execution of the more radical approach is essential to achieve salvage of the patient and his limbs even though many aspects of it may be difficult.

Again the approach consists of two phases: (1) removal of the infected graft with proximal and distal control of the artery or arteries at the anastomotic sites, and (2) restoration of distal arterial flow through a separate operative field. The latter phase, which is not difficult since the groins are uninvolved by sepsis, should be performed first if possible. This can best be accomplished by an axillobifemoral bypass or bilateral axillofemoral bypasses. In the rare instance when neither axillary artery is suitable to provide inflow, the thoracic or supraceliac aorta may be used [2, 21].

Removal of the infected graft and control of bleeding can be far more difficult, particularly if the proximal anastomosis is immediately below the renal arteries. It is helpful and usually possible to determine by angiography how much aorta remains between the renal arteries and the proximal anastomosis. This determination is important since it indicates whether there is enough aortic length to permit ligation of the infrarenal aortic stump or whether it will be necessary to oversew it. The former procedure, if feasible, is safer and more secure than the latter, since subsequent infection and aortic rupture is less likely. Wide drainage of this area and excision of all infected tissue also help to

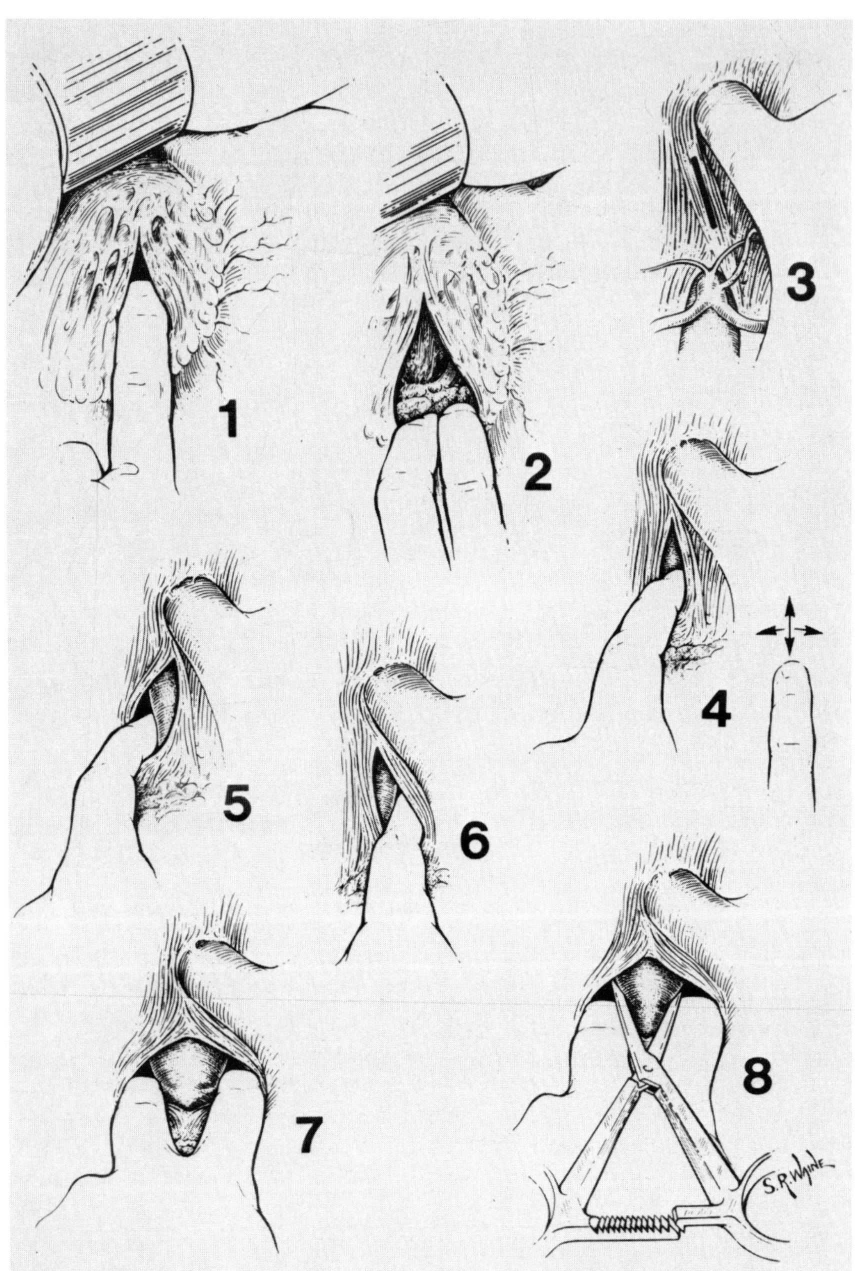

Fig. 2. Method for gaining control of the supraceliac aorta through the abdomen. The abdomen is opened with a long midline incision extending to the xiphoid, and the liver is retracted upward and to the right with a Deaver retractor. *1*, the index finger bluntly tearing the lesser omentum between the liver and the stomach. The caudate lobe of the liver is visualized through the upper portion of the lesser omentum. *2*, the opening in the lesser omentum

minimize the everpresent risk of hemorrhage from the infected aortic stump [19, 23].

Gaining control of the aorta distal to the renal arteries to permit ligation or oversewing may be difficult at best in a field obscured by previous operative scarring and infection. If the remaining infrarenal aortic segment is short and the anastomosis is disrupted, it may be impossible to gain this control without exsanguination. In such circumstances, we and others have found it beneficial to gain proximal control of the supraceliac aorta through the abdomen [6, 21].

This can safely be accomplished as shown in Fig. 2 [20]. The aorta may be occluded in this location as long as is necessary to gain effective control below the renal arteries so that debridement and oversewing or ligation can be performed. In our hands the supraceliac aorta has been occluded for more than an hour without causing serious impairment of hepatic, enteric, or renal function [20].

Another method has also been advocated by Diethrich and his co-workers to facilitate management of the infrarenal aortic segment in instances in which the proximal anastomosis is infected but intact [7]. According to this method, removal of the proximal graft is preceded by ligation of the graft limbs and several days delay to allow the infrarenal aorta to thrombose solidly. If feasible, this approach facilitates gaining aortic control, but whether it decreases the incidence of aortic stump infection as claimed remains to be shown.

After managing the proximal aortic anastomosis, the iliac arteries are controlled, debrided, and ligated or oversewn and the entire aortoiliac prosthesis removed. Aortic and iliac stumps are covered with any adjacent soft tissue, and wide retroperitoneal drainage through the left flank is established. The main

---

through which can be seen the peritoneum overlying the crura of the diaphragm superiorly and the upper border of the pancreas inferiorly. The celiac axis and its branches are intimately associated with the upper border of the pancreas and cannot be clearly distinguished from it without dissection. *3*, the position of these vessels diagramatically with the pancreas and other nonvascular structures omitted. The heavy line indicates the location of the incision in the posterior peritoneum overlying the diaphragmatic crura. This incision is made with the fingernail of the left index or middle finger. *4*, the method for digitally splitting and, with posteriorly directed pressure, transgressing the muscle fibers of the diaphragmatic crura to gain access to the periadventitial plane of the aorta. *5* and *6* show how this plane is widened medial and lateral to the aorta. No attempt is made to dissect the aorta circumferentially, since this can be difficult because of limited exposure and access. *7* and *8* illustrate how inferior traction with the fingers creates a space on either side of the aorta so that a totally occluding large clamp with slightly curved blades can be applied. [Reproduced from Veith FJ, Gupta S, Daly V: Technique for occluding the supraceliac aorta through the abdomen. Surg. Gynecol. Obstet. (in press). By permission of Surgery, Gynecology and Obstetrics.]

abdominal incision is then closed with a single layer of closely spaced retention-type monofilament sutures. If only the upper end of an aortofemoral graft is involved in the septic process, the distal uninfected graft will have previously been ligated and divided at the time of the axillofemoral bypass. The remaining graft can then be extracted at the time of the abdominal procedure.

Infection of an entire aortofemoral graft. Treatment in this situation is identical to that already outlined with two exceptions. First, graft removal usually would be preceded by bilateral axillopopliteal bypasses if limb viability is to be maintained. The course of these bypasses is lateral to the infected groin wounds. Second, the abdominal approach to remove the infected graft must also be accompanied by groin incisions and proximal and distal ligation of the femoral arteries involved in the distal anastomosis. Management and techniques in this area are similar to those already presented for infections restricted to groin wounds.

Although infected graft removal and securing of the involved remaining arteries in any of the above circumstances is best preceded by extraanatomic bypass in a clean field, this is not always possible. Exsanguinating hemorrhage from a disrupted anastomosis may require control and graft removal before any attempt is made to restore distal circulation. In an occasional instance, a patient's precarious condition following the graft removal and control of bleeding may force the surgeon to accept limb loss rather than perform the extra-anatomic bypass. However, this should be an extremely rare occurrence, particularly if treatment is not inadvisably delayed.

REFERENCES

1. Baker WH, Bodensteiner JA: The administration of antibiotics in vascular reconstructive surgery. A comparison of the effectiveness of systemic cephaloridine versus cephaloridine-soaked grafts in preventing graft infections in dogs. J. Thorac. Cardiovasc. Surg. 64:301, 1972
2. Blaisdell FW, DeMattei GA, Gauder PJ: Extraperitoneal thoracic aorta to femoral bypass graft as replacement for an infected aortic bifurcation prosthesis. Am. J. Surg. 102:583, 1961
3. Bradham RR, Cordle F, McIver FA: Effect of bacteria on vascular prostheses. Ann. Surg. 154:187, 1966
4. Burke JF: The effective period of preventive antibiotic action in experimental incisions and dermal lesions. Surgery 50:161, 1961
5. Carter SC, Cohen A, Whelan TJ: Clinical experience with management of the infected Dacron graft. Ann. Surg. 158:249, 1963
6. Crawford ES, Manning LG, Kelly TF: "Redo" surgery after operations for aneurysm and occlusion of the abdominal aorta. Surgery 81:41, 1977

7. Diethrich EB, Noon GP, Liddicoat JE, et al: Treatment of infected aortofemoral arterial prosthesis. Surgery 68:1044, 1970
8. Ehrenfeld WK, Wilbur BG, Olcott CN, et al: Autogenous tissue reconstruction in the management of infected prosthetic grafts. Surgery 85:82, 1979
9. Ernst CB, Campbell HC, Daugherty ME, et al: Incidence and significance of intra-operative bacterial cultures during abdominal aortic aneurysmectomy. Ann. Surg. 185:626, 1977
10. Fry WJ: Vascular prosthesis infections. Surg. Clin. North Am. 52:1419, 1972
11. Guida PM, Moore SW: Obturator bypass technique. Surg. Gynecol. Obstet. 128:1307, 1969
12. Jarrett F, Darling RC, Mundth ED, et al: Experience with infected aneurysms of the abdominal aorta. Arch. Surg. 110:1281, 1975
13. Kaiser AB, Clayson KR, Mulherin JL, et al: Antibiotic prophylaxis in vascular surgery. Ann. Surg. 188:283, 1978
14. Lindenauer SM, Fry WJ, Schaub G, et al: The use of antibiotics in the prevention of vascular graft infections. Surgery 62:487, 1967
15. Malone JM, Moore WS, Campagna G, et al: Bacteremic infectability of vascular grafts: The influence of pseudointimal integrity and duration of graft function. Surgery 78:211, 1975
16. Moore WS, Rosson CT, Hall AD: Effect of prophylactic antibiotics in preventing bacteremic infection of vascular prostheses. Surgery 69:825, 1971
17. Moore WS, Rosson CT, Hall AD, et al: Transient bacteremia: A cause of infection in prosthetic vascular grafts. Am. J. Surg. 117:342, 1969
18. Shaw RS, Baue AE: Management of sepsis complicating arterial reconstructive surgery. Surgery 53:75, 1963
19. Szilagyi DE, Smith RF, Elliott JP, et al: Infection in arterial reconstruction with synthetic grafts. Ann. Surg. 176:321, 1972
20. Veith FJ, Gupta S, Daly V: Technique for occluding the supraceliac aorta through the abdomen. Surg. Gynecol. Obstet. (in press)
21. Veith FJ, Hartsuck JM, Crane C: Management of aortoiliac reconstruction complicated by sepsis and hemorrhage. N. Engl. J. Med. 270:1389, 1964
22. Veith FJ, Moss CM, Fell SC, et al: New approaches to limb salvage by extended extra-anatomic bypasses and prosthetic reconstructions to foot arteries. Surgery 84:764, 1978
23. Vellar IDA, Doyle JC: Axillofemoral bypass in the management of infected aortic bifurcation Dacron graft. Aust. N. Z. J. Surg. 40:58, 1970
24. Wylie EJ: Discussion in Shaw RS, Baue AE [18]

Norris D. Johnson, M.D.
James S. T. Yao, M.D., Ph.D.
John J. Bergan, M.D.

Spinal Cord Ischemia After Abdominal Aortic Surgery

Spinal cord ischemia following thoracic aortic aneurysm resection is a known phenomenon. However, for surgery of the abdominal aorta, profound lower extremity neurological deficit with or without bowel and bladder paralysis is rare. DeBakey [9, 10] reported a 5% incidence of paraplegia following resection of thoracic aneurysms, but his group did not describe a single case of neurological deficit in 1400 patients who underwent resection of abdominal aortic aneurysms. Despite the infrequency of this condition, its occurrence remains a devastating experience for both the patient and the surgeon.

The present review examines the Northwestern University McGaw Medical Center experience in patients who had spinal cord ischemia following abdominal aortic surgery. In addition, a comprehensive review of the blood supply to the spinal cord and a survey of the current literature were made in an attempt to offer a better understanding of this rare but shocking complication.

HISTORICAL REVIEW

The first observation of spinal ischemia secondary to a procedure on the aorta was made in 1667, when Stennis [40] noted paralysis of the hindquarters of a rabbit following ligation of the abdominal aorta. This observation, which has been known for over 300 years, has only recently assumed clinical importance. In 1956, during a review of 24 instances of spinal cord ischemia associated with thoracic aortic surgery, Adams [3] did not observe a single case following infrarenal abdominal aortic procedures. He drew the following conclu-

---

Supported in part by the Dr. Scholl Foundation and the Northwestern University Vascular Research Fund.

sion: "The spinal cord is protected against damage during infrarenal aortic surgery either by the absence of infrarenal blood supply to the cord, or when present, by collateral supply from a constant and important low thoracic spinal vessel." In a discussion of Adams' report, the first cases of spinal ischemia following infrarenal abdominal aortic surgery were described [30].

Up to the present, there have been 35 reported cases in the medical literature. These have been comprehensively discussed in previous reports [14, 42]; 16 patients had spinal cord ischemia after repair of ruptured aortic aneurysms, whereas 13 cases occurred after elective resection of an intact infrarenal aortic aneurysm and 6 after aortofemoral reconstructions for aorto-iliac occlusive disease.

VASCULAR ANATOMY OF THE SPINAL CORD

The vascular supply of the spinal cord has been studied extensively [1, 2, 10, 12, 18, 25]. In fact, several of the more prominent studies are approaching the centennium. Adamkiewicz, in 1881, carried out and reported a study of the vascular supply of the spinal cord in an effort to substantiate a theory that tabes dorsalis might be a blood-borne disease [1, 2]. Kadyi, in 1889, reported that only one-fourth of nerve roots in man are accompanied by segmental arteries that contribute to the circulation of the spinal cord [26].

In embryonic development, each segment of the spinal cord receives paired radicular arteries from the aorta (reminiscent of the lower vertebrates), but in late fetal life many of these atrophy and disappear [3]. Consequently, the adult anatomic arrangement is a variable number of radicular arteries conveying blood to the spinal cord.

Initially, the proximal blood supply is quite abundant, consisting of posterior spinal segmental (rami) arteries from the costocervical, intercostal, lumbar, and ileolumbar arteries. The distribution of a typical spinal artery is illustrated in Fig. 1.

The anterior spinal artery is the largest spinal artery, is formed from the union of the anterior spinal rami from the intracranial portion of the vertebral artery, and lies in the vicinity of the anterior median fissure. The posterior spinal arteries, like the anterior spinal artery, originate as branches from the intracranial portion of the vertebral arteries [16].

The radicular arteries carry blood to the anterior spinal artery and two posterior spinal arteries. On reaching the surface of the spinal cord, each radicular artery divides into an ascending and descending branch which anastomose to form the anterior and posterior spinal arteries. The final anatomic arrangement of the radicular arteries is variable. Adamkiewicz described three to ten anterior radicular arteries; Kadyi, five to ten; Suh, six to eight; and Gillihan, seven to ten that anastomose with the anterior spinal artery.

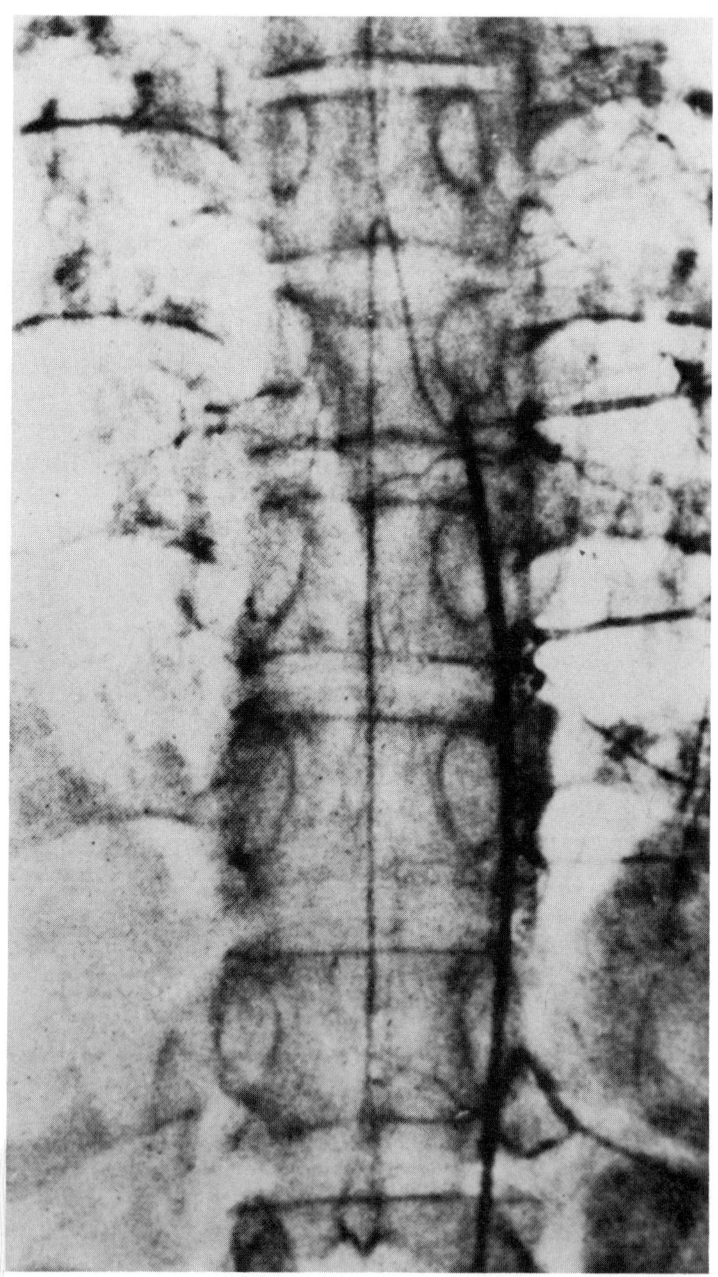

Fig. 1. Artery of Adamkiewicz (artery radicularis magna) demonstrated on selective arteriogram. [From Crocel L, Vincent A, Dereux JF: J. Sci. Med. Lille 91:155, 1973. Used with permission.]

The distribution is not symmetrical. According to Suh, there are usually one or two in the lumbar region, one in the lower thoracic region, none or one in the middle thoracic region, one or two in the lower cervical region, and one in the upper cervical region. The largest radicular has been named the artery radicularis magna, or the artery of Adamkiewicz (Fig. 1). Its origin is quite variable. Adamkiewicz described the arteria magna spinalis as originating from T-8 to L-3, most frequently being at T-9, T-10, or T-11. It is single and arises with equal frequency from the right or left side, with an average length of 2.5 cm [1, 2]. Kadyi described it as arising from T-9 to L-3. Suh observed it between T-8 and L-4, with L-2 being the most frequent site and occurring most frequently on the left. Doppman [11], on the basis of angiography, localized the origin from T-8 to L-2. Hilal, on the basis of angiographic evidence, found the anterior spinal artery receives a limited number of feeders not exceeding four throughout the thoracic region. Twenty-five percent (8/33) of patients who were studied had only one arterial feeder to the anterior spinal artery between T-4 and L-2 [22, 27].

According to Adams [3], at a certain point in development, there are two radicular arteries, one in the lower thorax and one in the lumbar region. In appproximately 50% of instances, the superior artery becomes more important and the inferior one regresses; in these cases, the lower thoracic aorta supplies about one-half of the spinal cord. In the other 50% of cases, the lower radicular artery predominates; in these instances, the lower thoracic aorta supplies one-fourth of the spinal cord.

The posterior radicular arteries that supply the posterior one-third of the spinal cord are similar in distribution to the anterior radicular arteries and anastomose to form the posterior spinal arteries [41]. According to Suh, there are 5-8 posterior radicular arteries, while others describe 10-20 [16, 26]. However, Hilal indicates that the posterior radicular arteries are much smaller and more numerous than the anterior radicular arteries and can be identified bilaterally at almost every level in the thoracic spine.

The caudal portion of the posterior spinal arteries receives an anastomotic loop from the anterior spinal artery at the crus medullaris. Consequently, in the lower portion of the spinal cord, there is greater interdependence on the anterior spinal artery for blood supply than in the other segments of the spinal cord [13]. Characteristically, the posterior spinal arteries supply the posterior one-third of the spinal cord and the anterior spinal artery supplies the anterior two-thirds of the cord (Fig. 2).

CLINICAL PRESENTATION AND DIAGNOSIS

Clinical manifestations of the spinal syndrome may be temporary or permanent. They may include sensory and motor aspects with or without bladder and bowel involvement. The classical anterior spinal artery syndrome is characterized

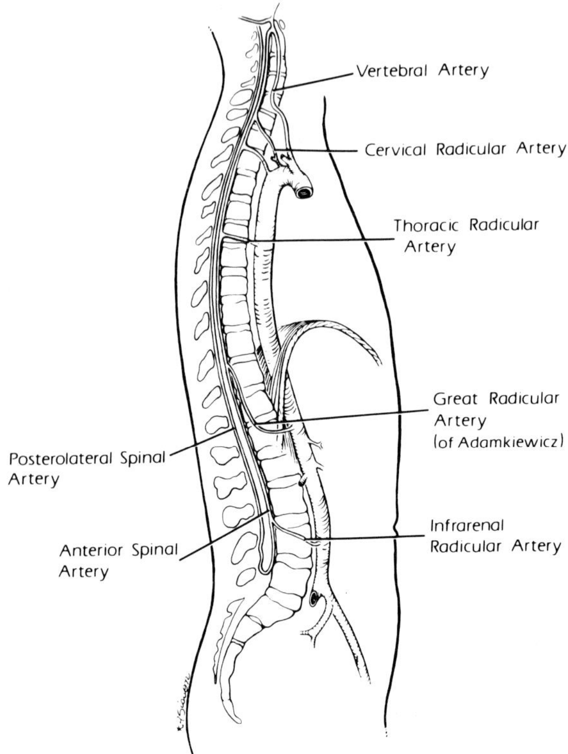

Fig. 2. Major blood supply of the spinal column.

by paraplegia, rectal and urinary incontinence, loss of pain and temperature sensation, but with sparing of vibration and proprioception sensation. Table 1 summarizes findings by various authors.

Immediately after surgery, the influence of anesthetics or muscle relaxants may hinder recognition of the symptoms and hence the diagnosis. However, careful observation of limb movements when the patient is being extubated may offer some clue to the problem. In reported cases, patients were found to have difficulty in moving their lower extremities and flaccid paralysis was noted.

Once spinal cord ischemia is suspected, establishing the diagnosis requires thorough knowledge of nerve supply from the cord. A meticulous examination of motor, sensory, bladder, and sphincter tone must be instituted to determine the extent of ischemia. In addition to testing tendon reflexes, a test of the cremasteric reflex may offer further information. The cremasteric reflex is one of the first to be lost in paraplegia and first to return in recovering cases. Because of the routine use of indwelling catheters in the bladder, disturbance of bladder function is the last to be recognized. Once motor and sensory examination is completed, a rectal examination must be done to examine the sphincter tone. If

Table 1
Summary of Spinal Cord Ischemia Following Abdominal Aortic Surgery

Author	Age/sex	Level	Neurological Deficit	Outcome
Abdominal aortic aneurysm — ruptured				
Couplund & Reeve [6]	79/M	T-12	Paraplegia developed 24 hours postoperatively	Death at 48 hours
Skillman et al. [38]	65/M	T-12	Paraplegia, flaccid anal sphincter, noted 48 hours postop.	Partial return
	73/M	L-2	Motor weakness, sensory level at L-2	Death at 6 weeks
Gump [20]	63/M	T-12	Paraplegia	Recovery at 12 months
Zuber et al. [43]	75/M	NI	Paraplegia, vesicorectal incontinence	Death at 1 month
	65/M	NI	Paraplegia, dissociated sensory loss	Permanent
	58/M	NI	Paraparesis, vesical incontinence	Recovery at 2 months
Hogan & Romanal [23]	76/M	L-2	Paraplegia, vesicorectal incontinence	Death at 24 hours
Mehrez et al. [31]	76/M	L-2	Paraplegia, vesicorectal incontinence	Death at 24 hours
	69/M	T-9	Paraplegia, rectal incontinence	Death at 36 hours
Sher & Healy [37]	82/F	T-12	Paraplegia, rectal incontinence	Death at 40 days
Golden et al. [18]	62/M	L-1	Paraplegia, vesicorectal incontinence	Partial return
Jorning & Brands [25]	58/F	T-12	Paraparesis, dissociated sensory loss	Recovery at 12 months
Michaels [32]	56/M	T-12	Loss of proprioception, motor function intact	Partial recovery
McCune [30]	NI	NI	Paraparesis	Death at 72 hours
	NI	NI	Spastic paralysis	No information

Abdominal aortic aneurysm — intact				
Couplund & Reeve [6]	59/M	T-12	Paralysis and sensory loss, developed 24 hours postoperatively	Permanent
Zuber et al. [43]	74/M	NI	Paraplegia	Death
Hara & Lipin [21]	64/M	S-2	Vesicorectal incontinence only	Recovery
Bates [4]	55/M	T-11	Paraplegia and sensory loss, developed 48 hours postoperatively	Death at 11 days
	60/M	L-3	Paraplegia, vesical incontinence	Death at 3 months
Golden et al. [17]	58/F	L-1	Paraplegia, vesical incontinence	Permanent
Reich [34]	71/M	T-12	Paraplegia, rectal incontinence	Death at 3 weeks
Pasternak et al. [33]	60/M	NI	Paraplegia	Recovery at 12 months
Edmondson & Giridin [12]	51/M	L-1	Paraplegia, sensory loss	Death at 10 days
Gensler & Hoffer [15]	72/M	L-2	Paraparesis	Recovery at 12 months
Lentin & Salis [29]	58/M	T-10	Paraplegia, sensory loss	Partial recovery
Aortoiliac occlusive disease				
Lake [28	46/F	T-10	Paraplegia, sensory loss	No information
Zuber et al. [43]	72/F	NI	Paraplegia, dissociated sensory loss	Death at 5 days
Scorza et al. [36]	62/M	L-3	Paraparesis	Permanent
Smith [39]	53/M	L-1	Paraplegia, complete sensory loss	Permanent

the sphincter is flaccid, the patient must be turned over for examination of the anal reflex. The latter is done by lightly stroking the perianal region and observing the contraction of the anal sphincter. Bowel involvement is indicated by relaxed sphincter tone and absence of the anal reflex.

In addition to establishing the diagnosis by the above examination, the level of spinal cord involvement can also be predicted. Table 2 outlines the level of spinal ischemia in relation to symptoms and signs.

Once the patient is completely awake and conscious, examination of vibratory sense and proprioception will determine whether the posterior column is involved. With involvement of the anterior spinal artery, one would expect that pain and temperature sensation would also be absent.

THE NORTHWESTERN UNIVERSITY EXPERIENCE

Previously, Ferguson et al. [14] have reported the Northwestern experience with spinal cord ischemia following aortic surgery. Table 3 summarizes the findings and outcome in five patients. The fifth case report is as yet unreported.

In order to illustrate the salient features of spinal cord ischemia, three cases will be described.

Case 1. A 68 year old diabetic male entered the Wesley Pavilion, Northwestern Memorial Hospital because of rest pain and gangrene in his left second toe. He was a maturity onset diabetic who had taken 55 U of NPH insulin daily for 12 years. He was also receiving digoxin and a diuretic following an episode of congestive heart failure 3 years prior to the present admission.

Physical examination showed him to be normotensive, blood pressure 140/90. No peripheral pulses were present in the lower extremities. Gangrene was present in the left second toe, and there were marked ischemic trophic changes bilaterally. The electrocardiogram showed old ischemic changes but no

Table 2
Determination of Level of Spinal Ischemia After Aortic Surgery

Symptom or Sign	Level of Innervation
Cremasteric reflex	L-2, L-3
Knee jerk	L-3, L-4
Quadriceps muscle	L-4
Ankle jerk	L-5, S-1
Plantar extension	L-5
Plantar flexion	S-1
Bladder control	S-2, S-3, S-4
Bowel control	S-2, S-3, S-4
Anal reflex	S-2, S-3, S-4

Modified from Ferguson et al: Spinal ischemia following abdominal aortic surgery. Ann. Surg. 181:267, 1975. By permission of the J.B. Lippincott Company.

Table 3
Northwestern University Experience With Spinal Cord Ischemia After Abdominal Aortic Surgery

Case	Age/Sex	Level	Neurological Loss	Operation	Outcome
1	66/M	L-2	Paresis, left greater than right, dissociated sensory loss	Intact abdominal aortic aneurysm	Recovered, 14 days
2	68/M	T-12	Paraplegia, complete sensory loss	Aortoiliac occlusive disease	Permanent
3	56/F	L-5	Paraplegia, complete sensory loss	Aortoiliac occlusive disease	Permanent
4	76/M	L-1	Paraplegia, complete sensory loss	Intact abdominal aortic aneurysm	Death in post-operative period
5	75/M	T-12	Paraplegia, complete sensory loss	Intact abdominal aortic aneurysm	Death in post-operative period

recent abnormalities. The arteriogram revealed bilateral common iliac artery occlusions.

Three days following angiography, a bilateral aortofemoral bypass graft was done using a Dacron prosthesis. A left lumbar sympathectomy was also performed. A large, patent midline lumbar artery was noted arising from the aorta at the level of the fourth lumbar vertebra. This was preserved but was temporarily occluded for 40 min during graft placement. During surgery and in the immediate postoperative period, blood pressure was normal. There was no period of hypotension. Urine output was adequate at all times.

In the recovery room and during the first postoperative day, the patient complained of complete loss of sensation below the umbilicus and total leg and thigh paralysis. The extremities showed a flaccid paraplegia, complete sensory level at T-12-L-1, flaccid anal sphincter, and areflexia in the lower extremities. Postoperative steroids were given to reduce spinal cord edema and subsequently a lumbar myelogram was done, which was negative.

The patient had virtually no neurologic recovery except that he had some control of the sartorius muscles bilaterally, thus demonstrating a degree of L-1 return. He remained paraplegic 3 years later, with incontinence and sensory status essentially as before.

Comment. This patient demonstrates the syndrome of irreversible lumbar and sacral ischemia with the areflexia to be expected in conus medullaris involvement.

After the stage of spinal shock passes, reflex activity of the spinal cord returns. Smooth muscle first regains function of activity. Rectal and urinary sphincter control is returned though the detrusor muscle may remain paralyzed. Skeletal muscle tone returns, but power does not. Deep tendon reflexes appear and may become exaggerated. Reflex defecation and urination become possible.

Case 2. A 66 year old white male was admitted to Northwestern Memorial Hospital because of an asymptomatic abdominal aortic aneurysm found on routine physical examination. Preoperative evaluation exclusive of the aneurysm, including laboratory data, was entirely normal.

An 8 cm abdominal aortic aneurysm was resected and a 20 mm bifurcation graft anastomosed end-to-end to the abdominal aorta below the renal arteries and end-to-end to the iliac arteries above their bifurcation. Total aortic clamping time was 1 hour. After the aneurysm was opened, a large midsacral artery was identified and oversewn within the aneurysm. At no time did hypotension occur during the procedure.

In the postoperative period, the patient complained of weakness of both lower extremities. Neurological examination revealed weakness of hip flexion and leg extension on the left, similar but not as profound weakness on the right. Deep tendon reflexes were increased at the knee and ankle bilaterally.

Rapid resolution of the process occurred during the next 5 days. As this occurred, a modified Brown-Sequard pattern was seen. There were decreased deep tendon reflexes on the left and decreased position sense with a contralateral decrease in pain sensation with weakness.

Total neurological recovery occurred in the 14 day period following graft placement. The patient remains well postoperatively. At no time was fecal incontinence noted, nor was urinary retention a significant problem in this patient.

Comment. This patient demonstrates a reversible lumbar spinal cord ischemia occurring after aneurysm surgery. The lack of vesicorectal disturbance suggests sparing of the conus medullaris and sacral fibers from the ischemic process. Similarly, the increased knee and ankle reflexes suggest upper motor neuron involvement, rather than the monosynaptic conus medullaris reflexes which would be demonstrated by hyporeflexia.

Case 3. A 74 year old white male presented to the emergency room of the Northwestern Memorial Hospital with sudden onset of severe lumbosacral and right lower quadrant pain of 6 hours duration. The patient had a history of previous myocardial infarction and congestive heart failure, hypertension, chronic bronchitis, and mild renal failure. Medications included digoxin and diuretics.

Physical examination revealed the patient to be normotensive and in mild distress. A 7 cm diameter tender abdominal aortic aneurysm was present, and the pedal pulses were absent bilaterally.

After evaluation, the patient underwent an urgent abdominal aortic aneurysmectomy. At the time of operation, an active infrarenal aortic aneurysm was discovered. There were edema and bullae of the aneurysmal wall, but a retroperitoneal hematoma was not present. A right common iliac artery aneurysm was also found. An aortobifemoral Dacron graft was inserted using end-to-end anastomoses at aorta and right femoral artery. The iliac artery orifices were oversewn, as was the proximal right femoral artery to exclude the right iliac artery aneurysm from the circulation.

During the operation and on the first postoperative day, the patient was normotensive with adequate urine output. The urine output rapidly diminished on the second postoperative day and did not respond to mannitol or escalating doses of furosemide. The patient remained responsive and had complete sensation and motor function of the lower extremities. Despite fluid restriction, the patient began to manifest clinical signs of biventricular heart failure. The electrocardiogram was diagnostic of acute myocardial infarction.

As the patient developed cardiogenic shock and resultant hypotension, lack of pain and temperature sensation and motor function of the lower extremities became evident. The rectal sphincter was patulous and the anal reflex was absent, as were proprioception and vibratory sensation. Despite cardiotonic drugs, the patient became increasingly unresponsive and died late on the second postoperative day. Permission was not granted for postmortem examination.

Comment. This patient demonstrates the phenomenon of neurological damage occurring after apparently successful and uneventful aneurysm repair. With the onset of hypotension from cardiogenic shock in the postoperative period, the ensuing neurological insult occurred. Most likely, spinal canal collateral blood supply from lumbar and hypogastric arteries was excluded from the circulation at operation. With hypotension, the remaining nutrient vessels in the upper lumbar and lower thoracic aorta either occluded or were unable to supply adequate blood flow to maintain viability of the lower spinal cord.

MANAGEMENT

Management of this devastating complication is largely supportive. Medications to reduce edema such as corticosteroids and mannitol are of little value. In the presence of bladder and bowel disturbance, great care must be exercised to avoid infection. Urogenic septicemia in postoperative patients with prosthetic graft insertion might be devastating. Both foot care and vigorous physical therapy are necessary to avoid pressure sores. The patient should remain in optimum condition, ready for recovery. In addition to physical therapy, counseling with the patient and family is necessary to ease the mental trauma. Because the sequelae are so unexpected, in some instances psychiatric care may become a necessity.

DISCUSSION

Three known mechanisms, hypotension and thrombosis, atheromatous emboli, or anomalies of the cord blood supply, may cause spinal cord ischemia. The last probably plays the most important role in the etiology of spinal cord ischemia.

The blood supply to the spinal cord is profuse but it is apparent that, with inadequate collateral circulation, disruption of the continuity of one radicular artery may have dire consequences. In abdominal aortic surgery, the artery of Adamkiewicz (or arteria radicularis magna) is of critical importance. This is jeopardized most frequently by aortic clamping between the diaphragm and renal arteries, but occasionally the artery may arise just below the renal arteries. The level of spinal ischemia will correspond to the level of this great radicular artery, which will usually lie between T-11 and L-1 [41]. The frequency at which there is an anomalously low position is unknown. Judging from the infrequency of spinal cord damage after infrarenal aortic clamping, it must be quite rare. Clinical experience shows that the chance of damaging the spinal cord on an anatomical basis alone is remote in abdominal aortic surgery.

The duration of time that the aorta can be clamped above the renal arteries but below the diaphragm without producing spinal cord damage is unknown. Usually, it is possible to interrupt aortic flow at this level for 20-25 min without renal damage. However, paraplegia has been reported following occlusion of the suprarenal aorta for as little as 10 min [43].

The individual pattern of blood distribution through the great radicular arteries will determine the chance for cord or conus damage. The greater frequency of spinal cord ischemia following surgery for ruptured aneurysms in which the clamp may be placed higher than usual (above the renal arteries, i.e., L-1 or T-12) is evidence for this. Other factors can be important. For example, atherosclerotic narrowing of the ostia of radicular arteries is common. Jellinger [24], in studying over 1000 autopsy cases, showed that spinal cord arteriosclerosis was a significant factor in medullary circulation disorders, although only about 5%-10% of cases of spinal cord infarction were caused by localized atheromas. The occurrence of atheromatous emboli, obstructing the collateral pathways or the spinal artery, may be another cause of spinal cord damage. This has been observed in other arteries, and Reich [34] reported an instance in which emboli were responsible for spinal cord damage.

Apart from anomalous blood supply and embolization, systemic hypotension has been proposed as a cause of spinal cord ischemia. This partly explains why cord ischemia is seen in patients after resection of a ruptured aortic aneurysm. The addition of encroachment by atherosclerotic plaque of the ostia of the vessels supplying the cord may further aggravate ischemia during the period of hypotension. Such impingement upon arterial supply is accentuated by unequal growth of the spinal column and the cord, which causes a greater than 90° angle of segmental arteries to the aorta. Jellinger [24] pointed out that the origins of vessels supplying the anterior spinal artery have an abrupt right angle takeoff from the aorta, and that partial stenosis or occlusion of the orifice has a profound effect upon lowering blood pressure in the arteria radicularis magna. Unequal growth has also been cited by Hilal [22, 27] to cause anterior spinal artery tributaries to form a hairpin curve from the major feeding vessels, thus

rendering these arteries susceptible to occlusion (Fig. 3). Lastly, arterial shunting of blood away from the main radicular tributaries could cause profound circulatory deficit in the distal spinal cord.

The neurological findings in our experience are of interest. In the anterior spinal artery syndrome, one would expect infarction of the anterior two-thirds of the cord (the area supplied by the anterior spinal artery) with preservation of the posterior one-third of the cord because of its better collateral blood supply. Neurological deficits should correspond to classical signs of anterior spinal artery syndrome (paraplegia, rectal and urinary incontinence, loss of pain and temperature sensation, but with sparing of vibration and proprioception sense). However, this was seldom seen in our five patients, nor was it encountered in published cases (Tables 1 and 3). Instead, there was a spectrum of neurological manifestations suggesting dysfunction occurring at various areas and levels of the cord. Patients sustaining neurological deficits in the lower extremities after

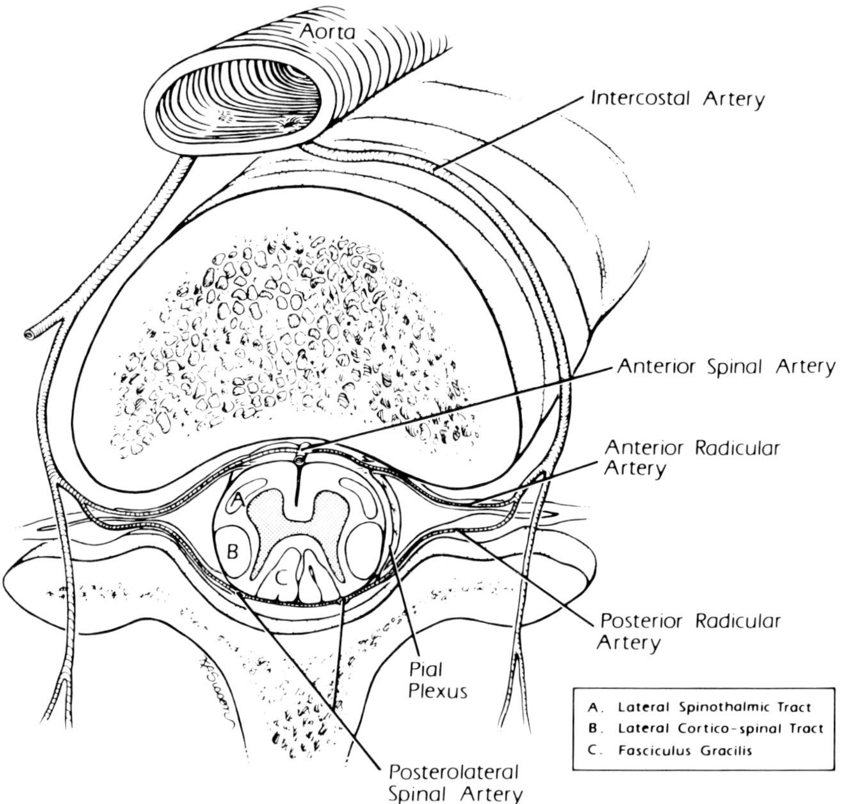

Fig. 3. Cross-sectional anatomy of the spinal cord depicting the major nerve tracts and blood supply.

abdominal aortic surgery commonly have loss of posterior column modalities. This is true because the low and midthoracic regions of the cord differ from proximal segments in that the posterior spinal artery receives a major contribution from the anterior spinal artery. Therefore the loss of proprioception in four of our five cases is completely compatible with anterior spinal artery occlusion. Alternatively, it has been suggested that position and vibration sensation are carried in dorsal spinocerebellar tracts that would be supplied by the anterior spinal artery [35]. With vesicorectal disturbance, only the conus medullaris and sacral fibers are damaged without more proximal cord damage.

Because of the magnitude of spinal cord ischemia, it might be thought that the neurological damage would be permanent. This is not the case, and complete recovery can be expected in one-half the patients. Of the 18 patients on whom information is available regarding recovery of neurological function, only 6 (33%) did not demonstrate any return. Of the remaining 12 patients (67%), 9 (50%) regained complete neurological function and 3 (17%) had partial return of neurological function. The recovery time varied from 14 days [14] to 12 months [33].

Unfortunately, there is not a single preoperative diagnostic technique available to predict the possibility of cord ischemia following abdominal aortic surgery. Study of blood flow of the spinal cord by isotopic technique is experimental and has yet to become applicable in clinical practice. The use of arteriography to visualize arteries supplying the cord is seldom practiced because the toxicity of the contrast medium itself may cause cord damage. Some investigators have suggested that arteriography may help to locate an anomalously low vessel to allow attempts to preserve it during aneurysmectomy [5, 7]. Such a maneuver seems to be impractical. With increasing use of arteriography in patients with abdominal aortic aneurysm, however, a consistent arteriographic pattern may emerge allowing a better knowledge of this tragic complication. At present, prevention of spinal cord ischemia lies in observing the basic vascular surgical principles of gentle dissection of the aorta, avoidance of hypotension and suprarenal aortic clamping, and adequate heparinization. Lastly, treatment is supportive together with physical and rehabilitation therapy.

REFERENCES

1. Adamkiewicz A: Die Blutge fasse des menschlichen Ruckenmankes. I. Thiel die Gefasse der Ruckenmarkssubstanz. Sitzunpb. Akad. Wirrensch. Math. Naturw. 84:469, 1882
2. Adamkiewicz A: Die Blutge fasse des menschlichen Ruckenmankes. II. Thiel die Defasse der Ruckenmarksoflache. Sitzunpb. Akad. Wirrensch. Math. Naturw. 84:101, 1882
3. Adams HD, van Geertruyden HH: Neurological complications of aortic surgery. Ann. Surg. 144:574, 1956

4. Bates T: Paraplegia following resection of abdominal aortic aneurysm. Br. J. Surg. 58:913, 1971
5. Connolly JE: In discussion of Szilagyi DE, et al. [42]
6. Coupland GAE, Reeve TS: Paraplegia: A complication of excision of abdominal aortic aneurysm. Surgery 64:878, 1968
7. Crawford ES, Fenstermacher JM, Richardson W, et al: Reappraisal of adjuncts to avoid ischemia in treatment of thoracic aneurysm. Surgery 67:182, 1970
8. Crawford ES: Thoraco-abdominal aortic aneurysms involving renal, superior mesenteric and celiac arteries. Ann. Surg. 179:763, 1974
9. DeBakey ME, Cooley DA, Crawford ES, et al: Analysis of 179 patients treated by resection. J. Thorac. Cardiovasc. Surg. 36:393, 1958
10. DeBakey ME, Crawford ES, Cooley DA, et al: Aneurysms of the abdominal aorta: Analysis of graft replacement. Ann. Surg. 160:622, 1964
11. Doppman JL, DiChina G, Morton DL: Arteriographic identification of spinal cord blood supply prior to aortic surgery. JAMA 204:174, 1968
12. Edmondson HT, Giridin RA: Paraplegia as a complication of abdominal aortic resection. Ann. Surg. 36:383, 1970
13. Fazio C, Agnoli A: The vascularization of the spinal cord – Anatomical and pathophysiological aspects. Vasc. Surg. 46:245, 1970
14. Ferguson LRJ, Bergan JJ, Conn J Jr, et al: Spinal ischemia following abdominal aortic surgery. Ann. Surg. 181:267, 1975
15. Gensler SW, Hoffer P: Paraparesis following resection of abdominal aortic aneurysm. N. Y. State J. Med. 71:2093, 1971
16. Gillihan LA: The arterial blood supply to the human spinal cord. J. Comp. Neurol. 110:75, 1958
17. Golden GT, Sears HF, Wellens HA Jr, et al: Paraplegia complicating resection of aneurysms of infrarenal abdominal aorta. Surgery 73:91, 1973
18. Golden GT, Wellens HA, Muller WH: Letter: Paraplegia after surgery for abdominal aortic aneurysms. JAMA 233:768, 1975
19. Grace RR, Mattox KL: Anterior spinal artery syndrome following abdominal aortic aneurysmectomy. Arch. Surg. 112:813, 1977
20. Gump FE: Paraplegia after resection of aneurysm. N. Engl. J. Med. 281:798, 1969
21. Hara M, Lipin RJ: Spinal cord injury following resection of abdominal aortic aneurysm. Arch. Surg. 80:419, 1960
22. Hilal SK, Keim HA: Selective spinal angiography on adolescent scoliosis. Radiology 102:319, 1972
23. Hogan EL, Romanal FCA: Spinal cord infarction occurring during insertion of aortic graft. Neurology 16:67, 1966
24. Jellinger K: Spinal cord arteriosclerosis and progressive vascular myelopathy. J. Neurol. Neurosurg. Psychiatr. 30:195, 1967
25. Jorning PG, Brands LC: Transient paraplegia after resection of an aneurysm of the abdominal aorta. Arch. Chir. Neerl. 26:354, 1974
26. Kadyi H: Uber die Blutgefasse des menschlichen Ruckensmarkes. Anat. Ang. 1:304, 1886
27. Keim HA, Hilal SK: Spinal angiography in scoliosis patients. J. Bone Joint Surg. 53A:904, 1971

28. Lake PA: Paraplegia after resection of aneurysm. N. Engl. J. Med. 281:798, 1969
29. Lentin M, Salis JS: Paraplegia as a complication of infrarenal aneurysmorrhaphy. Vasc. Surg. 6:224, 1972
30. McCune WS: Discussion in Adams HD, et al. [3]
31. Mehrez IO, Nabseth DC, Hogan EL, et al: Paraplegia following resection of abdominal aortic aneurysm. Ann. Surg. 156:890, 1962
32. Michales L: Case report: Spinal cord ischemia associated with repair of a ruptured abdominal aortic aneurysm. Stroke 3:238, 1972
33. Pasternak BM, Boyd DP, Ellis FH: Spinal cord injury after procedures on the aorta. Surg. Gynecol. Obstet. 135:29, 1972
34. Reich MP: Paraplegia following resection of an abdominal aortic aneurysm. Vasc. Surg. 2:230, 1968
35. Ross ED, Kirkpatrick JB, Lartimosa ACB: Position and vibration sensations: Functions of the dorsal spine cerebellar tracts. Ann. Neurol. 5:171, 1979
36. Scorza R, Berardinelli L, Odero A: Sur un caso di paraplegia succesivo a clampaggio dell'aorta sottorenale. Minerva Cardioangiol. 23:692, 1975
37. Sher MH, Healy EH: Paraplegia following infrarenal aneurysmorrhaphy. Vasc. Surg. 5:171, 1971
38. Skillman JJ, Zervas NT, Weintraub RM, et al: Paraplegia after resection of aneurysms of the abdominal aorta. N. Engl. J. Med. 281:422, 1969
39. Smith RA: Neurological complications of extraspinal arterial origin. Am. Surgeon 42:679, 1976
40. Stennis N [Stensen N]: Elementorum myologie specimen: Sur Musculi descriptio Geometrica. Ferdinandum II. Magnum Amstellodami Apud. Johan. Janssonium a Wrerberg und Viduam Elizei Weyerstraet, 1669 (cited by Adams HD, et al. [3])
41. Suh TH, Alexander L: Vascular system of the human spinal cord. Arch. Neurol. Psychiatr. 41:659, 1939
42. Szilagyi DE, Hageman JH, Smith RF, et al: Spinal cord damage in surgery of the abdominal aorta. Surgery 83:38, 1978
43. Zuber WF, Gaspar MR, Rothschild PO: The anterior spinal artery syndrome – A complication of abdominal aortic surgery. Ann. Surg. 172:909, 1970

Allan R. Downs, M.D., F.R.C.S.(C), F.A.C.S.

Management of Aortofemoral Graft Limb Occlusion

Aortoiliac and aortofemoral prosthetic bypass grafting have an established place in the management of aortoiliac occlusive and aneurysmal disease. The technique of operation has become fairly standardized, although there remain some individual variations. Most surgeons now perform aortobilateral femoral grafting for aortoiliac occlusive disease except in very localized disease or in very poor risk patients, when endarterectomy or extraanatomical bypass may be used. The long term results for aortofemoral grafting are well documented and vary from 60% to 90% patency [7, 8]. Critical patient selection, hemodynamic assessment, and complete preoperative angiography all contribute to better surgical management. The importance of the deep femoral artery in providing an adequate outflow has been properly emphasized. In spite of all of these improvements, graft occlusion continues to occur with a recurrence of symptoms. Graft limb obstruction is more common in patients with occlusive disease than in aneurysmal disease, but nevertheless occurs in both [5]. Not all occluded grafts require reoperation, since it depends on the symptomatology produced. The management of the occluded graft presents a challenge to the ingenuity of the surgeon.

This chapter describes our experience in reoperation for aortic graft limb occlusion.

CLINICAL MATERIAL

Seventeen patients had been subjected to 22 operations for reconstruction of graft limb occlusions. In two patients each limb of the graft occluded at different times, and in two patients reocclusion occurred requiring second and fourth operations. Hence there were 22 reconstructive procedures in 17 patients for 19 graft limb occlusions and 3 reocclusions. Four patients had rest pain

---

Supported in part by a research grant from Manitoba Medical Services Foundation.

before the primary operation, and 12 had rest pain following graft limb occlusion.

There were 13 males and 4 females, with an average age of 62 years. All patients were smokers, and 3 had late onset diabetes mellitus. Nine of the seventeen patients were hypertensive and six had documented coronary artery disease. Only two patients had cerebrovascular disease. Eleven patients had bilateral superficial femoral artery occlusions and four had unilateral superficial femoral occlusions on the side of the graft thrombosis. One patient had a popliteal artery obstruction on the side of the graft thrombosis. Only one patient did not have an outflow lesion, and he had originally been treated for a ruptured abdominal aortic aneurysm.

Original Operative Procedure

All patients had initially been treated for aortoiliac occlusive disease with the exception of one patient who had presented with a ruptured abdominal aortic aneurysm. Two patients had aneurysmal disease associated with their occlusive disease. Four of the seventeen patients had their first operation in another institution. All grafts extended from the infrarenal aorta to both femoral arteries, with the exception of one graft limb which was anastomosed to the external iliac artery. The original grafts in 15 patients were standard weight knitted Dacron, either 16 × 8 mm or 19 × 9.5 mm in diameter. There were one woven Dacron and one lightweight Dacron graft used. The interval between the original operation and the second operation varied from 2 to 120 months, with an average of 40.8 months. The interval between the time of graft occlusion as judged by the onset of symptoms varied from less than a week to 2 years, with an average of 14.9 weeks.

Causes of Graft Limb Occlusion

Femoral outflow occlusions were identified in all but three patients at the time of operation for graft limb thrombosis (Table 1). This was usually the result of progression of deep femoral artery disease in the presence of chronic superficial femoral artery occlusion (Figs. 1A and 1B). This was most commonly due

Table 1
Cause of Graft Limb Occlusion

OUTFLOW OCCLUSION	19
FALSE ANEURYSM	1
GRAFT PLEATING	1
TECHNICAL	1
TOTAL	22

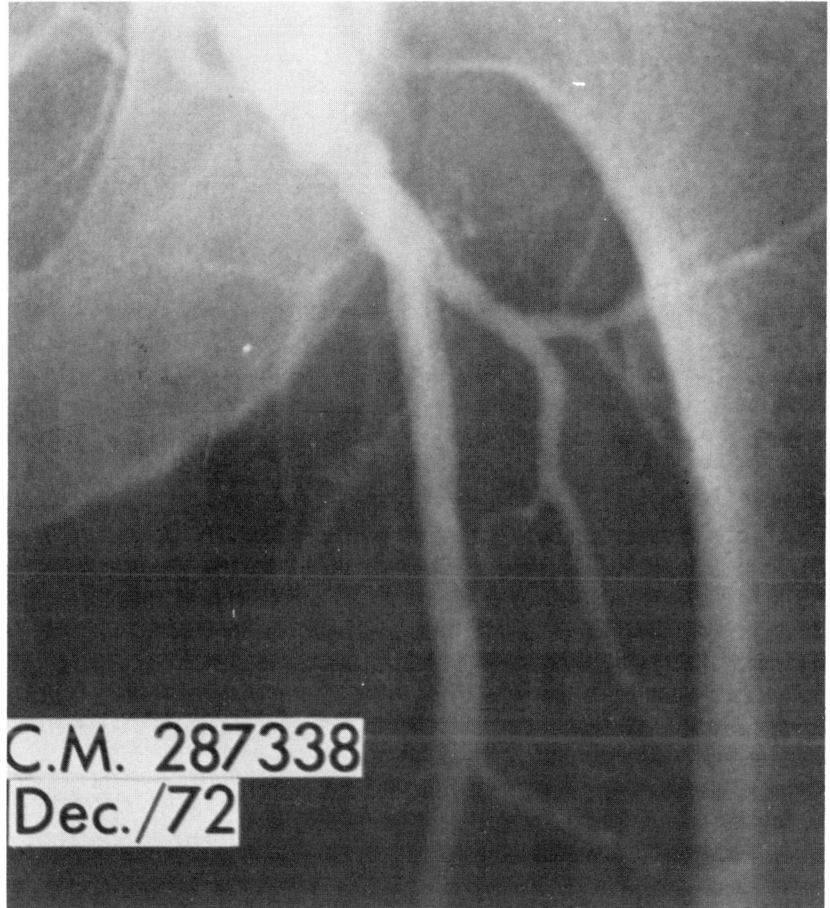

Fig. 1A. Deep femoral artery widely patent in 1972.

to stenosis at the orifice of the profunda artery and less commonly was due to extensive profunda disease. One occlusion was due to pleating in a woven Dacron graft. One occlusion was due to a false aneurysm (Fig. 2), and the third was probably technical due to graft rotation. The importance of identifying the cause of the graft limb thrombosis cannot be overemphasized, since the success of repair is dependent upon recognizing and correcting the causes of the occlusion.

Preoperative Assessment

Angiography is essential to identify the site of the occlusion and the outflow tract. Changes in the patent limb can also be assessed. Failure to visualize the deep femoral artery does not, however, exclude the possibility of reconstruction to this site. Since superficial femoral occlusion is nearly always present, it is

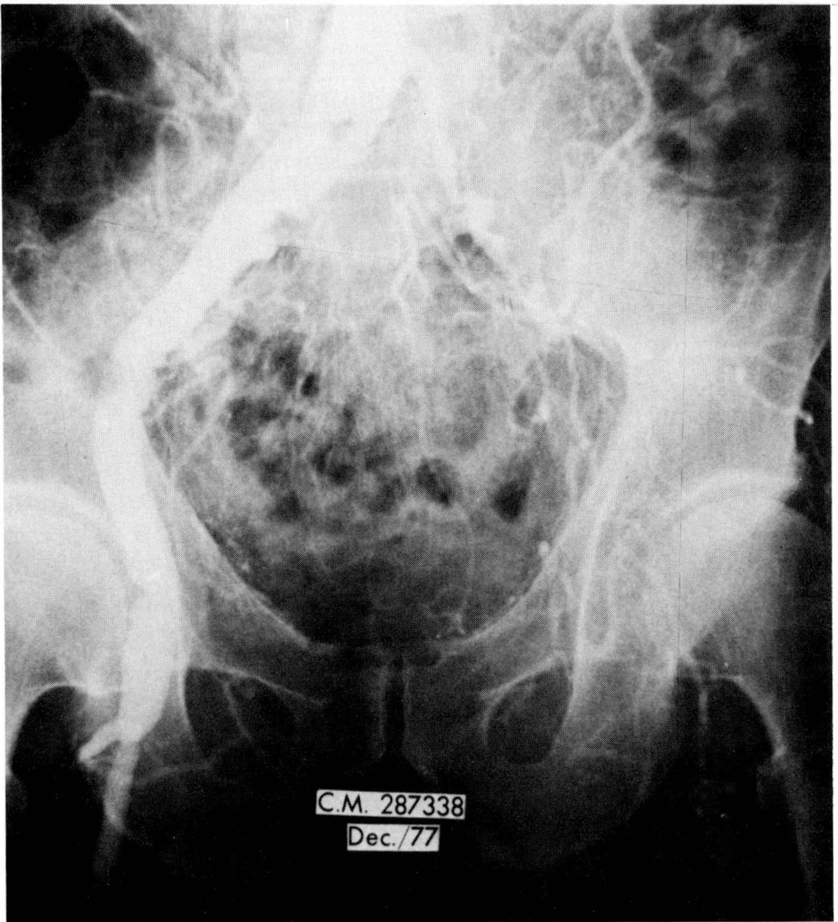

Fig. 1B. Occluded 1977 due to progression of disease.

essential to obtain popliteal visualization should distal reconstruction be necessary. All of our patients had preoperative translumbar aortography.

Operative Technique

The patient is prepared and draped for a standard transabdominal aortofemoral reconstruction. If there is doubt about the deep femoral artery outflow, the limb is draped free in readiness for a distal bypass.

Thrombectomy

The groin is explored through the previous incision. The prosthesis, common femoral, superficial, and deep femoral arteries are exposed and mobilized. Systemic heparinization is used in all patients. When the outflow disease is limited to the orifice of the deep femoral artery, a vertical arteriotomy is made

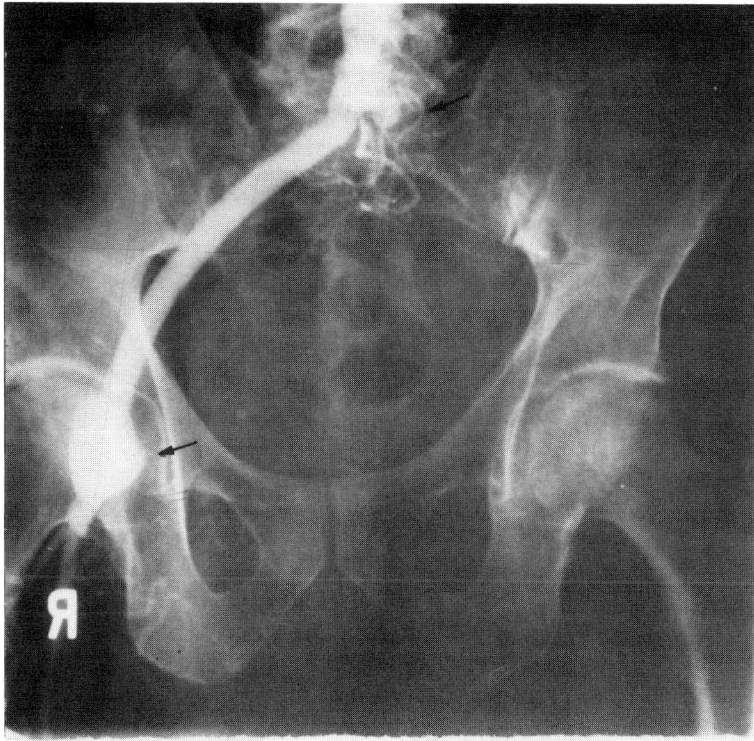

Fig. 2. Graft limb occlusion due to thrombosed false aneurysm. Reproduced by permission from Downs AR: Reoperation following failure of aortoiliofemoral arterial reconstruction. Can. J. Surg. 21:316, 1978.

across the orifice extending on to the common femoral artery. A local endarterectomy may then be necessary. A Fogarty catheter is then passed proximally into the prosthesis and a thrombectomy is performed as described by Bernhard et al. [1]. The arteriotomy is then closed with a patch graft of endarterectomized superficial femoral artery or saphenous vein (Fig. 3). When the outflow occlusion is at the anastomosis to the common femoral artery due to recurrent local atheroma, detachment of the graft, retrograde thrombectomy, and extension of the graft more distally on the common femoral artery will suffice (Fig. 4). In the presence of a false aneurysm with outflow occlusion, the deep femoral artery is divided at its origin and an extension graft placed from the thrombectomized limb to the deep femoral artery by end-to-end anastomosis (Fig. 5).

Cross Femoral Graft

On eight occasions in seven patients it was not possible to accomplish a thrombectomy through the limb of the prosthesis. On one occasion embolization to the open limb occurred. For that reason the patent limb from the

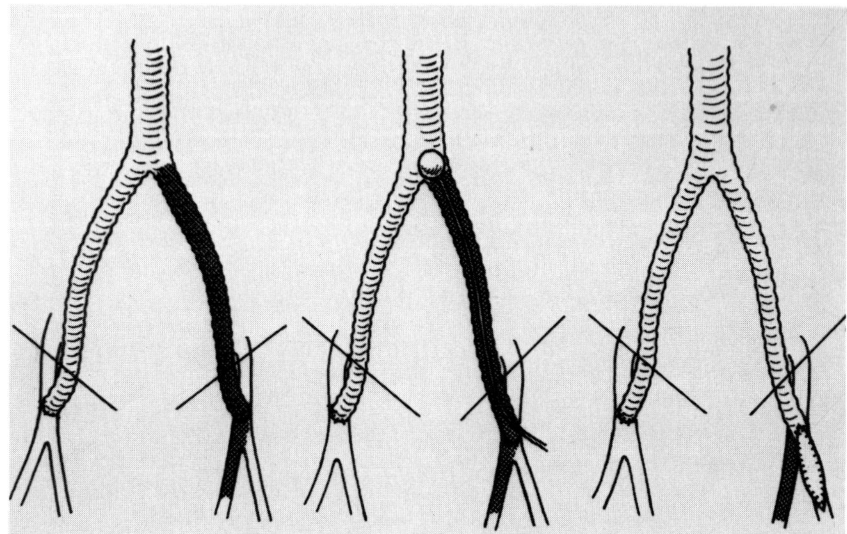

Fig. 3. Thrombectomy and patch profundaplasty.

opposite side was used for the inflow. Again it is essential to first establish an adequate deep femoral outflow. The donor limb graft is exposed by a vertical groin exposure and the graft is mobilized within its capsule proximal to the previous anastomosis. The prosthesis is clamped proximally and distally. An incision is made in the prosthesis and any free fragments of fibrin are removed. An 8 mm knitted Dacron or 6 mm Gortex graft is then anastomosed to this opening. Flow is reestablished to the open limb and the graft is tunneled

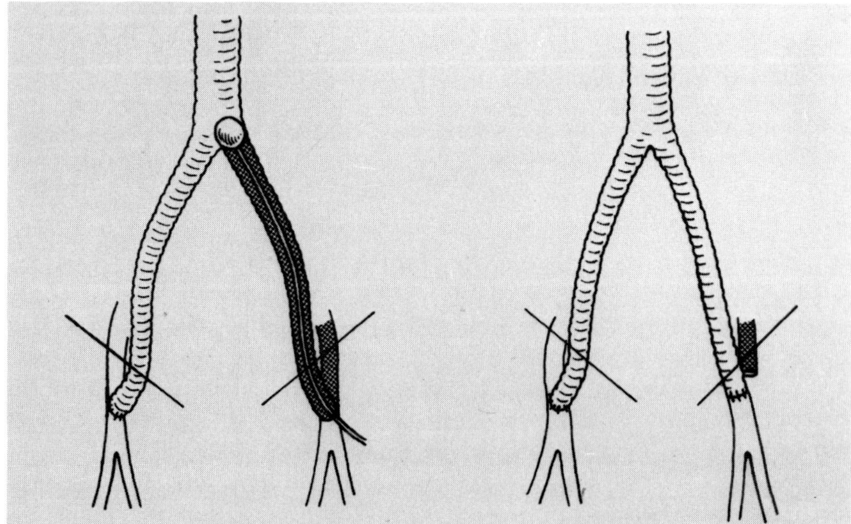

Fig. 4. Thrombectomy and reanastomosis to common femoral artery.

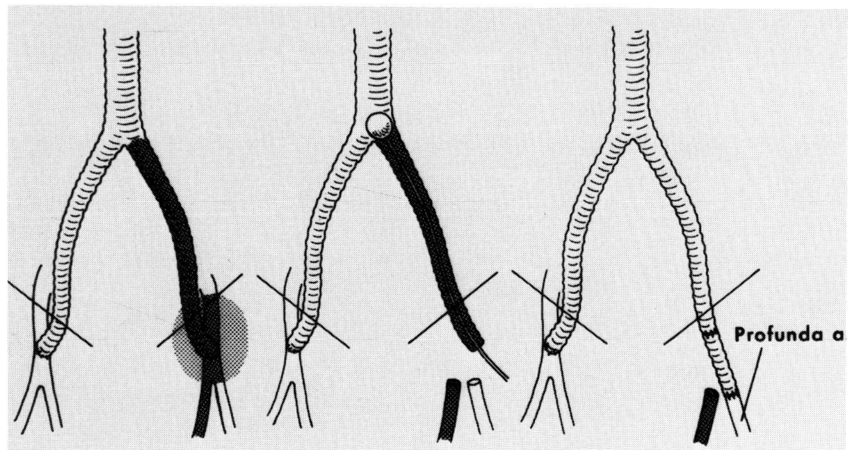

Fig. 5. Thrombectomy and extension graft in presence of false aneurysm.

subcutaneously to the opposite groin. Usually the anastomosis is performed to the divided end of the deep femoral artery (Fig. 6). If appropriate, the distal anastomosis may be made to the side of the deep femoral artery beyond the proximal disease. An excellent alternative to the groin exposure of the donor limb of the prosthesis is through an inguinal incision above and parallel to the inguinal ligament. The limb of the prosthesis is easily identified and the anastomosis is performed in a similar fashion. The prosthesis is then brought through the medial end of the incision and then subcutaneously to the opposite groin (Fig. 7). When there is extensive deep femoral artery disease a patch graft

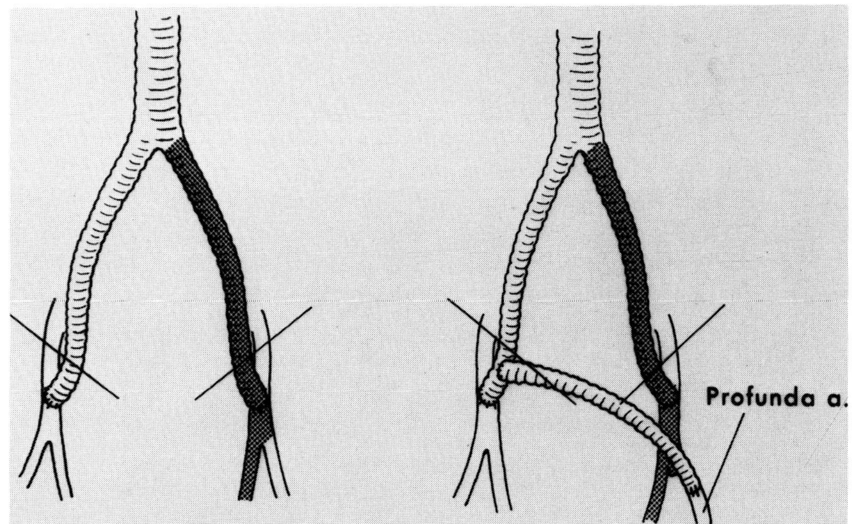

Fig. 6. Cross femoral graft to the orifice of the deep femoral artery. Reproduced by permission from Downs AR: Reoperation following failure of aortoiliofemoral arterial reconstruction. Can. J. Surg. 21:316, 1978.

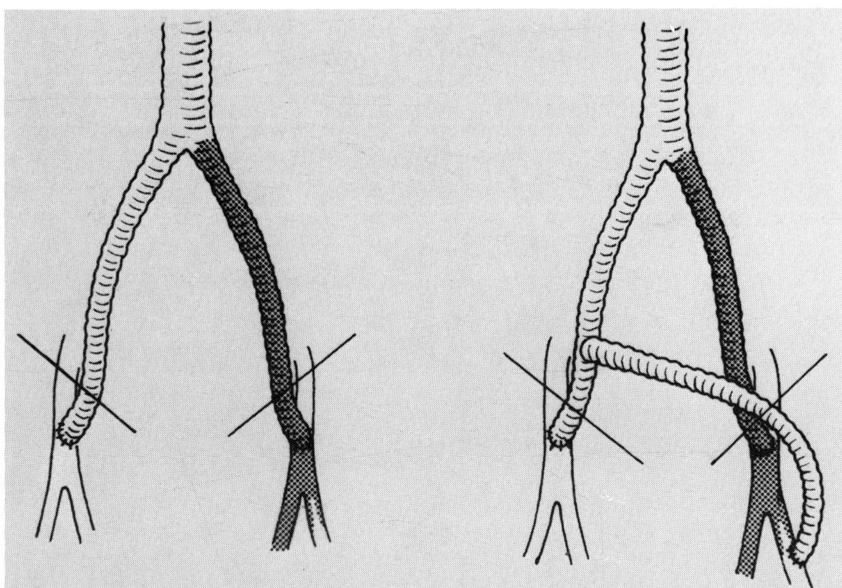

Fig. 7. Cross ilioprofunda showing the prosthesis arising proximal to the inguinal ligament from the patent limb.

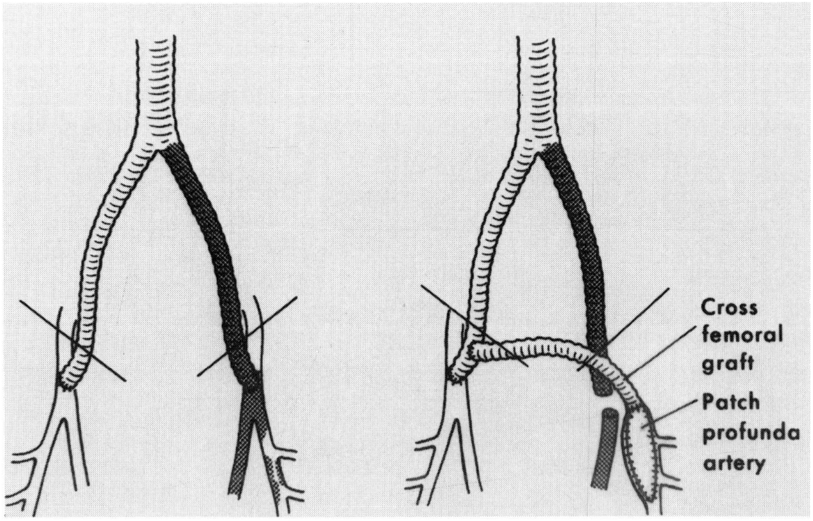

Fig. 8. Cross femoral prosthesis with an extended profundaplasty using either a saphenous vein patch or endarterectomized superficial femoral artery.

profundaplasty is necessary as described by Malone et al. [6] using autogenous tissue, either the endarterectomized superficial femoral artery or the saphenous vein (Fig. 8).

Alternative Procedures

On occasion a satisfactory femoral outflow cannot be established and it will then be necessary to take the graft to the popliteal artery. In each instance the donor limb has been exposed proximal to the inguinal ligament; the graft is tunneled subcutaneously to thc oppositc groin and then deep to the fascia of the sartorius muscle to the popliteal fossa either proximal to or distal to the knee joint (Fig. 9).

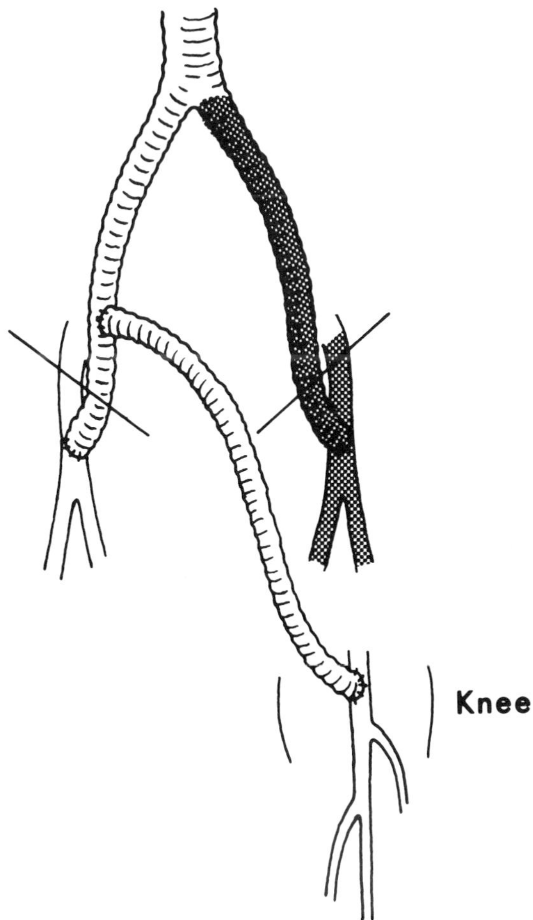

Fig. 9. Cross iliopopliteal graft.

On one occasion early in our experience, graft limb replacement was used as described by Najafi et al. [9] (Fig. 10). This was performed through a transabdominal approach. We no longer use this method of repair except when the whole graft is occluded. It may, however, be desirable to obtain proximal graft control when there is thrombus at the bifurcation of the graft extending into the open limb (Fig. 11). In this patient direct control and thrombectomy were accomplished with reanastomosis of the graft to the common femoral artery. This was the only instance in which there was no outflow obstruction and the occlusion appeared to be due to graft pleating as described by Szilagyi et al. [10]. Intraoperative angiography at the completion of the operation is essential to ensure a good inflow and a good outflow (Fig. 12).

RESULTS

Twenty-two operations were performed for 19 graft limb occlusions in 17 patients (Table 2). There were no operative deaths, and there have been no late deaths. All patients have been followed to within 6 months of the completion of the study. The followup varies from 1 to 96 months, for an average of 28.4 months. Seven patients have been followed for 12 months or less. There have been three early postoperative occlusions and four late occlusions. One patient has been successfully reoperated upon for late occlusion of a cross femoral graft. There remain 15 patent reconstructions in the 19 limb occlusions for a patency rate of 78.9%. Due to reocclusion, four above-knee amputations have been required in three patients.

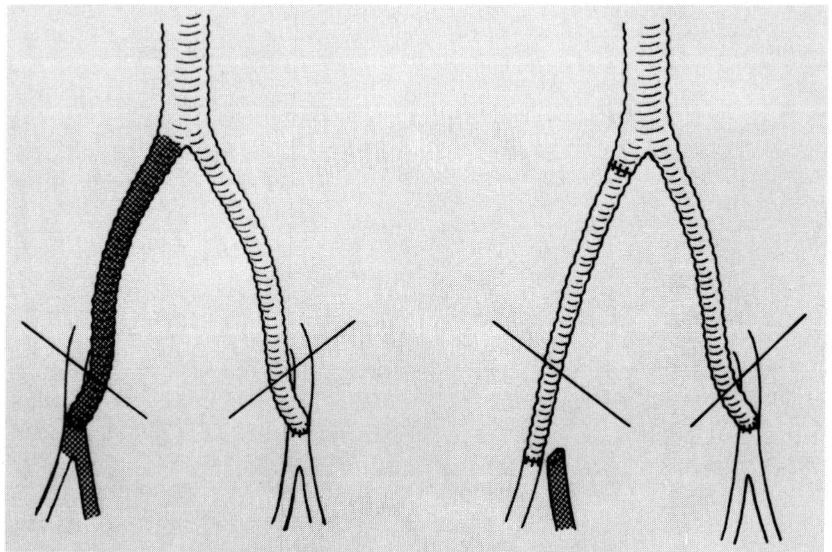

Fig. 10. Graft limb replacement.

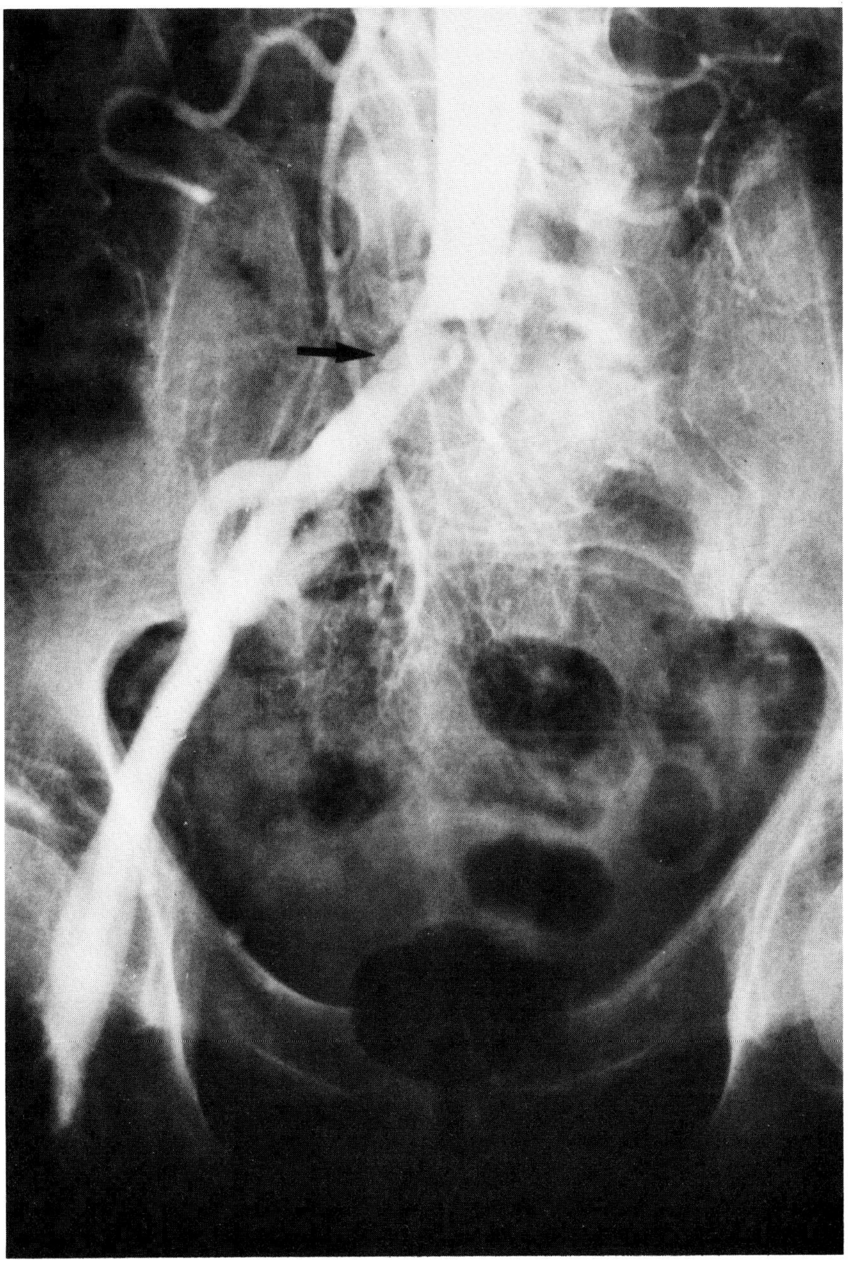

Fig. 11. Thrombosed graft limb showing thrombus extending into patent limb of graft. Reproduced by permission from Downs AR: Reoperation following failure of aortoiliofemoral arterial reconstruction. Can. J. Surg. 21:316, 1978.

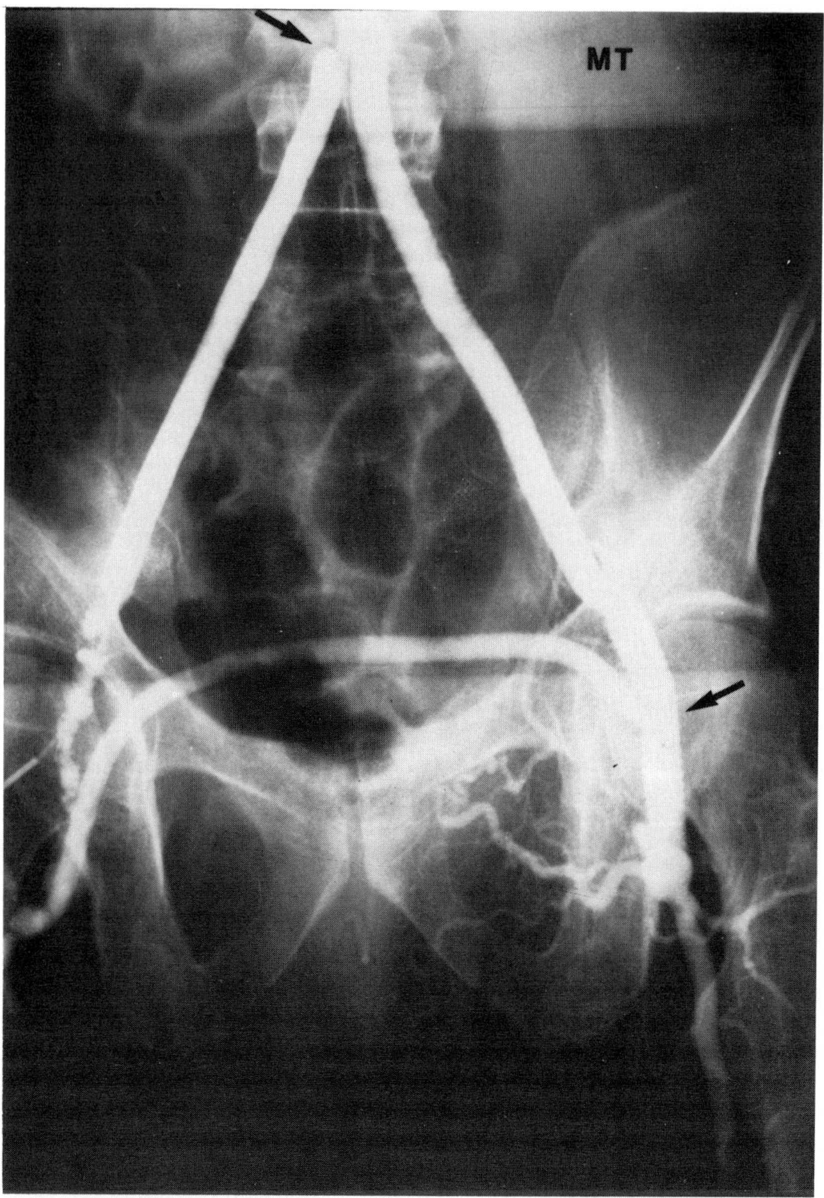

Fig. 12. Intraoperative angiogram shows residual thrombus at the bifurcation necessitating a cross femoral graft.

Table 2
Results

PROCEDURE	EARLY PATENCY	LATE PATENCY	OCCLUDED EARLY	OCCLUDED LATE	REOPERATED	TOTALS
Cross Femoral-Profunda	8	7	1	2	1	9
Cross Ilio-Profunda	1	1				1
Cross Ilio-Popliteal	5	2		3	3	5
Graft Replacement	2	2				2
Direct Thrombectomy	1	1				1
Retrograde Thrombectomy	0	0	1			1
Retrograde Thrombectomy & Profundaplasty	1	1	1			2
Retrograde Thrombectomy & Extension Graft	1	1				1
TOTALS	19	15	3	5	4	22

DISCUSSION

It is fundamental to recognize that graft thrombosis is best prevented or at least delayed by establishing a good femoral outflow at the first operation. Adequate angiographic assessment of the origin of the deep femoral artery prior to the initial reconstructive procedure is essential. Surgical techniques to accomplish the maximum femoral outflow have been previously described [4]. When the femoral outflow is inadequate, a femoropopliteal bypass should be combined with the proximal reconstruction. When symptoms recur following aortofemoral or aortoiliac bypass, early angiography may detect an outflow stenosis that can readily be corrected before graft limb occlusion occurs (Fig. 13). Although profundaplasty as described by Bernhard et al. [1] and Malone et al. [6] is recognized as an integral part of a successful reoperation for graft limb thrombosis, thrombectomy as advocated by these authors has not been universally accepted. It should be noted that in Bernhard's series [1] only 60% were treated by thrombectomy of the graft limb, and in Malone's series [6] 50% of the graft limbs had rethrombosed at 11 months. Other authors have used alternative procedures such as total graft replacement, reported by E. Crawford et al. [2], and graft limb replacement, reported by Najafi et al. [9]. It is apparent from our experience that no single procedure will be applicable to all patients. We have found the cross femoral graft as reported by F. Crawford et al. [3] to be very simple to perform, and it has not been associated with any morbidity affecting the donor limb. At the present time we suggest the cross femoral (Fig. 14) or cross iliac graft to be the procedure of choice in unilateral graft limb occlusion unless the thrombus is very recent and nonadherent to the inner wall of the graft.

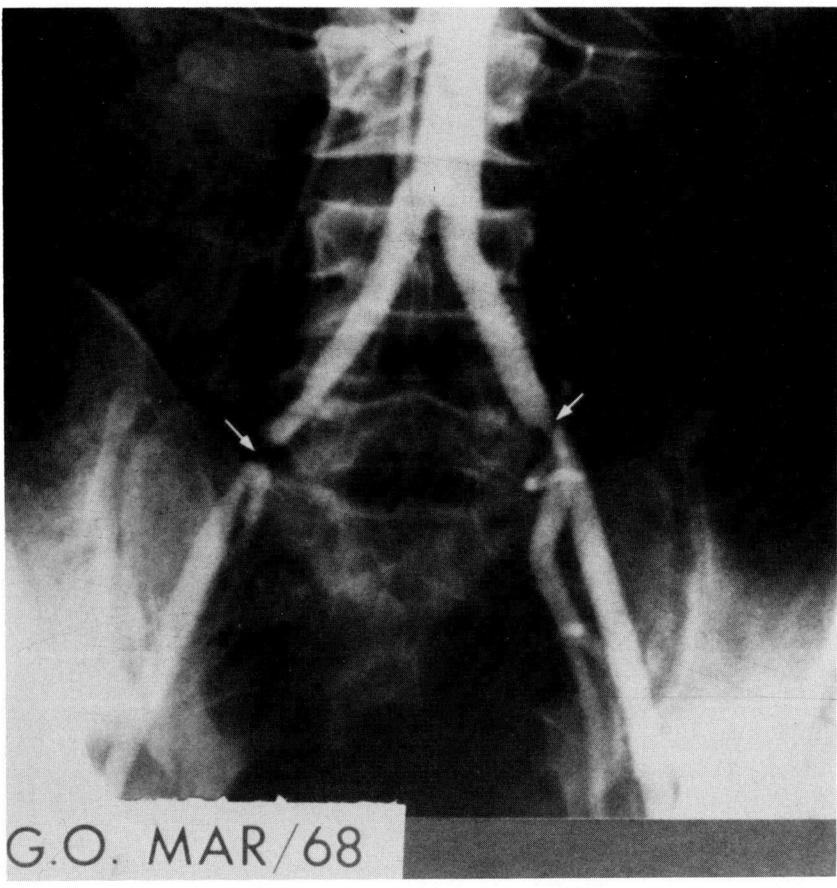

Fig. 13. Anastomotic stenosis in iliac arteries treated by graft extensions to femoral arteries. Reproduced by permission from Downs AR: Reoperation following failure of aortoiliofemoral arterial reconstruction. Can. J. Surg. 21:316, 1978.

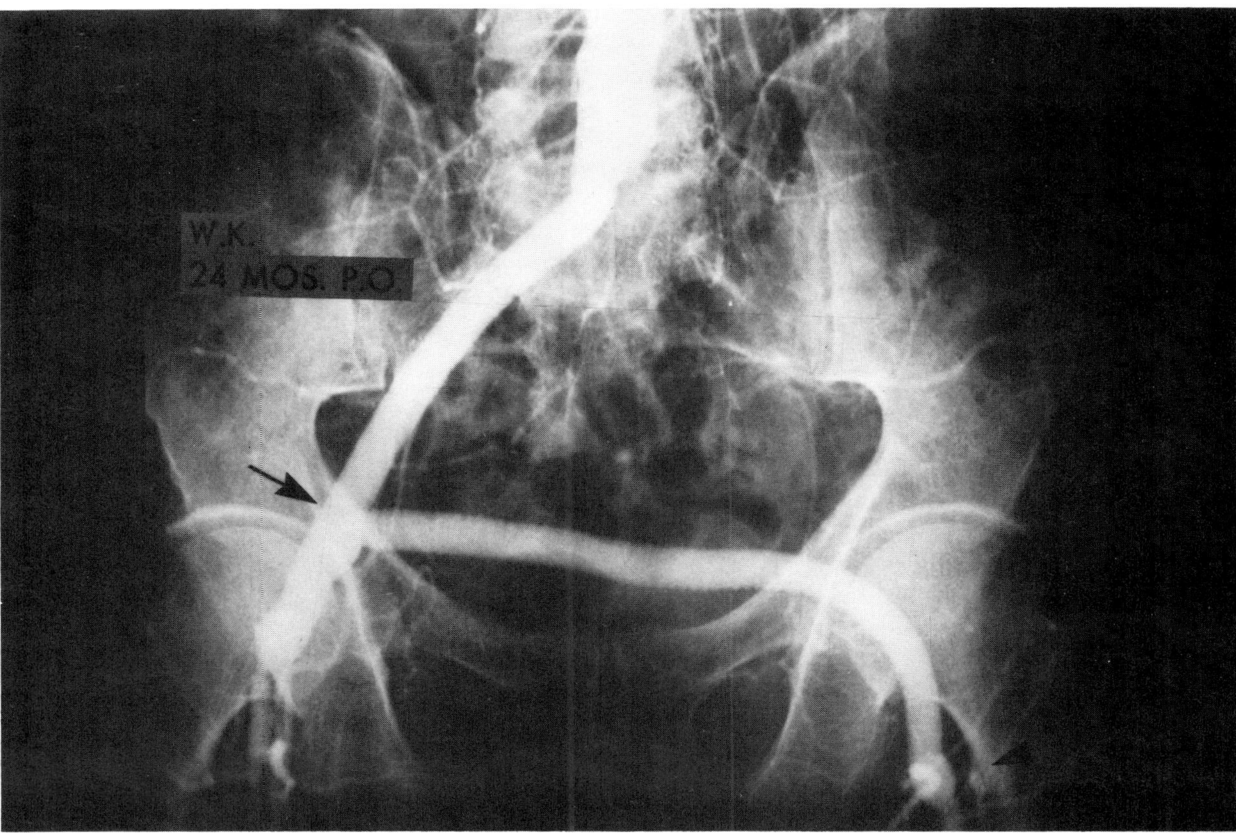

Fig. 14. Cross femoral to profunda graft using 8 mm Dacron.

REFERENCES

1. Bernhard MM, Ray LI, Towne JB: The reoperation of choice for aorto-femoral graft occlusion. Surgery 82:867-874, 1977
2. Crawford ES, Manning LG, Kelly TF: "Redo" surgery after operations for aneurysm and occlusion of abdominal aorta. Surgery 81:41-52, 1977
3. Crawford FA, Sethi GK, Scott SM, et al: Femoro-femoral grafts for unilateral occlusion of aortic bifurcation grafts. Surgery 77:150-153, 1975
4. Downs AR, Lye CR: Aorto-femoral prosthetic bypass grafting for aorto-iliac occlusive disease, in Bergan JJ, Yao JST (eds): Gangrene and Severe Ischemia of the Lower Extremities. New York, Grune & Stratton, 1978, pp 171-188
5. Knudson JA, Downs AR: Reoperation following failure of aorto-ilio-femoral arterial reconstruction. Can. J. Surg. 21:316-319, 1978
6. Malone JM, Goldstone J, Moore WS: Autogenous profundaplasty – The key to long-term patency in secondary repair of aorto-femoral graft occlusion. Ann. Surg. 188:817-823, 1978
7. Malone JM, Moore WS, Goldstone J: The natural history of bilateral aorto-femoral bypass grafts for ischemia of the lower extremity. Arch. Surg. 110:1300-1306, 1975
8. Mozersky DJ, Sumner DS, Strandness DE: Long-term results of reconstructive aorto-iliac surgery. Am. J. Surg. 123:503-509, 1972
9. Najafi H, Dye WS, Javid H, et al: Late thrombosis affecting one limb of aortic bifurcation graft. Arch. Surg. 110:409-412, 1975
10. Szilagyi DE, Elliott JP, Smith RP, et al: Secondary arterial repair – The management of late failures in reconstructive arterial surgery. Arch. Surg. 110:485-493, 1975

Richard H. Dean, M.D.
H. William Scott, Jr., M.D.

Subisthmic Aortic Coarctations

The term subisthmic aortic coarctation encompasses a wide variety of lesions that affect the descending thoracic and abdominal aorta. Since the term coarctation connotes a congenital origin, many of these lesions would best be called aortic constrictions, as they are acquired abnormalities. Few descriptions in the literature, however, make any effort for such a segregation of nomenclature. Even when each of the anatomic, etiologic, and functional subdivisions of subisthmic aortic coarctations are combined, they remain medical rarities and, cumulatively, only account for 2% of all aortic coarctations [50]. The remainder, 98%, are located at the aortic isthmus in juxtaposition to the ductus arteriosus or ligamentum arteriosum.

To date, less than 150 patients with subisthmic aortic coarctations have been described. Due to the infrequent occurrence, few centers have a large experience with their management, and cumulative reviews of the literature are necessary to define the spectrum of their clinical presentations. Review of the literature suggests that subisthmic aortic coarctations are either increasing in frequency or being identified more often during the past 15 years. Although the former explanation cannot be discounted, certainly the reduction in the risk of angiography during childhood has led to its more liberal use and subsequent, more frequent definition of anomalies of the cardiovascular system during this period.

HISTORICAL BACKGROUND

The first description of a subisthmic aortic coarctation is credited to Schlessinger [40]. His report in 1835 described a 15 year old female who died in congestive heart failure. The patient had a 2 year history of severe shortness of breath and grand mal seizures. At autopsy, he found the descending thoracic aorta to be almost completely obliterated 2 inches above the diaphragm. The aorta at that level was hypoplastic and appeared as a thin cordlike structure through which he could only pass a thin metal sound. The descending thoracic aorta above the coarctation had aneurysmal changes. The infradiaphragmatic aorta appeared normal.

The first case report of a subisthmic coarctation involving the abdominal aorta was described by Quain in 1847 [36]. His patient, a 50 year old male who died suddenly, had a 1 year history of epigastric pain on exertion. At autopsy, a coarctation of the aorta ½ inch in length, was found just below the level of the renal arteries. Although this is the first report of an abdominal aortic coarctation, Duncan [14], in 1843, suggested that knowledge of the entity existed. In describing a case of probable atherosclerotic obliteration of the infrarenal aorta he wrote, "Many cases are now on record in which the aorta has been found obliterated, some of them at the same point as in this specimen, some with gangrene, others not. Many of these have evidently been congenital." No references for such cases were given, however.

Power [35] described the second case of infrarenal aortic coarctation in 1861. The patient was a 17 year old male who had a prior history suggesting acute rheumatic fever with episodes of fever followed by epileptiform attacks. The child died following a seizure. At autopsy, aortic valvular stenosis and cardiomegaly were found. In addition, the internal mammary and epigastric arteries were enlarged and tortuous. Just below the origin of the inferior mesenteric artery the aorta became narrowed. This hypoplasia extended inferiorly to involve the iliac arteries also. Although Power felt the lesion was due to a developmental arrest, he did not discuss its etiology further.

Hasler's report [22], in 1911, of the autopsy findings in a 49 year old male who died of lobar pneumonia are of interest, for his case appears to be the first example of coarctations appearing at multiple sites. Postmortem examination in this patient revealed that the aorta was mildly narrowed just below the left subclavian artery, measuring 3.5 cm in circumference. Below that point it widened again to 4.5 cm. Three centimeters above the diaphragm it abruptly became obliterated for 7 cm and was represented only by a fibrous cord which measured 7 mm in diameter. Although he felt the lesion was from an acquired origin, he found no histologic evidence of scar tissue or inflammatory reaction.

Following these descriptions of subisthmic aortic coarctations, other sporadic reports of similar autopsied patients occurred over the next several decades [2, 20, 39]. Concomitant with the development of safe contrast arteriography, however, the number of reported cases increased dramatically. In a review of the literature in 1956, Inmon and Pollock [26] could only uncover 14 recorded cases. By 1959, Senning and Johansson [45] collected 29 cases of abdominal aortic coarctations and added 3 additional cases from their own center. They included both congenital lesions as well as lesions related to neurofibromatosis and other acquired diseases, however. Nevertheless, by 1972, Ben-Shoshan and his associates [4] reviewed 110 reported cases of congenital coarctations of the abdominal aorta alone, having excluded several cases caused by a variety of other diseases.

Although the historical background of the operative management of subisthmic aortic coarctations includes several early reports of the use of nephrectomy and sympathectomy [7, 13, 17, 26], its operative correction only spans the past 30 years. Six years following the independent reports of the correction of isthmic coarctation by Crafoord and Nylin [10] and Gross and Hufnagel [19], Beattie and his associates [3] described the first successful correction of an abdominal aortic coarctation in 1951. Their patient had a coarctation beginning at the level of the diaphragm and ending above the renal arteries. Correction was performed by creating an aortoaortic bypass around the coarctation using a homologous vessel graft. Less than 1 year later, Glenn et al. [17], in 1952, described the successful treatment of a similar lesion situated just below the celiac artery by swinging down the distal end of the splenic artery and thereby creating a bypass around the coarcted segment. Albanese and Barla [1] also attempted a graft replacement of a subisthmic aortic coarctation in 1952, but their patient died of renal failure in the early postoperative period. Patch angiography of the narrowed segment was performed first by Hanson and his associates [21] in 1959. Through refinement in operative techniques and greater use of angiography, increasing numbers of patients have undergone successful correction since these early reports. By 1966, DeBakey and his associates [12] reported a personal series of 16 patients treated by a variety of synthetic bypass grafts. To date, descriptions of over 85 patients who have had operative correction of subisthmic aortic coarctations have been reported.

ETIOLOGY

Lower thoracic and abdominal aortic coarctations may arise from a wide variety of causes. Early reports suggested that such coarctations were variations of a single entity but gave conflicting views of etiologic considerations responsible for their development. Currently, it is clear that quite a variety of acquired as well as congenital lesions are presented in the literature under the diagnosis of subisthmic or abdominal aortic coarctation.

Division of coarctations into congenital and acquired constrictions is useful for discussion of etiology. Certainly even congenital lesions may be secondary to maternal viral infections or drug ingestion and thereby also be considered acquired. Nevertheless, congenital lesions are depicted as those coarctations that lack any evidence of inflammatory infiltration or other evidence of injury such as irradiation or trauma. Grossly, congenital lesions lack an adventitial inflammatory reaction and appear as hypoplastic narrowings of the vessel. In contrast, acquired lesions are defined as conditions that effect a previously normal vessel with resulting constriction. Grossly, such lesions usually have evidence of a perivascular inflammatory response with neovascularity and/or fibrous proliferation in the periadventitial plane.

Congenital Coarctations

Several hypotheses explaining the development of congenital subisthmic coarctations have been suggested over the past 45 years. Maycock [30] proposed two possible causes of abdominal aortic coarctations. He felt that faulty or unequal fusion of the two omphalomesenteric arteries, dorsal aortae, might lead to the obliteration or loss of one of them with a resulting coarctate segment. Although he favored the first possibility, he alternatively suggested that abdominal coarctations might be due to a "kinking of the fused aortas with consequent localized increased longitudinal tension producing a permanent narrowing."

Costa [9] suggested a unified hypothesis to explain coarctations at all levels. According to his theory, implants of the embryonic aortic arches might produce the lesions. In this scheme, remnants of the fifth arch would cause infantile or preductal coarctations, remnants of embryonic tissue from the sixth aortic arch would produce adult or postductal isthmic coarctations, and remnants of tissue from the right aortic arch would result in coarctations at or below the first intercostal artery.

From the authors' experience, two basic causes of congenital subisthmic coarctations can be identified – (1) developmental arrest of the vessel and (2) anomalous maturation of the mesenchymal cell component. Developmental arrest can occur at any time during the maturation of the aorta and its branches. When the arrest occurs early in embryonic life, the involved segment becomes atretic and appears as a fibrous cord. The length and site of the atretic segment may vary widely. Figure 1 is the arteriogram and diagramatic representation of the isolated suprarenal abdominal coarctation in a 2 year old white male. The short, 2 cm long atretic segment in this child is in contrast to the lesion represented in Fig. 2. This latter example in a 2 month old white male shows diffuse atresia beginning just below the right renal artery with involvement of the entire left renal artery, the remaining aorta, and the proximal iliac arteries. In contrast to these examples of developmental arrest occurring early in embryonic life, development may stop later, after differentiation is complete. When arrest of aortic wall growth occurs late in embryonic life, arteriographic assessment will show no evidence of aortic coarctation during early childhood. As the adjacent uninvolved aorta expands with subsequent growth, however, the coarctate zone will be easily visualized. This is demonstrated in Figs. 3 and 4. Figure 3 is the arteriogram of a 2 month old infant with severe renovascular hypertension secondary to a left renal artery stenosis. At that age the abdominal aorta and right renal artery appeared normal. In contrast, an arteriogram performed 10 years later for evaluation of recurrent hypertension (Fig. 4) showed severe right renal artery stenosis and a moderate coarctation of the lower descending thoracic and abdominal aorta to the level of the inferior mesenteric artery. This patient not only demonstrates the occasional late appearance of abdominal aortic coarctation following subsequent growth of the normal adjacent aorta, but also underscores the importance of renal preservation in

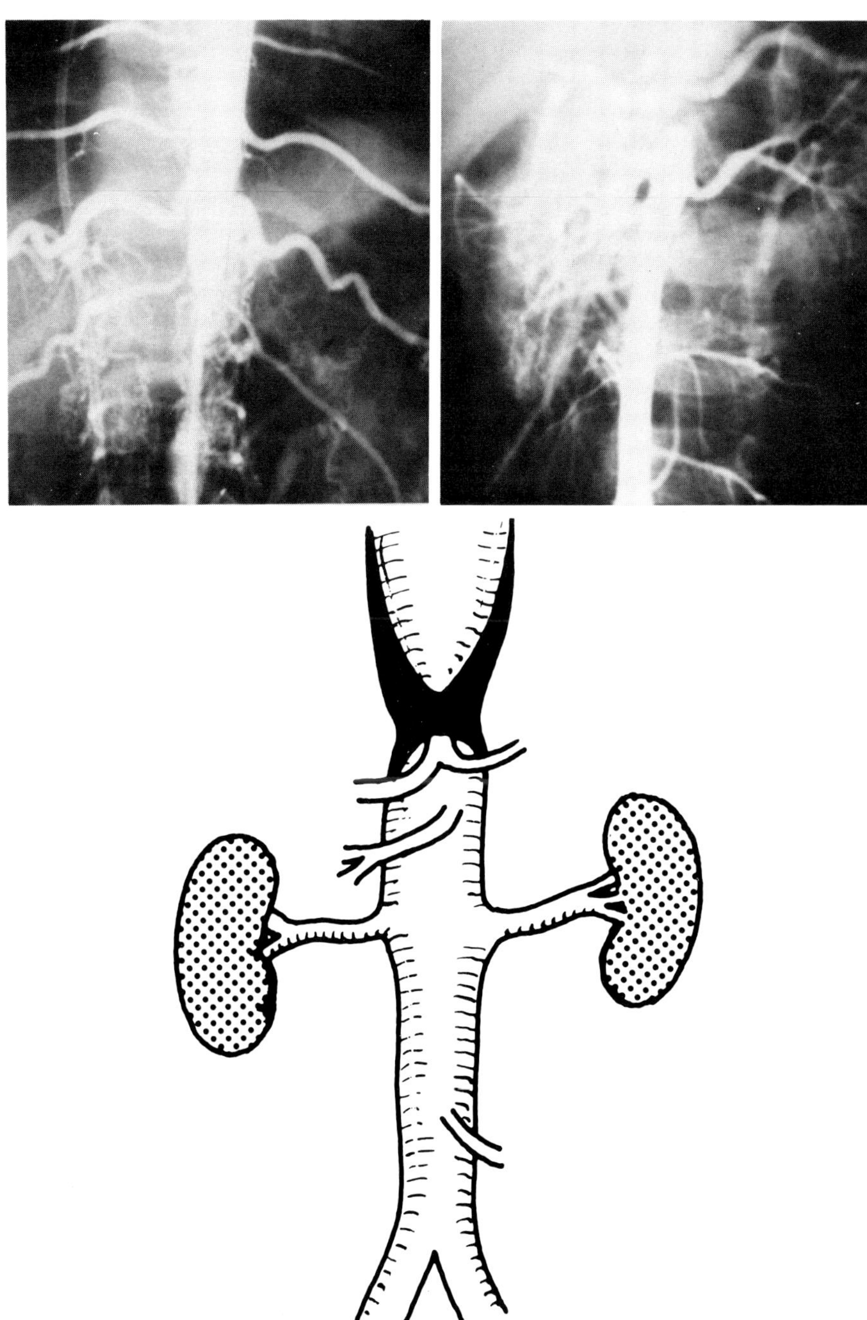

Fig. 1. Arteriogram in a 2 year old white male with severe hypertension demonstrating an isolated segmental aortic coarctation located just above the celiac axis.

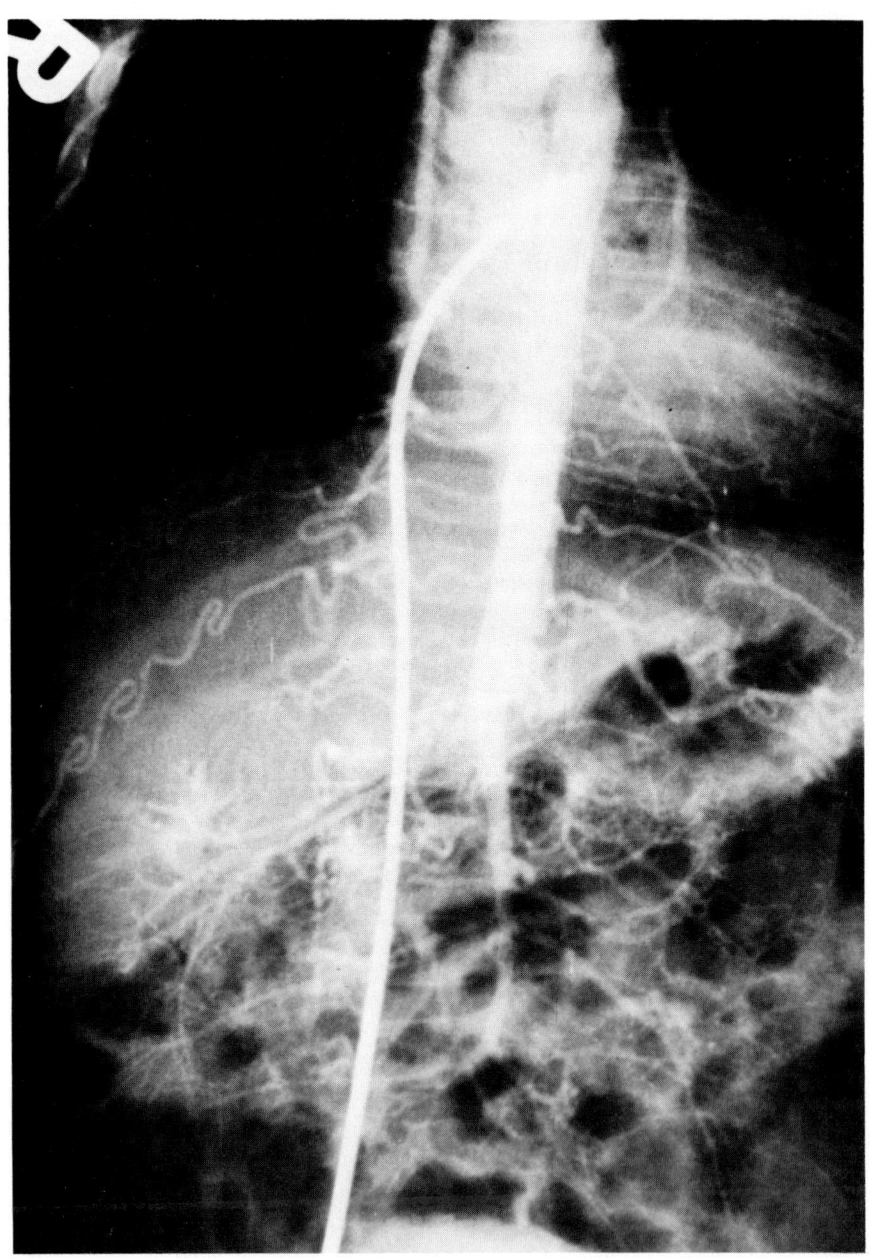

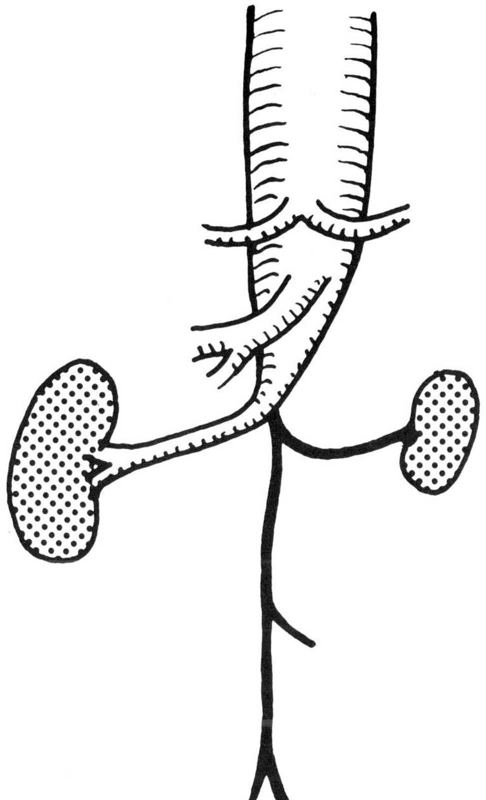

Fig. 2A (left) and B. Arteriogram in a 2 month old white male with severe hypertension showing diffuse atresia of the aorta beginning above the left but below the right renal artery. The drawing shows the extent of the atresia as identified at the time of left nephrectomy for control of hypertension.

treating renovascular hypertension during early childhood. Since subsequent contralateral renal artery involvement is not uncommonly identified, nephrectomy is only justified when revascularization is impossible and hypertension cannot be controlled with drug therapy.

Anomalous mesenchymal cell maturation of the developing aortic wall may also lead to coarctation of the aortic lumen. The macroscopic features of this type of coarctation include the finding of fibrous clefts and ridges obstructing flow through the aortic lumen. Figure 5 is an example of the arteriographic findings showing multiple eccentric ridges reducing flow through the aorta in an 11 year old white male with buttock claudication and hypertension. Microscopic examination of the aortic wall in this patient showed a disorganized media

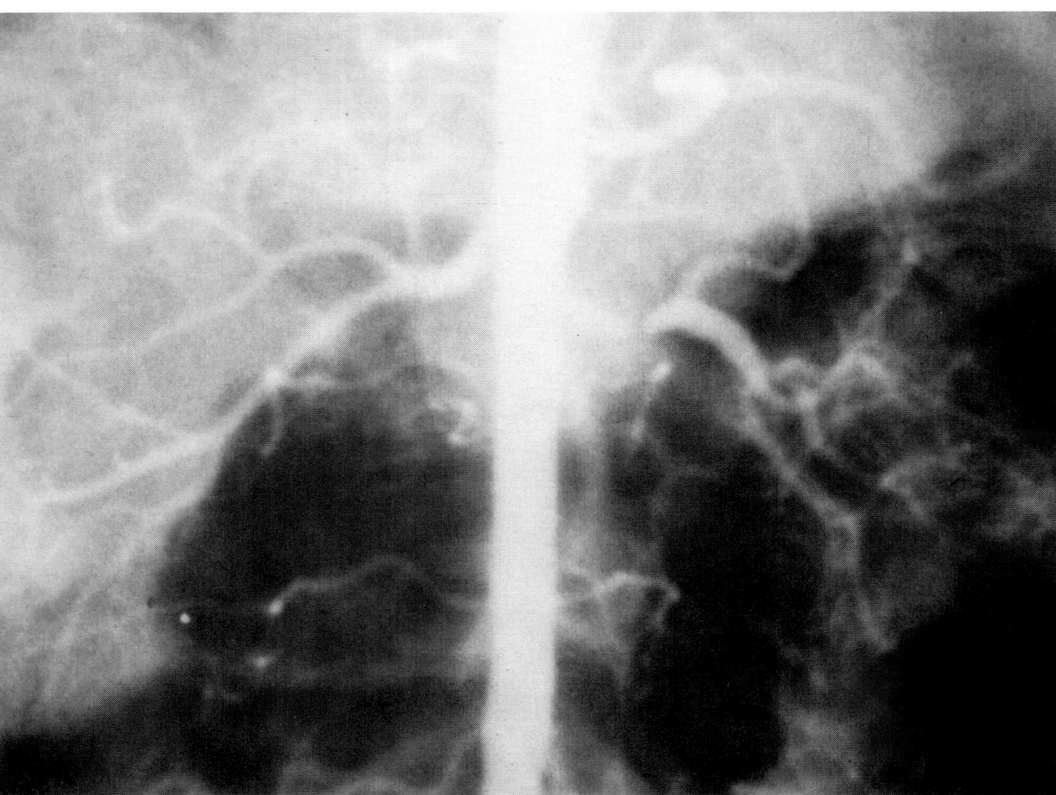

Fig. 3. Abdominal aortogram in a hypertensive 2 month old white male showing a severe left renal stenosis. Note that the abdominal aorta and right renal artery appear to have a normal caliber.

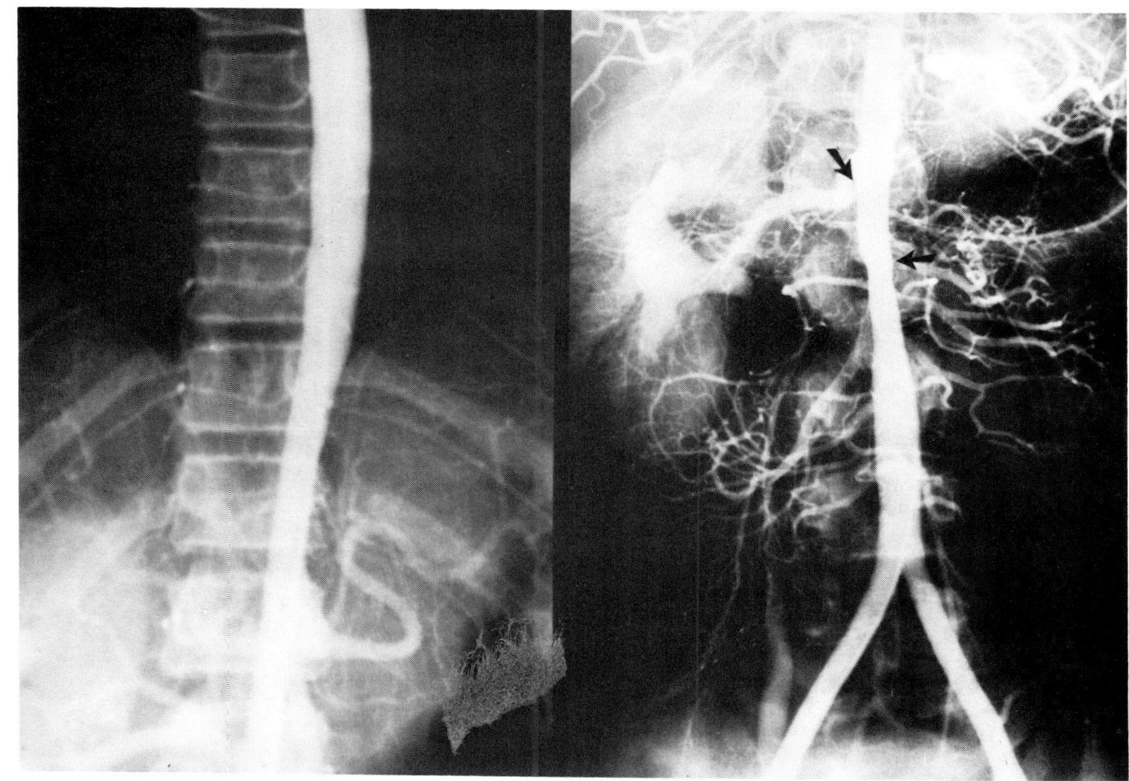

Fig. 4. Repeat thoracic and abdominal aortogram performed 10 years after the study shown in Fig. 3. Note the moderate narrowing of the distal descending thoracic and abdominal aorta and the severe right renal artery stenosis which has become apparent during followup.

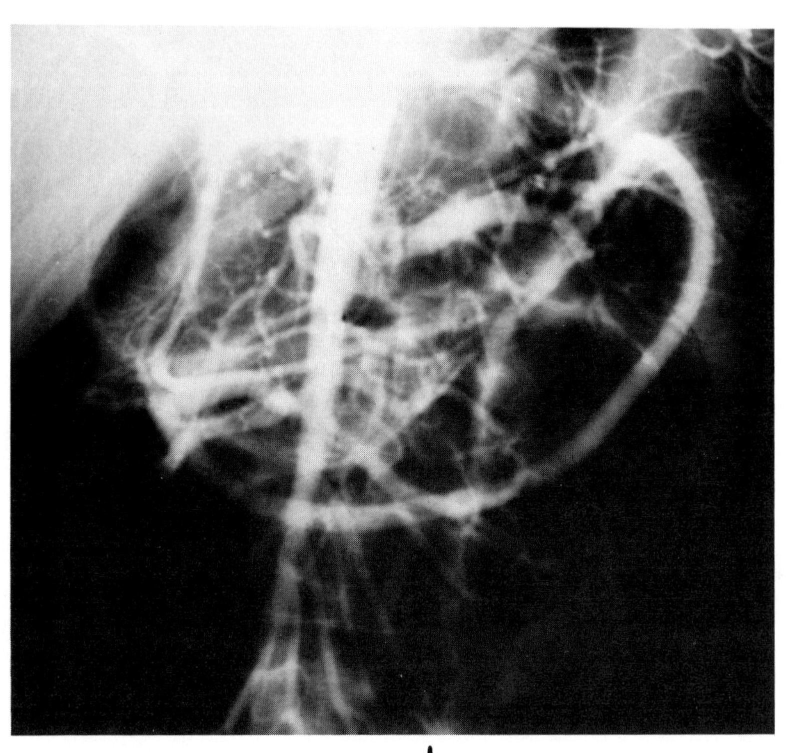

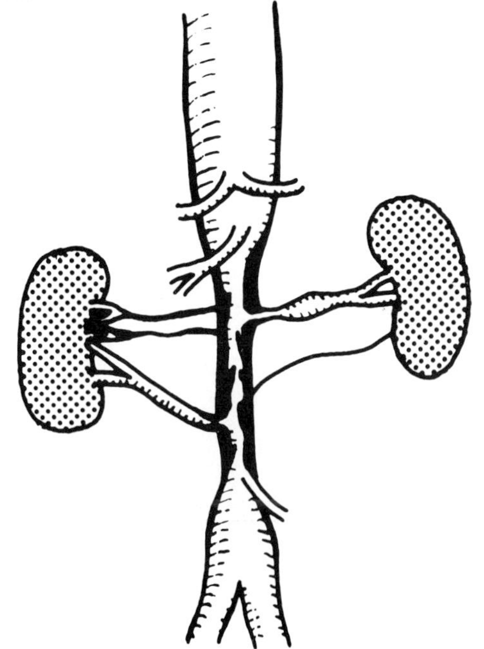

composed of dysplastic mesenchymal cell layers. Histologic study by Pierach [34] and others [23, 29] also confirms the presence of fibrous dysplasia in this variety of coarctation.

Acquired Coarctations

A wide variety of acquired lesions may involve the subisthmic aorta and produce constrictions of the lumen. Although many such lesions have easily identified causes, several forms of nonspecific arteritis also have been incriminated. Hickle [24] related diffuse descending thoracic coarctations to previous involvement by rheumatic fever. Likewise, Millay [30] suggested that rheumatic fever may have been an etiologic factor in his review of subisthmic aortic coarctation. In contrast, Fröig [16] suggested that many coarctations were forms of chronic nonspecific arteritis and believed that they were of an "allergic-hypergic" origin. Similarly, a relationship between stenosing lesions of the midabdominal aorta and Takayasu's disease or stenosing arteritis of the origins of the aortic arch branches has been noted by several authors [25, 41, 49]. Such a concomitant involvement at both sites is particularly prevalent in patients of Japanese descent. Although no acid-fact baccilli were identified, a previous history of tuberculosis led Sen [43] to suspect this as the etiology of subisthmic coarctation in 12 of the 16 patients he reviewed. Senning [45], Glenn [17], and others [6] have reported cases of abdominal aortic coarctation secondary to involvement by neurofibromatosis. Although this is a recognized cause of aortic and/or renal artery stenosis, one must identify the characteristic cafe au lait spots or extravascular involvement by the disease before this etiology can be supported in an individual case.

The multitude of potential causes of aortitis and secondary aortic constriction strongly suggest an autoimmune origin. Although the source of such a process remains obscure in most cases, the secondary coarctation is associated with an intense perivascular inflammatory response. Whereas the preoperative arteriogram may not define a congenital or acquired origin of the coarctation, the operative findings of periadventitial inflammatory and neovascularity strongly support an accquired source.

Fig. 5. Abdominal aortogram in a child, age 9 years, showing severe stenosis of the dominant left upper and right lower renal arteries and severe narrowing of the abdominal aorta. Total occlusion of two right upper and one left lower pole renal arteries is also present. The accompanying drawing shows the extent of aortic narrowing caused by fibrous clefts and ridges obstructing flow through the lumen.

CLASSIFICATION

Numerous methods of classifying congenital subisthmic aortic coarctations have been suggested in the literature [27, 37]. Likewise, acquired lesions are classified by etiology but also described by synonyms such as middle aortic syndrome [44], stenosing aortitis and abdominal aortic presentations of Martorell's syndrome [44], pulseless disease [46], or Takayasu's disease [48]. More appropriately, however, subisthmic aortic coarctations are best classified according to etiology (congenital versus acquired), relationship to the renal arteries (suprarenal, interrenal, or infrarenal) and the extent of involvement (diffuse hypoplasia versus segmental lesions). Using these criteria Ben-Shoshan et al. [4] reviewed the prevalence of each of the anatomic types in 105 congenital subisthmic aortic coarctations. Forty-seven cases were segmental lesions. By further subdividing these collected cases he found that 35% were segmental lesions, 21% had diffuse hypoplasia of the entire abdominal aorta, 15% were hypoplastic suprarenal lesions, 15% were hypoplastic infrarenal lesions, and 13% had a segmental infrarenal site. Similarly, in reviewing 35 patients with hypoplastic arterial anomalies, Nennhaus and his associates [31] found that 40% had involvement of the juxtarenal aorta and renal arteries. Interestingly, 34% had isolated involvement of the renal arteries without aortic involvement. The remaining 26% had either only suprarenal (13%) or infrarenal (13%) aortic involvement.

CLINICAL PRESENTATION

The sex predilection of patients with isthmic aortic coarctations varies in regard to the underlying cause. Although a 3:1 female:male ratio in Japanese with "stenosing midaortic syndrome" was noted in Onat's review [32], he found no sex difference in whites with congenital lesions.

The presenting symptoms and age of diagnosis of subisthmic aortic coarctations is primarily related to the site of the lesion. Whereas infrarenal coarctations usually present during the third or fourth decade with symptoms of lower extremity ischemia, interrenal and suprarenal lesions become manifest during the first or second decade. In contrast to infrarenal lesions, the latter varieties mimic isthmic coarctations as hypertension is the predominant symptom. Hypertension may be particularly severe, difficult to control, and present during infancy when both aortic and renal artery involvement are present. Figure 2 shows the arteriogram in such a patient who presented at 4 months of age with a blood pressure of 210/155 mm Hg having had five grand mal seizures. The admission chest x-ray showed cardiomegaly, and electrocardiography revealed left ventricular hypertrophy.

Occasionally, patients with intrarenal coarctations may present with both severe hypertension and claudication. The 9 year old child whose arteriogram is shown in Fig. 5 had both severe hypertension that required propranolol 160 mg/day, apresoline 100 mg/day, guanethidine 10 mg/day, and aldactazide for control and buttock claudication that occurred after walking 100 yards.

The symptoms of lower extremity ischemia associated with infrarenal aortic coarctations usually consist of thigh and buttock claudication but, at times, may be quite bizzare. Patients may have painful paresthesia at rest which is markedly increased by exercise and is associated with neurologic deficits. Sproul and Pinto [47] have suggested that these findings may result from spinal cord ischemia secondary to abnormal anatomic distribution of the lumbar and segmental neurospinal arteries. These neurologic sequellae are usually reversed following operative correction of the coarctation.

Physical examination is usually similar to the findings associated with isthmic coarctations. Absent or greatly diminished femoral pulses will suggest aortic occlusion. Infrequently, if collateral flow to the legs is extensive, femoral and pedal pulses may be palpable. In such circumstances, the measurement of lower extremity segmental pressures using Doppler ultrasound and comparison to upper extremity pressures will confirm the presence of lower extremity ischemia. Auscultation may help localize the coarctation to the subisthmic area, for the associated systolic-diastolic bruit will be heard best over the lower paravertebral area or epigastrium. Occasionally, an epigastric thrill will be noted.

DIAGNOSTIC EVALUATION

The chest x-ray may have a characteristic appearance in lower thoracic and upper abdominal aortic coarctations. The aortic knob, commonly notched or absent in the classical isthmic coarctation, is normal in the subisthmic variety. Rib notching, when present, is limited to the lower rather than the upper rib cage [32]. When hypertension has been severe the chest x-ray may show cardiac enlargement. Occasionally, cardiac decompensation may be present, producing roentgenographic signs of congestive heart failure with pulmonary edema.

The diagnosis is confirmed by contrast aortography. Selective catheterization and/or oblique views may be necessary if renal artery involvement is suspected on flush anteroposterior aortography. Since multiple locations have been reported [38], visualization of the entire thoracic and abdominal aorta is mandatory. This complete angiographic assessment is also useful during early childhood when the initial study reveals only renal artery involvement. Since late recurrence of hypertension has been noted secondary to previously undefined aortic and contralateral renal artery involvement (Figs. 3 and 4), an initially complete angiographic assessment is helpful in classifying the natural history of such lesions.

Diagnostic study of the source of hypertension is particularly important when renal artery involvement accompanies the aortic coarctation. Since either suprarenal aortic coarctation or renal artery stenosis can produce hypertension, diagnostic confirmation of the functional significance of the renal artery involvement is important in designing the operative management. This is particularly important when bilateral renal artery stenoses are present, for one side may be the predominant lesion having functional significance. We employ both split renal function studies and renal venous renin assays in older patients. Since split renal function studies require cystoscopy and ureteral catheterization, the risk of complication prohibits their use in pediatric patients. In contrast, renal venous renin assays can be performed safely in these patients and are helpful in discovering the necessity of simultaneous renal revascularization.

Renal venous renin assays have little diagnostic usefulness in patients with isolated suprarenal lesions. Preoperative identification of the origin of hypertension in such patients with aortic coarctation is more elusive. Recently, infusion of competitive inhibitors of angiotensin II have been used to confirm a renal origin of hypertension in these patients. The compound having greatest recognition in this regard is sar-^{8}-ala-angiotensin I (saralasin). By substitution of the aminoacids at the 1 and 8 positions in the angiotensin II molecule with sarcosine and alanine, respectively, saralasin loses most of the vasopressor properties of native angiotensin II. When given by infusion the drug acts as a competitive inhibitor of circulating angiotensin II if hypertension is of renal origin and is sustained by the renin-angiotensin pressor system. Therefore by showing a depressor response to saralasin infusion, cure of hypertension by aortic revascularization may be predicted. Unfortunately, such a positive response to saralasin infusion is not seen uniformly even in children with renovascular hypertension secondary to isolated renal artery stenosis [15].

NATURAL HISTORY

No studies evaluating sequential changes in the anatomic appearance of subisthmic aortic coarctation are available for review. Longitudinal arteriographic examination of two children in our series give some information, however. Figure 3 shows the arteriogram in one child, age 2 months, who required nephrectomy for control of hypertension secondary to an apparently isolated left renal artery stenosis. At that age, no evidence of aortic or right renal artery involvement was demonstrable. During the subsequent 10 years the distal descending thoracic aorta, proximal abdominal aorta, and proximal right renal artery apparently failed to enlarge normally when compared to the proximal thoracic and distal abdominal aorta. Through this lack of growth in these areas, a mild aortic coarctation with severe right renal artery stenosis ultimately developed leading to recurrent hypertension. Further, the late manifestation of coarctation in this child suggests that many children treated for apparently isolated renal artery stenosis may have a congenital lesion rather than an idiopathic fibromuscular dysplastic lesion. This underscores the necessity of long-term angiographic followup in children with single mural renal artery stenoses, for such lesions may be the initial manifestation of more diffuse abdominal aortic coarctation that occurs late during embryologic life.

Arteriographic followup in an additional child is also of interest. He was initially treated at age 2 months for an interrenal coarctation with the atresia beginning above the left renal artery but below the right renal artery (Fig. 2). Angiographic followup in this child 4 years postoperatively (Fig. 6) shows failure of growth of the proximal right renal artery. Also seen is the magnitude of collateral flow to the normal iliac arteries below the atretic segment. Palpable pedal pulses developed during this period of followup with excellent perfusion of the distal extremities.

The clinical course of untreated subisthmic coarctations depends upon the location of the narrowing. Infrarenal coarctations present late during adulthood and have no effect on life expectancy. Their late clinical manifestation suggests that they may become symptomatic only subsequent to secondary atherosclerotic involvement of the inflow collateral or outflow vessels in the lower extremities. In this regard, the patient's natural course would probably more closely parallel the extent of atherosclerotic disease in their cardiovascular system.

The clinical course of intrarenal and suprarenal subisthmic aortic coarctations is similar to that of isthmic coarctations. Certainly many children who present during infancy with malignant hypertension and cardiac decompensation have no life expectancy without operative treatment. In review of the natural history of 32 patients, Senning [32] found that 10 died before the age of 34 years. Most of these patients died from cerebral hemorrhage or cardiac failure as secondary manifestations of long-standing severe hypertension. Likewise, Bjork and Intonti [5] reviewed the course of 26 patients with untreated subisthmic coarctations and showed that 14 had died at an average age of 30 years.

OPERATIVE MANAGEMENT

Several innovative techniques of revascularization have been utilized in managing subisthmic coarctations. The selection of the most appropriate technique, however, depends primarily on the location and the extent of the coarctation. For this reason, discussion of the operative management will be directed to three general areas: (1) coarctations confined to a suprarenal location, (2) those involving the renal arteries, and (3) those limited to the infrarenal aorta.

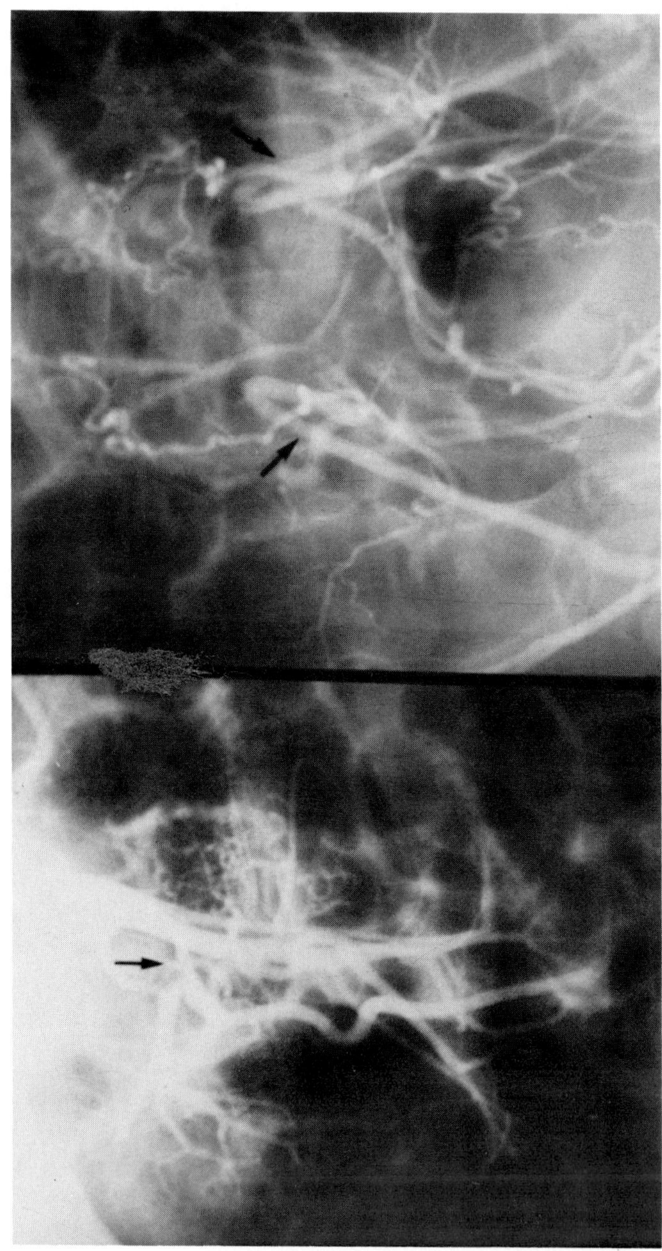

Fig. 6. Followup arteriogram performed 4 years after nephrectomy in the child shown in Fig. 2. Note the moderate narrowing of the proximal right renal artery and the collateral vessels to the distally patent iliac arteries.

Suprarenal Coarctations

Suprarenal coarctations are usually located in the descending thoracic aorta. They may be confined to the intrathoracic aorta but commonly extend to the level of the celiac axis. Aortography should be performed to define the proximal and distal extent of the lesion. Those confined to the upper or midportion of the descending thoracic aorta can be approached with a left lateral thoracotomy through the 5th or 6th interspace. If, however, the coarctation is more extensive and involves the descending thoracic aorta and the proximal intraabdominal aorta, a combined left thoracotomy and midline abdominal incision will give the most adequate exposure.

Morris [31] has recommended resection of isolated intrathoracic coarctations and favors graft interposition. Although this may be possible for short coarctations, the placement of a Dacron bypass graft is more expeditious, since there is no need to resect the lesion. This eliminates the time and risk of extensive dissection in an unusually vascular and fibrotic periaortic area. Tangential clamping of the proximal and distal aorta for the end-to-side anastomoses may be possible, thereby eliminating the necessity of total interruption of flow distally while performing the proximal anastomosis. Nevertheless, adequate visualization of the anastomotic site on the aorta is imperative. If this cannot be achieved with partial aortic occlusion, the aorta should be cross-clamped above and below the anastomotic area.

Those lesions which extend to the level of the celiac axis can best be corrected by creating the distal anastomosis at the infrarenal level. The graft can be brought through the left retroperitoneal space. This avoids a difficult exposure and anastomosis in the area of the celiac axis and superior mesenteric arteries. Retrograde perfusion of the kidneys and other viscera will be quite adequate from this infrarenal inflow site. Figure 1 shows the preoperative arteriogram of such a lesion. This 4½ year old white male presented with a history of a syncopal episode and was found to have a blood pressure of 170/100 mm Hg. Cure of hypertension was obtained by placing a 10 mm woven Dacron bypass graft from the descending thoracic aorta to the infrarenal aorta (Fig. 7).

Coarctations With Renal Artery Stenosis

Most coarctations involving the renal arteries have a characteristic pattern. The majority have a sharply defined area of involvement, usually arising in close proximity to the celiac axis and terminating at the level of the inferior mesenteric artery. Stenosis of the renal artery is usually limited to the orifice. Occasionally, however, the disease may extend further into the renal artery. Rarely, a diffuse hypoplasia is present. Although unilateral renal artery disease has been seen, bilateral involvement is the rule. Preoperative assessment of the relative functional severity of bilateral lesions is advantageous in older children

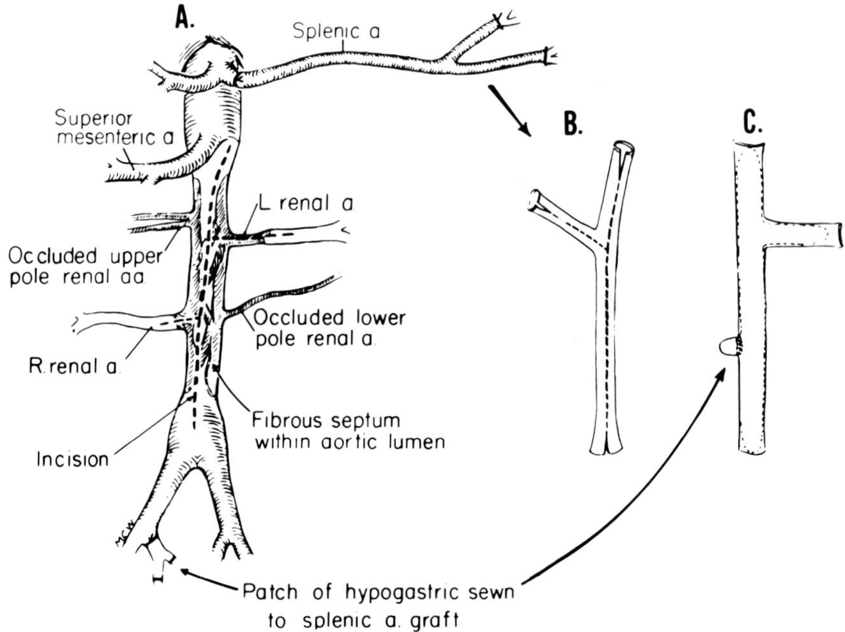

Fig. 7. Drawing of the Dacron aortoaortic bypass performed in the child shown in Fig. 1. This patient remains cured of hypertension 4 years postoperatively.

and adults. In this regard renal vein renin assays and split renal function study may be quite useful.

Since most lesions involve the proximal abdominal aorta, bypass grafting from the descending thoracic aorta to the distal abdominal aorta frequently is the safest and most expeditious method of aortic reconstruction. This can usually be performed through a left thoracic and midline abdominal incision as previously described. A lateral retroperitoneal approach with reflection of the spleen, pancreas, and left colon to the right gives the best exposure for simultaneous aortic and renal revascularization.

The decision to perform unilateral or bilateral renal artery reconstruction and the choice of graft material is more controversial. Renal venous renin assays and/or split renal function studies may be helpful in this regard. When severe bilateral stenoses are present, renal revascularization should be performed irrespective of the results of the functional studies.

The selection of the optimal conduit for renal revascularization is dependent on the age of the patients and the size of the renal artery. Autogenous saphenous vein, hypogastric or splenic artery, or Dacron can be used to revascularize the renal artery. Although preferable in adults, the saphenous vein is usually too small for use during the first decade. If uninvolved by the coarctation, either the splenic artery or hypogastric artery may be used in this group. When the distal renal artery is enlarged through poststenotic dilatation a 6 mm Dacron bypass graft may be equally acceptable for renal revascularization. The technique of renal artery bypass is discussed in detail elsewhere.

Although bypass grafting of the coarctate zone has been the most widely used method of operative management, patch angioplasty has been used sporadically. This method was first employed by Hanson in 1959 [21]. It has the advantage of allowing the greatest latitude should subsequent secondary procedures be required later in life. Similarly, it is useful when multiple renal arteries are involved in the coarctated segment.

Illustrative case. An example of such a case is shown in Figs. 5 and 8. This 9 year old white male with hypertension since age 1½ years also had a 1 year history of progressive thigh and buttock claudication. Abdominal aortography demonstrated an elongated abdominal aortic coarctation extending from the

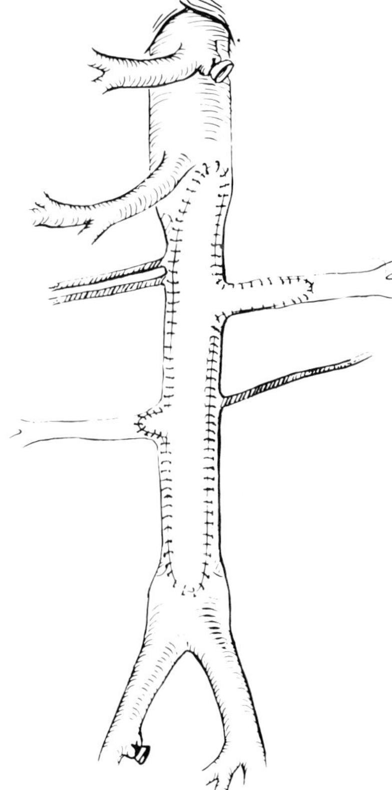

Fig. 8. Drawing of the operative technique used to accomplish both bilateral renal revascularization and aortic revascularization by patch angioplasty.

superior mesenteric artery to 3 cm above the aortic bifurcation. Further, there was severe stenosis of the dominant lower right and upper left renal arteries with total occlusion of one left lower pole and two right upper pole accessory renal arteries. At laparotomy, the aorta was found to be externally narrowed from the superior mesenteric artery to 3 cm above the aortic bifurcation. Operative management in this child is schematically represented in Fig. 8. The splenic artery and a portion of the right hypogastric artery were removed for use as aortic and bilateral renal artery patches. Upon entering the aorta, several clefts and ridges of fibrocollangenous tissue obstructing aortic flow were observed. These ridges of tissue were excised prior to application of the renal artery and aortic patches. Repeat angiography after operation showed continued patency of the reconstructed vessels. Residual occlusion of the accessory renal arteries, however, has led to mild residual hypertension. Three years after operation blood pressures range from 110/70 to 125/85 mm Hg on propranolol 10 mg twice daily and aldactazide one tablet per day. Since operation there has been complete resolution of previous symptoms of lower extremity claudication.

Infrarenal Coarctations

Coarctations limited to an infrarenal origin constitute the most benign variant of subisthmic lesions. They are usually limited to the distal aorta. They may, however, extend into the iliac arteries. Since the major symptoms are lower extremity claudication, any one of several standard techniques of lower extremity revascularization can be employed. Isolated lesions may be managed by resection with graft interposition, longitudinal incision and graft angioplasty, or by bypass grafting. The more extensive lesions are best managed by aortoiliac or femoral grafts. The technical aspects of these procedures are covered more extensively elsewhere.

RESULTS OF TREATMENT

The results of operation for subisthmic coarctations are dependent upon the site of aortic involvement. Infrarenal lesions have the most favorable prognosis. Since claudication rather than hypertension is the primary symptom, successful revascularization should give immediate relief of the symptoms without any residual sequellae. Interestingly, the bizarre neurologic findings occasionally seen preoperatively are also usually abolished by revascularization. Long-term patency and relief of symptoms should be obtained in over 90% of the cases.

Patients with suprarenal coarctations likewise have a favorable outlook following successful revascularization. The early postoperative course is similar to that of patients with isthmic lesions. Complete resolution or significant reduction in the level of hypertension should be expected in all patients. Like patients with isthmic coarctations, these individuals must be watched closely for evidence of paradoxical hypertension and bowel ischemia during the early postoperative period [42].

The fate of patients following revascularization for lesions involving the renal arteries might be expected to be less favorable. The risk of operation is probably greater, since the procedure itself is more extensive and involves aortic as well as renal revascularization. Nevertheless, in reviewing his operative experience with 16 patients, DeBakey [12] had no early or late deaths and all patients remained normotensive 5 or more years following operation. He also documented an improvement in renal function in these patients following successful revascularization.

Graham et al. [18] have reviewed the results of operative management in ten patients treated at the University of Michigan from 1961 to 1978. Although several techniques were employed for treatment of the lesions encountered in their series, they classified the results as excellent in six and good in four. In their review of the literature, they uncovered a total of 83 patients who had undergone concomitant renal revascularization or nephrectomy. Ten additional patients had been treated initially by renal revascularization alone or nephrectomy. Although the operative mortality in this collected series was 8%, among the survivors 89% had an excellent or good result.

The results in our experience with five patients underscores the need for long-term clinical and angiographic followup in these patients. A beneficial response in blood pressure control was seen in all four patients with suprarenal (one) or interrenal (three) coarctations. One patient initially cured by nephrectomy (Fig. 3) at age 2 months subsequently required contralateral renal revascularization and patch angioplasty of the infrarenal aorta 14 years later. Angiographic followup in an additional child has shown the development of progressive stenosis of the contralateral renal artery as the uninvolved proximal aorta and distal renal artery have enlarged with normal growth of the child (Fig. 4). Since many similar cases in the literature are reported without long-term followup, the ultimate results of operative therapy remain unknown. Clearly current operative techniques allow successful operative management of subisthmic aortic coarctations and concomitant renal revascularization. Nevertheless, the frequency of subsequent stenoses in initially normal appearing aortic branches and the durability of renal revascularization during 20-30 years of followup are unknown and require longer-term studies than are currently available.

REFERENCES

1. Albanese AR, Baila MR: Congenital coarctation of abdominal aorta. Bol. Trab. Acad. Argent. Circ. 37:211, 1953
2. Baylin GJ: Colateral circulation following obstruction of abdominal aorta. Anat. Rec. 75:405, 1939
3. Beattie EJ Jr, Cooke FN, Paul JS, et al: Coarctation of the aorta at the level of the diaphragm treated successfully with a preserved human blood vessel graft. J. Thorac. Surg. 21:506, 1951

4. Ben-Shoshan M, Rossi NP, Karns ME: Coarctation of the abdominal aorta. Arch. Pathol. 95:221, 1978
5. Bjork VO, Intoni F: Coarctation of abdominal aorta with right renal artery stenosis. Ann. Surg. 160:54, 1964
6. Bloor K, Williams RT: Neurofibromatosis and coarctation of the abdominal aorta with renal artery involvement. Br. J. Surg. 50:811, 1963
7. Brust AA, Howard JM, Bryant MR, et al: Coarctation of the abdominal aorta with stenosis of the renal arteries and hypertension. Am. J. Med. 27:793, 1959
8. Colquon J: Hypoplasia of the abdominal aorta following therapeutic irradiation in infancy. Radiology 86:454, 1966
9. Costa A: Obliterazione dell'aorta all'imbocco dell'aorta destra: Rottura della prima intercostale aortica. Classificazione e patogenesi delle atresia e stretture dell'aorta. Arch. Pat. Clin. Med. 9:305, 1930
10. Crafoord C, Nylin G: Congenital coarctation of the aorta and its surgical treatment. J. Thorac. Surg. 14:347, 1945
11. Dean RH, Foster JH: Criteria for the diagnosis of renovascular hypertension. Surgery 76:926, 1973
12. DeBakey ME, Garrett HE, Howell JF, et al: Coarctation of the abdominal aorta with renal arterial stenosis: Surgical considerations. Ann. Surg. 165:830, 1967
13. Doumer E, Lorriaux A, Steenhauwer B: Hypertension arterielle paraplasic de l'artere renale gauche avec malformation de l'aorte abdominale. Action passagere de la nephrectomie. Arch. Aml. Coeur 44:446, 1951
14. Duncan J: Case of spontaneous obliteration of the aorta. Lond. Edinb. Monthly J. Med. Sci. 3:781, 1843
15. Favre L, Boerth RC, Braren V, et al: Angiotensin II blockade by saralasin in the evaluation of hypertension in children. Kidney Int. 15:S-75, 1979
16. Frovig AG, Loken AC: The syndrome of obliteration of the arterial branches of the aortic arch, due to arteritis: Post-mortem angiographic and pathological study. Acta Psychiatr. Neurol. Scand. 26:313, 1951
17. Glenn F, Keefer EBC, Speer DS, et al: Coarctation of the lower thoracic and abdominal aorta immediately proximal to celiac axis. Surg. Gynecol. Obstet. 94:561, 1952
18. Graham LM, Zelenock GB, Erlandson EE, et al: Abdominal aortic coarctation and segmental hypoplasia. Thirty Sixth Annual Meeting of the Central Surgical Association, Omaha, 1979
19. Gross RE, Hufnagel CA: Coarctation of the aorta: Experimental studies regarding its surgical correction. N. Engl. J. Med. 233:287, 1945
20. Hahn M: Zur Frage tiefsitzender Stenosen der absteigenden Brustaorta. Inaug. Diss., Berlin, 1933
21. Hanson J, Ikkos D, Johansson L, et al: Coarctation of abdominal aorta – Case report and description of successful surgical treatment. Acta Chir. Scand. [Suppl.] 245:315, 1959
22. Hasler LH: Ueber ein Fall von Verschlauss der aorta in ungewohnert Stelle. Borna-Leipzig, R. Noske, 1911

23. Heberer G, Zumtobel V, Eigler FW, et al: Behandlung atypischer suprarenaler Stenosen der Aorta bei Hypertoniken. Dtsch. Med. Wochenschr. 96:615, 1971
24. Hickl W: Ueber zylindrische Aostoenverengerung im absteigenden Brustteil infolge von Mesaortitis. Z. Pathol. 41:176, 1931
25. Inada K: Atypical coarctation of the aorta with a special reference of its genesis. Angiology 16:608, 1965
26. Immon TW, Pollack BE: Coarctations of the abdominal aorta. Am. Heart J. 52:314, 1956
27. Lemmon WM, Bailey CP: A new classification for coarctations of the aorta. J. Thorac. Surg. 25:291, 1958
28. Martorell F, Fabre J: El Sindrome de Obliteration de los Trancos Supraorticos. Second Congress of the International Society of Angiology, Lisbon, 1954, p 271
29. Maycock W d'A: Congenital stenosis of the abdominal aorta. Am. Heart J. 13:633, 1967
30. Milloy F, Fell EH: Elongate coarctation of the aorta. Arch. Surg. 78:759, 1959
31. Nennhaus HP, Javis H, Hunter JA: Surgical treatment of renovascular hypertension in children, with a review of infradiaphragmatic arterial hypoplastic anomalies. J. Thorac. Cardiovasc. Surg. 54:246, 1967
32. Onat T, Zeren E: Coarctation of the abdominal aorta. Cardiologia 54:140, 1969
33. Pennington DG, Drapanas T: Acute post-traumatic coarctation of the abdominal aorta. Surgery 78:538, 1975
34. Pierach CA, Katkov H: Coarctation of the abdominal aorta. Vasc. Surg. 6:159, 1972
35. Power JH: Observations on disease of the aortic valves, producing both constriction of the aortic orifice, and regurgitation through it into the left ventricle, accompanied with abdominal enlargement of the two internal mammary arteries, and atrophy of the abdominal aorta and its iliac branches. Dublin J. Med. Sci. 32:314, 1861
36. Quain R: Partial contraction of the abdominal aorta. Trans. Pathol. Soc. London 1:244, 1847
37. Robicsek F, Sander PW, Daugherty HK: Coarctation of the abdominal aorta diagnosed by aortography. Ann. Surg. 162:277, 1965
38. Sautter RD, Myers WO, Smullen WA, et al: Tandem coarctations of thoracic and abdominal with intervening hypoplastic unilateral axillofemoral graft. Ann. Thorac. Surg. 23:582, 1977
39. Schleckat O: Angeeborene ringformige Stenose der Aorta descendens in Zwerchfellhohe. Z. Kreislaufforsch 25:417, 1933
40. Schlessinger: Merkwurdirge Verschkiessung der Aorta. Wenscher Ges. Heilkd. 31:489, 1835
41. Schire V, Asherson RA: Arteritis of the aorta and its major branches. Q. J. Med. 33:439, 1964
42. Sealy WC: Coarctation of the aorta and hypertension. Ann. Thorac. Surg. 3:15, 1967

43. Sen PK, Kinare SG, Kulkarni TP, et al: Stenosing aortitis of unknown etiology. Surgery 51:317, 1962
44. Sen PK, Kinare SG, Engineer SD, et al: The middle aortic syndrome. Br. Heart J. 25:610, 1963
45. Senning A, Johansson L: Coarctation of the abdominal aorta. J. Thorac. Cardiovasc. Surg. 40:517, 1960
46. Shimizu K, Sano K: Pulseless disease. J. Neuropathol. Exp. Neurol. 1:37, 1951
47. Sproul G, Pinto J: Coarctation of the abdominal aorta. Arch. Surg. 105:571, 1972
48. Takayasu M: A case with peculiar changes of the central retinal vessels. Acta Soc. Ophthalmol. Jpn. 12:554, 1908
49. Ueda H, Marooka S, Ito I, et al: Clinical observation of 52 cases of aortitis syndrome. Jpn. Heart J. 10:277, 1969
50. Wood PH: Diseases of the Heart and Circulation (ed. 2). London, Eyre & Spottiswoode, 1956

Victor M. Bernhard, M.D.
Leonard H. Kleinman, M.D.

Aortoenteric Fistulas

Erosion of the aorta into the adjacent gastrointestinal tract is a rare cause of gastrointestinal bleeding [1, 10, 21, 27, 41]. The fistula produced by this mechanism may be primary, originating from aneurysmal degeneration of the aorta [1, 14, 29-32, 41, 42, 47], or may be secondary to vascular reconstruction for either aneurysm or atherosclerotic obstruction disease [6-9, 13, 15, 16, 21, 27, 33-35, 45, 46, 52]. Secondary fistulas are almost invariably a late complication of prosthetic replacement or bypass of the abdominal aorta. Only one instance of fistula secondary to aortic endarterectomy has been recorded [11].

The first primary aortoenteric fistula was described by Sir Astley Cooper in 1817 [10]. Secondary fistulae began to appear shortly after the introduction of aortic reconstructive surgery by DuBost and his colleagues in 1952 [18]. Brock described the first aortoduodenal fistula due to aneurysmal degeneration of a homograft used to replace an abdominal aortic aneurysm [6]. Claytor reported the first fistula following the insertion of a synthetic (nylon) prosthesis [8]. The first successful repair of an aortoenteric fistula was accomplished by Herberer in 1957 [29].

Bleeding into the gastrointestinal tract from the aorta or one of its primary branches inevitably proceeds to exsanguination unless the disease process is treated surgically [15, 27, 33, 34, 36, 41, 45]. Unfortunately, by contrast with the more common causes of gastrointestinal blood loss, the presenting clinical pictures are indistinguishable [33]. This combination of infrequent occurrence and a clinical presentation similar to other, much less lethal processes has produced considerable confusion. As a result, the diagnosis is frequently overlooked and surgical intervention is significantly delayed until recurrent hemorrhage, shock, and death ensue [33].

PATHOGENESIS

The third portion of the duodenum lying directly over the infrarenal aorta or a suture line is the most frequent loop of bowel involved in primary fistulas [15, 19, 20, 27, 41, 49]. The aneurysm presses directly into the posterior wall of the duodenum as it enlarges, and a combination of pressure and pulsation produces an erosion of the bowel wall [27, 33, 40, 41, 46, 47]. Rupture into the bowel lumen is associated with infection of the aortic wall with enteric bacteria [33]. All four primary fistulae in our experience appeared to be the result of this sequence of events.

Infrequent causes of primary fistulas, especially in younger patients, include mycotic aneurysms [1, 24, 48], tuberculous degeneration of the aortic wall adjacent to bowel [25, 50], necrosis of bowel and aorta by infiltrating tumor masses [1, 28], false aneurysm secondary to trauma [45], and one case of possible idiopathic erosion of normal aorta into the duodenum [22]. Fistulization into other segments of the gastrointestinal tract, i.e., esophagus, stomach, proximal duodenum, jejunoileum, and colon, are usually the result of degenerative processes in the thoracic or upper abdominal aorta or one of the primary aortic branches [1, 32, 44].

Infectious factors [7, 33], in addition to anatomical and mechanical circumstances [16, 21, 27, 33], have been implicated in the formation of a secondary aortoenteric fistula. However, it is difficult to identify the precise initiating cause of a particular secondary fistula, since it is usually obliterated during maturation of the process. Nevertheless, in an analysis of 20 secondary fistulas presenting to our institutions [33], there were sufficient data recorded to ascribe a predisposing factor in 14 patients (Table 1). In five patients who required reoperation for some complication of the original aortic graft, the previous operative records described difficult dissections, extensive adhesions, and serosal tears in the bowel. Aneurysmal degeneration of a previous aortic homograft with silk suture anastomosis was noted in three. In three instances, the operative report from the original aortic surgery noted that no viable tissue had been interposed between the duodenum and the new graft, which correlated with the findings noted at the time of surgery for the fistula. Two patients demonstrated false aneurysms at the proximal aortic suture line. One individual had a septic course accompanied by renal infarction following a second aortic procedure. Angiography revealed a markedly redundant and kinked limb of a graft which at surgery was found to be pressing directly against a fixed loop of bowel.

We concur with the importance of mechanical factors emphasized by several investigators who recommend insertion of a layer of healthy tissue between the

Table 1
Factors Predisposing to the Development of an Aortoenteric Fistula

	No. of Patients
Reoperation for graft failure	5
Inadequate reperitonealization of graft	3
Use of aortic homograft	3
False aneurysm	2
Renal infarction and sepsis	1

intestine and the vascular structures at the time of retroperitoneal closure to protect bowel from foreign body reaction and pressure erosion due to a pulsatile graft [16, 21, 27, 33]. It has been suggested that mechanical injury may cause inapparent bowel perforation or development of a limited area of traumatic ischemia leading to secondary contamination of a graft [21].

Infection as the primary factor is obvious in mycotic aneurysms due to salmonella, tuberculosis, etc. Infections may arise secondary to bowel injury or hematogenous dissemination from a remote focus producing graft sepsis or false aneurysm formation of the suture line. The potential for exogenous infection at the time of primary or secondary operation of aortic disease must be considered in all patients. However, enteric pathogens were the primary flora encountered in all 9 of the 24 patients in our series who had cultures taken at surgery [33]. These findings indicate either secondary contamination from the bowel lumen after the fistula had developed or an enteric source for the infection initiating the fistulous process.

An animal study reported by Busuttil et al. [7] suggests that infection is the most important initiating factor in secondary aortoenteric fistulas. However, their failure to produce fistulas in those animals subjected to mechanical factors alone for 6 weeks may only indicate that time was insufficient for mechanical erosion to have taken place. Nevertheless, the importance of infection is highlighted by this study and suggests that a combination of factors produces fistula formation in most instances. Regardless of the pathogenesis, the presence and extent of infection must be considered in order to develop a satisfactory approach to therapy.

Two types of secondary fistulas have been described [16]. The most common type develops directly at a suture line with erosion into adjacent bowel. Infection at the suture line produces necrosis and intermittent gross intestinal hemorrhage which is temporarily controlled by formation of a thrombotic plug. Inevitably, the hole enlarges to permit exsanguination. When the graft erodes into bowel away from a suture line, the initial picture is one of sepsis and anemia with guiac positive stools due to minor bleeding through the interstices of the prosthesis. Eventually, infection travels along the graft to a suture line, producing anastomotic breakdown and gross hemorrhage into the bowel lumen [21]. The latter process, originally described by DeWeese [16], has been referred to as paraprosthetic fistula formation by Elliott [21] and has been recently reviewed in detail by O'Mara [38]. This type occurred in six of our patients, three of whom presented with anemia and fever. The other three did not come to our attention until the process had extended to a suture line producing gross bleeding.

CLINICAL PRESENTATION

Aortoenteric fistulas invariably present with some form of gastrointestinal bleeding. In all 4 of our primary fistulas and in 17 of 20 secondary fistulas, gross bleeding was the primary symptom. This appeared as hematemesis in 14 patients, melena in 4, and hematochezia in 3. A transient, self-limited, "herald bleed" was noted in 19 of 21 patients with gross gastrointestinal blood loss. One patient with a primary fistula and one with a secondary fistula were admitted to the hospital in hemorrhagic shock without an antecedent bleeding episode. It has been the universal experience that bleeding is usually intermittent during the early phases of fistula formation when the communication between the aorta and the bowel lumen is small and a plug of thrombus can temporarily prevent exsanguination [9, 14-16, 21, 27, 33, 34]. With enzymatic lysis of the plug and enlargement of the fistula, bleeding becomes progressively more severe and eventually exsanguinating.

Anemia with guiac positive stools was the presenting picture in four of our patients, three of whom had accompanying fever. In one patient, melena and shock developed subsequent to the demonstration of chronic anemia [33].

A pulsatile abdominal mass was noted in all four patients with primary fistulas produced by aortic aneurysms. This finding was also noted in the three patients with secondary fistulas due to homograft degeneration and in one patient with a false aneurysm at the proximal aortic suture line [33].

Pain in the abdomen, back, or flank has been frequently described with primary fistulas as a result of boney erosion or associated rupture. Except for cramps caused by sudden injection of blood into the bowel lumen, secondary fistulas are usually painless.

DIAGNOSIS

Any patient with gross or occult gastrointestinal bleeding and a history of prior aortic surgery or bleeding associated with a pulsatile abdominal mass should be considered to have an aortoenteric fistula until proven otherwise. An aggressive approach culminating in surgical exploration is required since the diagnosis is often obscure and difficult to prove, and the outcome without surgery is invariably lethal. Massive exsanguinating hemorrhage is rarely the presenting clinical picture. This occurred in only two patients in our series, one with secondary and one with a primary fistula. In the vast majority of cases, a period of at least a few hours is available to carry out appropriate diagnostic maneuvers to support a proper mode of therapy.

All of the standard diagnostic procedures to identify the source of gastrointestinal hemorrhage have been recommended [2, 13, 15, 21, 23, 36-38, 49]. However, their effectiveness for demonstrating a fistula is quite variable, and the findings are frequently inconclusive or confusing. The high incidence of peptic ulcer associated with abdominal aortic aneurysm [31] must be taken into consideration in evaluating any preoperative diagnostic maneuver. Barium contrast examination of the upper gastrointestinal tract may identify a filling defect or irregularity in the duodenum or an extraluminal paraprosthetic extravasation of contrast material [15-17, 23, 33]. In our experience [33], 11 patients were subjected to this study, with a clearly positive finding in only one instance. A large hiatal hernia was also noted in this patient, which might have erroneously been considered the source of bleeding. In two others, gastric ulcers were identified suggesting the need for nonoperative therapy. In the remaining eight patients, the study was entirely negative.

Aortography may demonstrate a true or false aneurysm or a perigraft extravasation of contrast material [15, 26, 27, 33, 45, 49]. This study was performed in six of our patients, in four of whom it was entirely negative and therefore of no value for establishing or ruling out the diagnosis of aortoenteric fistula. Extravasation of dye from the graft into the duodenal lumen in one patient and a false aneurysm at the proximal suture line in another supported the diagnosis and directed us to immediate surgical intervention.

Barium enema may be helpful by identifying neoplastic or diverticular disease of the colon, which may be the source of anemia and guiac positive stools or of continuing hematochezia. However, this study does not rule out fistula formation if positive for a primary colonic lesion and may delay surgery or incorrectly direct therapy. Although barium enema demonstration of graft erosion into the sigmoid has been reported [13], fistula formation into the colon is rare [3]. Nevertheless, identification of intrinsic colon pathology in patients with a picture of lower gastrointestinal bleeding permits preoperative bowel preparation so that a direct attack on the colon lesion can be carried out if a fistula is not found.

Upper gastrointestinal endoscopy is probably the most effective diagnostic modality for evaluating patients with aortoenteric fistulas [2, 33, 37, 38]. The findings of this study are important whether positive or negative. If the esophagus, stomach, and proximal duodenum are entirely normal or if a nonbleeding lesion is identified down to the level of the second portion of the duodenum, it can be assumed that an aortoenteric fistula is the most likely cause of gastrointestinal blood loss. Seventy-five percent of all fistulas are within the range of upper gastrointestinal endoscopic examination. Passage of the endoscope into the third and fourth duodenum or beyond the duodenojejunal flexure by a skilled endoscopist permits direct visualization of the intestinal side of the fistula.

Fiberoptic gastroduodenoscopy was accomplished in eight of our patients. A clot was demonstrated in the third portion of the duodenum in one patient with a primary fistula. In a second patient with a primary fistula, this study was performed when bleeding recurred following vagotomy and pyloroplasty for a chronic duodenal ulcer which was erroneously assumed to be the source of bleeding. The fistula was overlooked.

In six patients with secondary fistulas, endoscopy was negative in three and a nonbleeding gastric ulcer was noted in two. The absence of an actively bleeding lesion down to the level of the proximal duodenum in these cases was correctly interpreted as a positive indication for prompt laparotomy. A fistula was directly demonstrated in one patient; however, passage of the scope into the third portion of the duodenum induced massive hemorrhage with death of the patient during subsequent laparotomy. For this reason, we insist that endoscopy for patients who may have aortoenteric fistulas be performed in a readied operating room to minimize delay in controlling recurrent bleeding.

A gallium scan will support the diagnosis of paraprosthetic fistula by demonstration of an inflammatory process in the area of the graft. This was clearly helpful in one of our patients who presented with a 1 year history of recurring fever, anemia, and guiac positive stools.

Depending upon the nature of the clinical presentation, the following program of diagnostic intervention appears to be most effective from our experience. For the rare patient who appears with massive, continuing hemorrhage, there is no opportunity for any preoperative diagnostic workup and immediate laparotomy is required on the basis of history and clinical findings alone. In the vast majority of patients with a "herald bleed," upper gastrointestinal endoscopy should be carried out immediately. If possible, the scope should be passed into the third and fourth portions of the duodenum to directly visualize the fistula when an actively bleeding lesion is not noted in the more proximal segments of the upper gastrointestinal tract. If this study is negative and the patient is stable, aortography should be performed immediately to search for a false aneurysm, paraprosthetic leakage of dye, or demonstration of a primary aneurysm which was not obvious by abdominal examination. Obviously, in all patients over age 50 with gastrointestinal bleeding, routine abdominal films should be obtained to search for an aneurysm which may have been overlooked on physical examination. When a pulsatile aneurysm is palpable and if the patient is clinically stable, preoperative aortogram may be helpful during the subsequent operative procedure.

In patients who present with hematochezia or guiac positive stools with anemia, upper gastrointestinal endoscopy should be performed and, if negative, should be followed by an aortogram. Aortography should always be done before barium study so that visualization of vascular structures will not be obscured. If this is also negative, barium enema should be performed to identify a primary colon lesion which may require surgical management if exploration is negative for aortoenteric fistula. Although massive hemorrhage will eventually occur in these patients who are most likely to have a paraprosthetic erosion, there is usually sufficient time for mechanical and antibiotic bowel preparation prior to abdominal exploration.

Because surgical intervention for aortoenteric fistula is an urgent matter, the various elements of the diagnostic workup should be accomplished within a few hours of hospital admission. The studies should be followed by immediate laparotomy to search for a fistula even if all studies, including direct visualization of the distal duodenum, are negative. None of the diagnostic studies will demonstrate a fistula into the jejunum or ilium except for the occasional indirect findings on aortography.

Upper gastrointestinal x-rays are unnecessary, time wasting, and confusing in the presence of satisfactory upper endoscopy. The finding of a potentially bleeding lesion by barium contrast study does not insure that it is the source of bleeding and does not rule out fistula formation [33].

SURGICAL MANAGEMENT

Surgical intervention is mandatory in all cases of aortoenteric fistula, since exsanguinating gastrointestinal hemorrhage is inevitable [33]. All patients should be prepared for immediate laparotomy whenever the diagnosis is suspected, and surgery should be delayed only long enough for essential diagnostic maneuvers.

Identification of the fistula requires exploration of the entire retroperitoneal area with mobilization of the third and fourth portion of the duodenum, the duodenojejunal flexure, and separation of any loops of bowel adhering to the anterior aspect of the aorta and iliac arteries or the bed of a graft. Preliminary gastrotomy is an unnecessary and time wasting maneuver especially if a prior gastroscopy was negative.

Before dismantling the fistula, the aorta must be controlled. This can frequently be accomplished by the dissection of the aorta inferior to the renal arteries [19]. However, in patients who are actively bleeding or in whom there is considerable scarring in this area, temporary aortic control should be promptly carried out proximal to the celiac axis. This can be accomplished with external compression or more effectively by slitting the aortic hiatus to expose the distal end of the thoracic aorta for temporary clamp application [12]. The infrarenal aorta can now be exposed in a more leisurely and precise manner, following which the clamp is replaced in the infrarenal position and the fistula tract entered. A search for other sources of bleeding should be considered only after full mobilization of the duodenum, jejunoileum, and colon fails to reveal a fistula.

The defect in the small intestine is usually small and in most instances can be readily repaired with simple suture techniques. Occasionally, extensive destruction of the wall of the distal duodenum is produced by a paraprosthetic fistula. In this circumstance, it may be wise to resect this segment of bowel, close the proximal end of the duodenum where tissues are healthy, and then anastomose the jejunum to the free anterolateral margin of the second portion of the duodenum [33].

In patients with primary fistula associated with abdominal aortic aneurysm, resection of the aneurysm and graft replacement in the retroperitoneal position appears to be satisfactory [14]. Infection is usually limited to a narrow area around the fistula which can be readily excised, and the retroperitoneal tissues are not extensively involved. Contamination from the upper duodenum after opening the bowel is minimal and can be controlled with local and systemic antibiotic therapy. The retroperitoneal graft should be covered by viable tissue. If sufficient aortic wall remains after resection of the portion involved in the fistula, this may be satisfactory; otherwise, a tongue of omentum can be brought down to surround the graft and its anastomoses. Daugherty and his associates [14] presented three patients and reviewed 11 cases reported by others managed in this manner. All 14 did well initially. Ten were followed over the long term, of which nine patients followed for an average of 9.8 years had no further problems and only one succumbed to recurrent aortointestinal fistula 2 years postoperatively.

In our series, one patient died from exsanguination before laparotomy could be performed. A second patient developed exsanguinating hemorrhage during search for an upper gastrointestinal bleeding point through a gastrotomy, and in a third patient the fistula was overlooked and lethal hemorrhage occurred 1 week following vagotomy and pyloroplasty. In one patient, the diagnosis was made by preoperative endoscopy. The aneurysm was resected and the lower extremities revascularized by axillobifemoral bypass. This patient did well in the initial postoperative period but succumbed to a pulmonary embolism on the 8th postoperative day (Table 2).

The surgical approach to a secondary fistula requires excision of all previously inserted prosthetic materials [20, 33]. It is extremely difficult to eradicate infection from the interstices of the graft wall, and the presence of a foreign body during the maturation of the fistula promotes more extensive infection in the retroperitoneal tissues. Although small series and isolated case reports have documented short and long term success with direct closure of the aortic defect [19], vein or Dacron patch angioplasty [5, 39, 40], or resection of all or

Table 2
Surgical Treatment of Aortoenteric Fistula

	No. of Patients	Survival *No.*	Survival %	Cause of Death
Primary				
Resection AAA, ax-fem bypass	1	0	0	Pulmonary embolism
Exploration only	1	0	0	Hemorrhage
Ulcer operation	2	0	0	(2) Hemorrhage
Secondary				
Resection graft, ax-fem bypass	7	5	71.4	Myocardial infarction, (1) Renal failure
Resection of graft, no revascularization	4	2	50	(2) Extremity and colon ischemia
Repair fistula, graft retained or replaced	4	0	0	(4) Recurrent fistula
Exploration only, fistula overlooked	3	0	0	(3) Fistula hemorrhage
Operative death	2	0	0	(2) Hemorrhage

part of the previous graft and retroperitoneal replacement of a new prosthesis [27], recurrent sepsis and fistulization have been frequent lethal complications of these techniques. This was the unfortunate outcome in all four of our patients in whom a portion of the old prosthesis was retained or a new graft was replaced in the retroperitoneal space [33]. Therefore we strongly favor complete removal of all Dacron material from the retroperitoneum.

Prior to closing the abdomen, every effort should be made to buttress the oversewn aortic stump with viable periaortic tissue. A strip of anterior spinal ligament can be incorporated into the aortic suture line. If major infection or abscess formation is present, retroperitoneal drains should be brought out through stab wounds on the side of the abdomen opposite to the anticipated axillofemoral bypass.

Revascularization of the lower extremity should be carried out immediately in all patients unless the graft is thrombosed and adequate collaterals have had an opportunity to form [3], or when prior amputation has eliminated the need for revascularization. We elected to omit this step in two patients with patent grafts because the limbs appeared to be viable after graft excision and abdominal closure. Unfortunately, both of these patients developed progressive buttock, extremity, and left colon ischemia and died from sepsis [33]. On the other hand, graft excision without revascularization was tolerated in one of our patients with bilateral above knee amputations and in another with unilateral amputation and bilateral graft occlusion prior to development of their fistulas. Normal limb perfusion was obtained in all of the eight patients in whom an axillobifemoral bypass was performed after graft excision (Table 2).

Fistulas associated with aortobifemoral grafts pose the additional problem of infection or contamination of subsequent groin incisions required for removal of the distal limbs of the graft and subsequent extraanatomic bypass. If infection is confined to the aortic portion of the graft, the limbs of the graft can be ligated and transected just proximal to the inguinal ligament with removal of the graft. The tracts of the graft limbs should be plugged with healthy intraabdominal tissues to seal them from the groins. After closure of the abdomen and reprepping and draping, the distal portions of the graft which have sustained only minimal contamination are brought down into the field through fresh groin incisions and the previous femoral anastomoses are dismantled. After thorough antibiotic irrigation and under adequate systemic antibiotic coverage, the axillobifemoral graft is inserted. This maneuver, of course, should not be performed if the intraabdominal infection has extended down the limb of the graft into the groin.

RESULTS

A high mortality has been associated with aortoenteric fistulas due to missed diagnosis, unwarranted operative delay, or an inappropriate surgical procedure [15, 16, 20, 21, 33, 38, 41]. The overall survival rate for our entire series was 7 of 24 patients (29%). All of our patients with primary fistulas succumbed; however, only one patient had the diagnosis made preoperatively and was promptly subjected to a reliable surgical procedure. He did well until his death from a pulmonary embolism on the eighth postoperative day. In Daugherty's collected series, all patients survived immediate resection and retroperitoneal placement of a graft, and only one patient succumbed to anastomotic leak at 5 months [14].

Seven patients in our group of 20 secondary fistulas survived (35%). Two died from exsanguination during surgery due to delay in making the diagnosis and three from subsequent hemorrhage due to the fact that the fistula was overlooked. Four succumbed to recurrent fistula formation due to residual prosthetic material in the retroperitoneal space and two due to failure to revascularize the lower extremities. However, of nine patients who were correctly diagnosed preoperatively and had appropriate surgery, seven survived (78%). One died at 7 months due to hemorrhage from aneurysmal degeneration of the aortic stump. The remaining 6 patients were alive and well 3-88 months postoperatively. Similar results have been recorded by Ehrenfeld [20] and O'Mara [38].

CONCLUSION

Proper management of an aortoenteric fistula requires prompt recognition and expeditious surgical intervention. This diagnosis should be made in all patients who present with any form of gastrointestinal bleeding associated with clinical or x-ray evidence of an abdominal aneurysm or who have had previous aortic surgery. Upper gastrointestinal endoscopy is the most useful maneuver for establishing the diagnosis by direct demonstration of the lesion or by ruling out the more common causes of bleeding. Aortography is helpful only if it is positive. Barium contrast studies are of little value and frequently confuse the issue. Thorough retroperitoneal exploration is required to verify or rule out the presence of a fistula. Aneurysm resection and standard graft replacement is the proper mode of therapy for patients with primary fistulas in the absence of extensive retroperitoneal infection. In patients with secondary fistulas, all retroperitoneal graft material should be excised and lower extremity revascularization provided by axillofemoral bypass unless the patient is an amputee or major collaterals have developed due to prior graft occlusion. Morbidity and mortality have been significantly reduced when these principles have been applied.

REFERENCES

1. Bagnuolo WG, Bennett HD: Non-traumatic aortic perforations into the gastrointestinal tract. Am. Heart J. 40:784, 1950

2. Baker MS, Fisher JH, van der Reis L, et al: The endoscopic diagnosis of an aortoduodenal fistula. Arch. Surg. 111:304, 1976
3. Beach PM, Risley TS: Aortico sigmoid fistula following aortic resection. Arch. Surg. 92:805, 1966
4. Becker RM, Blundell PE: Infected aortic bifurcation grafts: Experience with fourteen patients. Surgery 80:544, 1976
5. Brenner WI, Richman H, Reed GE: Roof patch repair of an aorto-duodenal fistula resulting from suture line failure in an aortic prosthesis. Am. J. Surg. 127:762, 1974
6. Brock RC: Aortic homografting: A report of six successful cases. Guy's Hosp. Rep. 102:204, 1953
7. Busuttil RW, Rees W, Baker JD, et al: Pathogenesis of aortoduodenal fistula: Experimental and clinical correlates. Surgery 85:1, 1979
8. Claytor H, Birch L, Cardwell ES, et al: Suture-line rupture of a nylon aortic bifurcation graft into the small bowel. Arch. Surg. 73:947, 1956
9. Cohn R, Angell WW: Late complications from plastic replacement of aortic abdominal aneurysms. Arch. Surg. 97:696, 1968
10. Cooper A: Notes taken from lectures on surgery delivered by Astley Cooper at St. Thomas' Hospital in London 1817-1818. Taken by Dr. John M. Sterling, London, 1822, p 57
11. Cordell AR, Wright RH, Johnston FR: Gastrointestinal hemorrhage after abdominal aortic operations. Surgery 48:997, 1960
12. Crawford ES, Manning LG, Kelly TF: "Redo" surgery after operations for aneurysms and occlusion of the abdominal aorta. Surgery 81:41, 1977
13. Dalinka MK, Goehl VK, Schaffer B, et al: Gastrointestinal complications of aortic bypass surgery. Clin. Radiol. 27:255, 1975
14. Daugherty M, Shearer GR, Ernst CG: Primary aortoduodenal fistula: Extra-anatomic vascular reconstruction not required for successful management. Surgery 86:399, 1979
15. Dean RH, Allen TR, Foster JH, et al: Aortoduodenal fistula: An uncommon but correctable cause of upper gastrointestinal bleeding. Am. Surgeon 44:37, 1978
16. DeWeese MS, Fry WJ: Small-bowel erosion following aortic resection. JAMA 179:882, 1962
17. Donovan TJ, Bucknam TJ: Aorto-enteric fistula. Arch. Surg. 95:810, 1967
18. Dubost C, Allary M, Oeconomos N: Resection of an aneurysm of the abdominal aorta: Reestablishment of the continuity by a preserved human arterial graft with result after five months. Arch. Surg. 64:405, 1952
19. Eastcott HHG: Discussion of paper by Kleinman LH, Towne JB, Bernhard VM. A diagnostic and therapeutic approach to aorto-enteric fistulas: Clinical experience with 20 patients. Presented at the meeting of The Society for Vascular Surgery, June 1979
20. Ehrenfeld WK, Lord RSA, Stoney RJ, et al: Subcutaneous arterial bypass grafts in the management of fistulae between the bowel and plastic arterial prostheses. Ann. Surg. 168:29, 1968
21. Elliott JP Jr, Smith RF, Szilagyi DE: Aortoenteric and paraprosthetic-enteric fistulas: Problems of diagnosis and management. Arch. Surg. 108:479, 1974

22. Evans DM, Webster JHH: Spontaneous aortoduodenal fistula. Br. J. Surg. 59:368, 1972
23. Ferris EJ, Szego Koltay MR, Koltay OP, et al: Abdominal aortic and iliac graft fistulae: Unusual roentgenographic findings. Am. J. Roentgenol. 94:416, 1965
24. Foa P: Aneurisma spurio-periaortic d'origine infettiva. G. Reale Accad. Med. Torino 3.S 43:374, 1895
25. Frosch HL, Horowitz W: Rupture of the abdominal aorta into duodenum (through a sinus tract created by a tuberculous lymphadenitis). Ann. Intern. Med. 21:481, 1944
26. Gardner TJ, Brawley RK, Gott VL: Anastomotic false aneurysms. Surgery 72:474, 1972
27. Garrett HE, Beall AC Jr, Jordan GL Jr, et al: Surgical considerations of massive gastrointestinal tract hemorrhage caused by aortoduodenal fistula. Am. J. Surg. 105:6, 1963
28. Geary SR, Walunth EZ: Aortoduodenal fistula secondary to metastatic carcinoma angiographic demonstration. JAMA 235:2510, 1976
29. Heberer G: Diagnosis and treatment of aneurysms of the abdominal aorta. Ger. Med. Monthly 2:203, 1957
30. Hirst AE, Affeldt J: Abdominal aortic aneurysm with rupture into the duodenum: A report of eight cases. Gastroenterology 17:504, 1951
31. Jones AW, Kirk RS, Bloor K: The association between aneurysm of the abdominal aorta and peptic ulceration. Gut 11:679, 1970
32. Kane JM, Meyer KA, Kozoll DD: An anatomical approach to the problem of massive gastrointestinal hemorrhage. Arch. Surg. 70:570, 1955
33. Kleinman LH, Towne JB, Bernhard VM: A diagnostic and therapeutic approach to aorto-enteric fistulas: A clinical experience with 20 patients. Surgery (in press)
34. Levy MJ, Todd DB, Lillehei CW, et al: Aorticointestinal fistulas following surgery of the aorta. Surg. Gynecol. Obstet. 120:992, 1965
35. Long L, Hunter JA, Dye WS: Migration of aortic prosthesis into the duodenum: Case report and review. Ann. Surg. 157:560, 1968
36. Mehta AI, McDowell DE, James EC: Hemorrhage from aorto-enteric fistula. Surg. Gynecol. Obstet. 145:59, 1978
37. Mir-Madjlessi SH, Sullivan BH Jr, Farmer RG, et al: Endoscopic diagnosis of aortoduodenal fistula. Gastrointest. Endosc. 19:187, 1973
38. O'Mara C, Imbembo AL: Paraprosthetic enteric fistula. Surgery 81:556, 1977
39. Pinkerton AJ Jr: Aortoduodenal fistula. JAMA 225:1196, 1973
40. Ray FS, McAfee RE, Hiebert CA, et al: Aortoduodenal fistula: Primary repair with saphenous vein patch graft. JAMA 236:2423, 1976
41. Reckless JPD, McColl I, Taylor GW: Aorto-enteric fistulae: An uncommon complication of abdominal aortic aneurysms. Br. J. Surg. 59:458, 1972
42. Rosata FE, Barker C, Roberts B: Aorto-intestinal fistula: Three cases of successful management. J. Thorac. Cardiovasc. Surg. 53:511, 1967
43. Scribner R, Baker MS, Towes RL, et al: Recurrent aortoduodenal fistula. Arch. Surg. 112:1265, 1977

44. Shaigany A, Gillespie L, Mock JP, et al: Aortoenteric fistula: A complication of renal artery bypass graft. Arch. Intern. Med. 136:930, 1976
45. Sheil AGR, Reeve TS, Little JM, et al: Aorto-intestinal fistulas following operations on the abdominal aorta and iliac arteries. Br. J. Surg. 56:840, 1969
46. Sheranian LO, Edwards JE, Kirklin JW: Late results in 110 patients with abdominal aortic aneurysm treated by resectional placement of aortic homograft. Surg. Gynecol. Obstet. 109:309, 1959
47. Skromak SJ, O'Neill JF, Ciccone EF, et al: Aneurysm of the abdominal aorta. Two cases with rupture into the intestinal tract. Gastroenterology 33:575, 1957
48. TenEyck FW, Wellman WE: Salmonellosis associated with abdominal aortic aneurysm and edema of the lower extremities: Case report. Postgrad. Med. 26:334, 1959
49. Thompson WM, Johnsrude IS, Jackson DC: Late complications of abdominal aortic surgery: Roentgen evaluation. Ann. Surg. 185:326, 1977
50. Tozer EA: A case of tuberculosis aneurysm of the abdominal aorta with rupture into the duodenum. Br. Med. J. 2:1022, 1914
51. Voyles WR, Moretz WH: Rupture of aortic aneurysms into the intestinal tract. Surgery 43:666, 1958
52. Wierman WH, Straham RW, Spencer JR: Small bowel erosion by synthetic aortic grafts. Am. J. Surg. 112:791, 1962

Fred N. Littooy, M.D.
William H. Baker, M.D.

Major Arteriovenous Fistulas of the Aortic Territory

The rare occurrence of a fistula between the aorta or a major branch of the aorta and a major venous channel presents a major challenge to the vascular surgeon. These fistulas are usually high volume fistulas because of their central location; consequently, they may present in dramatic ways, such as refractory congestive heart failure, severe venous hypertension, or end organ ischemia. Despite the rarity of occurrence there are numerous etiologies which can further confuse the inexperienced vascular surgeon.

Arteriovenous fistulas as an entity were first described by Hunter [10] in 1757, but Syme [24] was the first to describe an aortovenous fistula in 1831 when he reported on a 22 year old man who died as a result of this condition 3½ months after the onset of symptoms. In 1935 Lehman [13] made the first, albeit unsuccessful, attempt to repair an aortocaval fistula. A successful repair was first reported by Cooley [3] in 1955, and several other reports of successful repairs quickly followed. Proper treatment depends on recognition, an understanding of the pathophysiology, and a thoughtful surgical approach. This chapter attempts to place these essentials in perspective.

ETIOLOGY

Major arteriovenous fistulas are classified as acquired or congenital. This chapter will not review congenital lesions but will only deal with acquired arteriovenous fistulas (Table 1). Spontaneously acquired fistulas are secondary to processes which weaken the wall of the aorta or its major branches and lead to rupture into the adjacent venous channel.

The major cause of spontaneous, acquired aortovenous fistulas is erosion of arteriosclerotic abdominal aortic aneurysms into an adjacent vein. Syphilitic

Table 1
Causes of Acquired Arteriovenous Fistulas of the Abdominal Aortic Territory

Spontaneous rupture of abdominal aortic aneurysm
Arteriosclerotic aneurysms
Syphilitic aneurysms
Mycotic aneurysms
Penetrating trauma
Gunshot wounds and other missiles (low velocity)
Stab wounds
Iatrogenic
Post Iaminectomy — primarily in area of bifurcation
Inadvertent intraoperative injury to adjacent artery and vein

aneurysms can lead to the same consequences, and indeed Syme's first description of an aortocaval fistula was secondary to a syphilitic aneurysm. To put the incidence of spontaneous aortocaval fistulas in perspective, Mohr [17] reviewed the literature in 1975 and found only 69 reported cases. Baker et al. [1] noted in their series of all abdominal aortic aneurysms over a 15 year period that aortocaval fistula secondary to ruptured aortic aneurysms accounted for 1.25% of all aneurysms operated upon and 4.3% of all ruptured aneurysms operated upon. In addition, Suzuki [23] reported on a case of aorta-left renal vein fistula and reviewed the other six cases in the literature. Of anatomical interest, six of the seven reported aorta-left renal vein fistulas occurred into a retroaortic left renal vein. This is logical, since retroaortic left renal veins tend to enter the vena cava at a lower level and consequently lie at the favored site of rupture of an abdominal aortic aneurysm.

Other spontaneously acquired major arteriovenous fistulas are extremely rare, but include erosions of tumors, such as mesenchymal tumors or hypernephromas into adjacent arterial and venous structures, and erosions of infected false aneurysms into adjacent venous channels.

Major arteriovenous fistulas may also be caused by trauma, either low velocity missile wounds or stab wounds. However, in the overall picture of traumatic arteriovenous fistulas, communications between the abdominal aorta and major venous channels occur infrequently. This infrequent occurrence may be due to the somewhat protected position of the structures, but more likely there is major hemorrhage and death before treatment can be initiated. Simultaneous injury to the aorta and a major vein, such as the inferior vena, common iliac veins, or left renal vein may result in a pulsating hematoma and later a fistula. The patient population tends to be younger, and because of better overall cardiovascular status the diagnosis is often delayed if major hemorrhage does not occur. Recognition of this type of traumatic aortovenous fistula may be overlooked at exploratory laparotomy for the initial injury (Fig. 1). Nonexpanding retroperitoneal hematomas are often not explored, as the consequences of retroperitoneal exploration of major venous injuries may be more deleterious than observation. This is the usual history in the patients seen subsequent to their injury when they develop signs and symptoms of a chronic arteriovenous fistula.

Postlaminectomy arteriovenous fistulas were first recognized in 1945 [15]. Jarstfer [11] reported on a collective review of 73 cases in 1976, thus underlining the importance of this iatrogenic complication. Although most of these cases involve the common iliac arteries and veins, about 10% involve the aorta and a major vein. Fistulas between the lumbar arteries and veins have also been reported. The causative factors are many. The prone positioning of the patient tends to push the viscera and vessels against the vertebral column. A fear of leaving disc material behind that may cause later neurologic symptoms may lead to an overaggressive use of the pituitary rongeur and perforation of the anterior spinal ligament with subsequent vascular injury. Anatomically the aorta and vena cava bifurcate at the level of most disc surgery, i.e., L_{4-5}.

The surgeon contributes to acquired arteriovenous fistulas by mass ligatures of adjacent arteries and veins, such as the renal or splenic pedicles, and by inadvertent injuries of nearby vascular structures such as the portal vein or mesenteric veins and adjacent arteries.

PATHOPHYSIOLOGY

Prior to embarking on the diagnosis and management of aortovenous fistulas, a brief trip to the physiology lab will be helpful to gain an understanding of the hemodynamic and other effects of large arteriovenous fistulas in the aortic region. Holman [8] in 1937 emphasized at least three factors as major determinants of the hemodynamic effect of an arteriovenous fistula – size, location, and distensibility of the vascular rim. Larger fistulas allow greater flow, as do more centrally located fistulas where the normal flow is greater. A stiff rimmed fistula is less likely to enlarge, but a more pliable rim may increase in size with time and lead to greater flow. The hemodynamic effects of aortovenous fistulas tend to be dramatic because at least two of the three determinants, size and location, favor high flows.

An arteriovenous communication provides a direct diversion of blood from the higher pressure arterial system into the low resistance venous system. This short circuit decreases the mean systemic arterial pressure and the effective systemic blood flow to vital organs. Then, primarily due to modification by the kidneys in response to this decreased perfusion and pressure, sodium and water are retained to increase circulating volume. Lewis [14] demonstrated the dilatation of the entire circulatory system, i.e., veins, arteries, and chambers of the heart, in response to the fistula. This dilatation is gradual and is accompanied by

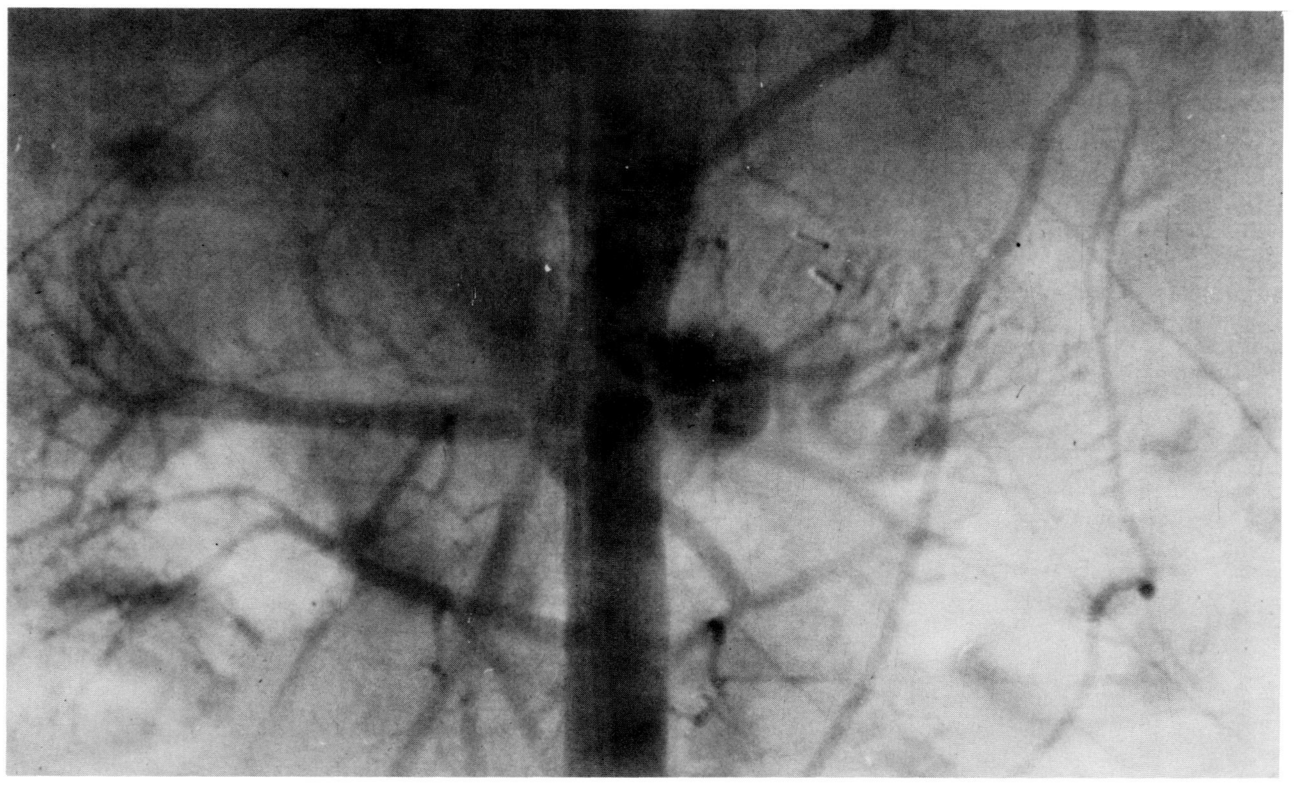

Fig. 1. Aortogram obtained after previous laparotomy for gunshot wound. Injury sheared off the left renal artery, leaving a false aneurysm and traversed on to the right causing an aortocaval fistula.

an increased blood volume. Although the heart rate increases in response to the stimulated baroreceptors and to increasing circulating volume, cardiac output increases primarily by increased stroke volume [18].

Eventually the heart cannot further accommodate the increased blood volume with increasing cardiac output and congestive heart failure develops. This failure may occur acutely in both young and old patients but tends to occur earlier in diseased hearts and later with a younger, healthier myocardium.

Increased venous pressure develops in the pelvis, lower extremities, and renal veins in aortocaval fistulas. Several sequelae follow. Increased venous pressure in the pelvis is transmitted to the venous plexus of the bladder and rectum and can lead to bleeding from friable distended veins in either organ. Increased venous pressure in the lower extremities often leads to leg edema, varicosities, and even a picture indistinguishable from chronic venous insufficiency. Renal venous hypertension may add to effects of the decreased renal perfusion and lead to decreased renal function, oliguria, and azotemia. An aorta-left renal vein fistula [22] produces an even more dramatic increase in renal venous pressure and usually leads to hematuria and markedly decreased function of the affected kidney.

In addition to renal ischemia, cerebrovascular and lower extremity ischemia may develop. Stenotic carotid or cerebral vessels may not maintain adequate cerebral perfusion in the face of the low diastolic and decreased mean systemic pressures in patients with a large aortocaval fistula. Similarly, advanced atherosclerosis in the lower extremities may not permit adequate distal perfusion in the face of this decreased systemic pressure; moreover, the flow distal to an arteriovenous fistula is even further decreased. In patients with a large fistula, the resistance on the venous side will be less than the resistance of the distal arterial tree, leading to reversed flow in the distal arterial segment. At some point distal in the extremity, depending upon collateral flow and pressure, these relationships change and antegrade flow resumes. It is easy to understand that flow may be inadequate under such circumstances in a normal vascular bed, even more so in an atherosclerotic peripheral bed.

But as Holman [9] pointed out in 1940, these hemodynamic changes are for the most part reversible if not allowed to go too long, thus emphasizing the necessity for prompt recognition. Once the diagnosis has been made, the vascular surgeon can then expedite the necessary treatment.

SIGNS AND SYMPTOMS

Although the clinical diagnosis of a large arteriovenous fistula should be relatively easy, the literature is replete with incorrect diagnoses and surprise findings at operation. Certainly the rarity of this disorder contributes to missed diagnoses. In addition, patients often present in an atypical manner.

The classical presentation for an aortovenous fistula includes high output congestive heart failure, peripheral edema, venous hypertension, distal arterial insufficiency, cyanosis of lower extremities, and pain. Coupling these signs and symptoms with physical findings of a widened pulse pressure, pulsatile abdominal mass, and a continuous loud abdominal bruit makes the diagnosis relatively straightforward.

In spontaneous aortocaval fistulas, sudden pain is characteristic; however, the distribution or location of the pain takes on many forms. Classical lumbar back pain of a ruptured aneurysm may be present. The basis for the pain is an associated retroperitoneal hemorrhage, or in the absence of hemorrhage, it may be on the basis of the acute distention of the caval system. The pain may be abdominal or flank in location or radiate into the groin or legs. The flank pain and pain radiating to the groin or testicle can mislead the observer into diagnoses of genitourinary disorders. In the report by Reckless [19] 88% presented with pain of some kind.

Signs and symptoms of congestive heart failure developed in 37% of patients reviewed by Reckless [19] and in 68% of patients in Jarstfer's review of postlaminectomy arteriovenous fistulas. In traumatic aortovenous fistulas congestive heart failure may develop, although usually at a time remote from the injury, probably because the patients tend to be younger. Obviously the size of the fistula and preexisting cardiac status governs the onset and presentation of congestive heart failure. Certainly congestive heart failure responding poorly to medical therapy or congestive heart failure in a young patient should alert the physician to this diagnosis when there is a proper antecedent history or other associated findings for aortovenous fistula.

Leg edema or lower body edema was seen in 56% in Reckless's review. In postlaminectomy arteriovenous fistulas the edema may be unilateral if the fistula is unilateral. In the collection of seven aorta-left renal vein fistulas, leg edema was noted in two patients. Causative factors for the peripheral edema are venous hypertension, congestive heart failure, and compression of the vena cava by the abdominal aortic aneurysm. The regional distribution of the edema may help differentiate it from anasarca associated with congestive heart failure, renal failure, etc. The leg edema and oft-associated superficial varicosities can lead to the mistaken diagnosis of deep venous thrombosis or insufficiency.

Pelvic or renal venous hypertension produces other significant findings. The congested dilated rectal plexus of veins may lead to rectal bleeding. Of more significance, however, is hematuria, which is seen in only 1 of 1000 elective aneurysmectomy patients but in 17%-23% of patients with spontaneous aortocaval fistulas [2]. Aorta-left renal vein fistulas produced hematuria of either renal or bladder origin in six of seven reported cases. Therefore hematuria associated with an abdominal aortic aneurysm should alert the diagnostician.

The other classic finding that deserves detailed discussion is an abdominal bruit. Reckless found that 83% presented with an abdominal bruit. Vander Veer et al. [24] point out that the bruit may be absent due to clot occluding the fistula. Additionally, hypotension and low flow diminish the bruit. Depending on the anatomic location of the thrombus, the bruit may come and go.

The onset of symptoms of spontaneous aortocaval fistulas may be acute or insidious. Acutely the most frequent presentation is high output cardiac failure that is characterized as being difficult to control medially. Hypotension may present acutely with oliguria due to decreased renal flow or with a symptomatic aneurysm that has leaked retroperitoneally in addition to rupturing into the vena cava. Any of the other prominent signs or symptoms of rectal bleeding, hematuria, altered cerebral status, regional edema, or ischemic extremities may accompany these syndromes.

However, postlaminectomy and posttraumatic arteriovenous fistulas and more rarely fistulas secondary to aneurysms in the aortic territory may have an insidious onset of fatigue, malaise, shortness of breath, and other signs of congestive heart failure. The other prominent signs previously mentioned may also accompany this chronic presentation.

Evaluating any constellation of signs and symptoms without associating other constellations produces a greater number of errors in diagnosis and management. Onset of cardiac failure in a young patient with a remote history of trauma or lumbar disc surgery puts one on the right trail early. A continuous abdominal bruit in a patient with a pulsating abdominal mass and back pain is an important association to recognize in preparation for a technically safe operation. These are but two of many examples that could be made.

EVALUATION

A careful history and physical examination are the hallmark of the proper evaluation of these patients. The nuances of the signs and symptoms have been presented. What laboratory and radiological tests are necessary or helpful? A simple urinalysis may reveal hematuria, and as noted earlier this is important information. An IVP may be helpful when evaluating a possible aorta-left renal vein fistula to establish the function of each kidney as a baseline for later comparison and to help establish the diagnosis. Aortography is rarely needed to make the diagnosis, but in chronic cases or difficult cases aortography is diagnostic. If the patient is stable and does not require an immediate operation for associated hemorrhage such as in trauma or retroperitoneal rupture of an aneurysm, aortography can give valuable information about the precise location of the fistula (Figs. 2 and 3).

PRINCIPLES OF THERAPY

The treatment of aortocaval fistulas is surgical. An accurate preoperative diagnosis permits a thoughtful surgical approach. Fluid management in any major arteriovenous fistula may be complicated compared to the usual aneurysmectomy patient. Technical aspects of the operation become especially critical in aortovenous fistulas. These include the possible need for extended incisions, autotransfusion, and deep hypothermia with circulatory arrest. A surprise diagnosis at the time of operation does not allow for any of these preparations.

Fluid management in general is difficult in these patients. Patients with acute fistulas with associated hemorrhage due to trauma or rupture are hypovolemic. Patients with chronic arteriovenous fistulas are hypervolemic as a consequence of their fistula. Proper recognition of the patient's volume status requires sophisticated monitoring to allow judicious use of fluids and blood both before and after closure of the fistula. The Swan-Ganz catheter is likely the most

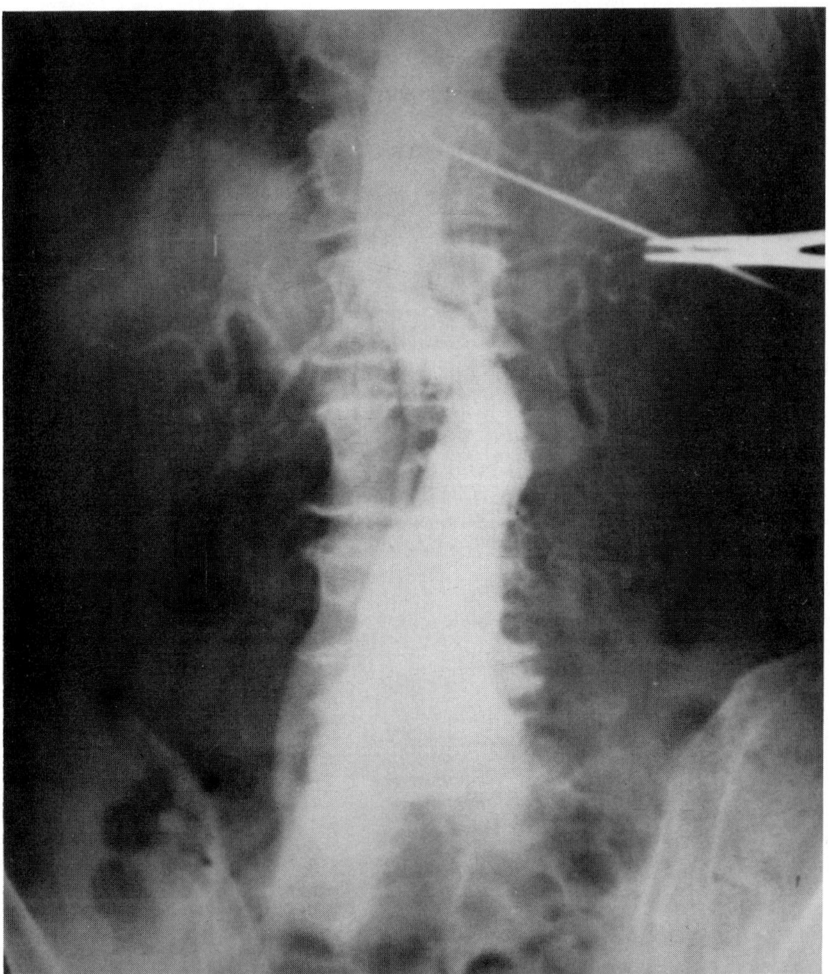

Fig. 2. Early phase of a translumbar aortogram shows an abdominal aortic aneurysm with filling of the inferior vena cava.

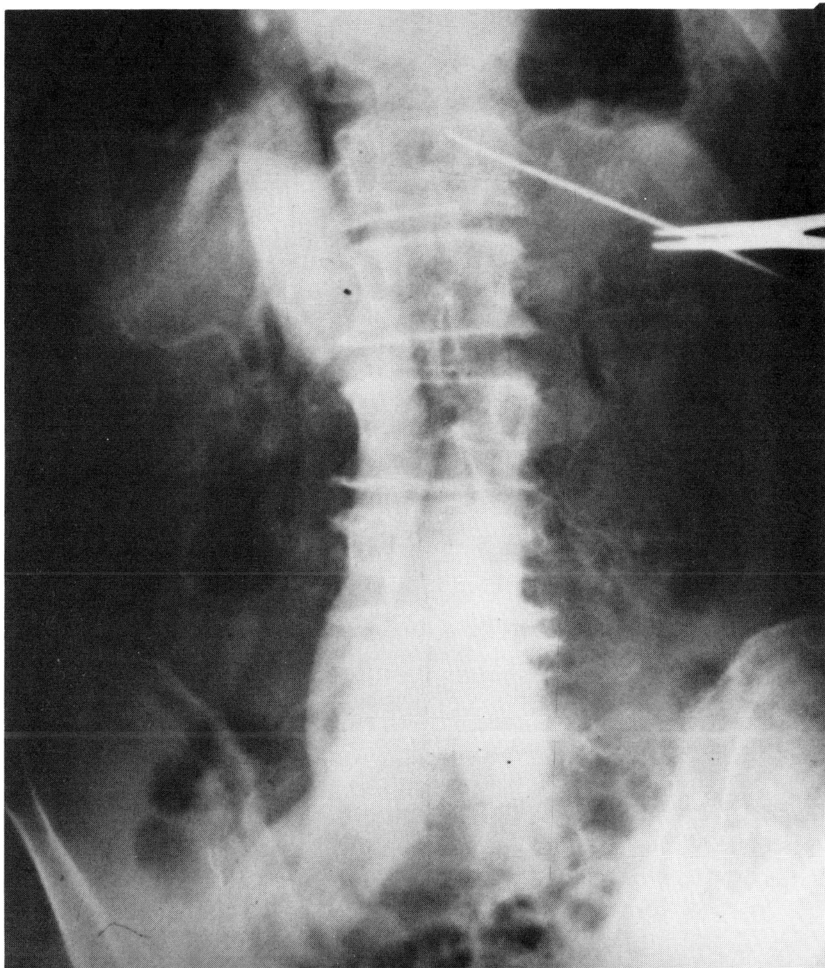

Fig. 3. Later phase of the same translumbar aortogram shows continued prograde filling of the inferior vena cava and retrograde filling of the right iliac vein. [From Baker WH, Sharzer LA, Ehrenhaft JL: Aortocaval fistula as a complication of abdominal aortic aneurysms. Surg. 72:933-938, 1972.]

important advance in recent years in monitoring such delicate fluid management problems. Kwann et al. [12] even advocated its use in the preoperative evaluation and diagnosis of any patient with an abdominal aortic aneurysm and congestive heart failure. With the Swan-Ganz catheter concurrent measurements of CVP, pulmonary artery pressure, pulmonary wedge pressures, and cardiac output are available. These measurements monitor right and left heart mechanics and dictate proper fluid therapy. Thus the blood loss during the initial dissection in a hypervolemic patient may actually be therapeutic and proper monitoring will check the improper replacement of volume.

Schumacker [20] states the goals of surgical therapy: "It has long been recognized that the ideal method of treating aneurysms and AV fistulae involving important arteries is the extirpation of the lesion combined with some procedure which permits maintenance or reestablishment of the continuity of the affected artery." Within the context of timing, he advocated that the best time for this repair is on an immediate basis. The modern approach is so based to provide an easier technical approach to the problem and to avoid irreversible hemodynamic problems. When quadruple ligation was all that was available, a 2-6 month waiting period was deemed helpful so that collaterals might develop to save the distal circulation after ligation. The waiting period often proved fatal.

The patient with an aortovenous fistula and congestive heart failure needs urgent operation. In all likelihood the patient's myocardium will not respond to digitalis preparations but will only improve performance once the fistula is closed. This problem is vastly different from the usual patient with atherosclerotic heart disease. Operation should not be delayed "to get the patient in better shape," but medical manipulation should be performed en route to the operating room.

The actual technical approach to the major arteriovenous fistulas is well described by several authors [1, 2, 5-7, 22]. Extensive prepping enables the surgeon to make extraordinary incisions necessary to control major bleeding. Proximal and distal control of the involved artery away from the fistula is axiomatic, and when feasible similar control of the involved vein is helpful. For instance, high abdominal aortovenous fistulas may require supradiaphragmatic control of the aorta; therefore prepping of the thorax is essential. Clamping of the suprarenal aorta may induce significant hypertension and increased cardiac afterload. This may require pharmacological afterload reduction during aortic cross clamping and careful titration as aortic declamping ensures. Arterial control some distance away from the area may also be necessary to avoid premature rupture of an associated false aneurysm. In addition, placement of arterial clamps should allow for the resection of damaged or diseased artery should this be present.

Actual control of the vein away from the fistula may be very difficult due to the venous distention. Intermittent clamping of the isolated proximal and distal artery to reduce venous pressure facilitates this dissection. When the involved venous channel is the vena cava, control or clamping of the vena cava may lead to markedly diminished venous return with reduced filling of the ventricles and serious cardiac effects. Therefore it is essential that open lines of communication with the anesthesiologists are established. If hypotension occurs either volume must be restored before clamping or an alternate technique employed.

Although complete venous control is ideal it is sometimes technically impossible to achieve. With good proximal and distal arterial control most types of aortovenous fistulas can then be opened from the aortic side and the fistula controlled with direct finger control or by sponge stick compression above and below the fistula from within the aneurysm. This maneuver is especially applicable in spontaneous aortocaval fistula secondary to abdominal aortic aneurysms (Fig. 4).

With the fistula exposed, direct repair through the opened artery is usually feasible. After fistula repair is completed, then arterial continuity is restored. In the case of an abdominal aortic aneurysm, the usual Dacron graft replacement is

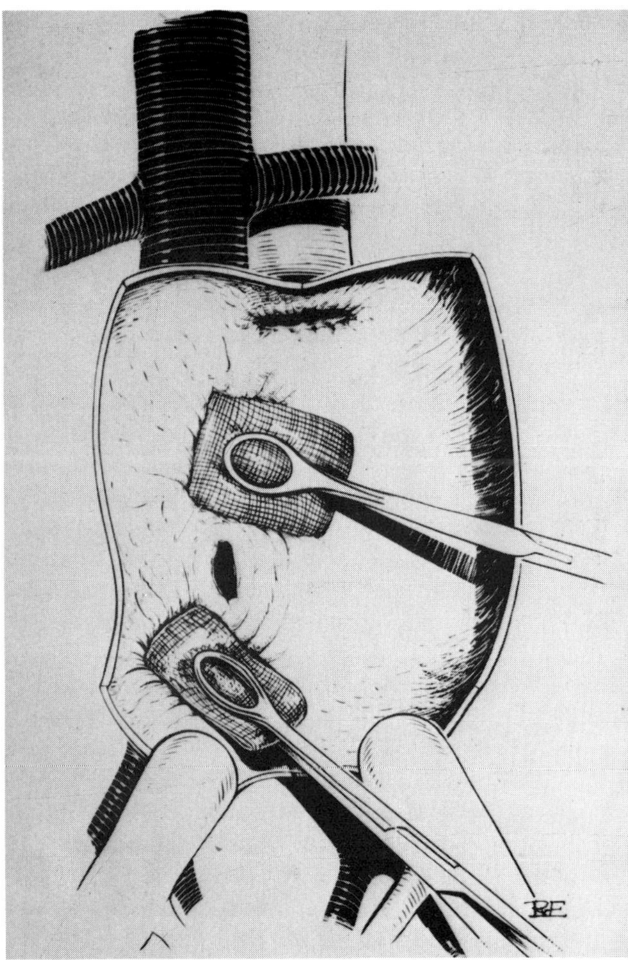

Fig. 4. Demonstration of the maneuver to control bleeding from the inferior vena cava from within the opened aneurysmal sac. [From Baker WH, Sharzer LA, Ehrenhaft JL: Aortocaval fistula as a complication of abdominal aortic aneurysms. Surg. 72:933-938, 1972.]

carried out. In trauma, the arterial repair may be a simple lateral suture repair, division and end-to-end reanastomosis or replacement with interposition graft. If contamination from associated bowel injuries or an infected false aneurysm is present, the artery may require in situ ligation and an extraanatomic bypass through a clean surgical field after closure of the wound.

Similar to the restoration of arterial flow, all reasonable attempts at venous reconstruction should be made. In certain instances ligation of the vein may be safer. In large or difficult aortocaval fistulas, the vena cava may be ligated, although Marcelletti et al. [16] did replace the vena cava with a synthetic graft on one occasion with success. Certainly the left renal vein can be safely divided if the adrenal and gonadal veins are intact.

An additional note of caution is pertinent to the dissection of the aorta in aortocaval fistulas secondary to abdominal aortic aneurysm. Because of the associated mural thrombus in the aneurysm sac, minimal careful dissection of the neck of the aneurysm is essential. If mural thrombus is dislodged it may exit through the fistula and lead to a paradoxical pulmonary embolus [1, 4] (Fig. 5).

A special problem in management is noted by Griffen et al. [6] in their review of four traumatic aorta-renal vein fistulas, one of which was their own. At operation they were unable to conventionally approach the fistula safely due to the massive distention of regional vessels, especially the thin walled distended veins, and the anatomical distortion from the previous injury. Their solution to this problem was to place the patient on cardiopulmonary bypass, employ deep hypothermia to 17°C, and under circulatory arrest carry out a successful repair.

Massive blood loss despite the method of repair is a distinct possibility. Even when aortovenous fistulas are correctly identified, operative blood loss is reported at 3-5 liters. To reduce heterologous blood replacement and possible related respiratory and renal dysfunction, Doty et al. [5] advocate the use of autotransfusion in conjunction with proper monitoring. In their experience with two patients total blood replacement with autotransfusion was 2000 and 2500 ml.

MORBIDITY AND MORTALITY OF MAJOR ARTERIOVENOUS FISTULA REPAIR

The determinants of the morbidity and mortality of arteriovenous fistulas are not only those associated with uncomplicated aortic surgery but are dependent upon the unusual hemodynamic disturbances. These include congestive heart failure, reduced renal function, and altered third space fluid shifts. Nonetheless, morbidity and mortality from the surgical intervention become quite acceptable, especially when the diagnosis is appreciated preoperatively and proper steps are taken.

Mohr [17] reported on 69 cases of spontaneous aortocaval fistulas in his literature review. Fifty-seven had surgical intervention, and 55% were successful.

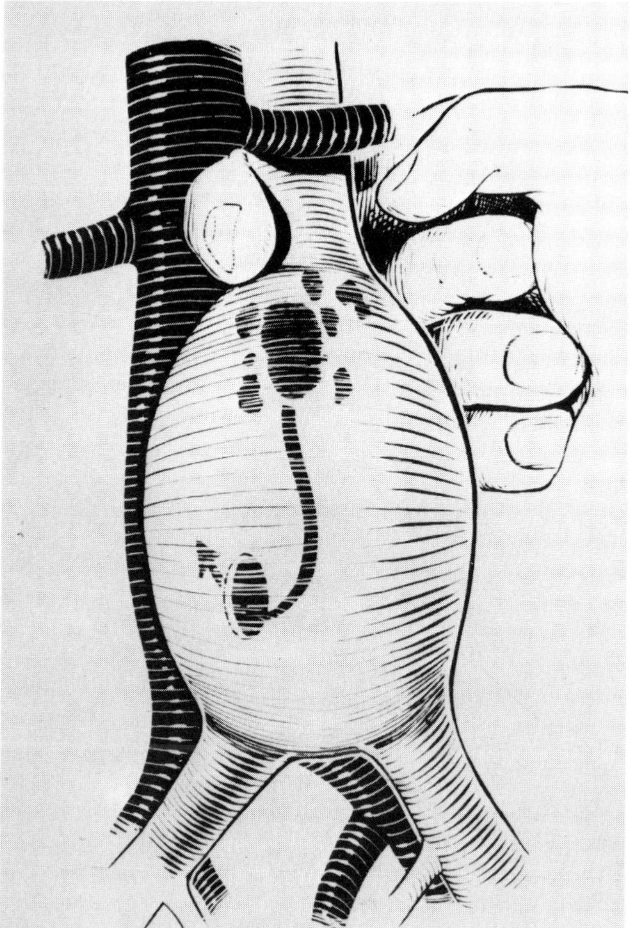

Fig. 5. Undue manipulation of the aneurysm or the neck of the aneurysm may dislodge atheromatous debris and clot, which then may course through the fistula to the pulmonary artery. [From Baker WH, Sharzer LA, Ehrenhaft JL: Aortocaval fistula as a complication of abdominal aortic aneurysms. Surg. 72:933-938, 1972.]

The associated aneurysmal disease in an atherosclerotic elderly patient with other cadiovascular complications make this a high risk situation. Still, proper recognition and prompt repair with careful monitoring should improve this mortality rate. The reported seven cases of spontaneous aorta-left renal vein fistulas were all successfully treated [22].

Patients with postlaminectomy arteriovenous fistulas fare much better. This is likely due to the younger age of the patients and the somewhat smaller size of the fistulas. The operative mortality in Jarstfer's review [11] of 73 patients was 6.9%. Morbidity was increased in those patients who underwent ligation procedures. Among five patients undergoing quadruple ligation two developed claudication. Of four patients requiring ligation of the artery only, one developed claudication and one required a transmetatarsal amputation. Venous complications including one case each of postphlebitic syndrome, pulmonary embolization, lower extremity edema, thrombophlebitis, and venous insufficiency were noted, and most of these followed quadruple ligation procedures.

CONCLUSIONS

Arteriovenous fistulas of the abdominal aortic territory require sharp clinical acumen for recognition, as they are rare. The proper evaluation of these patients then leads to prompt and proper preoperative and operative management to reverse the hemodynamic disturbances and to reestablish arterial and venous continuity. Ideally the already acceptable morbidity and mortality of surgical intervention can be improved with modern technical capabilities. Without surgical treatment the outcome is a morbid patient within a few days to a few months.

REFERENCES

1. Baker WH, Sharzer LA, Ehrenhaft JL: Aortocaval fistula as a complication of abdominal aortic aneurysms. Surgery 72:933-938, 1972
2. Brewster DC, Ottinger LW, Darling RC: Hematuria as a sign of aortocaval fistula. Am. J. Surg. 186:766-771, 1977
3. Cooley DA: Discussion of "Resection of ruptured aneurysms of abdominal aorta" by Javid H, Dye WS, Grove WJ, Julian OC. Ann. Surg. 142:613-624, 1955
4. Cooperman M, Deal KF, Wooley CF, et al: Spontaneous aortocaval fistula with paradoxical pulmonary embolization. Am. J. Surg. 134:647-649, 1977
5. Doty DB, Wright CB, Yambreth WC, et al: Aortocaval fistula associated with aneurysm of the abdominal aorta: Current management using autotransfusion techniques. Surgery 84:250-251, 1978
6. Griffen LH Jr, Fishback ME, Galloway RF, et al: Traumatic aortorenal fistula: Repair using total circulatory arrest. Surgery 81:480-483, 1977
7. Hildreth DH, Turcke DA: Post-laminectomy arteriovenous fistulas. Surgery 81:512-520, 1977
8. Holman E: Arteriovenous Aneurysms: Abnormal Communication Between the Arterial and Venous Circulations. New York, MacMillan, 1937
9. Holman E: Clinical and experimental observations on arteriovenous fistulae. Ann. Surg. 112:840, 1940
10. Hunter W: The history of an aneurysm of the aorta, with some remarks on aneurysms in general. Med. Obs. Soc. Physiol. Lond. 1:323, 1757

11. Jarstfer BS, Rich NM: The challenge of arteriovenous fistula formation following disc surgery: A collective review. J. Trauma 16:726-733, 1976
12. Kwaan JHM, McCart PM, Jones SA, et al: Aortocaval fistula detection using a Swan-Ganz catheter. Surg. Gynecol. Obstet. 144:919-921, 1977
13. Lehman EP: Spontaneous arteriovenous fistula between the abdominal aorta and the inferior vena cava. Ann. Surg. 108:694, 1938
14. Lewis T: The adjustment of blood flow to the affected limb in arteriovenous fistula. Clin. Sci. 4:277, 1940
15. Linton RR, White PD: Arteriovenous fistula between the right common iliac artery and the inferior vena cava. Arch. Surg. 50:6, 1945
16. Marcelletti C, Astolfi D, DePinto F, et al: Abdominal aortocaval fistula: Treatment with aortic and caval synthetic grafts. (One-year followup.) J. Cardiovasc. Surg. 18:137-140, 1977
17. Mohr LL, Smith LL: Arteriovenous fistula from rupture of abdominal aortic aneurysm. Arch. Surg. 110:806-812, 1975
18. Nakano J, DeSchryver C: Effects of arteriovenous fistula on systemic and pulmonary circulations. Am. J. Physiol. 207:1319, 1964
19. Reckless JPD, McColl I, Taylor GW: Aorto-caval fistulae: An uncommon complication of abdominal aortic aneurysms. Br. J. Surg. 59:461, 1972
20. Schumacker HB Jr: The problem of maintaining the continuity of the artery in the surgery of aneurysms and arteriovenous fistulas: Notes on the development and clinical application of methods of arterial suture. Ann. Surg. 127:207, 1948
21. Strandness DE Jr, Sumner DS: Arteriovenous Fistula in Hemodynamics for Surgeons. New York, Grune & Stratton, 1975, p 632
22. Suzuki M, Collins GM, Bassinger GT, et al: Aorto-left renal vein fistula: An unusual complication of abdominal aortic aneurysm. Ann. Surg. 184:31-34, 1976
23. Syme J: Case of spontaneous varicose aneurysm. Edinb. Med. Surg. 36:104, 1931
24. Vander Veer JB, Robinson HJ, Blake AD: Abdominal aortic aneurysm with vena caval fistula. Arch. Intern. Med. 114:551, 1964

R. M. Greenhalgh, M.A., M.Chir., F.R.C.S.

Dilation and Stretching of Knitted Dacron Grafts Associated With Failure

Failure in three aortic Dacron grafts by aneurysmal dilatation, one with fatal rupture, was reported by Cooke et al. [1]. Ottinger et al. [3] had further reported 11 occasions in which ultralightweight knitted Dacron grafts were complicated by dilatation. The ultralightweight Dacron grafts have not been marketed in Great Britain, and in this series of patients standard, normal weight knitted Dacron bifurcation grafts have been employed throughout. Over the many years during which this type of graft has been imported to Britain, remarkably few arterial reconstruction failures have been attributed to mechanical failure in the fabric.

PATIENTS

Ten patients are described, eight of whom had aortic bifurcation grafts performed between December 1971 and September 1975 (Table 1). Seven of the patients had a bypass to the femoral vessels and the eighth to the iliac vessels. Six of these were men and two were women. The ages ranged between 49 and 77 years. Standard techniques were used for these operative procedures. On each occasion the standard weight knitted Dacron bifurcation graft was preclotted using approximately 80 ml of unheparinized blood, syringing it through until the Dacron became "tight." The patients were then given approximately 5000 units of heparin intravenously and the aortic bifurcation grafts anastomosed to the front of the infrarenal aorta, using Mersilene. The limbs were tunneled behind the peritoneum to either the iliac or femoral vessels and again anastomosed to the front of these vessels. The lower anastomoses were performed with Tevdek.

Table 1
Patient Data

Patient		Operation			Dacron Failure			
Number	Age (Years)/ Sex	Date	Type	Dacron Size (mm)	Date	Time to Failure (Years)	Dacron Limb Size Then (mm)	How Measured
1	72/M	Dec. 1971	Aortobifemoral	19 × 9.5	Jun. 1976	4.5	30	At reoperation
2	77/F	Oct. 1972	Aortobifemoral	16 × 8	Jul. 1976	3.75	20	At reoperation
3	52/M	Feb. 1973	Aortobiiliac	16 × 8	Mar. 1976	3.0	20	At reoperation
4	49/M	Jun. 1973	Aortobifemoral	20 × 10	Apr. 1975	1.75	18	At reoperation
5	65/M	Aug. 1973	Aortobifemoral	16 × 8	Dec. 1976	3.5	20	From aortogram
6	49/M	Apr. 1974	Aortobifemoral	16 × 8	Jan. 1976	1.75	16	At reoperation
7	53/M	Apr. 1974	Aortobifemoral	19 × 9.5	Nov. 1975	1.5	15	At reoperation
8	71/F	Sept. 1975	Aortobifemoral	13 × 6.5	Oct. 1978	3.00	12	At reoperation
9	53/M	Nov. 1976	R. Ilioprofunda	8 mm velour	Aug. 1978	1.75	16	At reoperation
10	71/M	Feb. 1976	L. Iliopopliteal	6 mm velour	Feb. 1978	2.00	15	At reoperation

Patients 9 and 10 had more recent procedures, and the rather newer internal velour tube of Dacron was used. On one occasion an 8 mm tube was used for a right ilioprofunda bypass, and on the other a 6 mm internal velour Dacron tube was used for an iliopopliteal bypass. These Dacron tubes were preclotted in a similar way to the bifurcation grafts and the patients were then heparinized, while the anastomosis was taking place.

LATE DACRON FAILURE

Over a period of time ranging between 1.5 and 4.5 years after the operation, one of the Dacron limbs of these ten patients failed. Either after aortography and at reoperation (nine patients) or from aortography alone (one patient), the diameter of the failed Dacron limb was measured. It was found that the Dacron limbs had stretched to twice and sometimes three times the original sizes (mean 2.24 times). Patient 3 (Fig. 1) had a 16 × 8 mm knitted bifurcation graft

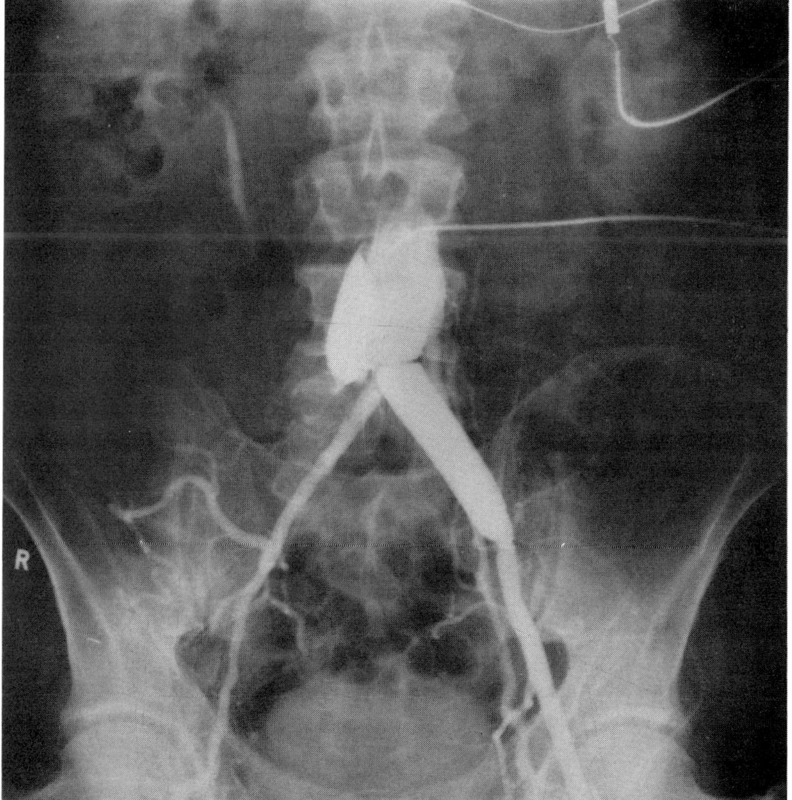

Fig. 1. Patient 3. In 3 years this man's knitted Dacron limb stretched from 8 to 20 mm and one limb occluded.

inserted for severe intermittent claudication of the left buttock and calf, in association with a left iliac stenosis. In view of the significant disease in the right iliac system at that time, a bifurcation graft was performed from the front of the infrarenal aorta to the external iliac arteries. The operation was performed in February 1973. Figure 1 shows the translumbar aortogram of March 1976 after the right limb of the Dacron graft had occluded. During this 3 year period, the 8 mm limb had enlarged to 20 mm. Also, quite clearly, the Dacron had elongated, allowing a kink to appear on the aortogram at the upper end of the left Dacron limb. The main stem of the Dacron had enlarged to be double the width of the aorta. Quite clearly the dimensions of this Dacron in March 1976 were totally inappropriate for this man's requirements. It was necessary to take it out and put in another bifurcation graft.

Patient 6 was a 49 year old laborer who in April 1974 received a Dacron bifurcation graft to the femoral vessels for severe bilateral intermittent claudication of the calves. A translumbar aortogram was performed in January 1976 (Fig. 2). This shows that the left Dacron limb of the bifurcation graft had occluded at its origin and that the right Dacron limb had expanded. At operation, this right Dacron limb was found to be 16 mm in diameter, exactly twice the diameter when it was inserted 21 months before. The tube of Dacron was now comparable in diameter to the aorta itself and it was quite clearly totally inappropriate for the patient's requirements. Shortly after this aortogram, the right Dacron limb shown in Fig. 2 occluded.

DISCUSSION

Biochemical causes of late arterial reconstruction failure have been described [2]. In these ten patients, biochemical factors might clearly have played a part in causing the late reconstruction failure; in other words, the disease process may have continued and the runoff or input to the grafts may have altered during the period of time that the graft was working. However, in all of these patients, a limb of Dacron failed, and this failure was associated with an inappropriate stretching of Dacron. This increase in diameter would bring about a drastic reduction in linear flow, and it is clearly possible that the linear velocity of blood fell below the necessary level to keep the graft open. It is possible therefore that in these ten patients the stretching of Dacron predisposed to thrombosis of the grafts and that this had nothing to do with a continuing atherosclerotic disease process in the usual sense.

These conclusions are in no way meant to criticize the knitted Dacron grafts, which have served so many of our patients very well for many years. It is remarkable that more mechanical graft failure does not occur. From December 1971 to February 1976 approximately 1000 Dacron bypasses were inserted; this is an estimate, but if it is correct, it would assess the incidence of Dacron failure associated with stretching at approximately 1%.

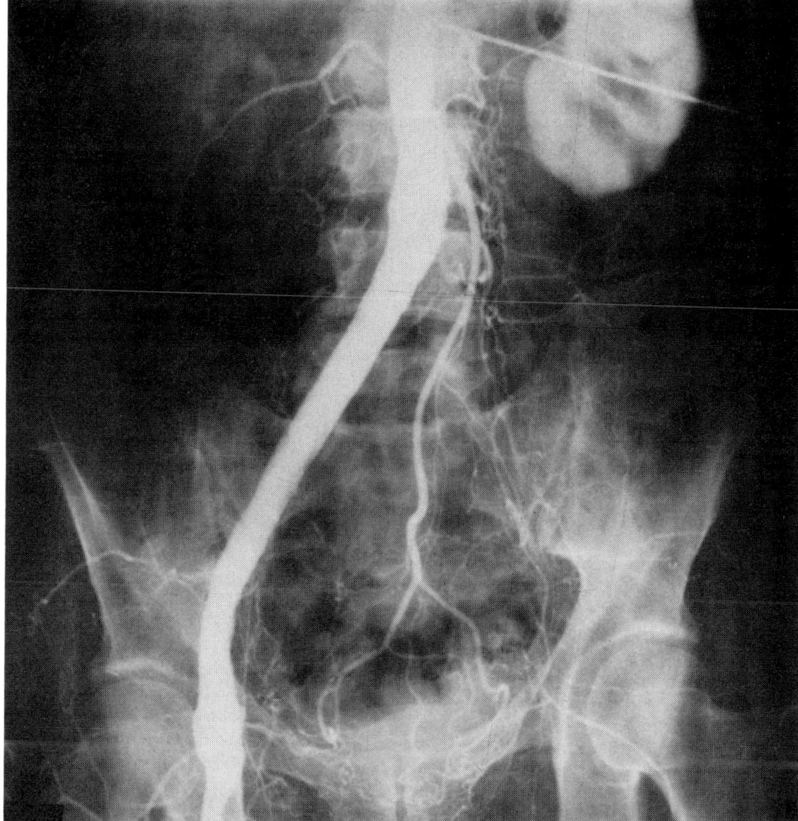

Fig. 2. Patient 6. In 21 months this man's Dacron limb had doubled its size from 8 to 16 mm. Clearly now it has a diameter comparable to the aorta, which is totally inappropriate.

The purpose of drawing attention to this stretching concerns the development of new graft materials. Clearly, attention should be paid to the ability of new graft materials to maintain the dimensions which these grafts have when they are selected by the surgeon at the time of operation. Much research has been performed in determining the best dimensions of graft materials. Clearly, many of the conclusions made on dimensions are irrelevant if the graft materials stretch and the graft alters its dimensions within months of its insertion.

Another conclusion to be made from this series is that when the surgeon is in doubt, he might be more inclined to choose a graft a size smaller than he might otherwise accept to allow for some distension. It seems that the fast linear velocity down a graft may be a rather important factor necessary to keep the graft open.

REFERENCES

1. Cooke PA, Nobis PA, Stoney RJ: Dacron aortic graft failure. Arch. Surg. 108:101-103, 1974
2. Greenhalgh RM: Biochemical abnormalities and smoking in arterial ischemia, in Bergan JJ, Yao JST (eds): Gangrene and Severe Ischemia of the Lower Extremities. New York, Grune & Stratton, 1978, pp. 39-60
3. Ottinger LB, Darling RC, Wirthlin LS, et al: Failure of ultralightweight knitted Dacron grafts in arterial reconstruction. Arch. Surg. 111:146-149, 1976

Index